Encyclopedia of Atrial Fibrillation

Encyclopedia of Atrial Fibrillation

Edited by **Ruth Brown**

hayle medical

New York

Published by Hayle Medical,
30 West, 37th Street, Suite 612,
New York, NY 10018, USA
www.haylemedical.com

Encyclopedia of Atrial Fibrillation
Edited by Ruth Brown

International Standard Book Number: 978-1-63241-121-1 (Hardback)

Printed in China.

Contents

Preface

Atrial Fibrillation; a common heart disorder, is the focus of this book. The book is intended to give a complete evaluation and introduction of Atrial Fibrillation. This book contains several chapters divided into distinct parts according to its respective functions. It explains the fundamental mechanisms of initiation and maintenance of atrial fibrillation. Then, it discusses mapping of atrial fibrillation and new techniques of signal detection. Clinical prognostic and remodeling is also revised thoroughly within the book. Furthermore, it describes universal evaluations of catheter-based/surgical dealing and treatment of the disorder. Finally, it deals with atrial fibrillation in precise situation and its difficulties.

This book is a comprehensive compilation of works of different researchers from varied parts of the world. It includes valuable experiences of the researchers with the sole objective of providing the readers (learners) with a proper knowledge of the concerned field. This book will be beneficial in evoking inspiration and enhancing the knowledge of the interested readers.

In the end, I would like to extend my heartiest thanks to the authors who worked with great determination on their chapters. I also appreciate the publisher's support in the course of the book. I would also like to deeply acknowledge my family who stood by me as a source of inspiration during the project.

Editor

Part 1

Mechanisms and Pathophysiology

1

Atrioventricular Conduction in Atrial Fibrillation: Pathophysiology and Clinical Implications

Attila Roka
Hospital of St. Raphael,
USA

1. Introduction

The atrioventricular (AV) node is the only conduction pathway between the atria and ventricles, it is located at the base of the right atrium. The conduction through the atrioventricular node is slow to allow the atria to pump blood into the ventricles before they contract. It also acts as a backup pacemaker, in case the sinoatrial node fails and limits the number of action potentials conducted to the ventricles during atrial fibrillation (AF). Despite this filtering function, adequate ventricular rate control in atrial fibrillation often requires utilization of pharmacological and/or non-pharmacological treatment modalities.

2. Functional anatomy of the atrioventricular junction

The AV node is part of the cardiac pacemaker and conduction system. It develops from the embryonic myocardium that maintains essential features of its primitive phenotype, while the adjacent myocardium differentiates into working myocardium (Bakker et al., 2010). The AV node is a heterogenous structure, histologically consists of 3 layers: superficial/subendocardial, intermediate/midpart and deep innermost. A central fibrous body surrounds the distal structures (compact node and penetrating bundle), while the proximal part merges with the atrial myocardium via the inferior nodal extension and the transitional zone (Figure 1).

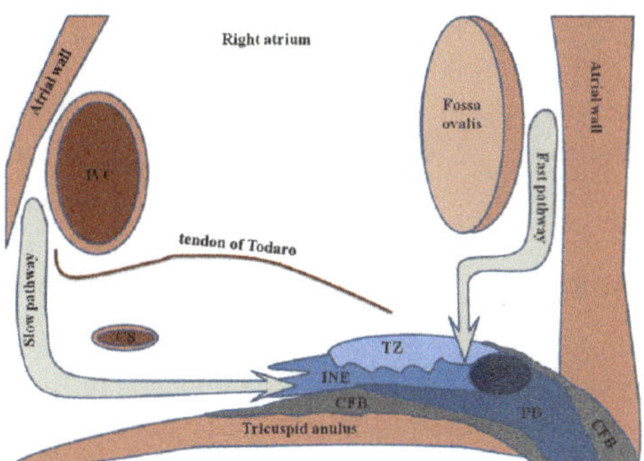

Fig. 1. Schematic anatomy of the AV node. View from the right atrium. IVC: inferior vena cava. CS: ostium of the coronary sinus. CFB: central fibrous body. INE: inferior nodal extension. TZ: transitional zone. PB: penetrating bundle. CN: compact node.

Based on the morphology of the recorded action potentials, there are 3 distinct regions: atrionodal, compact nodal and nodo-His. At least 6 different cell types have been described so far based on action potential morphology, excitability and refractory period. The correlation between histologic, microstructural and electrophysiological properties is still not fully elucidated despite recent advances in this field using voltage-sensitive fluorescent dyes. The slow and fast pathways of AV nodal activation involve extranodal areas in the right atrium, in posteroinferior (crista terminalis) and anterosuperior (interatrial septum) locations, respectively. The AV node receives both sympathetic and parasympathetic innervation (Meijler & Janse, 1988; Kurian et al., 2010).

3. Ion channels, currents and their modulation in the atrioventricular node

The electrical activity is determined by the expression of ion channels in the myocytes making up the conduction system. The ion channel expression in the AV node is specialized, similar to the sinoatrial node. There is very little expression of $K_{ir}2$ channels, responsible for the $I_{K,1}$ K^+ current, the main current to keep working cardiomyocytes at a negative resting potential. Other K_{ir} channel subunits ($K_{ir}3.1$, $K_{ir}3.4$, $K_{ir}6.2$ and SUR2) are also poorly expressed in the nodal tissues. The hyperpolarization-activated cyclic nucleotide-gated Na^+ channels, responsible for the pacemaker current I_f, are highly expressed in the sinoatrial and atrioventricular node. Conduction through the AV node is slow in order to introduce a delay between atrial and ventricular systole, which is due to the lack of connexin Cx43 expression and Na^+ channel Nav1.5. The upstroke of the nodal action potential is Ca^{2+} -dependent, but instead of the myocardial L-type Ca^{2+} channel, Cav1.2, the alternative Cav1.3 is expressed, which has a more negative activation threshold, thus more appropriate for a Ca^{2+} -dependent action potential. Data regarding the presence and distribution of T-type Ca^{2+} channel is less consistent. Ion channel expression is plastic and may change with aging, heart failure, diabetes or athletic training (Boyett et al., 2009; Greener et al., 2011).

Neurohormonal stimuli have a significant role in the behavior of the AV node during atrial fibrillation. Sympathetic activity (increased sympathetic nerve activation or release of circulating catecholamines) acts via β_1-receptors/increased cAMP/protein kinase A activation, enhances the T-type Ca^{2+} and I_f currents, increases the slope of diastolic depolarization (which plays no significant role during atrial fibrillation in the AV node), increases the rate and completeness of I_K deactivation (which decreases the effective refractory periods, thus decreasing the efficacy of the filtering function of the AV node in AF). Parasympathetic stimuli act via M_2 muscarinergic receptors/G_i protein activation, which activate the $I_{K/Ach}$ K^+ current, leading to membrane hyperpolarization, and inhibition of I_{Ca} Ca^{2+}- and I_f Na^+ currents via reducing cAMP and protein kinase A activity (Boyett et al., 2009).

4. Activation of the atrioventricular node in atrial fibrillation

In sinus rhythm, the action potential enters the AV node via the penetrating bundle (and then passes to the ventricles) via a fast pathway (formed partly by the transitional zone) and a slow pathway (formed partly by the inferior nodal extension). During AF, the node is continuously bombarded from different directions with varying degrees of penetration. Propagation is dependent on the relative timing of the septal inputs to the AV node at the crista terminalis and interatrial septum, and also depends on atrial input frequency (Garrigue et al., 1999). The constant bombardment of atrial impulses creates varying degree of concealed conduction, when most stimuli enter the AV node but do not conduct to the ventricle, creating a wake of refractoriness encountered by subsequent impulses (Fujiki et al., 1990). This generally slows down the resulting ventricular rate, which becomes irregularly irregular. The atrial cycle length also changes continuously and may not be the same between different atrial regions (Duytschaever et al., 2001). As electrophysiological remodeling of the atrial myocardium occurs early during AF, with changes in effective refractory period and excitability, the input signals arriving to the AV node may vary significantly. Results from experimental studies are heterogenous as various methods for AF induction have been used, that affect the resulting atrial electrical activity and atrioventricular conduction (Roka et al., 2008) (Figure 2). The randomness of the ventricular rhythm is still debated (van den Berg et al., 1995; Stein et al., 1999; Roka & Merkely, 2008).

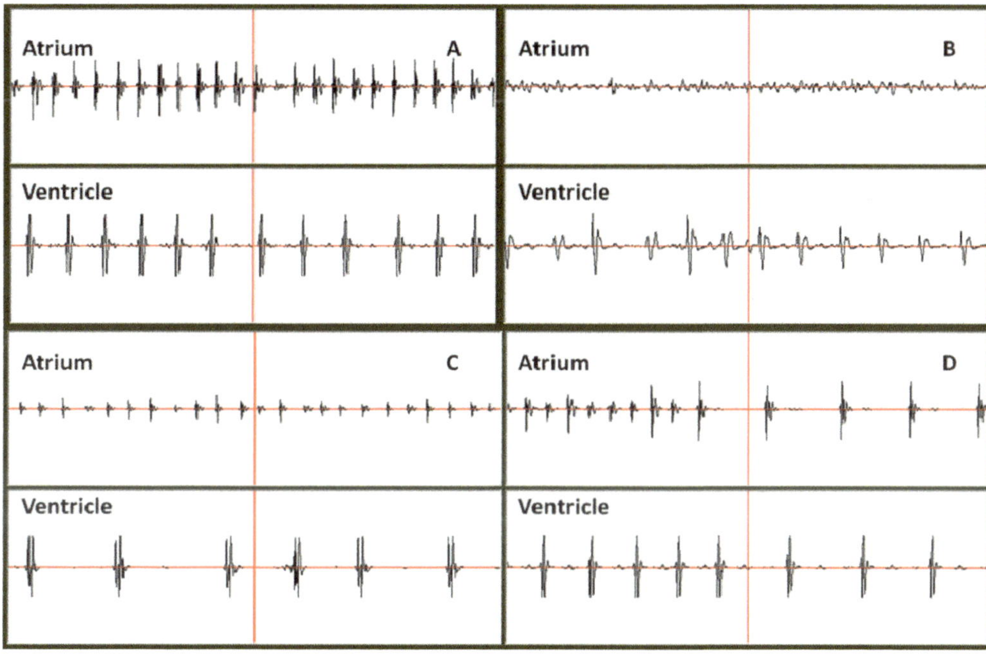

Fig. 2. Intracardiac recordings from healthy dogs with atrial fibrillation, induced by 50 Hz alternating current stimulation of the atria. Signals are recorded near the bundle of His (Ventricle) and near the AV node (Atrium). Atrial signal morphology is highly variable even in similar subjects with similar induction methods. A: discrete high frequency atrial signals with rapid, irregular ventricular rate. B: high frequency atrial signals without identifiable isoelectric baseline. C: discrete atrial signals with slower ventricular rate. D: spontaneous cardioversion of atrial fibrillation.

Main factors affecting the ventricular rate in AF are the electrophysiological properties of the AV node, rate and organization of atrial inputs, autonomic tone and effect of medications on the AV node. Increased parasympathetic and reduced sympathetic tone exert negative dromotropic effects on AV nodal conduction, while the opposite is true in states of decreased parasympathetic and increased sympathetic tone. Vagal tone also enhances the negative chronotropic effects of concealed conduction in the AV node (van den

Berg et al., 1997). Fluctuations in autonomic tone can produce wide variations in ventricular rate - slow ventricular rate during sleep but accelerated ventricular response during exercise. Several other factors also play a significant role, such as exercise (Bootsma et al.,, 1970), retrograde conduction after premature or ventricular paced beats (Greenhut et al., 1996), drugs, age and gender (Hnatkova et al., 1998).

5. Clinical relevance of AV node function in atrial fibrillation

If untreated, the ventricular rate is generally 90-170/minute in AF. Rates below 60/minute are seen with intrinsic AV node disease, high vagal tone or due to medications. Rates higher than 200/minute may be due to hyperthyroidism, presence of an accessory pathway or high catecholaminergic state. Regular ventricular rate during AF may indicate AV block with junctional or ventricular escape, or accelerated junctional activity. Occasionally, regularly irregular or group beating may be observed if the lower nodal pacemaker activity has a Wenckebach type exit block (Figure 3).

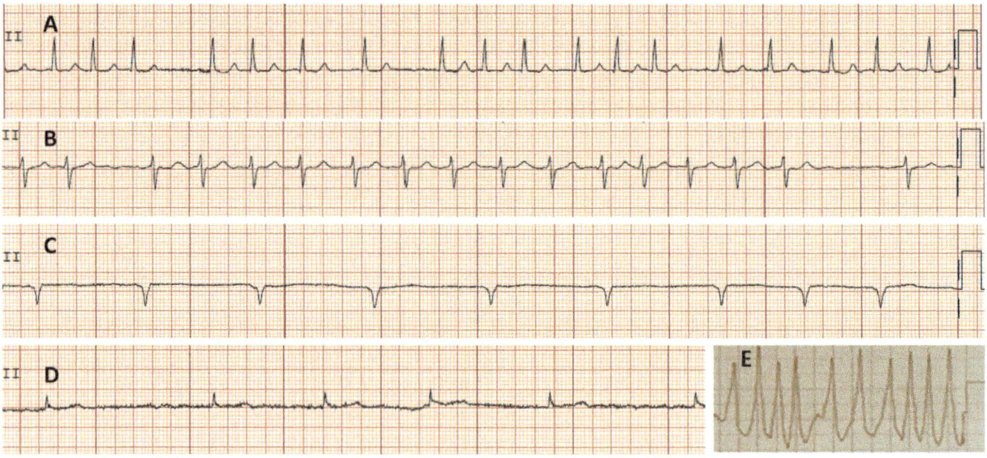

Fig. 3. Atrial fibrillation - variations of rate response. A: "typical" irregularly irregular rhythm. B: quasi-regular rhythm with occasional longer RR cycles. C: slow ventricular response, with junctional rhythm for most of the tracing. D: slow, irregular ventricular response. E: atrial fibrillation with preexcitation, "FBI tachycardia" - fast, broad, irregular.

A conventional 12-lead electrocardiogram is usually enough to establish the diagnosis. In paroxysmal forms Holter monitoring, event- or loop recording may be necessary (Fuster et al., 2011). In most cases, atrial fibrillation is easily diagnosed by the absence of P waves, presence of f waves and irregularly irregular RR intervals. QRS complexes are narrow unless there is fixed or rate-dependent bundle-branch block or preexcitation. Aberrant conduction is common and facilitated by the irregularity of the ventricular response. When a long interval is followed by a relatively short interval, the QRS complex following the short interval is often aberrantly conducted (Ashman phenomenon). In case of severely decreased AV conduction, junctional escape may lead to a regular rhythm (Figure 4). This may be often observed with digoxin toxicity, due to impaired AV conduction and enhanced junctional automaticity.

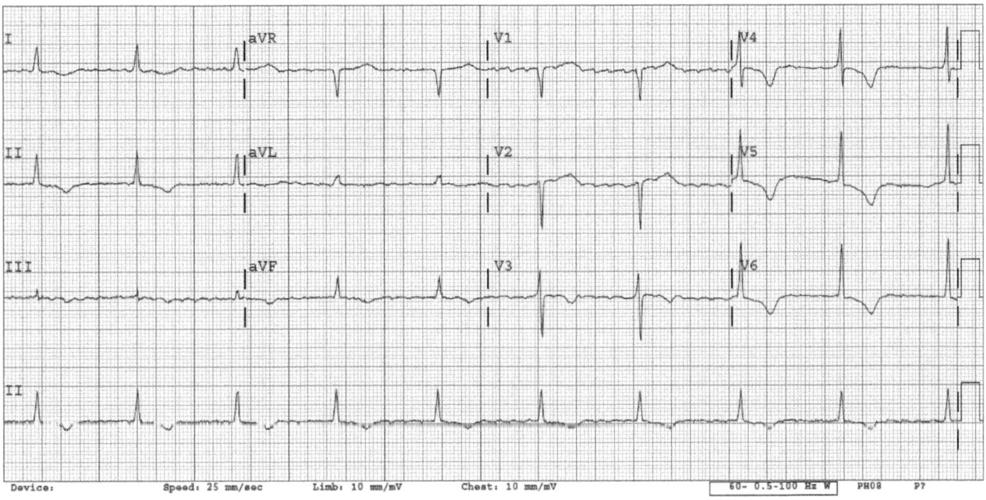

Fig. 4. Atrial fibrillation with junctional escape rhythm – the RR intervals are regular.

Atrial fibrillation may lead to irregular wide QRS tachycardia when it is associated with intraventricular conduction abnormalities, such as bundle branch block (Figure 5). Despite the irregular RR intervals, the QRS morphology shows little variation in these cases and is generally consistent with typical bundle branch block, occasionally showing rate-dependency. The differential diagnosis should include atrial fibrillation with preexcitation (QRS morphology is variable, delta waves are present) and polymorphic ventricular tachycardia (highly variable QRS morphology usually not typical for bundle branch block, atrioventricular dissociation, fusion or capture beats may be visible).

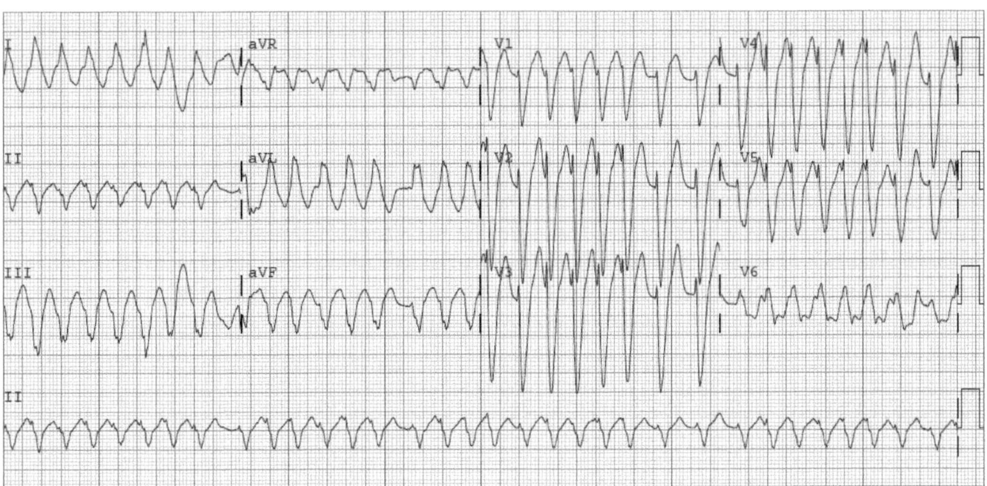

Fig. 5. Atrial fibrillation with rapid ventricular rate and left bundle branch block.

Multiple supraventricular arrhythmias may mimic the irregularly irregular ventricular activation seen in AF, either due to irregular atrial rate or variable atrioventricular conduction. Multifocal atrial tachycardia may be difficult to distinguish from atrial fibrillation if the P wave amplitude is low. In this case, each QRS should be preceded by a P wave, the atrioventricular delay may be slightly variable (Figure 6). In case of very high atrial rate or use of AV-nodal blocking agents non-conducted P waves may be also observed.

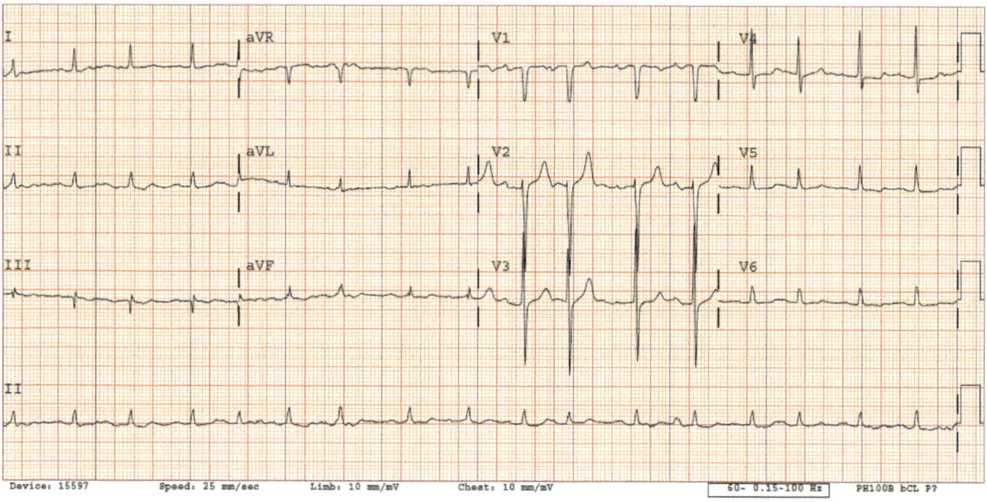

Fig. 6. Multifocal atrial tachycardia with irregularly irregular RR intervals similar to atrial fibrillation, however, each QRS is preceded by a P wave.

Atrial flutter may lead to irregular ventricular rate if the atrioventricular conduction does not follow a fixed ratio. Atypical flutters may lack the typical negative F waves in the inferior leads (Figure 7). In certain cases, serial electrograms may show evidence of both atrial fibrillation and flutter in the same patient.

Occasionally, even sinus or atrial tachycardia may be difficult to distinguish from AF, if the P waves are hidden in the QRS-T complex due to high heart rate or prolonged atrioventricular delay and frequent premature beats lead to irregular rate.

Persistently elevated ventricular rate during AF may lead to tachycardia-induced cardiomyopathy. It is important to recognize this condition, in which heart failure is a consequence rather than the cause of AF as control of the ventricular rate may lead to reversal of the myopathic process (Grogan et al., 1992). The time and heart rate required to develop tachycardia-induced cardiomyopathy is less clear, however, heart rate above 130/minute seems to be necessary in most cases (Shinbane et al., 1997).

Irregular ventricular rate itself decreases the cardiac output (Clark et al., 1997) and coronary blood flow (Wichmann et al., 1983). Myocardial contractility is not constant during AF because of force-interval relationships associated with variations in cycle length, this contributes to the largely variable pulse pressures and stroke volumes (Brookes et al., 1998).

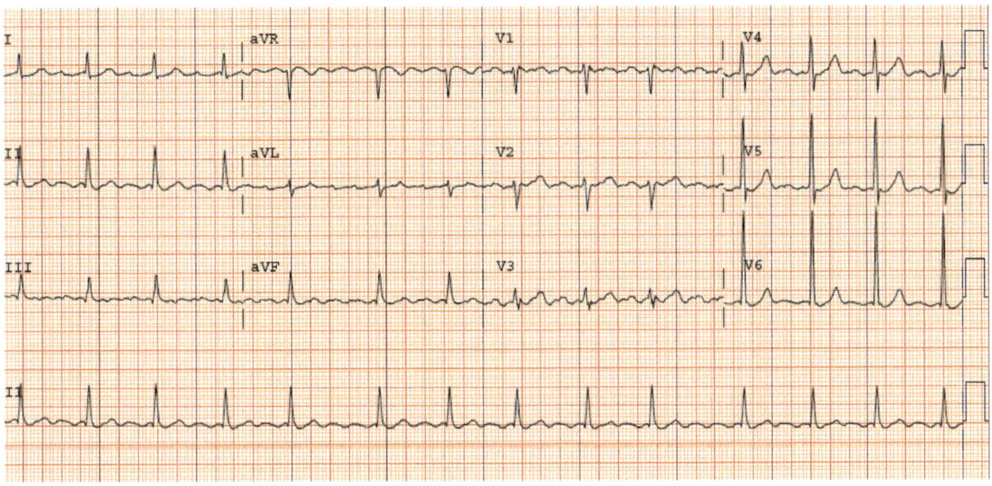

Fig. 7. Atypical atrial flutter with irregular RR intervals due to variable atrioventricular conduction.

Rapid ventricular rate during AF may adversely impact mitral valve function, increasing mitral regurgitation, due to the relationship between left atrial and left ventricular pressures. In addition, rate-related intraventricular conduction delay (such as left bundle-branch block) may further compromise the synchrony of LV wall motion and reduce cardiac output. Such conduction disturbances may further exacerbate mitral regurgitation and limit ventricular filling. Controlling the ventricular rate and regularity may reverse these adverse hemodynamic effects, however, the changes can persist for a prolonged time even after cardioversion (Upshaw, 1997). Tachycardia-induced cardiomyopathy tends to resolve within 6 months of rate or rhythm control; when tachycardia recurs, LV ejection fraction declines and HF develops over a shorter period, this is associated with a relatively poor prognosis (Nerheim et al., 2004). Although it would be clinically important to identify patients where high ventricular rate plays the major role in the development of heart failure, thus may benefit from aggressive rate and/or rhythm control, prospective identification of these cases is difficult, so far heart failure associated with relatively small left ventricular size seems to be predictive (Fujino et al., 2007).

6. Pharmacological rate control

Several complications of atrial fibrillation are due to high, irregular ventricular rate: palpitations, heart failure, and tachycardia-induced cardiomyopathy. The ventricular rate may increase excessively during exercise even when it is well controlled at rest. Medications used to control ventricular rate generally work by increasing the refractory period of the $I_{ca,\,L}$ Ca^{+} current, thus increasing the filtering function of the AV node. Non-dihydropyridine (non-DHP) calcium channel inhibitors, such as verapamil and diltiazem, directly inhibit the $I_{ca,\,L}$, while adrenergic β-blockers work indirectly through the adrenergic receptors. Digoxin increases parasympathetic vagal activity and is ineffective in situations when vagal tone diminishes, such as exercise. Antiarrhythmic medications, such as amiodarone or dronedarone may also be used for rate control due to their pluripotent effects. When Na^{+} channel blockers are used for cardioversion or maintenance of sinus rhythm, increase in ventricular rate may occasionally be observed due to vagolytic effects (quinidine, disopyramide) or regularization of atrial activity (such as atrial flutter), which in turn decreases the filtering effect of concealed conduction. Adenosine binds to A1 receptors and activates $I_{K/Ado}$, a subtype of I_k similar to $I_{K/Ach}$, increasing outward K^+ current, similar to parasympathetic stimuli; it also inhibits I_f.

The definition of adequate rate control has been based primarily on short-term hemodynamic studies and mostly refers to ventricular rate below a certain limit, but has not been well studied with respect to regularity of the ventricular response. Initial rate control criteria varied with patient age, usually involved achieving ventricular rates between 60-80/minute at rest and between 90-115/minute during moderate exercise. For the AFFIRM trial, adequate control was defined as an average heart rate up to 80/minute at rest and either an average rate up to 100/minute over at least 18 hour ambulatory Holter monitoring with no rate above 100% of the maximum age-adjusted predicted exercise heart rate or a maximum heart rate of 110/ minute during a 6-minute walk test (Olshansky et al., 2004). The RACE trial used heart rate less than 100/minute at rest. In the rate control arm, no differences were observed in terms of cardiovascular morbidity, mortality, and quality of life between the patients who achieved resting heart rate <80/minute, compared to those with higher resting heart rate (Groenveld et al., 2009). A comparison of the rate control arms of the AFFIRM and RACE studies (mean heart rate 76.1 vs. 83.4/minute) showed no significant difference in the primary composite endpoint of mortality, cardiovascular hospitalization and myocardial infarction. However, patients with mean heart rates during AF within the AFFIRM (≤80/minute) or RACE (<100/minute) criteria had a better outcome than patients with heart rates ≥100/minute (hazard ratios 0.69 and 0.58, respectively, for ≤80/minute and <100/minute compared with ≥100/minute, van Gelder et al., 2006).

The large randomized, prospective RACE II trial compared lenient rate-control (resting heart rate <110/minute) vs. strict rate-control strategy (resting heart rate <80/minute and heart rate during moderate exercise <110/minute), in 614 patients with permanent atrial fibrillation. The primary outcome was a composite of death from cardiovascular causes, hospitalization for heart failure, and stroke, systemic embolism, bleeding, and life-threatening arrhythmic events. The duration of follow-up was at least 2 years, with a maximum of 3 years. The estimated cumulative incidence of the primary outcome at 3 years was 12.9% in the lenient-control group and 14.9% in the strict-control group (p<0.001 for the prespecified non-inferiority margin). The frequencies of the components of the primary outcome were similar in the two groups. More patients in the lenient-control group met the target heart rate: 97.7% vs. 67.0% (p<0.001), with fewer total visits (median 0 vs. 2 per patient, p<0.001). The frequencies of symptoms and adverse events were similar in the two groups (van Gelder et al., 2010). The study population was 66% male with an average age of 68±8 years, body mass index of 29±5, left ventricular ejection fraction of 52±12%, 65% in NYHA functional class I. Lenient rate control with a resting heart rate <110/minute may be adequate for these patients. Patients with moderate to severe heart failure were underrepresented in this study (NYHA III in 4.7%, left ventricular ejection fraction <40% in 15% of patients), the optimal heart rate for these patients is less clear.

The clinical outcomes (mortality, morbidity), that can be achieved with focusing on rate control and anticoagulation were similar to those with aggressive rhythm control using antiarrhythmic drugs and cardioversion in the large randomized AFFIRM and RACE trials (Olshansky et al., 2004; Hagens et al., 2005). However, this may be due to the relative inefficacy and poor side effect profile of current antiarrhythmic medications and may change in the near future as new medications are developed and indications of atrial fibrillation ablation evolve. Patients who actually stayed in sinus rhythm in the AFFIRM trial, independent of treatment strategy, had better outcomes (Corley et al., 2004).

The practice guidelines on the management of atrial fibrillation, including rate control, have recently been updated by the American College of Cardiology Foundation, American Heart Association, and, and the European Society of Cardiology (Fuster et al., 2011, Table 1 and 2).

Recommendations	Class of recommendation	Level of evidence
General		
Measurement of the heart rate at rest	I	B
In patients with AF-related symptoms during activity, heart rate control should be assessed during exercise	I	B
Use of pharmacological rate control for persistent of permanent AF	I	B
Acute setting		
Iv. beta-blocker or non-DHP calcium channel antagonist to slow down ventricular rate (caution in hypotensive patients)	I	B
Iv. digoxin or amiodarone for patients with AF and heart failure, without preexcitation	I	B
Iv. amiodarone when other measures are unsuccessful or contraindicated	IIa	C
Iv. procainamide or ibutilide in AF with preexcitation, if electrical cardioversion is not indicated	IIa	C
Iv. procainamide, disopyramide, ibutilide, or amiodarone for hemodynamically stable AF with accessory pathway	IIb	B
Chronic pharmacological rate control		
Oral digoxin for rate control at rest in patients with HF, LV dysfunction, or sedentary lifestyle	I	C
Oral digoxin + beta blocker or non-DHP calcium channel antagonist for rate control at rest and during exercise. Medication choice and doses should be individualized to avoid bradycardia.	IIa	B
Oral amiodarone alone or in combination if adequate rate cannot at rest and during exercise cannot be achieved with beta-blocker, non-DHP calcium channel antagonist, or digoxin	IIb	C
Non-pharmacological rate control		
Ablation of the AV node or accessory pathway when pharmacological therapy is insufficient or associated with side effects	IIa	B
Catheter ablation of the AV node if rate control cannot be achieved by pharmacological agents or tachycardia-mediated cardiomyopathy is suspected	IIb	C

Table 1. Recommended procedures and interventions for ventricular rate control in atrial fibrillation. Levels of recommendation: class I - generally recommended. Class IIa - should be considered. Class IIb - may be considered. Levels of evidence: B - single randomized trial or nonrandomized studies. C - consensus opinion of experts, case studies or standard of care. *AF: atrial fibrillation. DHP: dihydropyridine. Iv.: intravenous. HF: heart failure. LV: left ventricular. AV: atrioventricular.*

Contraindicated procedures and interventions	Class of recommendation	Level of evidence
Digoxin alone in paroxysmal atrial fibrillation	III	B
Catheter ablation of the AV node without prior attempt of pharmacological rate control	III	C
Iv. non-DHP calcium channel antagonist in decompensated HF	III	C
Iv. digoxin or non-DHP calcium channel antagonist in AF with preexcitation	III	C

Table 2. Contraindicated procedures and interventions for ventricular rate control in atrial fibrillation. Levels of recommendation: class III – generally contraindicated as there is no benefit or may be harmful. Levels of evidence: B – single randomized trial or nonrandomized studies. C – consensus opinion of experts, case studies or standard of care. *AF: atrial fibrillation. DHP: dihydropyridine. Iv.: intravenous. HF: heart failure. LV: left ventricular. AV: atrioventricular.*

6.1 Acute rate control

Patients who are symptomatic with rapid ventricular rates during AF require prompt medical management, and cardioversion should be considered if symptomatic hypotension, angina, or heart failure is present. The pharmacological agent of choice depends on the presence of comorbidities, such as heart failure/hemodynamic instability and preexcitation (Fuster et al., 2011; Table 3).

Medication	Dose in acute setting	Class of recommendation	Level of evidence
No heart failure or accessory pathway			
Esmolol	500 μg/kg slow iv. bolus, 60-200 μg/kg/min infusion	I	C
Metoprolol	2.5-5 mg slow iv. bolus	I	C
Diltiazem	0.25 mg/kg slow iv. bolus, 5-15 mg/h infusion	I	B
Verapamil	75-150 μg/kg slow iv. bolus	I	B
Heart failure			
Digoxin	0.25 mg iv. every 2 hours, up to 1.5 mg; followed by 0.125-0.375 mg/day iv. or po., slow onset of action	I	B
Amiodarone	150 mg iv. over 10 minutes, 0.5-1 mg/min infusion	IIa	C
Accessory pathway			
Amiodarone	150 mg iv. over 10 minutes, 0.5-1 mg/min infusion	IIa	C
Accessory pathway and heart failure			
-	Urgent electrical cardioversion	I	B

Table 3. Recommendations for acute rate control in atrial fibrillation. Instead of esmolol and metoprolol, similar beta-blocking agents may be used with same class of recommendation. Levels of recommendation: class I – generally recommended. Class IIa – should be considered. Levels of evidence: B – single randomized trial or nonrandomized studies. C – consensus opinion of experts, case studies or standard of care. *Iv.: intravenous.*

Intravenous non-DHP calcium channel antagonists are effective for ventricular rate control (Boudonas et al., 1995), although these agents should be avoided in patients with heart failure due to systolic dysfunction because of their negative inotropic effects. A randomized trial comparing intravenously administered diltiazem, digoxin and amiodarone found that patients presenting to the emergency department with AF and heart rate >120/min achieved shorter time to rate control (rate <90/minute), largest reduction in AF symptom frequency and severity scores and significantly shorter hospital stay if they were assigned to the diltiazem group, versus digoxin or amiodarone (Siu et al., 2009). Beta blockers may be particularly useful in states of high adrenergic tone, such as postoperative AF, but more data is available for rhythm control in this situation: intravenous esmolol produced more rapid conversion to sinus rhythm than diltiazem after noncardiac surgery, ventricular rates after 2 and 12 hours were similar with both treatments (Balser et al., 1998).

Combinations may be necessary to achieve rate control, which requires careful dose titration. Although intravenous digoxin may slow down the ventricular response in AF at rest, the onset is delayed for at least 60 minutes in most patients and the peak effect does not develop for up to 6 hours. There is lack of evidence whether a second agent should be added early (to avoid possible dose-related side effects of medications) or only after administration the maximum recommended dose of the first agent. Wide variations in clinical practice exist, however, the outcomes were similar in observational studies (Buccelletti et al., 2011; Stiell et al., 2011).

6.2 Chronic rate control

There is no evidence that long-term pharmacological rate control would adversely influence left ventricular function, although bradycardia and heart block may occur as an unwanted effect of beta blockers, amiodarone, digoxin, or non-DHP calcium channel antagonists. Elderly patients and those with paroxysmal AF are more likely to experience side effects. Some patients develop symptomatic bradycardia that requires permanent pacing, while still having episodes of rapid ventricular rate. Non-pharmacological therapy should be considered when pharmacological measures fail.

Beta-blockers are safe and effective for rate control and superior to placebo. They should be initiated cautiously in patients with heart failure who have reduced ejection fraction. Most data are available for nadolol and atenolol. Patients may experience slow rates at rest, or exercise tolerance may be compromised when the rate response is blunted excessively (Segal et al., 2000). Sotalol, in addition to its antiarrhythmic effects, also provides excellent rate control (Anderson & Prystowsky, 1999). Atenolol, metoprolol, and sotalol provide better control of exercise-induced tachycardia than digoxin (Lewis et al., 1989). Carvedilol is similarly effective. Beta blockers were the most effective drug class for rate control in the AFFIRM trial (with or without digoxin), achieving rate control endpoints in 70% of patients, compared to 54% with use of calcium channel blockers (Olshansky et al., 2004).

Non-DHP calcium channel antagonist agents (verapamil and diltiazem) are the only agents that were shown to improve quality of life and exercise tolerance. Direct comparisons of verapamil and diltiazem have demonstrated similar effectiveness (Lundström & Rydén, 1990). These agents may be preferred for long-term use over beta blockers in patients with bronchospasm or chronic obstructive pulmonary disease.

The efficacy of digoxin is reduced in states of high sympathetic tone or in paroxysmal AF. The combination of digoxin and atenolol is effective for rate control (Farshi et al., 1999). In contrast to its limited effect in patients with paroxysmal AF, digoxin is moderately effective in those with persistent AF, particularly when HF is present. Digoxin administered alone slows the resting heart rate, but it does not slow heart rate during exercise (Segal et al., 2000). Given the multiple interactions and side effects, digoxin should not be considered as first line therapy for rate control. The combination of digoxin and a beta blocker appears more effective than the combination of digoxin with a calcium channel antagonist (Farshi et al., 1999).

Amiodarone has both sympatholytic and calcium antagonist properties, which depresses AV conduction. Intravenous amiodarone is generally well tolerated in critically ill patients who develop rapid atrial tachyarrhythmias refractory to conventional treatment, but efficacy has not been sufficiently evaluated in this indication. It may be considered when first line agents are ineffective or contraindicated (Clemo et al., 1998). The potential toxicity must be carefully weighted (Fuster et al., 2011, Table 4).

Medication	Maintenance dose	Class of recommendation	Level of evidence
	No heart failure or accessory pathway		
Metoprolol	25-100 mg twice a day	I	C
Diltiazem	120-360 mg daily, divided doses or slow release	I	B
Verapamil	120-360 mg daily, divided doses or slow release	I	B
	Heart failure, no accessory pathway		
Digoxin	0.5 mg po. loading, 0.125-0.375 mg/day po. maintenance; slow onset of action (2 days)	I	C
Amiodarone	800 mg daily for 1 week, 600 mg daily for 1 week, 400 mg daily for 4-6 week, maintenance 200 mg po. daily; slow onset of action (1-3 weeks)	IIb	C
	Accessory pathway		
-	Ablation should be considered	-	-

Table 4. Recommendations for chronic rate control in atrial fibrillation. Instead of metoprolol, similar beta-blocking agents may be used with same class of recommendation. Levels of recommendation: class I - generally recommended. Class IIb - may be considered. Levels of evidence: B - single randomized trial or nonrandomized studies. C - consensus opinion of experts, case studies or standard of care. *po.: oral.*

Oral amiodarone decreases the ventricular rate without affecting exercise capacity, quality of life or AF symptoms, even if it is unable to cardiovert the patient (Tse et al., 2001). Dronedarone has also good rate control characteristics in addition to its antiarrhythmic effects, with a side effect profile more favorable than amiodarone (Page et al., 2011). However, excess mortality and morbidity in elderly patients with permanent AF lead to early discontinuation of the PALLAS trial, so dronaderone is contraindicated in permanent AF.

In patients with paroxysmal atrial flutter and fibrillation, propafenone or flecainide used for rhythm control may promote 1:1 AV conduction during the flutter, leading to excessive ventricular rate. These agents must be coadministered with AV nodal blocking agents, unless ablation has been performed without recurrence of the flutter.

7. Non-pharmacological rate control

The efficacy of pharmacological interventions designed to achieve rate control in patients with AF has been about 80% in clinical trials (Weerasooriya et al., 2003). Non-pharmacological measures should be considered in patients who are still symptomatic or in whom adequate rate control cannot be achieved.

Ventricular pacing at approximately the mean ventricular rate during AF may regularize the ventricular rhythm during AF by eliminating longer ventricular cycles and reducing the number of short ventricular cycles due to retrograde block (Wittkampf et al., 1988). This may be useful for patients with marked variability in ventricular rates or resting bradycardia during pharmacological treatment. However, frequent right ventricular pacing may lead to left ventricular dysfunction. Patients with paroxysmal AF indicated a preference for the paced regularization strategy in a study, while patients with permanent AF showed no preference despite a 29% improvement of irregularity (Simpson et al., 2001). However, another study showed no benefit in any group (Tse et al., 2004).

AV node ablation in conjunction with permanent pacemaker implantation provides effective control of the heart rate and improves symptoms in selected patients with AF. Patients most likely to benefit from this strategy are those with symptoms or tachycardia mediated cardiomyopathy related to rapid ventricular rate during AF, that cannot be controlled adequately with antiarrhythmic or negative chronotropic medications (Wood et al., 2000). In the Ablate and Pace Trial, 25% of patients with AF who had an ejection fraction below 45% displayed a greater than 15% increase in ejection fraction after ablation (Kay et al., 1998).

The slow pathway of the AV node has a short effective refractory period that may be responsible for maintaining rapid ventricular rate during AF. Catheter ablation of this area (inferior atrial inputs to the AV node) slows the ventricular rate during AF and improves symptoms without pacemaker implantation (Williamson et al., 1995). However, the ventricular rate rises over the 6 months following ablation.

Complete AV nodal ablation and permanent pacemaker implantation demonstrated better symptom relief than AV node modification alone. The 1-year mortality rate after AV nodal ablation and permanent pacemaker implantation is approximately 6.3%, with 2.0% risk of sudden death. Although a causal relationship between the procedure and sudden death still remains controversial, the pacemaker is routinely set to a high basic rate, such as 90/minute for the first month after ablation, to avoid bradycardia-induced tachyarrhythmias after a prolonged period of rapid ventricular rate (Evans et al., 1991). Although the symptomatic benefits of AV nodal ablation are clear, limitations include the persistent need for anticoagulation, loss of AV synchrony, and lifelong pacemaker dependency.

As the adverse hemodynamic effects of right ventricular apical pacing are well known, biventricular devices should be considered in these patients, especially in those with left ventricular dysfunction or heart failure. The PAVE trial showed better exercise tolerance with biventricular pacing, but no mortality benefit was realized over the relatively short follow up period of 6 months (Doshi et al., 2005). A subgroup analysis suggested that functional improvements were confined to patients with left ventricular ejection fraction below 35% before ablation. Upgrade to a biventricular device should be considered after AV node ablation in patients with heart failure and a right ventricular pacing system (Leon et al., 2002).

In patients with heart failure and AF, undergoing cardiac resynchronization therapy, ablation of the AV node should be considered as rapid ventricular rate may lead to suboptimal biventricular stimulation. Biventricular stimulation should be at least 98% to achieve optimal benefits from resynchronization, which may be difficult to achieve in AF without AV node ablation (Hayes et al., 2011; Figure 8). In addition, the irregular rhythm alone adversely affects the hemodynamic function.

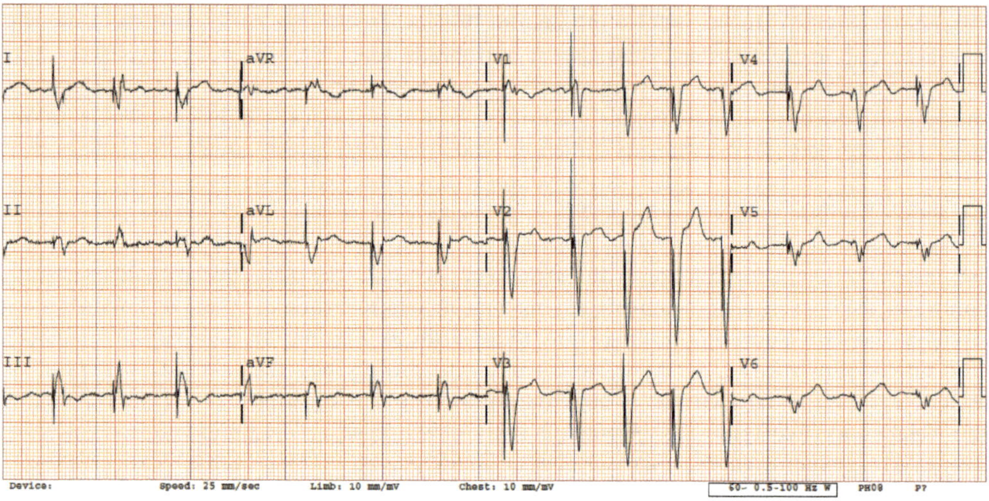

Fig. 8. Importance of rate control in patients with cardiac resynchronization devices. These devices improve hemodynamics in patients with severe left ventricular dysfunction and intraventricular conduction delay by simultaneously pacing the right and left ventricle. In case the ventricles get activated before the delivery of the pacing stimuli, such as in atrial fibrillation with suboptimal rate control, the only option left for the device is to pace simultaneously with the sensed beat (sense response pacing). However, this fusion beat may be hemodynamically inferior to the biventricular paced beat. In addition, irregularity of the rhythm adds to the hemodynamic derangement.

Parasympathetic nerve stimulation is an experimental method to achieve rate control via selective stimulation of the parasympathetic nerves supplying the AV node. This may be accomplished with a coronary sinus electrode or an active fixation electrode positioned near the AV node (Vago et al., 2004). This method may be an option in the future for patients with highly symptomatic paroxysmal atrial fibrillation, when medications or ablation are not desired, tolerated or effective. However, in some cases, atrial fibrillation may be vagally mediated and this method of stimulation may potentially increase the incidence of arrhythmias or increase the duration of the episodes.

8. Preexcitation in atrial fibrillation

A bypass tract with non-decremental conduction and short effective refractory period may allow the almost unfiltered propagation of AF to the ventricles, resulting in an extremely high ventricular rate, even >300/minute. Variable QRS morphology and irregular rate may be useful clues for identification and differentiation from ventricular tachycardia. Prompt recognition and treatment is important as this entity may rapidly degenerate to ventricular fibrillation (Fuster V., 2011). In hemodynamically stable patients with preexcitation, type I antiarrhythmic agents or amiodarone may be administered intravenously. AV nodal blocking drugs are contraindicated as the heart rate increases when the ventricles are activated solely through the bypass tract. The potential for beta blockers to facilitate conduction across the accessory pathway is controversial. In unstable cases, prompt electrical cardioversion is the treatment of choice. Beta blockers and calcium channel blockers may be considered for chronic oral use (Petri et al., 1983).

9. Conclusion

Ventricular rate in atrial fibrillation is determined by a complex interaction between the atrial electrical activity and properties of the AV node. Although the hemodynamic consequences of the rapid and irregular ventricular rate are well known, details of electro-pathophysiology still need to be elucidated.

Rate control is one of the most important aspects in the treatment of patients with atrial fibrillation, with substantial evidence supporting the use of pharmacological agents in both acute and chronic settings. Effective non-pharmacological treatment options may be used in refractory cases.

10. Acknowledgments

Dr. Erika Toth's contribution to the manuscript is appreciated.

The publication was supported by TAMOP 4.2.2-08/1/KMR-2008-0004, TAMOP-4.2.1.B-09/1/KMR and TAMOP 4.2.2./B10/1.-2010-0013 grants provided by the National Development Agency of Hungary.

11. References

Anderson, J.L. & Prystowsky, E.N. (1999). Sotalol: An important new antiarrhythmic. *Am Heart J*, Vol. 137, No. 3, pp. 388-409.

Bakker, M.L., Christoffels, V.M. & Moorman, A.F.M. (2010). The cardiac pacemaker and conduction system develops from embryonic myocardium that retains its primitive phenotype. *J Cardiovasc Pharmacol*, Vol. 56, No. 1, pp. 6-15.

Balser, J.R., Martinez, E.A., Winters, B.D., Perdue, P.W., Clarke, A.W., Huang, W., Tomaselli, G.F., Dorman, T., Campbell, K., Lipsett, P., Breslow, M.J. & Rosenfeld, B.A. (1998). Beta-adrenergic blockade accelerates conversion of postoperative supraventricular tachyarrhythmias. *Anesthesiology*, Vol. 89, No. 5, pp. 1052-1059.

Bootsma, B.K., Hoelen, A.J., Strackee, J. & Meijler, F.L. (1970). Analysis of R-R intervals in patients with atrial fibrillation at rest and during exercise. *Circulation*, Vol. 41, No. 5, pp. 783-794.

Boudonas, G., Lefkos, N., Efthymiadis, A.P., Styliadis, I.G. & Tsapas, G. (1995). Intravenous administration of diltiazem in the treatment of supraventricular tachyarrhythmias. *Acta Cardiol*, Vol. 50, No. 3, pp. 125-134.

Boyett, M.R. (2009). 'And the beat goes on' The cardiac conduction system: the wiring system of the heart. *Exp Physiol*, Vol. 94, No. 10, pp. 1035-1049.

Brookes, C.I., White, P.A., Staples, M., Oldershaw, P.J., Redington, A.N., Collins, P.D., Noble, M.I. (1998). Myocardial contractility is not constant during spontaneous atrial fibrillation in patients. *Circulation,* Vol. 98, No. 17, pp. 1762-1768.

Buccelletti, F., Di Somma, S., Galante, A., Pugliese, F., Alegiani, F., Bertazzoni, G., Silveri, N.G., Legramante, J.M. & Franceschi, F. (2011). Disparities in management of new-onset atrial fibrillation in the emergency department despite adherence to the current guidelines: data from a large metropolitan area. *Intern Emerg Med,* Vol. 6, No. 2, pp. 149-156.

Clark, D.M., Plumb, V.J., Epstein, A.E. & Kay, G.N. (1997). Hemodynamic effects of an irregular sequence of ventricular cycle lengths during atrial fibrillation. *J Am Coll Cardiol,* Vol. 30, No. 4, pp. 1039-1045.

Clemo, H.F., Wood, M.A., Gilligan, D.M. & Ellenbogen K.A. (1998). Intravenous amiodarone for acute heart rate control in the critically ill patient with atrial tachyarrhythmias. *Am J Cardiol,* Vol. 81, No. 5, pp. 594-598.

Corley, S.D., Epstein, A.E., DiMarco, J.P., Domanski, M.J., Geller, N., Greene, H.L., Josephson, R.A., Kellen, J.C., Klein, R.C., Krahn, A.D., Mickel, M., Mitchell, L.B., Nelson, J.D., Rosenberg, Y., Schron, E., Shemanski, L., Waldo, A.L., Wyse, D.G. & AFFIRM Investigators. (2004). Relationships between sinus rhythm, treatment, and survival in the Atrial Fibrillation Follow-Up Investigation of Rhythm Management (AFFIRM) Study. *Circulation,* Vol. 109, No. 12, pp. 1509-1513.

Doshi, R.N., Daoud, E.G., Fellows, C., Turk, K., Duran, A., Hamdan, M.H., Pires, L.A. & PAVE Study Group. (2005). Left ventricular-based cardiac stimulation post AV nodal ablation evaluation (the PAVE study). *J Cadiovasc Electrophysiol,* Vol. 16, No. 11, pp. 1160-1165.

Duytschaever, M., Mast, F., Killian, M., Blaauw, Y., Wijffels, M. & Allessie, M. (2001). Methods for determining the refractory period and excitable gap during persistent atrial fibrillation in the goat. *Circulation,* Vol. 104, No. 8, pp. 957-962.

Evans, G.T.Jr., Scheinman, M.M., Bardy, G., Borggrefe, M., Brugada, P., Fisher, J., Fontaine, G., Huang, S.K., Huang, W.H. & Josephson, M. (1991). Predictors of in-hospital mortality after DC catheter ablation of atrioventricular junction. Results of a prospective, international, multicenter study. *Circulation,* Vol. 84, No. 5, pp. 1924-1937.

Farshi, R., Kistner, D., Sarma, J.S., Longmate, J.A. & Singh, B.N. (1999). Ventricular rate control in chronic atrial fibrillation during daily activity and programmed exercise: a crossover open-label study of five drug regimens. *J Am Coll Cardiol,* Vol. 33, No. 2, pp. 304-310.

Fujiki, A., Tani, M., Mizumaki, K., Yoshida, S. & Sasayama S. (1990). Quantification of human concealed atrioventricular nodal conduction: relation to ventricular response during atrial fibrillation. *Am Heart J,* Vol. 120, No. 3, pp. 598-603.

Fujino, T., Yamashita, T., Suzuki, S., Sugiyma, H., Sagara, K., Sawada, H., Aizawa, T., Igarashi, M. & Yamazaki, J. (2007). Characteristics of congestive heart failure accompanied by atrial fibrillation with special reference to tachycardia-induced cardiomyopathy. *Circulation Journal,* Vol. 71, No. 6, pp. 936-940.

Fuster, V., Rydén, L.E., Cannom, D.S., Crijns, H.J., Curtis, A.B., Ellenbogen, K.A., Halperin, J.L., Kay, G.N., Le Huezey, J.Y., Lowe, J.E., Olsson, S.B., Prystowsky, E.N., Tamargo, J.L. & Wann, L.S. (2011). 2011 ACCF/AHA/HRS focused updates incorporated into the ACC/AHA/ESC 2006 guidelines for the management of patients with atrial fibrillation: a report of the American College of Cardiology Foundation/American Heart Association Task Force on Practice Guidelines. *J Am Coll Cardiol,* Vol. 57, No. 11, pp. e101-e198.

Kurian, T., Ambrosi, C., Hucker, W., Fedorov, V.V. & Efimov, I.R. (2010). Anatomy and electrophysiology of the human AV node. *Pacing Clinc Electrophysiol,* Vol. 33, No. 6, pp. 754-762.

Leon, A.R., Greenberg, J.M., Kanuru, N., Baker, C.M., Mera, F.V., Smith, A.L., Langberg, J.J. & DeLurgio, D.B. (2002). Cardiac resynchronization in patients with congestive heart failure and chronic atrial fibrillation: effect of upgrading to biventricular pacing after chronic right ventricular pacing. *J Am Coll Cardiol,* Vol. 39, No. 8, pp. 1258-1263.

Lewis, R.V., McMurray, J. & McDevitt, D.G. (1989). Effects of atenolol, verapamil, and xamoterol on heart rate and exercise tolerance in digitalised patients with chronic atrial fibrillation. *J Cardiovasc Pharmacol,* Vol. 13, No. 1, pp. 1-6.

Garrigue, S., Tchou, P.J. & Mazgalev, T.N. (1999). Role of the differential bombardment of atrial inputs to the atrioventricular node as a factor influencing ventricular rate during high atrial rate. *Cardiovasc Res,* Vol. 44, No. 2, pp. 344-355.

Greener, I.D., Monfredi, O., Inada, S., Chandler, N.J., Tellez, J.O., Atkinson, A., Taube, M.A., Billeter, R., Anderson, R.H., Efimov, I.R., Molenaar, P., Sigg, D.C., Sharma, V., Boyett, M.R. & Dobrzynski, H. (2011). Molecular architecture of the human specialised atrioventricular conduction axis. *J Mol Cell Cardiol,* Vol. 50, No. 4, pp. 642-651.

Greenhut, S.E., Fraser, J., Steinhaus, B., Feld, G. & Hughes, W. (1996). Optimized standby rate reduces the ventricular rate variability in pacemaker patients with atrial fibrillation. *Pacing Clin Electrophysiol,* Vol. 19, No. 11, pp. 1780-1785.

Groenveld, H.F., Crijns, H.J., Rienstra, M., van den Berg, M.P., van Veldhuisen, D.J., van Gelder, I.C. & RACE investigators. (2009). Does intensity of rate control influence outcome in persistent atrial fibrillation? *Am Heart J,* Vol. 158, No. 5, pp. 785-791.

Grogan, M., Smith, H.C., Gersh, B.J. & Wood, D.L. (1992). Left ventricular dysfunction due to atrial fibrillation in patients initially believed to have idiopathic dilated cardiomyopathy. *Am J Cardiol,* Vol. 69, No. 19, pp. 1570-1573.

Hagens, V.E., Crijns, H.J., van Veldhuisen, D.J., van den Berg, M.P., Rienstra, M., Ranchor, A.V., Bosker, H.A., Kamp, O., Tijssen, J.G., Veeger, N.J., van Gelder, I.C. & RACE study group (2005). Rate control versus rhythm control for patients with persistent atrial fibrillation with mild to moderate heart failure: results from the RAte Control versus Electrical cardioversion (RACE) study. *Am Heart J,* Vol. 149, No. 6, pp. 1106-1111.

Hayes, D.L., Boehmer, J.P., Day, J., Gilliam, F.R.3rd, Heidenreich, P.A., Seth, M., Jones, P.W. & Saxon, L.A. (2011). Cardiac resynchronization therapy and the relationship of percent biventricular pacing to symptoms and survival. *Heart Rhythm,* in press.

Hnatkova, K., Waktare, J.E., Murgatroyd, F. D., Guo, X., Camm, A.J. & Malik M. (1998). Age and gender influences on rate and duration of paroxysmal atrial fibrillation. *Pacing Clin. Electrophysiol,* Vol. 21, No. 11, pp. 2455-2458.

Kay, G.N., Ellenbogen, K.A., Giudici, M., Redfield, M.M., Jenkins, L.S., Mianulli, M. & Wilkoff, B. (1998). The Ablate and Pace Trial: a prospective study of catheter ablation of the AV conduction system and permanent pacemaker implantation for treatment of atrial fibrillation. APT Investigators. *J Interv Card Electrophysiol,* Vol. 2, No. 2, pp. 121-135.

Lundström, T. & Rydén, L. (1990). Ventricular rate control and exercise performance in chronic atrial fibrillation: effects of diltiazem and verapamil. *J Am Coll Cardiol,* Vol. 16, No. 1, pp. 86-90.

Meijler, F.L. & Janse, M.J. (1988). Morphology and electrophysiology of the mammalian atrioventricular node. *Physiol Rev,* Vol. 68, No. 2, pp. 608-647.

Nerheim, P., Birger-Botkin, S., Piracha, L. & Olshansky, B. (2004). Heart failure and sudden death in patients with tachycardia-induced cardiomyopathy and recurrent tachycardia. *Circulation,* Vol. 110, No. 3, pp. 247-252.

Olshansky, B., Rosenfeld, L.E., Warner, A.L., Solomon, A.J., O'Neill, G., Sharma, A., Platia, E., Feld, G.K., Akiyama, T., Brodsky, M.A., Greene, H.L. & AFFIRM Investigators. (2004). The Atrial Fibrillation Follow-up Investigation of Rhythm Management (AFFIRM) study: approaches to control rate in atrial fibrillation. *J Am Coll Cardiol,* Vol. 43, No. 7, pp. 1201-1208.

Page, R.L., Connolly, S.J., Crijns, H.J., van Eickels. M., Gaudin, C., Torp-Pedersen, C., Hohnloser, S.H. & ATHENA Investigators. (2011). Rhythm- and rate-controlling effects of dronedarone in patients with atrial fibrillation (from the ATHENA trial). *Am J Cardiol,* Vol. 107, No. 7, pp. 1019-1022.

Petri, H., Kafka, W., Rudolph, W. (1983). Discrepant effects of oral and intravenous verapamil on A-V conduction in patients with ventricular preexcitation and atrial fibrillation. *Herz,* Vol. 8, No. 3, pp. 144-152.

Roka, A., Toth, E., Szilagyi, S. & Merkely, B. (2008). Electrical atrial fibrillation induction affects the characteristics of induced arrhythmia. *J Electrocardiol,* Vol. 41, No. 2, pp. 131-137.

Roka, A. & Merkely, B. (2008). Development and validation of a model of atrioventricular conduction in atrial fibrillation based on junctional intracardiac electrograms. *Comp Cardiol,* Vol. 35, No. 1, pp. 405-408.

Segal, J.B., McNamara, R.L., Miller, M.R., Kim, N., Goodman, S.N., Powe, N.R., Robinson, K., Yu, D. & Bass, E.B. (2000). The evidence regarding the drugs used for ventricular rate control. *J Fam Pract,* Vol. 49, No. 1, pp. 47-59.

Shinbane, J.S., Wood, M.A., Jensen, D.N., Ellenbogen, K.A., Fitzpatrick, A.P. & Scheinman MM. (1997). Tachycardia-induced cardiomyopathy: a review of animal models and clinical studies. *J Am Coll Cardiol,* Vol. 29, No. 4, pp. 709-715.

Simpson, C.S., Yee, R., Lee, J.K., Braney, M., Klein, G.J., Krahn, A.D. & Skanes, A.C. (2001). Safety and feasibility of a novel rate-smoothed ventricular pacing algorithm for atrial fibrillation. *Am Heart J,* Vol. 142, No. 2, pp. 294–300.

Siu, C.W., Lau, C.P., Lee, W.L., Lam, K.F. & Tse, H.F. (2009). Intravenous diltiazem is superior to intravenous amiodarone or digoxin for achieving ventricular rate control in patients with acute uncomplicated atrial fibrillation. *Crit Care Med*, Vol. 37, No. 7, pp. 2174–2179.

Stein, K.M., Walden, J., Lippman, N. & Lerman, B.B. (1999). Ventricular response in atrial fibrillation: random or deterministic? *Am J Physiol*, Vol. 277, No. 2, pp. H452–H458.

Stiell, I.G., Clement, C.M., Brison, R.J., Rowe, B.H., Borgundvaag, B., Langhan, T., Lang, E., Magee, K., Stenstrom, R., Perry, J.J., Birnie, D. & Wells, G.A. (2011). Variation in management of recent-onset atrial fibrillation and flutter among academic hospital emergency departments. *Ann Emerg Med*, Vol. 57, No. 1, pp. 13–21.

Tse, H.F., Lam, Y.M., Lau, C.P., Cheung, B.M. & Kumana, C.R. (2001). Comparison of digoxin versus low-dose amiodarone for ventricular rate control in patients with chronic atrial fibrillation. *Clin Exp Pharmacol Physiol*, Vol. 28, No. 5-6, pp. 446–450.

Tse, H.F., Newman, D., Ellenbogen, K.A., Buhr, T., Markowitz, T., Lau, C.P. & Atrial Fibrillation SYMPTOMS investigators (2004). Effects of ventricular rate regularization pacing on quality of life and symptoms in patients with atrial fibrillation (Atrial fibrillation symptoms mediated by pacing to mean rates [AF SYMPTOMS study]). *Am J Cardiol*, Vol. 94, No. 7, pp. 938–941.

Upshaw, C.B.Jr. (1997). Hemodynamic changes after cardioversion of chronic atrial fibrillation. *Arch Intern Med*, Vol. 157, No. 10, pp. 1070–1076.

Vago, H., Roka, A., Acsady, G. & Merkely, B. (2004). Parasympathetic cardiac nerve stimulation with implanted coronary sinus lead. *J Cardiovasc Electrophysiol*, Vol. 15, No. 5, pp. 588-590.

van den Berg, M.P., de Langen, C.D., Haaksma, J., Bel, K.J., Crijns, H.J., Dijk, W.A. & Lie, K.I. (1995). Analysis of randomness of atrial and ventricular rhythm in atrial fibrillation. *Eur Heart J*, Vol. 16, No. 7, pp. 971-976.

van den Berg, M.P., Brouwer, J., Tieleman, R.G., Mulder, G & Crijns H.J. (1997). Heart rate variability in patients with atrial fibrillation is related to vagal tone. *Circulation*, Vol. 96, No. 4, pp. 1209-1216.

van Gelder, I.C., Wyse, D.G., Chandler, M.L., Cooper, H.A., Olshansky, B., Hagens, V.E., Crijns, H.J. & RACE and AFFIRM Investigators. (2006). Does intensity of rate-control influence outcome in atrial fibrillation? An analysis of pooled data from the RACE and AFFIRM studies. *Europace*, Vol. 8, No. 11, pp. 935-942.

van Gelder, I.C., Groenveld, H.F., Crijns, H.J., Tuininga, Y.S., Tijssen, J.G., Alings, A.M., Hillege, H.L., Bergsma-Kadijk, J.A., Cornel, J.H., Kamp, O., Tukkie, R., Bosker, H.A., van Veldhuisen, D.J., van den Berg, M.P. & RACE II Investigators. (2010). Lenient versus strict rate control in patients with atrial fibrillation. *New Eng J Med*, Vol. 362, No. 15, pp. 1363-1373.

Weerasooriya, R., Davis, M., Powell, A., Szili-Torok, T., Shah, C., Whalley, D., Kanagaratnam, L., Heddle, W., Leitch, J., Perks, A., Ferguson, L. & Bulsara, M. (2003). The Australian Intervention Randomized Control of Rate in Atrial Fibrillation Trial (AIRCRAFT). *J Am Coll Cardiol*, Vol. 41, No. 10, pp. 1697-1702.

Wichmann, J., Ertl, G., Höhne, W., Schweisfurth, H., Wernze, H. & Kochsiek, K. (1983). Alpha-receptor restriction of coronary blood flow during atrial fibrillation. *Am J Cardiol,* Vol. 52, No. 7, pp. 887-892.

Williamson, B.D., Man, K.C., Daoud, E., Niebauer, M., Strickberger, S.A. & Morady, F. (1995). Radiofrequency catheter modification of atrioventricular conduction to control the ventricular rate during atrial fibrillation. *New Eng J Med,* Vol. 331, No. 14, pp. 910-917.

Wittkampf, F.H., de Jongste, M.J., Lie, H.I. & Meijler, F.L. (1988). Effect of right ventricular pacing on ventricular rhythm during atrial fibrillation. *J Am Coll Cardiol,* Vol. 11, No. 3, pp. 539-545.

Wood, M.A., Brown-Mahoney, C., Kay, G.N. & Ellenbogen, K.A. (2000). Clinical outcomes after ablation and pacing therapy for atrial fibrillation : a meta-analysis. *Circulation,* Vol. 101, No. 10, pp. 1138-1144.

2

Changes in the Atrial Substrate Alters the Spatiotemporal Organization and Characteristics of Atrial Fibrillation

Thomas H. Everett
Division of Cardiology, Department of Medicine, University of California San Francisco, San Francisco, California, USA

1. Introduction

Atrial fibrillation (AF) is the most common cardiac arrhythmia (Nattel and Opie 2006) and can occur in a variety of clinical settings. Several animal models have been developed to mimic the clinical settings in which AF occurs (Everett et al. 2000; Li et al. 1999; Morillo et al. 1995; Neuberger et al. 2006; Schuessler et al. 1992; Verheule et al. 2003; Wijffels et al. 1995). These models have individually addressed different types of atrial structural remodeling which leads to conduction abnormalities and acute and chronic atrial electrical remodeling. AF vulnerability in structurally normal hearts is very low and rarely propagates in this setting (Guerra et al. 2006; Lee et al. 2006). However, any changes in the atrial substrate either through structural or electrical remodeling can increase AF vulnerability and can create an environment in which not only can AF be initiated, but can propagate.

Advancements in the technologies available for atrial activation mapping have increased our understanding of cardiac arrhythmias and action potential propagation. In addition, several signal processing tools have been utilized to study the spatiotemporal organization of AF, and to gain insight into its characteristics and mechanisms. These tools include cross correlation (Botteron and Smith 1995), wavelet analysis (Lee et al. 2004), entropy (Akar et al. 2002; Richman and Moorman 2000), chaos theory (Garfinkel et al. 1997; Gray and Jalife 1998), signal linearity (Sih et al. 1999), and frequency domain analysis using the FFT (Everett, Kok, et al. 2001; Skanes et al. 1998; Ryu et al. 2006). All of these analyses are being used to help find organization within a seemingly chaotic rhythm, identifying and study mechanisms which could possibly be used to identify ablation sites (Pachon et al. 2004; Sanders et al. 2005), and to time defibrillation and pacing for AF termination (Everett et al. 2002; Everett, Moorman, et al. 2001). In addition, activation mapping and signal processing tools have demonstrated that the AF that occurs in within different atrial substrates has different spatiotemporal and mechanistic properties (Everett et al. 2010; Everett et al. 2006).

2. Basics of signal processing and analysis

Several parameters have been used to measure the spatiotemporal organization of AF in different animal models to aid in understanding of the different characteristics and mechanisms of the AF. One simple method is either endocardial or epicardial activation mapping of the atrial fibrillation. For each atrial activation, the time at which the maximum first derivative (dV/dT) occurs is determined and isochronal maps are constructed. From these maps, several behavior characteristics of the AF can be determined. These characteristics include wavefront direction and propagation, the number of wavefronts, and the number of sites that exhibit early activation. However, this type of analysis if highly dependent on where the beginning and end points of the analysis window are placed, the size of the analysis window, and the accuracy of marking local activation (often determined by the maximum dV/dT). (Ideker et al. 1989) Because of these limitations, other analyses have been developed that are more objective measurements of the spatiotemporal organization of the AF. These analyses include cross correlation (Botteron and Smith 1995), frequency domain analysis using the FFT (Everett, Kok, et al. 2001; Ryu et al. 2006; Skanes et al. 1998), measuring the linking of wavefronts (Gerstenfeld, Sahakian, and Swiryn 1992), sample entropy (Richman and Moorman 2000), and wavelet analysis (Lee et al. 2004).

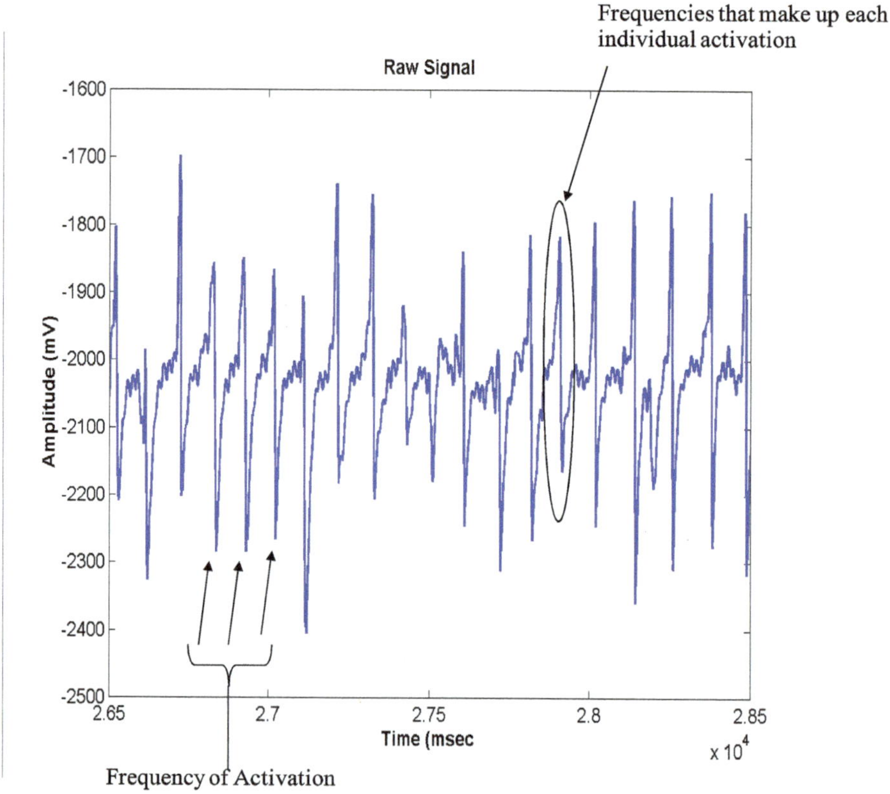

Fig. 1. An example of a raw unipolar atrial fibrillation signal. The frequencies that compose the cycle length of the fibrillation are different from the frequencies that compose the unipolar deflection that indicates an atrial activation. (Reproduced with permission from Everett TH, Olgin JE. Signal processing of fibrillatory electrograms. Aliot EE, Haissaguerre M, Jackman WM editors. Catheter Ablation of Atrial Fibrillation. Blackwell Publishing, Malden, Massachusetts.2008; 85-101.)

When performing signal analysis, some degree of signal processing is performed via filtering. In general, filtering of signals is employed to eliminate or reduce any signal components that would interfere with the analysis such as 50 or 60 Hz noise, any unwanted cardiac activation such as QRS complexes, and any far-field artifacts. Filtering is also used to enhance the signal generated by a cardiac activation. Specific signal processing aimed at signal analyses can be employed to uncover fundamental characteristics of the recorded signal and to aid in understanding the characteristics of the fibrillatory signals.

When filtering and analyzing fibrillatory electrograms, there are two types of frequency components within the signal that we need to be concerned with, and these are shown in figure 1. One is the frequency of the fibrillation which can vary from 3 - 15 Hz. The other type of frequency component of the signal is the frequencies that compose each individual activation spike. These frequencies can be greater than 20 Hz. This becomes important when performing signal analysis. One common type of signal analysis is frequency domain analysis using a fast Fourier transform (FFT) the results of which indicate the frequencies that compose the signal. The high frequency content that composes each atrial activation can dominate the FFT masking the frequency of the fibrillation. Filtering the electrograms can bring the frequency of the actual atrial activation frequency to the foreground (Botteron and Smith 1995; Everett, Kok, et al. 2001). Filtering can also increase the probability that an atrial activation occurred at that point in time, and reduce the influence of low frequency far field artifacts such as far-field QRS complexes or low frequency respiration that can create unwanted noise in the recording (Botteron and Smith 1995).

2.1 Frequency domain analysis

In order to generate a signal, Jean Babtist Fourier, a French mathematician, first claimed that any repetitive signal could be composed of sums of sinusoids. Figure 2 shows two examples, one of a square wave (Panel A) and the corresponding sinusoids that are added together to generate this signal, and one of a triangle wave (Panel B) and its corresponding sinusoids. This same theory can also be applied to cardiac signals. Fourier also developed what is known as the Fourier transform which is based on the concept that signals can be approximated by a sum of sinusoids, each at a different frequency. The Fourier transform is then a description of what frequencies are present and how much of each frequency composes the signal. The results of a FFT are either given as a magnitude spectrum or a power spectrum as a graph of peaks at the frequencies that are present within the signal. The more a certain frequency is influencing a signal, the higher the peak. The highest peak of a magnitude spectrum is considered the dominant frequency (DF), which indicates the main frequency that composes the signal. The magnitude spectrum also composes peaks at frequencies which are integer multiples of the dominant peak called the harmonic peaks. The FFT is now being applied to cardiac electrograms during fibrillation to study the spatiotemporal characteristics of the signals. Studies have shown that the resulting magnitude spectrum from FFT calculations can vary from the recording location, and over time (Everett, Moorman, et al. 2001; Everett et al. 2006). From the results of the frequency domain analysis a couple of simple methods to quantitate differences in magnitude spectrums have been devised. A measurement of the organization of the AF signal can be obtained through either the regularity index (RI) which is defined as the ratio of the area under the dominant peak to the total area of the spectrum (Kalifa et al. 2006) or the organization index (OI) which is defined as the ratio of the area under the dominant peak *and* its harmonics to the total area of the spectrum. (Everett, Kok, et al. 2001)

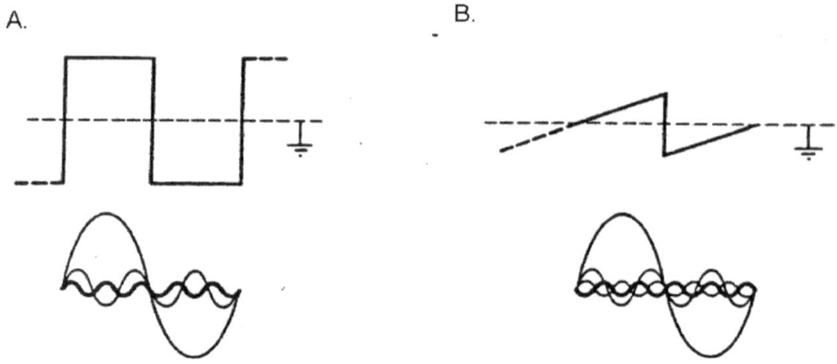

Fig. 2. Every repetitive signal can be represented by adding sine waves of different frequencies together. An example of a square wave and a triangle wave are shown with their corresponding sine waves that added together compose that particular signal. (Reproduced with permission from Everett TH, Olgin JE. Signal processing of fibrillatory electrograms. Aliot EE, Haissaguerre M, Jackman WM editors. Catheter Ablation of Atrial Fibrillation.Blackwell Publishing, Malden, Massachusetts.2008; 85–101.)

In addition to measuring the organization of a signal, FFT analysis can also be used to detect areas of conduction block. Areas of block, alter the frequency of the fibrillation at that site. The recording electrodes then record a signal that is influenced by other frequencies. These other frequencies then appear in the resulting FFT as peaks that are not associated with the dominant one as a harmonic. When compared to an isochronal map of activation during AF, the signals that result in FFTs that have secondary peaks within their magnitude spectrum were located in and around areas of conduction block (Evans et al. 1999). These extra peaks within the magnitude spectrum would also decrease the organization of the signal as measured from the resulting FFT by the OI.

3. Substrate differences among models of Atrial Fibrillation

Atrial fibrillation occurs in a variety of clinical settings, and investigators have developed several animal models to mimic those settings in which AF occurs. The most widely studied canine models include congestive heart failure (CHF), mitral regurgitation (MR), rapid atrial pacing (RAP), and a cholinergically mediated model induced with acetylcholine or methylcholine. The structural and electrical characteristics of each of these models are outlined below.

3.1 Congestive Heart Failure (CHF)

The most studied model of heart failure involves pacing the right ventricle of canine hearts at 220-240 beats per minute for 4 weeks. Although other heart failure models are being developed that show a similar atrial substrate as described below. (Lau et al. 2011; Shimano et al. 2008) As figure 3 shows, the ventricular tachycardia pacing produces a significant increase in atrial interstitial fibrosis. In addition, as figure 4 shows, there is an increase in conduction anisotropy produced by localized conduction slowing which has correlated to an increase in AF vulnerability (Li et al. 1999), and a propensity for long durations of AF

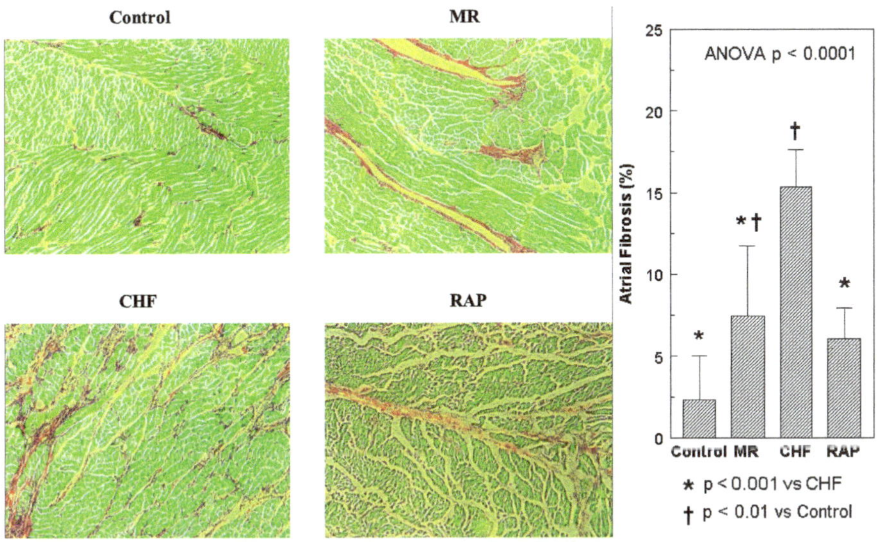

Fig. 3. Amount and distribution of fibrosis from atrial tissue samples from the canine models of Control, MR, CHF, and RAP. Each tissue sample is stained with Sirus red and magnified 100X. The CHF group had a significantly larger amount of fibrosis as compared to the other groups. (Reproduced with permission from **Everett TH**, Wilson EE, Verheule S, Guerra JM, Foreman S, Olgin JE. Structural atrial remodeling alters the substrate and spatiotemporal organization of atrial fibrillation: a comparison in canine models of structural and electrical remodeling. Am J Physiol Heart CircPhysiol 2006; 291: H2911 - H2923.

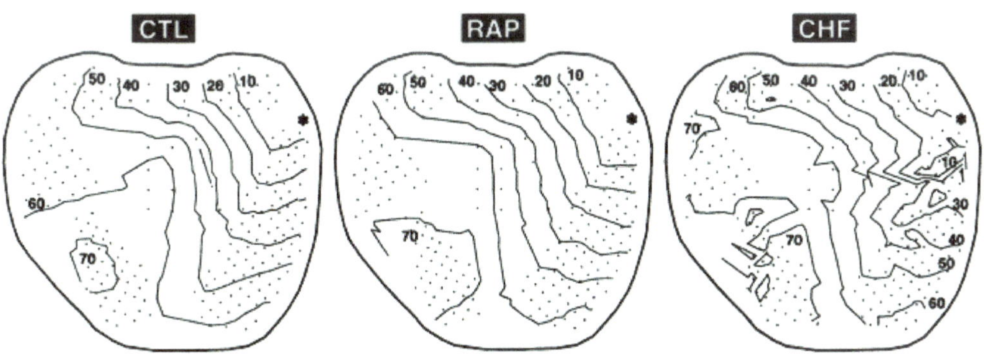

Fig. 4. Isochronal activation maps for control (CTL), rapid atrial pacing (RAP), and congestive heart failure (CHF). The CHF model, which is assocatied with structural atrial remodeling, had an increase in conduction heterogeneity as compared to the other models. The RAP model, which is associated with electrical atrial remodeling, had homogeneous conduction that was similar to control. (Reproduced with permission from Li D, Fareh S, Leung TK, Nattel S. Promotion of atrial fibrillation by heart failure in dogs: atrial remodeling of a different sort. Circulation 1999; 100:87-95.)

(Lee et al. 2006). An investigation into the ion currents in this model has shown a decrease in I_{to}, I_{Ks}, and I_{Ca}along with an up regulation of the Na^{+}-Ca^{+2} exchange current. (Cha, Ehrlich, Zhang, and Nattel 2004) This remodeling in ionic currents results in an increased atrial effective refractory period (AERP). In this model, AF vulnerability has been shown to remain even after a 5 week recovery period in which the heart failure resolves (Shinagawa et al. 2002) and there is recovery of the ionic remodeling. (Cha, Ehrlich, Zhang, Shi, et al. 2004) This model has shown that structural remodeling alone can promote a substrate that enhances AF initiation and propagation.

3.2 Mitral Regurgitation (MR)

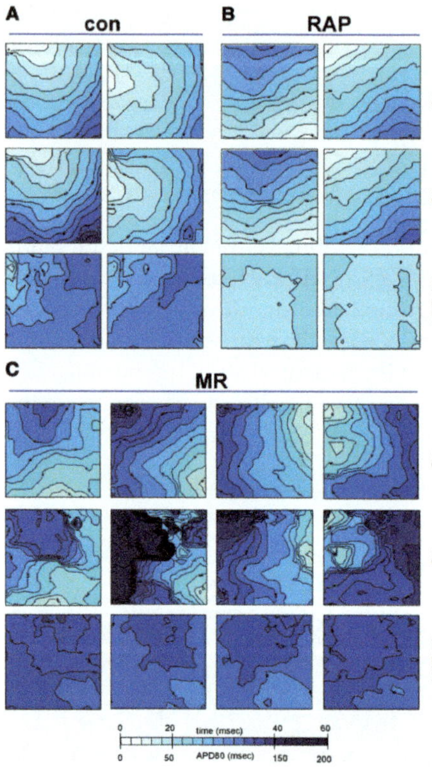

Fig. 5. Conduction patterns recorded with optical mapping during pacing at 350ms (S1) and with an extrastimulus (S2) in the LA along with the APD_{80} during the S1. For the control and RAP, 2 stimulus sites are shown and similar conduction is seen at each site. For the MR group, 4 stimulus sites are shown as the conduction was more variable, and depended on the stimulation site. The MR model, which is associated with structural atrial remodeling, had an increase in conduction heterogeneity as compared to the other models. The RAP model, which is associated with electrical atrial remodeling, had homogeneous conduction that was similar to control. (Reproduced with permission from Verheule S, Wilson E, Banthia S, Everett T, Shanbhag S, Sih H, Olgin J.Direction-dependent conduction abnormalities in a canine model of atrial fibrillation due to chronic atrial dilatation. Am J Physiol Heart CircPhysiol 2004;287: H634-H644).

Similar to the CHF model, structural changes are seen with chronic MR and these animals are more susceptible to AF. (Verheule et al. 2003) The MR model is created through catheter avulsion of the mitral chordae. After 4 weeks, structural remodeling is observed which includes LA enlargement, inflammation, fiber separation, (Verheule et al. 2003) and with only a moderate increase in interstitial fibrosis as shown in figure 3. (Everett et al. 2006) These structural changes correlated to increased conduction heterogeneity and anisotropy in the LA as shown in figure 5 (Verheule et al. 2004). Electrophysiologically, this model has demonstrated a homogeneous increase in AERP in both the RA and LA *in vivo* (Verheule et al. 2003) while figure 6 shows that with optical mapping no differences were seen in the action potential duration as compared to structurally normal hearts (Verheule et al. 2004). This model again shows that structural remodeling can increase AF vulnerability.

3.3 Rapid Atrial Pacing (RAP)

A commonly used large animal model of AF is the RAP model. This model is usually developed by placing an endocardial pacing lead into the RA and pacing the atria at 400-600 beats per minute for at least 6 weeks (Morillo et al. 1995; Verheule et al. 2004; Wijffels et al. 1995). The atrial pacing at high rates results in electrophysiological remodeling which includes a decrease in the atrial effective refractory period (AERP) (Morillo et al. 1995; Wijffels et al. 1995), action potential duration (APD) (Verheule et al. 2004; Yue et al. 1997), and an increase in the dispersion of refractoriness (Fareh, Villemaire, and Nattel 1998).

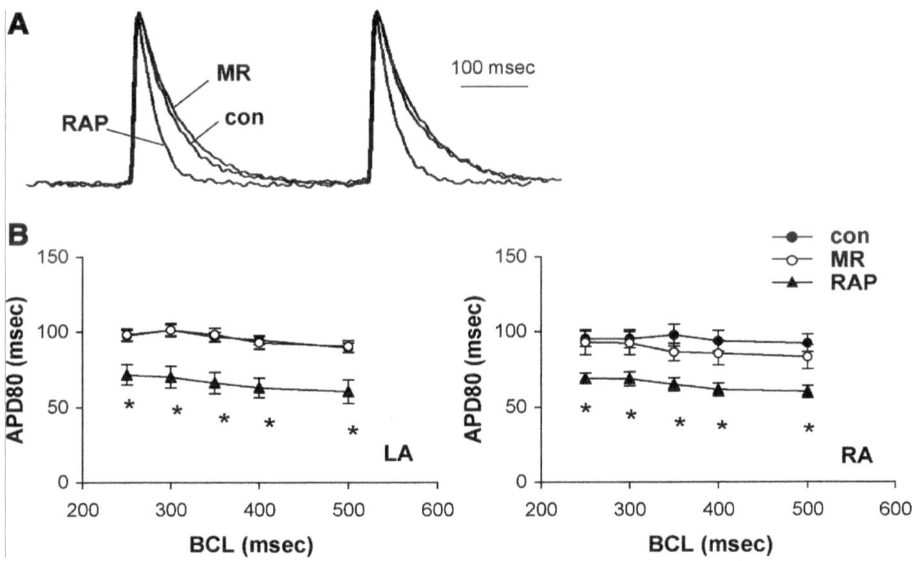

Fig. 6. Action potential duration and conduction velocity. A) Representative examples of optical action potentials at a BCL of 350 msec recorded in control, MR and RAP LA. B) APD80 as a function of the BCL in the LA (left panel) and RA (right panel). Data are mean ± s.e.m. Asterisks indicate significant difference compared to control. (Reproduced with permission from Verheule S, Wilson E, Banthia S, Everett T, Shanbhag S, Sih H, Olgin J.Direction-dependent conduction abnormalities in a canine model of atrial fibrillation due to chronic atrial dilatation. Am J Physiol Heart CircPhysiol 2004;287: H634-H644).

Figure 6 shows an example of action potentials recorded with optical mapping and a significant decrease in APD80 is seen as compared to control atria (Verheule et al. 2004). This type of remodeling has been shown to create a substrate that increases AF vulnerability. Continued pacing promotes longer durations of AF until it eventually becomes self-sustained ("AF begets AF") (Wijffels et al. 1995).

Structurally, this model has resulted in cellular hypertrophy, altered mitochondrial morphology, loss of myofibrillar structure, glycogen accumulation, and an increase in extracellular matrix protein expression (Ausma et al. 1997; Morillo et al. 1995). However, as shown in Figure 3, these structural changes occur without a significant increase in fibrosis as compared to the CHF model. In addition, Figure 7 shows that atrial dilation does not occur in the RAP as there was no difference in atrial size between the RAP model and the structurally normal hearts of the control group. This was in contrast to the CHF and MR models which showed significant atrial dilatation. Finally, the RAP model shows homogeneous conduction as shown in Figures 4 and 5 similar to structurally normal hearts (Verheule et al. 2004).

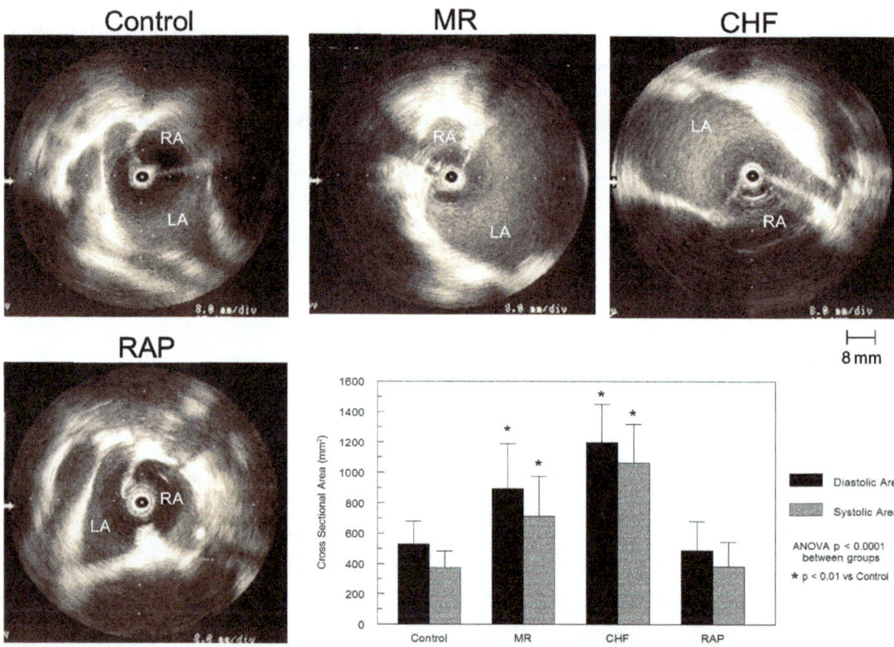

Fig. 7. Intracardiac Echo (ICE) images of the LA from each of the models studied during diastole. The ICE probe was placed at the septal wall at the level of the fossa ovalis such that the LA appendage and the mitral valve annulus were in the field of view. The cross sectional area of the LA was then measured. Also shown is summary data of the average left atrial cross sectional area for each canine AF model. A cross-sectional area was measured during both diastolic (solid bars) and systolic contractions (hatched bars.) (Reproduced with permission from Everett TH, Wilson EE, Olgin JE. The effects of atrial fibrillation substrate and spatiotemporal organization on atrial defibrillation thresholds. Heart Rhythm 2007; 4:1048-1056.)

3.4 Cholinergic agnonist

An acute model of AF that is created through infusion of drugs such as acetylcholine or methylcholine which activates K_{Ach} channels and results in a dose-dependent shortening of the action potential duration. Cholinergic agonists are given to structurally normal hearts and have shown to have little or no effect on atrial conduction properties. (Schuessler, Bromberg, and Boineau 1990; Rensma et al. 1988) In addition, no structural remodeling occurs however, an increase in AF vulnerability has been shown.

4. Characteristics of Atrial Fibrillation in the different models

In order to study the characteristics of the AF within each of the models described, several different recording devices and technologies have been utilized. For *in vivo* studies, these include plaques or ribbons of electrodes that are placed on the epicardial surface of the atria (Everett et al. 2006; Okuyama et al. 2003), and/or catheters with various arrays of electrodes that are inserted into a chamber of the atria to record endocardial signals (Everett et al. 2010; Akar et al. 2002; Lazar et al. 2004). An endocardial array that is used is non-contact mapping using the Ensite 3000 mapping system (Everett et al. 2010; Earley et al. 2006; Kadish et al. 1999; Schilling, Peters, and Davies 1999). A non-contact balloon mapping catheter is positioned in a chamber of the heart along with a standard EP catheter. Using the location algorithm in the ESI, the EP catheter can be detected as it moves around the chamber thus creating a three dimensional rendering of the atria. The catheter records 64 cavitary potentials and then inversely applies them through the Laplace equation in real time generating more than 3,000 unipolar "virtual" electrograms that are then projected on the geometry of the heart chamber. For *in vitro* studies, optical mapping is a technology which uses voltage sensitive dyes to record the activation and repolarization of cardiac tissue from several sites simultaneously which provides an increase in the spatial resolution over traditional electrode recordings (Ding and Everett 2010). Activation mapping and signal analysis techniques described above can then be performed on the signals recorded during AF to measure the spatiotemporal organization and to provide insights into the characteristics and mechanisms of the AF in each model.

4.1 Congestive Heart Failure

The CHF model is associated with structural remodeling with a significant increase in atrial fibrosis which leads to conduction abnormalities and increased AF vulnerability. Several studies have mapped the atria during AF in this model and evidence exists for both reentry and discrete, stable foci. Li et al showed that conduction abnormalities increased AF vulnerability in this model and epicardial mapping showed that the resulting AF had a mechanism of macroreentry which could be terminated with dofetilide, an I_{Kr} channel blocker (Li, Benardeau, and Nattel 2000). In a separate study, this same group when comparing endocardial versus epicardial activation again showed an AF mechanism of macrorentry which supported their previous findings (Derakhchan et al. 2001). Everett et al also performed endocardial and epicardial mapping in the CHF canine model and 5/6 dogs studied had AF characterized by stable focal mechanisms on the endocardial surface with non-contact mapping. Epicardial plaque mapping showed 4/6 dogs with focal AF (Everett et al. 2010). Figure 8C shows an example of this focal activation on the endocardial surface with non-contact mapping. From the focal source, the wave front rotates counterclockwise on both sides of the LA. A focal mechanism of AF was also reported by Stambler et al which was terminated by calcium channel blockers (Stambler et al. 2003). In a later study this group performed biatrial mapping in the CHF dogs and again showed a focal mechanism of

AF. Radiofrequency catheter ablation of the focal site terminated the AF in 67% of the animals studied (Fenelon, Shepard, and Stambler 2003). In the CHF model, there is also evidence that suggests that focal sources of AF activation can be found in the pulmonary veins. High resolution mapping of the pulmonary veins by Okuyama et al showed that half of the AF episodes were characterized by focal sources in the pulmonary veins versus none in structurally normal hearts (Okuyama et al. 2003).

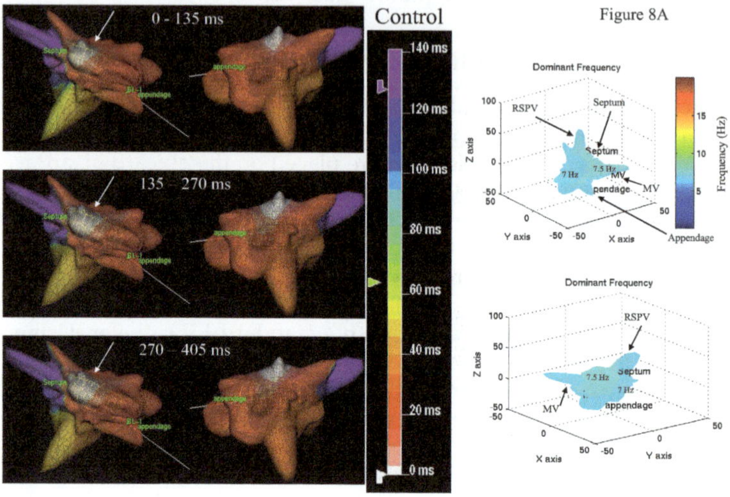

Fig. 8a. (continuation)

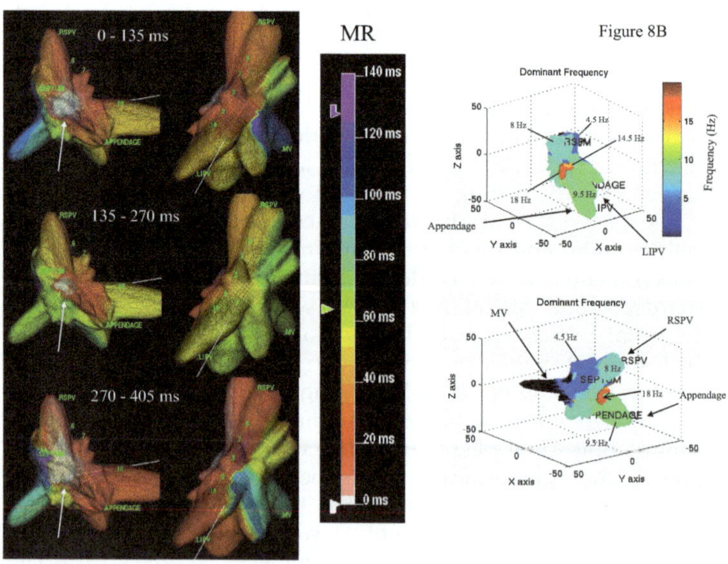

Fig. 8b. (continuation)

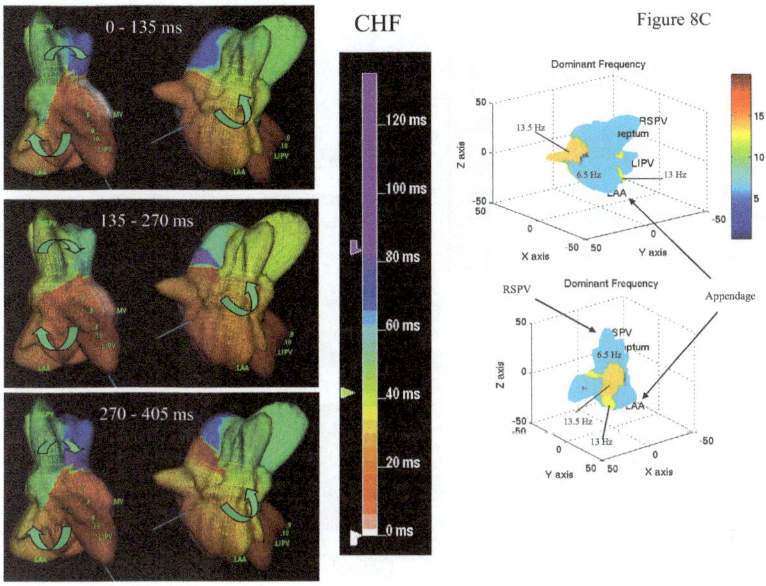

Fig. 8c. (continuation)

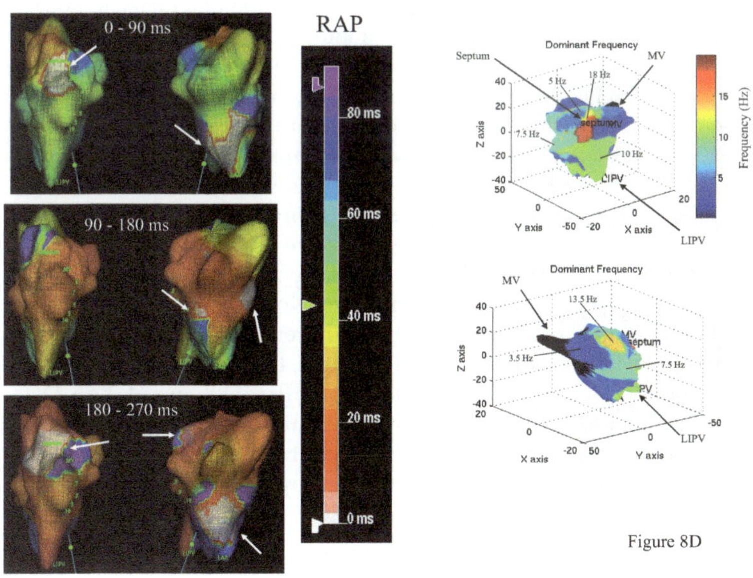

Fig. 8d. (continuation)

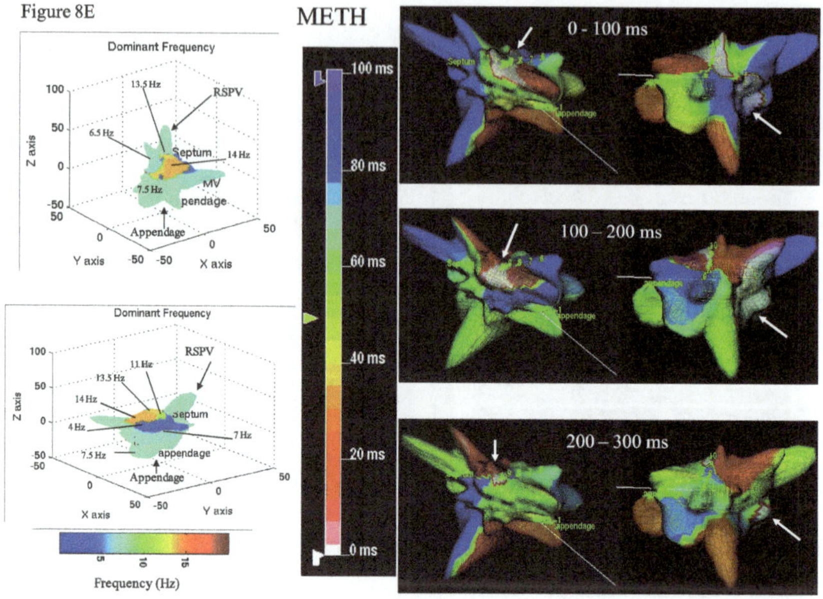

Fig. 8e. Isochronal maps of AF activation along with static DF maps in each of the canine models of Control (A), MR (B), CHF (C), RAP (D), and cholinergic stimulation (Meth) (E). On the isochronal maps, the colors indicate the timing of activation, with white representing the earliest activation and purple representing the latest. Curved arrows indicate the direction of reentry; straight arrows, the earliest activation of a focus. Reentry is determined by areas of earliest activation meeting areas of latest activation. In the example from the control group (A), 3 sequential maps are shown at 135-ms intervals. A stable, focal site is seen in each map. Two DF maps are shown of different views of the 3-D geometry from the same 2-second window. In the MR example, maps are shown at 135 ms intervals. A focal area of activation is seen near the RSPV. Two DF maps are shown of different views of the 3-D geometry from the same 2-second window showing a high DF area at the site of focal activation. In the CHF example, maps are also shown at 135 ms intervals and a stable, focal reentrant wavefront is seen in every map. Again, two DF maps are shown of different views of the 3-D geometry from the same 2-second window. The RAP model had AF characterized by multiple wavelets. In this example, each 90 ms window shows a different site of early activation. Two DF maps are shown from two different time periods showing the transient nature of the high DF areas. For the METH example, two stable focal sites of activation are seen in each window. Two DF maps are shown of different views of the 3-D geometry from the same 2-second window. (Reproduced with permissiom from Everett TH, Wilson EE, Hulley GS, Olgin JE. Transmural characteristics of atrial fibrillation in canine models of structural and electrical atrial remodeling assessed by simultaneous epicardial and endocardial mapping. Heart Rhythm 2010;7:506-517.)

Frequency domain analysis of electrograms recorded during AF has demonstrated that the AF is characterized by stable, high-frequency regions. Using FFT analysis, Ryu et al demonstrated that the AF had stable drivers in either the RA, LA, or both (Ryu et al. 2005). Everett et al also reported AF in the CHF model characterized by stable, high-frequency regions. However these regions were singular and appeared in either the RA or LA with steep frequency gradients away from these sites (Everett et al. 2006). Figure 9 shows an example of a dominant frequency map during AF recorded with epicardial plaques. A singular high-frequency area is seen in the RA.

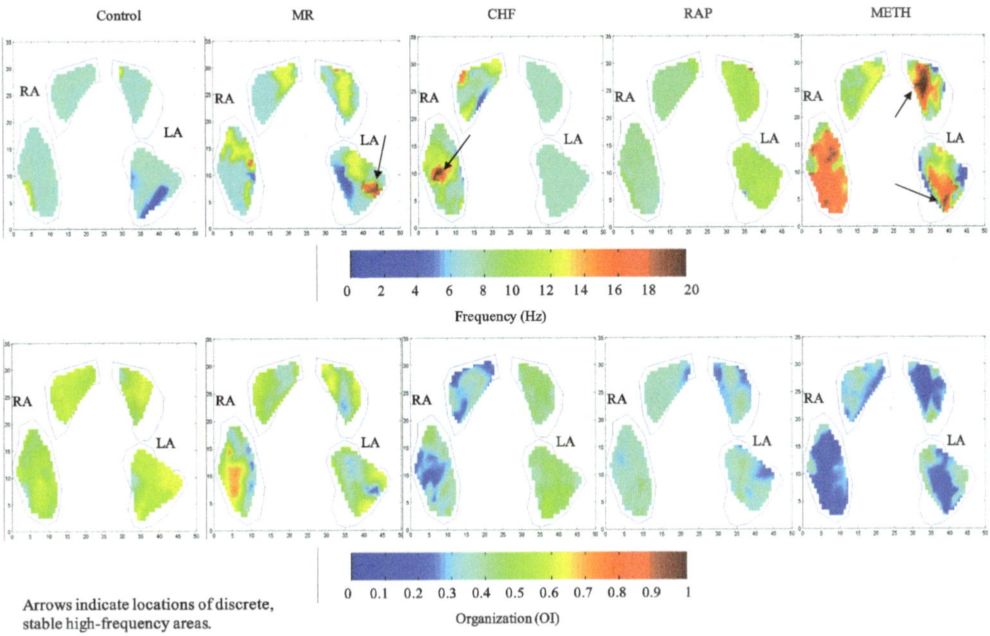

Fig. 9. Examples of static dominant frequency maps (top panels), and organization maps (bottom panels) for the canine models both structural atrial remodeling (CHF and MR) and electrical atrial remodeling (RAP and METH) along with control. DFs and OIs are shown from an FFT performed on a 2-second window of AF. Arrows indicate the location of stable, discrete high DF areas. (Reproduced with permission from Everett TH, Wilson EE, Olgin JE. The effects of atrial fibrillation substrate and spatiotemporal organization on atrial defibrillation thresholds. Heart Rhythm 2007; 4:1048-1056).

4.2 Mitral Regurgitation

The MR model is associated with structural remodeling with LA dilatation, inflammation, and fiber separation (Verheule et al. 2003), however, this model has significantly less fibrosis than the heart failure model (Everett et al. 2006), but still shows an increase in conduction heterogeneity and an increase in AF vulnerability (Verheule et al. 2004; Verheule et al. 2003). AF activation patterns on the epicardial surface have shown either stable wavefronts or focal sources. Focal sources or reentrant wavefronts were consistently seen on the endocardial surface with non-contact mapping (Everett et al. 2010). Figure 8B shows an example of the focal activation seen on the endocardial surface in MR dogs. Similar to the CHF model, the MR model had very stable activation patterns. Using linking to measure stability, it has been shown that AF in the MR model has a high degree of linked beats in both the RA and LA (Everett et al. 2006). In three separate studies, Everett et al performed frequency domain analysis of AF signals recorded from epicardial plaques and have reported the presence of stable, high-frequency areas although they were not seen in every experiment (Everett et al. 2010; Everett, Wilson, and Olgin 2007; Everett et al. 2006). However, they were consistently seen in the LA with optical mapping (Everett et al. 2004). An example of a dominant frequency map with a discrete, high-frequency area in the LA is seen in Figure 9.

4.3 Rapid atrial pacing

The rapid atrial pacing model is associated with electrical remodeling, with a shortening of the atrial effective refractory period and action potential duration (Morillo et al. 1995; Wijffels et al. 1995). When analyzing the mechanism of AF in this model, most data points towards a mechanism of multiple wavelets. In addition, it has been shown that the longer the pacing continues, the more disorganized the AF becomes with more wavelets, shorter cycle lengths, and shorter AERPs promoting AF propagation and leading to the term "AF begets AF." (Wijffels et al. 1995)

In the persistent AF RAP models, epicardial plaque mapping by Sih et al and Everett et al has shown AF characterized by multiple wavelets with twice as many sites of early activation than other models (MR or CHF) (Everett, Wilson, and Olgin 2007) or control (Sih et al. 2000). However, one study by Wu et al showed that the pulmonary veins and ligament of Marshall were the sources of the highest frequency of activation during AF in this model (Wu et al. 2001). Endocardial non-contact mapping also showed a mechanism of multiple wavelets (Everett et al. 2010). An example of this type of activation is shown in Figure 8D. When linking is used to analyze the stability of the AF wavefronts by quantifying the number of continuous beats traveling in the same direction, the RAP model had the lowest percentage of linked beats when compared to control or the CHF and MR models.

Frequency domain analysis did not show any discrete, stable high-frequency areas with either epicardial plaque mapping (Everett et al. 2010; Everett, Wilson, and Olgin 2007; Everett et al. 2006), endocardial non-contact mapping (Everett et al. 2010), or optical mapping (Everett et al. 2004). Any high frequency areas were transient and not stable. FFT analysis of plaque AF electrograms and optical mapping signals did show that the RAP model was the only one in which the LA had consistently higher dominant frequencies than the RA (Everett et al. 2004; Everett et al. 2006).

4.4 Cholinergic induced AF

An acute model of electrical remodeling, studies using cholinergic stimulation of AF have shown a variety of AF mechanisms. It was using this model in a sheep that AF characterized by a discrete region of stable, high-frequencies was shown (Skanes et al. 1998). These areas would consist of frequencies that were higher than any other in the atrium, thus considered to be responsible for driving the AF. Further experiments showed that these discrete, stable high-frequency areas resulted from microreentrant sources (Mandapati et al. 2000), and that at a critical frequency threshold, a frequency gradient developed between the LA and RA (Mansour et al. 2001).

In a canine heart, discrete, stable-high frequency areas were seen in the LA, but they were also observed in the RA, and no LA-RA frequency gradient existed (Everett et al. 2006). Figure 9 shows an example of a dominant frequency map with 2 stable high-frequency areas in the LA. AF recordings with epicardial plaques showed AF characterized by multiple sites with early activation and a low degree of stability as quantified by measuring the number of linked beats. Everett et al also showed that AF induced with methylcholine had varying mechanisms of multiple wavelets, multiple foci, and in some cases organized stable wavefronts were seen on the epicardial surface (Everett et al. 2010). Non-contact mapping on the endocardial surface showed different mechanisms in different experiments from multiple wavelets, multiple foci, and reentry. The example in Figure 8E shows 2 stable focal sites of activation. These differences in AF characteristics between species may be due to differences in the distribution of I_{kAch} (Sarmast et al. 2003) channels, thus varying the influence of cholinergic drugs on the atria.

5. Transmural characteristics

A couple of recent studies have shown that the atrial substrate also plays a role in the transmural characteristics of AF. In the left atrium of 5 different canine models, Everett et al simultaneously recorded AF signals from the endocardial and epicardial surfaces (Everett et al. 2010). Virtual endocardial signals (Ensite®, Endocardial Solutions, Inc. St. Paul, Minnesota) were directly compared with contact signals from plaques placed on the epicardial surface. Figure 10 shows the maximum dominant frequency on both the epicardial and endocardial surfaces for each model of Control, MR, CHF, RAP, and methylcholine. As the graph shows, the endocardial surface had significantly higher maximum dominant frequencies than the epicardial surfaces for each model. Figure 11 shows the summary data from directly comparing individual endocardial to epicardial

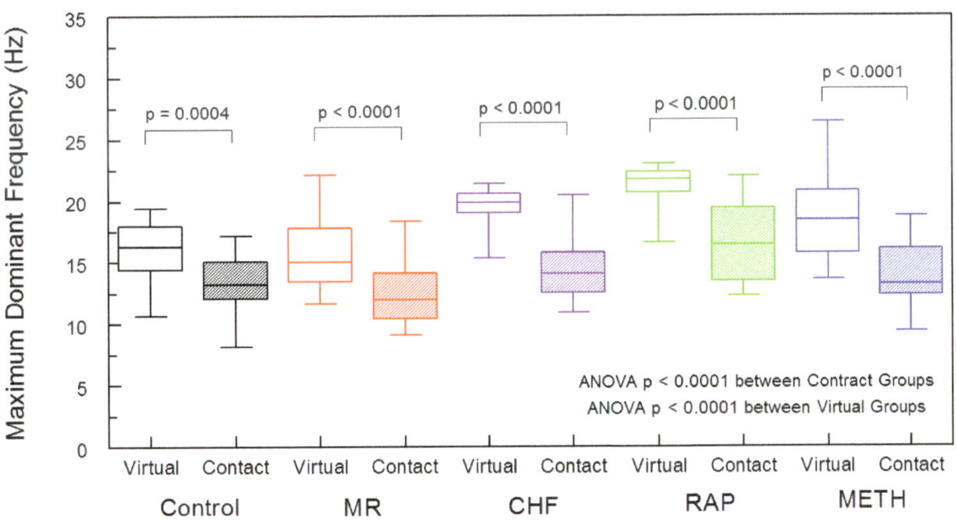

Fig. 10. Maximum dominant frequency for both the epicardial (hatched box) and endocardial (open box) surfaces for each model of Control, mitral regurgitation, heart failure, rapid atrial pacing, and cholinergic stimulation (meth). As the graph shows, the endocardial surface had significantly higher maximum dominant frequencies than the epicardial surfaces for each model.

signals. The panel on the left indicates the percentage of paired electrograms that had a cross correlation coefficient above 0.8. The panel on the right represents the percentage of paired electrograms that had matching dominant frequencies. As both of these graphs show, the structurally remodeled AF models of CHF and MR had the highest percentage of correlation coefficients above 0.8 and similar dominant frequencies. The electrically remodeled rapid atrial pacing model had the lowest percentage of both metrics. When the mechanisms on both surfaces were compared, AF characterized by multiple wavelets was seen on both the endocardial and epicardial surfaces of the RAP model which had the lowest degree of transmural similarities. The majority of the AF in the CHF model was characterized by focal sources and the highest amount of transmural similarities, however half of the CHF dogs studied had different endocardial/epicardial AF activation patterns.

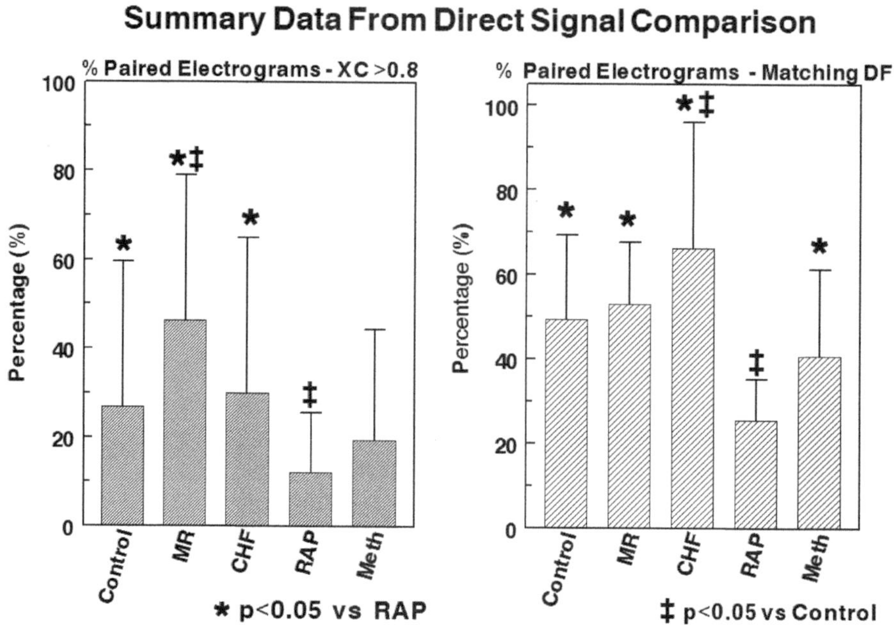

Fig. 11. Summary data from directly comparing individual endocardial to epicardial signals. The panel on the left indicates the percentage of paired electrograms that had a cross correlation coefficient above 0.8. The panel on the right represents the percentage of paired electrograms that had matching dominant frequencies. As both of these graphs show, the structurally remodeled AF models of CHF and MR had the highest percentage of correlation coefficients above 0.8 and similar dominant frequencies. The electrically remodeled rapid atrial pacing model had the lowest percentage of both metrics.

In another recent study, Eckstein et al performed simultaneous endocardial/epicardial AF recordings in the left atrium in goats divided into 3 groups: acute AF, 3 weeks of rapid atrial pacing, and 6 months of rapid atrial pacing (Eckstein et al. 2011). What was shown was an increase in the electrical dissociation between the endocardial and epicardial surfaces after 3 weeks of rapid atrial pacing which increased further with 6 months of pacing. Dissychony was demonstrated by differences in epicardial/endocardial activation times and local conduction vectors. An increase in the electrical dissociation between the endocardial and epicardial surfaces was theorized to provide a substrate for AF propagation.

6. Comparisons among models

Each animal model discussed here represents a different substrate that results in an increased AF vulnerability. While AF can be reliably initiated in any of these substrates, the mechanisms and spatiotemporal characteristics of the AF in each differs. However, some common features can be perceived from models that share common substrate properties, especially structural remodeling. The models that experienced structural remodeling known to result in alterations in conduction, (Li et al. 1999; Verheule et al. 2004; Verheule et al. 2003) had stable, discrete high frequency areas in the DF maps. Steep frequency gradients, and large areas of similar frequencies were seen away from the high frequency areas. These frequency characteristics remained stable from epoch to epoch as the stable high-frequency areas remained consistently spatially located from episode to episode. The structural changes seen in the MR and CHF models likely contribute to the frequency gradient that occurs outward from the high-frequency area as the structural remodeling promotes conduction delay and block as well as wave break. Based on the spatiotemporal data, this would suggest a stable rotor in these models with highly organized wavefronts in the other areas of the atria, which would correlate with the 'mother-rotor' theory as an AF mechanism in these models. An AF mechanism of focal reentry dominates the AF activation patterns in these models, especially in the CHF model. The CHF model also had a high degree of quantifiable transmural similarities between the endocardial and epicardial surfaces (Everett et al. 2010).

As described above, both the RAP and cholinergic models are characterized primarily by atrial electrical changes. However, how this remodeling is achieved is different for each model. The RAP model uses 6 weeks of rapid atrial pacing to achieve the desired effects. During this time, some cellular changes will occur. However, in both whole heart and optical mapping studies, no conduction abnormalities are observed (Li et al. 1999; Verheule et al. 2004). For the cholinergic model, the remodeling occurs acutely on the ionic level with no other cellular changes. While both of these models had higher dominant frequencies, lower organization levels, and lower degrees of transmural similarities when compared to the CHF and MR models (Everett et al. 2010; Everett, Wilson, and Olgin 2007; Everett et al. 2006), the similarities between the RAP and cholinergic models don't continue.

In the RAP model, no AF episodes were characterized with stable, discrete high-frequency areas or frequency gradients within the LA. However, the RAP model was also the only model in which every animal studied showed a consistent frequency gradient between the right and left atria with the LA always having significantly higher frequencies than the RA. This could be due to the smaller degree of structural changes and lack of remodeling that affects conduction in the RAP model, so that the entire LA is activated at a similar frequency masking a potential high frequency site. The AF activation patterns in the RAP model are consistently characterized by multiple wavefronts (Everett et al. 2010; Sih et al. 2000). This type of mechanism is also seen in the cholinergic model, but multiple focal sources have also been observed. Frequency domain analysis has also shown multiple stable, high-frequency areas could exist in this model (Everett et al. 2010; Everett et al. 2006).

7. Clinical data

In the clinical setting, different atrial substrates and altering the substrate through catheter ablation can alter the mechanism and spatiotemporal characteristics of the AF. As discussed with the canine heart failure model, atrial fibrosis creates a substrate that promotes AF (Guerra et al. 2006; Li et al. 1999; Lee et al. 2006). In patients with heart failure and no history of AF, atrial fibrosis was shown to alter the electrophysiological properties of the atria by increasing atrial effective refractory periods, prolonging conduction times, and decreasing bipolar voltage signal amplitudes (Sanders et al. 2003). Studies examining atrial structure in patients with AF as opposed to those in sinus rhythm have seen increased amounts of fibrosis (Boldt et al. 2004; Kostin et al. 2002; Luo, Li, and Yang 2006).

Most clinical studies comparing AF in different substrates either occurs between persistent /permanent and paroxysmal AF or before and after catheter ablation. Sanders et al performed FFT analysis on AF signals from patients with paroxysmal AF and from patients with permanent AF (Sanders et al. 2005). High frequency areas were seen in both groups, but paroxysmal AF was more likely to have the high frequency sites in the pulmonary veins compared to permanent AF which had more atrial high frequency sites. Sanders et al also looked at the effects of pulmonary vein isolation on the AF frequencies (Sanders et al. 2006). Pulmonary vein isolation resulted in a significant decrease in the dominant frequencies in patients with paroxysmal AF, but not permanent. In another study by Lazar et al, it was shown that a LA to RA frequency gradient disappears with pulmonary vein isolation (Lazar et al. 2006). Takahashi et al used signal processing techniques to show that the organization of AF increases after catheter ablation of the pulmonary veins (Takahashi et al. 2006). It was also shown that a high OI value was associated with AF termination.

Lin, et al used FFTs to study the spatial distribution of frequencies during different types of paroxysmal AF. (Lin et al. 2006) The location of the initiating foci was determined, and the area from which the AF originated had the highest dominant frequency. When the AF originated from the pulmonary veins, a LA to RA frequency gradient existed. A gradient was not seen when the AF originated from the SVC. In a study by Lazar et al, recordings were made in both the RA and LA in patients with paroxysmal and persistent AF (Lazar et al. 2004). A LA to RA frequency gradient was observed, but this gradient was only seen in patients with paroxysmal AF but not those with persistent AF.

8. Conclusions

Several different canine models have been developed to study AF. Even though each model shows an increase in AF vulnerability, the substrate that is created (either through structural or electrical remodeling) in each model that allows the AF to occur is different. These differences in substrate lead to different characteristics of the AF spatiotemporal organization and mechanisms of AF. Models that were characterized by structural remodeling had AF associated with stable, high-frequency areas and a focal source as the AF mechanism. Models that were characterized by electrical remodeling had AF associated with multiple wavefront or multiple foci. Structural remodeling may promote the stability of AF drivers that have been shown to be characterized by stable, high-frequency areas.

9. References

Akar, J. G., T. H. th Everett, L. C. Kok, J. R. Moorman, and D. E. Haines. 2002. "Effect of electrical and structural remodeling on spatiotemporal organization in acute and persistent atrial fibrillation." *J Cardiovasc Electrophysiol* no. 13 (10):1027-34.

Ausma, J., M. Wijffels, F. Thone, L. Wouters, M. Allessie, and M. Borgers. 1997. "Structural changes of atrial myocardium due to sustained atrial fibrillation in the goat." *Circulation* no. 96 (9):3157-63.

Boldt, A., U. Wetzel, J. Lauschke, J. Weigl, J. Gummert, G. Hindricks, H. Kottkamp, and S. Dhein. 2004. "Fibrosis in left atrial tissue of patients with atrial fibrillation with and without underlying mitral valve disease." *Heart* no. 90 (4):400-5.

Botteron, G. W., and J. M. Smith. 1995. "A technique for measurement of the extent of spatial organization of atrial activation during atrial fibrillation in the intact human heart." *IEEE Trans Biomed Eng* no. 42 (6):579-86.

Cha, T. J., J. R. Ehrlich, L. Zhang, and S. Nattel. 2004. "Atrial ionic remodeling induced by atrial tachycardia in the presence of congestive heart failure." *Circulation* no. 110 (12):1520-6.

Cha, T. J., J. R. Ehrlich, L. Zhang, Y. F. Shi, J. C. Tardif, T. K. Leung, and S. Nattel. 2004. "Dissociation between ionic remodeling and ability to sustain atrial fibrillation during recovery from experimental congestive heart failure." *Circulation* no. 109 (3):412-8.

Derakhchan, K., D. Li, M. Courtemanche, B. Smith, J. Brouillette, P. L. Page, and S. Nattel. 2001. "Method for simultaneous epicardial and endocardial mapping of in vivo canine heart: application to atrial conduction properties and arrhythmia mechanisms." *J Cardiovasc Electrophysiol* no. 12 (5):548-55.

Ding, C., and T. H. th Everett. 2010. "Assessment of cardiac conduction: basic principles of optical mapping." *Methods Mol Biol* no. 660:239-52. doi: 10.1007/978-1-60761-705-1_15.

Earley, M. J., D. J. Abrams, S. C. Sporton, and R. J. Schilling. 2006. "Validation of the noncontact mapping system in the left atrium during permanent atrial fibrillation and sinus rhythm." *J Am Coll Cardiol* no. 48 (3):485-91.

Eckstein, J., B. Maesen, D. Linz, S. Zeemering, A. van Hunnik, S. Verheule, M. Allessie, and U. Schotten. 2011. "Time course and mechanisms of endo-epicardial electrical dissociation during atrial fibrillation in the goat." *Cardiovasc Res* no. 89 (4):816-24. doi: 10.1093/cvr/cvq336.

Evans, F. G., J. M. Rogers, W. M. Smith, and R. E. Ideker. 1999. "Automatic detection of conduction block based on time-frequency analysis of unipolar electrograms." *IEEE Trans Biomed Eng* no. 46 (9):1090-7.

Everett, T. H. th, J. G. Akar, L. C. Kok, J. R. Moorman, and D. E. Haines. 2002. "Use of global atrial fibrillation organization to optimize the success of burst pace termination." *J Am Coll Cardiol* no. 40 (10):1831-40.

Everett, T. H. th, L. C. Kok, R. H. Vaughn, J. R. Moorman, and D. E. Haines. 2001. "Frequency domain algorithm for quantifying atrial fibrillation organization to increase defibrillation efficacy." *IEEE Trans Biomed Eng* no. 48 (9):969-78.

Everett, T. H. th, H. Li, J. M. Mangrum, I. D. McRury, M. A. Mitchell, J. A. Redick, and D. E. Haines. 2000. "Electrical, morphological, and ultrastructural remodeling and reverse remodeling in a canine model of chronic atrial fibrillation." *Circulation* no. 102 (12):1454-60.

Everett, T. H. th, J. R. Moorman, L. C. Kok, J. G. Akar, and D. E. Haines. 2001. "Assessment of global atrial fibrillation organization to optimize timing of atrial defibrillation." *Circulation* no. 103 (23):2857-61.

Everett, T. H. th, S. Verheule, E. E. Wilson, S. Foreman, and J. E. Olgin. 2004. "Left atrial dilatation resulting from chronic mitral regurgitation decreases spatiotemporal organization of atrial fibrillation in left atrium." *Am J Physiol Heart Circ Physiol* no. 286 (6):H2452-60.

Everett, T. H. th, E. E. Wilson, G. S. Hulley, and J. E. Olgin. 2010. "Transmural characteristics of atrial fibrillation in canine models of structural and electrical atrial remodeling assessed by simultaneous epicardial and endocardial mapping." *Heart Rhythm* no. 7 (4):506-17. doi: 10.1016/j.hrthm.2009.12.030.

Everett, T. H. th, E. E. Wilson, and J. E. Olgin. 2007. "Effects of atrial fibrillation substrate and spatiotemporal organization on atrial defibrillation thresholds." *Heart Rhythm* no. 4 (8):1048-56.

Everett, T. H. th, E. E. Wilson, S. Verheule, J. M. Guerra, S. Foreman, and J. E. Olgin. 2006. "Structural atrial remodeling alters the substrate and spatiotemporal organization of atrial fibrillation: a comparison in canine models of structural and electrical atrial remodeling." *Am J Physiol Heart Circ Physiol* no. 291 (6):H2911-23.

Fareh, S., C. Villemaire, and S. Nattel. 1998. "Importance of refractoriness heterogeneity in the enhanced vulnerability to atrial fibrillation induction caused by tachycardia-induced atrial electrical remodeling." *Circulation* no. 98 (20):2202-9.

Fenelon, G., R. K. Shepard, and B. S. Stambler. 2003. "Focal origin of atrial tachycardia in dogs with rapid ventricular pacing-induced heart failure." *J Cardiovasc Electrophysiol* no. 14 (10):1093-102.

Garfinkel, A., P. S. Chen, D. O. Walter, H. S. Karagueuzian, B. Kogan, S. J. Evans, M. Karpoukhin, C. Hwang, T. Uchida, M. Gotoh, O. Nwasokwa, P. Sager, and J. N. Weiss. 1997. "Quasiperiodicity and chaos in cardiac fibrillation." *J Clin Invest* no. 99 (2):305-14.

Gerstenfeld, E. P., A. V. Sahakian, and S. Swiryn. 1992. "Evidence for transient linking of atrial excitation during atrial fibrillation in humans." *Circulation* no. 86 (2):375-82.

Gray, R. A., and J. Jalife. 1998. "Ventricular fibrillation and atrial fibrillation are two different beasts." *Chaos* no. 8 (1):65-78.

Guerra, J. M., T. H. th Everett, K. W. Lee, E. Wilson, and J. E. Olgin. 2006. "Effects of the gap junction modifier rotigaptide (ZP123) on atrial conduction and vulnerability to atrial fibrillation." *Circulation* no. 114 (2):110-8.

Ideker, R. E., W. M. Smith, S. M. Blanchard, S. L. Reiser, E. V. Simpson, P. D. Wolf, and N. D. Danieley. 1989. "The assumptions of isochronal cardiac mapping." *Pacing Clin Electrophysiol* no. 12 (3):456-78.

Kadish, A., J. Hauck, B. Pederson, G. Beatty, and C. Gornick. 1999. "Mapping of atrial activation with a noncontact, multielectrode catheter in dogs." *Circulation* no. 99 (14):1906-13.

Kalifa, J., K. Tanaka, A. V. Zaitsev, M. Warren, R. Vaidyanathan, D. Auerbach, S. Pandit, K. L. Vikstrom, R. Ploutz-Snyder, A. Talkachou, F. Atienza, G. Guiraudon, J. Jalife, and O. Berenfeld. 2006. "Mechanisms of wave fractionation at boundaries of high-frequency excitation in the posterior left atrium of the isolated sheep heart during atrial fibrillation." *Circulation* no. 113 (5):626-33.

Kostin, S., G. Klein, Z. Szalay, S. Hein, E. P. Bauer, and J. Schaper. 2002. "Structural correlate of atrial fibrillation in human patients." *Cardiovasc Res* no. 54 (2):361-79.

Lau, D. H., P. J. Psaltis, L. Mackenzie, D. J. Kelly, A. Carbone, M. Worthington, A. J. Nelson, Y. Zhang, P. Kuklik, C. X. Wong, J. Edwards, D. A. Saint, S. G. Worthley, and P. Sanders. 2011. "Atrial remodeling in an ovine model of anthracycline-induced nonischemic cardiomyopathy: remodeling of the same sort." *J Cardiovasc Electrophysiol* no. 22 (2):175-82. doi: 10.1111/j.1540-8167.2010.01851.x.

Lazar, S., S. Dixit, D. J. Callans, D. Lin, F. E. Marchlinski, and E. P. Gerstenfeld. 2006. "Effect of pulmonary vein isolation on the left-to-right atrial dominant frequency gradient in human atrial fibrillation." *Heart Rhythm* no. 3 (8):889-95.

Lazar, S., S. Dixit, F. E. Marchlinski, D. J. Callans, and E. P. Gerstenfeld. 2004. "Presence of left-to-right atrial frequency gradient in paroxysmal but not persistent atrial fibrillation in humans." *Circulation* no. 110 (20):3181-6.

Lee, K. W., T. H. Everett, H.T. Ilhan, I. Linscott, and J. Olgin. 2004. Feature Extraction of the Atrial Fibrillation Signal Using the Continuous Wavelet Transform. Paper read at Proceedings of the 26th Annual International Conference of the IEEE EMBS, September, at San Francisco, CA.

Lee, K. W., T. H. th Everett, D. Rahmutula, J. M. Guerra, E. Wilson, C. Ding, and J. E. Olgin. 2006. "Pirfenidone prevents the development of a vulnerable substrate for atrial fibrillation in a canine model of heart failure." *Circulation* no. 114 (16):1703-12.

Li, D., A. Benardeau, and S. Nattel. 2000. "Contrasting efficacy of dofetilide in differing experimental models of atrial fibrillation." *Circulation* no. 102 (1):104-12.

Li, D., S. Fareh, T. K. Leung, and S. Nattel. 1999. "Promotion of atrial fibrillation by heart failure in dogs: atrial remodeling of a different sort." *Circulation* no. 100 (1):87-95.

Lin, Y. J., C. T. Tai, T. Kao, H. W. Tso, S. Higa, H. M. Tsao, S. L. Chang, M. H. Hsieh, and S. A. Chen. 2006. "Frequency analysis in different types of paroxysmal atrial fibrillation." *J Am Coll Cardiol* no. 47 (7):1401-7.

Luo, M. H., Y. S. Li, and K. P. Yang. 2006. "Fibrosis of Collagen I and Remodeling of Connexin 43 in Atrial Myocardium of Patients with Atrial Fibrillation." *Cardiology* no. 107 (4):248-253.

Mandapati, R., A. Skanes, J. Chen, O. Berenfeld, and J. Jalife. 2000. "Stable microreentrant sources as a mechanism of atrial fibrillation in the isolated sheep heart." *Circulation* no. 101 (2):194-9.

Mansour, M., R. Mandapati, O. Berenfeld, J. Chen, F. H. Samie, and J. Jalife. 2001. "Left-to-right gradient of atrial frequencies during acute atrial fibrillation in the isolated sheep heart." *Circulation* no. 103 (21):2631-6.

Morillo, C. A., G. J. Klein, D. L. Jones, and C. M. Guiraudon. 1995. "Chronic rapid atrial pacing. Structural, functional, and electrophysiological characteristics of a new model of sustained atrial fibrillation." *Circulation* no. 91 (5):1588-95.

Nattel, S., and L. H. Opie. 2006. "Controversies in atrial fibrillation." *Lancet* no. 367 (9506):262-72. doi: 10.1016/S0140-6736 (06)68037-9.

Neuberger, H. R., U. Schotten, Y. Blaauw, D. Vollmann, S. Eijsbouts, A. van Hunnik, and M. Allessie. 2006. "Chronic atrial dilation, electrical remodeling, and atrial fibrillation in the goat." *J Am Coll Cardiol* no. 47 (3):644-53.

Okuyama, Y., Y. Miyauchi, A. M. Park, A. Hamabe, S. Zhou, H. Hayashi, M. Miyauchi, C. Omichi, H. N. Pak, L. A. Brodsky, W. J. Mandel, M. C. Fishbein, H. S. Karagueuzian, and P. S. Chen. 2003. "High resolution mapping of the pulmonary vein and the vein of Marshall during induced atrial fibrillation and atrial tachycardia in a canine model of pacing-induced congestive heart failure." *J Am Coll Cardiol* no. 42 (2):348-60.

Pachon, M. Jc, M. Ei Pachon, M. Jc Pachon, T. J. Lobo, M. Z. Pachon, R. N. Vargas, D. Q. Pachon, M. Fj Lopez, and A. D. Jatene. 2004. "A new treatment for atrial fibrillation based on spectral analysis to guide the catheter RF-ablation." *Europace* no. 6 (6):590-601.

Rensma, P. L., M. A. Allessie, W. J. Lammers, F. I. Bonke, and M. J. Schalij. 1988. "Length of excitation wave and susceptibility to reentrant atrial arrhythmias in normal conscious dogs." *Circ Res* no. 62 (2):395-410.

Richman, J. S., and J. R. Moorman. 2000. "Physiological time-series analysis using approximate entropy and sample entropy." *Am J Physiol Heart Circ Physiol* no. 278 (6):H2039-49.

Ryu, K., J. Sahadevan, C. M. Khrestian, B. S. Stambler, and A. L. Waldo. 2006. "Use of fast fourier transform analysis of atrial electrograms for rapid characterization of atrial activation-implications for delineating possible mechanisms of atrial tachyarrhythmias." *J Cardiovasc Electrophysiol* no. 17 (2):198-206.

Ryu, K., S. C. Shroff, J. Sahadevan, N. L. Martovitz, C. M. Khrestian, and B. S. Stambler. 2005. "Mapping of atrial activation during sustained atrial fibrillation in dogs with rapid ventricular pacing induced heart failure: evidence for a role of driver regions." *J Cardiovasc Electrophysiol* no. 16 (12):1348-58. doi: 10.1111/j.1540-8167.2005.00266.x.

Sanders, P., O. Berenfeld, M. Hocini, P. Jais, R. Vaidyanathan, L. F. Hsu, S. Garrigue, Y. Takahashi, M. Rotter, F. Sacher, C. Scavee, R. Ploutz-Snyder, J. Jalife, and M. Haissaguerre. 2005. "Spectral analysis identifies sites of high-frequency activity maintaining atrial fibrillation in humans." *Circulation* no. 112 (6):789-97.

Sanders, P., J. B. Morton, N. C. Davidson, S. J. Spence, J. K. Vohra, P. B. Sparks, and J. M. Kalman. 2003. "Electrical remodeling of the atria in congestive heart failure: electrophysiological and electroanatomic mapping in humans." *Circulation* no. 108 (12):1461-8. doi: 10.1161/01.CIR.0000090688.49283.67.

Sanders, P., C. J. Nalliah, R. Dubois, Y. Takahashi, M. Hocini, M. Rotter, T. Rostock, F. Sacher, L. F. Hsu, A. Jonsson, M. D. O'Neill, P. Jais, and M. Haissaguerre. 2006.

"Frequency mapping of the pulmonary veins in paroxysmal versus permanent atrial fibrillation." *J Cardiovasc Electrophysiol* no. 17 (9):965-72.

Sarmast, F., A. Kolli, A. Zaitsev, K. Parisian, A. S. Dhamoon, P. K. Guha, M. Warren, J. M. Anumonwo, S. M. Taffet, O. Berenfeld, and J. Jalife. 2003. "Cholinergic atrial fibrillation: I (K,ACh) gradients determine unequal left/right atrial frequencies and rotor dynamics." *Cardiovasc Res* no. 59 (4):863-73.

Schilling, R. J., N. S. Peters, and D. W. Davies. 1999. "Noncontact mapping of cardiac arrhythmias." *J Electrocardiol* no. 32 Suppl:13-5.

Schuessler, R. B., B. I. Bromberg, and J. P. Boineau. 1990. "Effect of neurotransmitters on the activation sequence of the isolated atrium." *Am J Physiol* no. 258 (6 Pt 2):H1632-41.

Schuessler, R. B., T. M. Grayson, B. I. Bromberg, J. L. Cox, and J. P. Boineau. 1992. "Cholinergically mediated tachyarrhythmias induced by a single extrastimulus in the isolated canine right atrium." *Circ Res* no. 71 (5):1254-67.

Shimano, M., Y. Tsuji, Y. Inden, K. Kitamura, T. Uchikawa, S. Harata, S. Nattel, and T. Murohara. 2008. "Pioglitazone, a peroxisome proliferator-activated receptor-gamma activator, attenuates atrial fibrosis and atrial fibrillation promotion in rabbits with congestive heart failure." *Heart Rhythm* no. 5 (3):451-9. doi: 10.1016/j.hrthm.2007.12.010.

Shinagawa, K., Y. F. Shi, J. C. Tardif, T. K. Leung, and S. Nattel. 2002. "Dynamic nature of atrial fibrillation substrate during development and reversal of heart failure in dogs." *Circulation* no. 105 (22):2672-8.

Sih, H. J., D. P. Zipes, E. J. Berbari, D. E. Adams, and J. E. Olgin. 2000. "Differences in organization between acute and chronic atrial fibrillation in dogs." *J Am Coll Cardiol* no. 36 (3):924-31.

Sih, H. J., D. P. Zipes, E. J. Berbari, and J. E. Olgin. 1999. "A high-temporal resolution algorithm for quantifying organization during atrial fibrillation." *IEEE Trans Biomed Eng* no. 46 (4):440-50.

Skanes, A. C., R. Mandapati, O. Berenfeld, J. M. Davidenko, and J. Jalife. 1998. "Spatiotemporal periodicity during atrial fibrillation in the isolated sheep heart." *Circulation* no. 98 (12):1236-48.

Stambler, B. S., G. Fenelon, R. K. Shepard, H. F. Clemo, and C. M. Guiraudon. 2003. "Characterization of sustained atrial tachycardia in dogs with rapid ventricular pacing-induced heart failure." *J Cardiovasc Electrophysiol* no. 14 (5):499-507.

Takahashi, Y., P. Sanders, P. Jais, M. Hocini, R. Dubois, M. Rotter, T. Rostock, C. J. Nalliah, F. Sacher, J. Clementy, and M. Haissaguerre. 2006. "Organization of frequency spectra of atrial fibrillation: relevance to radiofrequency catheter ablation." *J Cardiovasc Electrophysiol* no. 17 (4):382-8. doi: JCE414 [pii] 10.1111/j.1540-8167.2005.00414.x.

Verheule, S., E. Wilson, S. Banthia, T. H. th Everett, S. Shanbhag, H. J. Sih, and J. Olgin. 2004. "Direction-dependent conduction abnormalities in a canine model of atrial fibrillation due to chronic atrial dilatation." *Am J Physiol Heart Circ Physiol* no. 287 (2):H634-44.

Verheule, S., E. Wilson, T. th Everett, S. Shanbhag, C. Golden, and J. Olgin. 2003. "Alterations in atrial electrophysiology and tissue structure in a canine model of chronic atrial dilatation due to mitral regurgitation." *Circulation* no. 107 (20):2615-22.

Wijffels, M. C., C. J. Kirchhof, R. Dorland, and M. A. Allessie. 1995. "Atrial fibrillation begets atrial fibrillation. A study in awake chronically instrumented goats." *Circulation* no. 92 (7):1954-68.

Wu, T. J., J. J. Ong, C. M. Chang, R. N. Doshi, M. Yashima, H. L. Huang, M. C. Fishbein, C. T. Ting, H. S. Karagueuzian, and P. S. Chen. 2001. "Pulmonary veins and ligament of Marshall as sources of rapid activations in a canine model of sustained atrial fibrillation." *Circulation* no. 103 (8):1157-63.

Yue, L., J. Feng, R. Gaspo, G. R. Li, Z. Wang, and S. Nattel. 1997. "Ionic remodeling underlying action potential changes in a canine model of atrial fibrillation." *Circ Res* no. 81 (4):512-25.

3

Modeling Mother Rotor Anchoring in Branching Atrial Tissue*

Gerald Fischer[1], Leonhard Wieser[1] and Florian Hintringer[2,†]
[1]*Institute of Electrical, Electronic and Bioengineering, University for Health Sciences, Medical Informatics and Technology (UMIT), Hall i.T.*
[2]*Department for Cardiology, Medical University Innsbruck*
Austria

1. Introduction

Background: It has been hypothesized that stable mother rotors may increase the stability of atrial fibrillation. Local shortening of action potential duration due to vagotonic activity may promote the formation of mother rotors. However, prior studies have shown that meandering rotors typically drift out of the region of short action potential duration (APD), making the formation of stable rotors unlikely. Thus, for the formation of mother rotors in vagotonic AF a mechanism must be involved which increases rotor stability.
Hypothesis: Local variation of electrotonic load due to branching muscle sleeves in the atrial tissue may avoid rotor drift and ease the formation of stable vagotonic AF. In this chapter the underlying mechanisms are illustrated by means of computer modeling.
Model formulation: Anchoring is illustrated in a square patch of tissue and a monolayer model of the atria. Vagotonic activity was modeled by increasing ACh-concentration in the vicinity of the pulmonary veins (PVs). Close to the right lower PV, a muscle sleeve branching into the vein was included in the model. A model of canine atrial membrane kinetics was used providing detailed data on electrical remodeling and vagal activity. AF was analyzed computing dominant frequency (DF) maps and phase singularities (PSs).
Model predictions: In the case of a missing anchor site AF was self terminating within 2 s of simulated activity. The rotor drifted out of the short APD region. After including a branching tissue structure, mother rotor formation was observed (anchoring and almost periodic activity over the entire simulated interval of 4.2 s). Pull and push currents were identified as the mechanism stabilizing the rotor trajectory. Push currents in the bundle reduced the DF at the branching by about 10% with respect to the highest DF (15 Hz). The computed DF map mainly reflected the underlying ACh concentration (correlation 0.9).
Summary: Branching tissue structures in regions of high ACh-concentration may constitute the substrate underlying vagotonic AF. Future experimental studies are needed to further confirm motor rotor anchoring in branching tissue.

---

*Research on cardiac arrhythmia is supported by the Standortagentur Tyrol within the K-Regio Projekt Kryotipkatheter.
†Disclosures: G. Fischer and F. Hintringer are partners at AFreeze GmbH.

2. Background

Several mechanisms are involved in the onset and the maintenance of atrial fibrillation (AF), Nattel (2002). Beside the conceptual models of multiple self-maintaining wavelets and fast firing ectopic foci, also mother rotors have become subject of basic and applied research. A mother rotor is thought to be a locally very organized and fast micro-reentry circuit driving AF. While the original concept of a single driving reentry underlying AF goes back to the early twentieth century, high resolution optical mapping, Chen et al. (2000) and micro-electrode recordings, Mandapati et al. (2000) in the Langendorff-perfused sheep heart led to an increased interest in mother rotors in this century. Recently, electro-anatomical mapping displayed regions of high dominant frequency (DF) in humans, Sanders et al. (2005). Several DF sites were found per patient.

In computer models of atrial and ventricular fibrillation mother rotors are associated with regions of local shortening of the action potential duration (APD), Samie et al. (2001). Such shortening is obtained by heterogeneous membrane properties which can arise for instance from a locally increased concentration of the vagal neurotransmitter acetylcholine (ACh), Kneller et al. (2002). However, a single region of short APD does not guarantee the formation of a mother rotor. Any heterogeneity in membrane properties causes a rotor or spiral wave drift. As has been shown by Ten Tusscher & Panfilov (2002), the rotor typically tends to drift towards regions of long APD. This hampers the formation of mother rotors. In Kneller et al. (2002) a multiple number of properly sized ACh-regions was needed for creating a stable rotor of high frequency.

3. Hypothesis

The central hypothesis of this chapter is to illuminate a mechanism which reverses the direction of rotor drift and, thus, supports anchoring of mother rotors. The anchor site is formed by a branching tissue structure in the region of short APD. There are multiple branchings in the atria such as inter-atrial connections (e.g., the Bachmann's bundle [BB]), muscle sleeves branching from the left atrium into the pulmonary veins (PVs), the pectinate muscles, etc. Normal conduction in branching tissue is well investigated, Fast & Kléber (1995), Kucera & Rudy (2001). If a wavefront activates a bundle an increased current is drawn by the increased load of the branching tissue. This causes slowing of conduction or even functional block. Kucera and Rudy named this the pull-effect. Once the bundle is activated, current is re-injected back into the branching bringing the cells burdened by the pull currents back to a normal plateau level. This effect reduces the window of vulnerability and is named the push effect. For fibrillatory conduction it has been shown that a branching can create wave breaks but also an anchor site and that pull and push currents are involved in these phenomena, Wieser et al. (2007).

The hypothesis was tested as follows: first, a square patch of tissue was investigated for demonstrating rotor drift out of the ACh-region in the absence of an anchor site. This lead to spontaneous termination of fibrillation. The same finding was obtained for a model of the atrial geometry. Second, an anchor point was included in the ACh-region of the square patch by a branching tissue structure. It was shown that the direction of drift is reversed and a mother rotor was formed. Also, for the model of atrial geometry an anchor site increased the rotor stability.

4. Model formulation

4.1 Bioelectric activity

The membrane kinetics were described by the ionic current model of the atrial canine cell developed by Ramirez et al. (2000). As described in Xie et al. (2002) Na^+ and Cl^- concentrations were set to a fixed predefined value. Vagal actions were included by the acetylcholine (ACh) sensitive K^+-current as formulated by Kneller et al. (2002). Heterogeneous membrane properties were introduced into the models by spatially varying the ACh concentration. An adaptive time step scheme was used for solving the ordinary differential equations, Wieser et al. (2007).

Cell to cell coupling in atrial tissue was described by the monodomain equation. The finite element method was used for spatial discretization. The approximate edge length of a cell element was 200 μm. Time integration of the monodomain equation was performed using an explicit Euler scheme, treating the ionic current part and the diffusion part separately. Further details can be found in Wieser et al. (2007). Tissue properties were described by the following parameters: surface to volume ratio of the cell (100 mm^{-1}), cell capacitance per unit area (0.01 μFmm^{-2}) and conductivity (values given below).

Fibrillatory conduction was simulated for a time interval of 4.2 s duration. This interval is identical as for the recorded data in Sanders et al. (2005) and Fischer et al. (2007).

4.2 Square model

A $60 \times 60 \times 1$ mm^3 block of cardiac tissue including a bundle of cylindrical shape (diameter 3 mm) in the tissue center was constructed. Fibers were included within the bundle running along its axis (longitudinal and transversal conductivity are 0.3 S/m and 0.1 S/m, respectively). For the rest of the tissue an isotropic conductivity of 0.1 S/m was assumed. This yields a propagation velocity of about 47 cm/s in the bulk tissue and a velocity of about 83 cm/s along the bundle. In order to study the effective role of the bundle in the simulations it was also possible to remove the bundle from the model. An ACh concentration was assigned to a circular region (diameter 50 mm) centered at the tissue center (i.e. the bundle insertion). Here, the maximal ACh concentration was 0.003 μM. Similar as in Kneller et al. (2002), a harmonic function was used for assigning a smooth transition of the concentration to zero (no ACh outside the region). Electrical remodeling was considered by reducing the Ca^{2+} current to 20% of its original value.

4.3 Atrial model

A detailed description of our atrial model and the model validation for sinus rhythm and paced beats can be found in Wieser, Richter, Plank, Pfeifer, Tilg, Nowak & Fischer (2008). Briefly, a monolayer representation of the atria (curved surfaces in space) was created based on magnetic resonance (MR) imaging data of a female patient (50 kg body weight) with a supraventricular arrhythmia but a structurally normal atrium, Berger et al. (2006). The left and the right atrium (LA, RA, resp.) are electrically connected via three conductive structures: Bachmann's bundle (BB), a coronary sinus (CS) muscle sleeve and the rim of the fossa ovalis (FO). In the monolayer representation BB and the CS muscle sleeve are strip-like structures with insertions in either atrium. The FO itself is non-conductive except for the rim. Thus, it is represented as a hole in the atrial septum. A ring-like structure represents the conducting rim and connects the FO orifices to each of the atria.

The atrial monodomain conductivity was assumed to be isotropic with 0.08 S/m (reference value). For all fibrous structures in the model (BB, CS muscle sleeve, crista terminalis) the longitudinal conductivity was increased to a 3–6 fold of the reference. The transversal conductivity is identical to the reference (0.08 S/m). For the FO (poor conduction) one fourth of the reference conductivity was chosen. The conduction velocity obtained by the reference conductivity was 43 cm/s. The maximum diameter of the atrial geometry was 3.8 cm [RA] and 4.3 cm [LA].

Atrial remodeling was considered by reducing the Ca^{2+} current to 31% and the fast transient outward K^+-current to 35% of the original value. According to experimental data for the normal and remodeled canine atrial cell, Ramirez et al. (2000), this corresponds to a degree of electrical remodeling obtained after 42 days of persistent atrial tachycardia. The ACh concentration was increased around the PVs as vagal nerve endings can be found in this region Armour et al. (1997). From the MR data only one common left pulmonary vein (LPV) ostium was identified. In a circular region around each ostium the ACh concentration was interpolated by a harmonic function. The maximal concentration was 0.02 μM. The diameters of the three ACh-regions were 50 mm. In the area between the two right PVs the regions were overlapping in part. Here, the higher of the two concentration values was taken.

For our study an anchoring bundle could be introduced close to the right lower PV. The bundle was mimicking a muscle sleeve extending into the PV. Due to the monolayer representation of the atrium the bundle had a strip like structure with a width of 2 mm. The bundle branched off from the atrial tissue about 4 mm peri-ostial from the PV. Its longitudinal conductivity was the six-fold of the reference conductivity while the transversal conductivity was equal to the reference.

4.4 Phase information and dominant frequency

Phase information is computed as described in Iyer & Gray (2001) using two independent variables of each cell, namely the action potential V (reference value -40 mV) and the h-gate (sodium inactivation gate, reference value 0.4). On the triangulated atrial geometry phase singularities (PSs) are determined by applying the concept of topological charge as described in Rantner et al. (2007).

The direct current (dc) component was removed from the action potential prior to spectral analysis. This has a similar effect as appling a high pass filter component in clinicaly recorded data and enables the comparision of the spectral analysis with the the data shown in Sanders et al. (2005), Fischer et al. (2007). Furthermore, the data was was down-sampled to 250 Hz. Two different spectral estimators were used for computing the spectral profile of the action potential. First, the Fast Fourier Transform (FFT) was used which is a kind of standard for computing dominant frequency (DF), Kneller et al. (2002), Sanders et al. (2005), Fischer et al. (2007). For the simulated time interval of 4.2 s the obtained frequency resolution is 0.24 Hz. Second, a spectral estimator based on autoregressive (AR) modeling (Yule-Walker method), Signorini et al. (2003) was used for improving the spectral resolution. The Yule-Walker method performs well if the spectrum is expected to contain pronounced peaks. However, this spectral estimator looses accuracy if the sampling frequency is too high. Thus, a two point moving average low-pass filter was applied and the sampling frequency was halved to 125 Hz (about the ten-fold of the expected DFs). The AR-model order was fixed to twelve, which means that not more than six prominent peaks are expected to appear in the spectral profile. The spectrum was computed with a resolution of 0.01 Hz and the maximum of the power spectral density was taken as the DF.

Action potential data and phase singularities were continuously displayed for all computer simulations with a temporal resolution of 1 ms as described in Rantner et al. (2007) using the computer visualization package AmiraDev 2.3. Note that each PS is automatically detected by the computer program and directly linked to statistical evaluation removing any observer depended bypass. Furthermore, also the DF maps have been displayed with AmiraDev 2.3 and computer supported detection of low and high sites.

5. Model predictions

5.1 Missing anchor

A spiral wave was initiated in the square model with its tip close to the tissue center. First, the bundle was removed (missing anchor site). Within the first second of simulated activity the spiral wave formed a meandering rotor. A DF of 12.5 Hz (FFT) was obtained in the region of high ACh concentration (short APD). Outside this region the tissue could not follow the rapid activation and wave breaks gave rise to chaotic activity at a lower DF (8.5 Hz). In total 28 new phase singularities were generated with a relatively short life span (3 ms to 759 ms, mean 128 ms). As expected, the original rotor was slowly drifting out of the region of short APD and terminated after 1314 ms by a collision with a PS of opposite chirality. After 1866 ms fibrillation terminated spontaneously by the collision of the last two PSs.

A similar behavior was observed for the atrial geometry in the absence of an anchor site. The APD was shortened in the proximity of the pulmonary veins by an increased ACh concentration. Fibrillation was induced by cross shock protocol. Two PSs were created by a wave break in the region of short APD close to the right lower pulmonary vein. Similar as in the square model, one PS became a rotor of a long life time meandering with a slow drift towards regions of longer APD. After 932 ms it died out by collision (see Fig. 1). Again, wave breaks occurred in the border zone of the short APD regions. Furthermore, wave breaks were observed at the left atrial insertion of the Bachmann's bundle due to load effects in branching tissue. In total 125 PSs of relatively short life time (4 ms to 468 ms, mean 60 ms) were counted. Again fibrillation terminated spontaneously after 1528 ms by collision of the last PS with border of the anterior lateral mitral annulus.

5.2 Mechanism of anchoring

Again, a spiral wave was initiated in the square model with its tip close to the center. This time, the bundle was included in the model. Thus, APD was prolonged at the branching site due to the push currents drawn in the plateau phase. This effect locally reversed the APD gradient produced by the acetylcholine distribution. Thus, the meandering spiral wave tip displayed a slow drift towards the bundle. After 220 ms, the rotor attached to the bundle for the first time and then displayed a repeatable activation pattern.

One cycle (one full PS rotation) of the repeatable activation pattern is shown in Fig. 2. At 300 ms the PS reached the bundle in an eleven o'clock position. Due to the push currents of the previous cycle the cells in the branching were not yet recovered. Thus, the rotor was forced to circumvent the bundle along its right border. Strong pull currents were drawn from the area right to the bundle, as the activation front traveled close to an increased and unexcitable load (refractory tissue branching). The bundle became conductive when the rotor reached a six o'clock position (321 ms). Now the excitable region was inside the bundle and the refractory tissue was outside the right border (due to the strong pull currents the tissue had already recovered to about −65 mV). The rotor traveled the same way back along the border and detached again in an eleven o'clock position (folding of the trajectory). Due to the small area of the excitable gap the rotor was accelerated when traveling back (traveling down takes about 20 ms, while traveling back up takes only 10 ms). As the rotor was drifting away from the bundle the push currents prolonged the plateau phase in the bundle. At 345 ms it can be clearly seen in the color coding that the action potential within the bundle was higher ('push region') than within the right vicinity of the bundle ('pull region'). Then the rotor meandered back towards the bundle (360 ms). The pull region recovered first and attracted the rotor. Thus, the rotor moved again towards the right bundle border where the strongest pull currents were observed. This time the bundle was reached in a twelve o'clock position. The cycle was then repeated which a pattern slightly rotated in a clockwise fashion. Due to this slight

rotation in each cycle a rosette like trajectory of the rotor is obtained for the entire simulated time interval of 4.2 s.
Within the bundle region the DF was 11.3 Hz (FFT). Interestingly, the DF in the surrounding of the bundle was somewhat increased with a value of 12.3 Hz. Outside the ACh region the DF ranged from 8.0 Hz to 8.5 Hz. The mother rotor persisted for the entire simulated time. The remaining 117 PSs had a short life span (6 ms to 296 ms, mean 46 ms) and were all created by wave breaks.

5.3 Mother rotor in the atrium

A bundle was included close to the right lower pulmonary vein of the atrial geometry. Fibrillation was induced as before by a cross shock protocol applied close to the bundle. Two phase singularities were created by a wave break and the one closer to the bundle drifted in a meandering fashion towards the bundle and reached the bundle 4 ms after its initiation for the first time. It detached again, and after three rotations taking another 212 ms it anchored again. Then, similar as in the square model, it attached and detached repeatedly forming a mother rotor which lasted for the entire simulated time interval (4.2 s). The rotor trajectory is shown in Fig. 3 together with a the action potential in a cell near the bundle (mother rotor area) and the spectra obtained by the FFT and the AR-model.
The remaining 744 PSs were of relatively short life span (4 ms to 536 ms, mean 45 ms). The majority was created in the border zones of the acetylcholine areas near the PVs. Furthermore, frequent wave breaks were observed at the left atrial insertion of the Bachmann's bundle (increased load at the tissue branching). To a smaller degree wave breaks were also observed at the right atrial insertion of the Bachmann's bundle and at the two connections of the coronary sinus muscle sleeve with both atria. Also unstable anchoring of PSs at the Bachmann's Bundle was observed. As there is no acetylcholine (long APD) in this region no stable rotor was formed. Typically, the PSs attached only once or twice at the Bachmann's bundle and died out in the meandering phase when traveling away from the bundle by collision with other PSs. Only 122 PSs (16%) were observed in the right atrium. Figure 4 shows three sample snapshots of chaotic conduction in a left anterior oblique view.
The dominant frequency map was computed by the FFT and the AR-model. Some results are listed in Tab. 1. The DF map obtained for the AR-model is shown in Fig. 5. For all cell elements the correlation between the two spectral estimators is 0.97. Similar as for the square model the highest frequency (15.4 Hz, AR) is obtained in the tissue surrounding the bundle. Again in the bundle itself the frequency is slightly reduced (13.8 Hz, AR). Here, comparisons are based on AR-model data due to the better spectral resolution.
Interestingly, also at the common left pulmonary vein (14.9 Hz) a higher DF is obtained than at the bundle itself. As can been from Fig. 5, the DF distribution closely matched the ACh concentration. The DF map shows a high correlation with the ACh concentration (0.89 FFT, 0.90 AR-model). The lowest DF in the left atrium is found at the left atrial appendage (6.4 Hz). In the right atrium the DF is almost constant (6.5 Hz to 7.2 Hz). The transition from high DF regions (blue) to low DF regions (red) occurs in a narrow region. Note the effect of the Bachmann's bundle on the left atrial DF map in Fig. 5. The low frequency region in the basal anterior left atrium extends up to the bundle insertion. This can be explained by push currents prolonging the APD in the tissue branching.

6. Summary

6.1 Anchoring

The major scope of this study was the investigation of load effects fixing a mother rotor pathway in a region of short APD. Before anchoring, the push currents prolong the APD at the

branching. Thus, a spiral wave in the vicinity drifts towards the bundle and anchors. Strong pull currents are drawn by the large unexcitable load (refractory bundle). When the bundle becomes excitable, the phase singularity travels back. Within the bundle the push currents prolong the APD (push region). This is a major difference to normal conduction where the pull currents drawn from a cell are later injected back by push currents into the same cell.
It has been shown previously by Wieser et al. (2007) that for a rectangular patch of tissue with homogeneous membrane properties anchoring is mainly determined by the load of the branching structure. Varying the shape of the bundle the rotor trajectory changes too, but the basic effect that the trajectory is fixed at the bundle is still observable. Even for the idealized situation of a flat strip in the monolayer model anchoring takes place. Several effects stabilize the rotor. First, the interaction of pull and push currents cause a folding of the trajectory at the bundle border. This lengthens the rotor pathway. Second, in the pull phase (wavelet outside the bundle) the strong load decreases the speed of the rotor. This contributes to a short wavelength. Third, the pull currents produce a zone which recovers early and attracts the rotor.
Interestingly, the interaction of APD prolongation in the bundle (push effect) and folding of the rotor trajectory makes it possible that the DF at the anchor site is somewhat below the DF of the surrounding tissue. At this point its should be stressed that the slight local decrease in DF (around 10%) is biophysically reasonable as push currents prolong the APD in the branching. Furthermore, the slight local decrease in DF was confirmed by two independent spectral estimators (FFT and AR-model). For the FFT the decrease was only four digits of the spectral resolution (1 Hz). Thus, a second spectral estimator (AR-model) with a theoretically infinite spectral resolution (but still a limited accuracy) was used. With this method a continuous decrease of DF was observed when zooming into the region around the bundle (data not shown). To our experience the AR-model is more accurate than the FFT for stationary signals (no termination of AF in the investigated time interval).
It must be stressed that permanent anchoring needs both local APD shortening and a branching tissue structure. Short time anchoring was observed at the left atrial insertion of the BB. Due to the long APD in this region the rotor was forced to travel far away from the bundle when detaching. This provoked a collision with PSs originating from the ACh-border zone. Another effect frequently observed in branching tissue is a wave break (Fig. 4) caused by the transition of an intact wave front, Wieser et al. (2007).

6.2 Left atrial AF

Induction of AF by a cross shock near one of the PVs can be interpreted as a critically timed extrasystole originating from a pulmonary vein. One of the two created PSs anchored within 0.2 s and became the mother rotor. Also within 0.2 s the first wave breaks occurred at the border of the ACh-region creating a completely chaotic activation pattern for large parts of the left atrium. In the right atrium the first PSs were observed 1.3 s after induction of AF. They were created by a wave break caused by the irregular stimuli across the interatrial connections in combination with steep restitution curve of the right atrial cells, Virag et al. (2002). Wave breaks at the right atrial insertions of the interatrial connections (BB, CS, FO) created PSs of only a few milliseconds life span. In the left atrium the number of PSs counted was the five-fold compared to the right atrium.
For the constructed model (the anchor site and the ACh-regions are near to the PVs) AF is a left atrial disease. We do not claim that this is true for all types of AF. However, it is an interesting observation that reasonable assumptions can be made (muscle sleeves and ACh-regions close to the PVs) which make the left atrium the source and the right atrium the innocent bystander.

6.3 Clinical implications

In the past decade catheter ablation of AF was mainly focusing on the left atrium and here in particular on the ostia of the PVs, Cappato et al. (2005). Originally, the attention paid to the anatomical structure of the PVs was motivated by a report identifying muscle sleeves from the PVs as triggers of AF, Haïssaguerre et al. (1998). To a smaller degree also other left and right atrial structures can host triggers. In the performed computer simulations a muscle sleeve branching from the atrial muscle could also constitute the substrate of the arrhythmia.
From a clinical point of view the understanding of paroxysmal AF is dominated by the picture of rapidly firing foci triggering the onset of the arrhythmia. Interestingly, the results of the presented computer model and other simulation studies, Wieser, Nowak, Tilg & Fischer (2008), Kneller et al. (2002), Kneller et al. (2005) suggest that fibrillation terminates within very few seconds without additional involved stabilizing mechanisms. For the investigated model of vagotonic AF the interplay of electrical remodeling, vagotonic activity and conduction in branching tissue structures stabilizes the reentry pathway. They constitute, thus, the substrate of the arrhythmia. This enables the development of longer, haemodynamically relevant episodes of AF. Thus, muscle fibers branching from the left atrium into the PVs do not only constitute the triggers of paroxysmal AF but may form also its substrate. In the computer model AF terminates within less than two seconds when removing the bundle from the vein. Similarly, AF often terminates during catheter ablation due to a modification of the underlying substrate. Here, future experimental work is needed for confirming the predictions of the computer model.
Guided ablation of AF needs signal parameters which identify the maintaining substrate(s). Here, two signal types are considered marking potential ablation targets: high DF sites, Sanders et al. (2005) and locations with fractionated potentials, Rostock et al. (2006).
It has been shown for patients with paroxysmal AF that ablation at a high DF site can terminate AF, Sanders et al. (2005). In our computer model the anchor site did not display the highest DF but a slightly reduced value (in the order of the spectral resolution obtained by the FFT). This discrepancy could be explained by keeping in mind that different signal types are used in clinical routine and computer modeling. A computer model yields the action potential (containing the intracellular potential) with a submillimeter spacial resolution. In contrast to this, mainly bipolar electrocardiograms (extracellular potentials) are assessed during an electrophysiological study. For the typical electrode spacing in the order of a few millimeters the catheter signal is sensitive to electric activity in a patch of tissue with several millimeters of diameter. Thus, the limited spatial and spectral resolution of current clinical technology can easily mask the small local decrease of DF predicted by our model.
The DF map computed by our computer model closely approximates the ACh-distribution in the atrial model (correlation coefficient 0.9). Branching tissue structures like the left atrial BB insertion and the PV muscle sleeve have only a minor influence on the DF map. It appears that the DF map in our model gives primely a picture of ACh-concentration. Also at the PVs without an anchor structure the computed DF was high. Interestingly, the computed DF map is in good qualitative agreement (high DF near the PVs, low DF in the right atrium and the basal anterior left atrium) with the DF map shown in Sanders et al. (2005) for paroxysmal AF. One might speculate that for paroxysmal AF the DF map displays mainly a picture of the vagal tonus.

6.4 Model simplifications

Every model is per definition a simplified and abstract approximation of a true system. The developed model is no exception from this rule.
The actual size and dimensions of the included branchings are not based on detailed anatomical data. They were assumed in the range of a few millimeters Wieser et al. (2007).

	FFT	AR-model
	Hz	Hz
maximum left atrium	15.5	15.4
minimum left atrium	6.0	6.4
maximum right atrium	7.9	7.2
minimum right atrium	6.0	6.5
mean of both atria	9.9	9.4
anchor site	14.3	13.8
left pulmonary vein	15.2	14.9

Table 1. Dominant Frequency computet by the FFT and AR-modeling

This seems reasonable for the largest muscle bundles in the atria. Also the distribution of ACh was assumed similarly as suggested in earlier computer models Kneller et al. (2002), Kneller et al. (2005) and in agreement with anatomical studies on atrial vagal innervation Armour et al. (1997). With the variation of these parameters also the strength of the observed rotor stabilization might change. However, the principal observation that tissue branchings in regions of short APD can contribute to mother rotor anchoring should remain valid. Having in mind that for example in the proximity of the PV ostia we find both, APD shortening and branching muscle fibers, the observed mechanisms could yield a contribution to mother rotor stabilization in humans.

We do not claim that the described mechanism of rotor stabilization is the sole or most important mechanism contributing to the formation of sustained AF. A plurality of other mechanisms is well investigated which contribute to stable AF. These mechanisms involve locally organized activity Kneller et al. (2005) but also entirely random activation which might be facilitated structural and mechanical remodeling Wijffels et al. (1995). The chapter presents a model of vagotonic AF based on reasonable assumptions.

We do also not claim that the stability observed for the short time span of a few seconds can be generalized to significantly longer periods of hour and days. However, it has been shown that the described mechanism can significantly prolong the live time of a fibrillatory episode. Thus, it might contribute to the formation of long periods of AF.

The atrial membrane kinetics were approximated by a computer model of the canine atrial cell. It was chosen as it contains detailed data for electrical remodeling by Ramirez et al. (2000) and vagal modulation of function Kneller et al. (2002). The atrial anatomy was human. The canine atrial cell has a relatively short APD Ramirez et al. (2000). This explains the relatively high DF (6 Hz to 15 Hz) predicted by our model. In humans the DF remains in the range of 4 Hz to 10 Hz in patients with paroxysmal AF. Sanders et al. (2005).

The use of a monolayer approximation of the atrium yields a significant save in computation time Wieser, Richter, Plank, Pfeifer, Tilg, Nowak & Fischer (2008), Virag et al. (2002), Vigmond et al. (2001). However, the variation of wall thickness cannot be included in the model. Furthermore, it has been shown that load effects are slightly over-estimated Wieser, Richter, Plank, Pfeifer, Tilg, Nowak & Fischer (2008). The predictions of the described model are consistent with a prior studies where bundle dimensions/geometry and ACh concentration have been varied, Wieser, Nowak, Tilg & Fischer (2008).

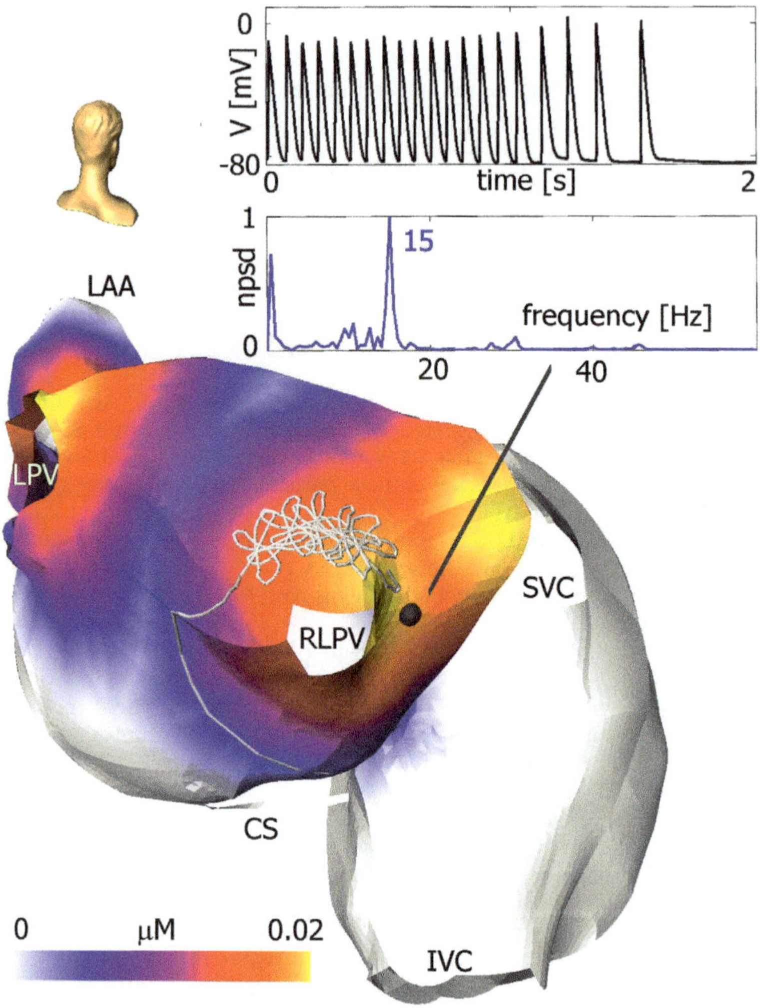

Fig. 1. Rotor drift in the case of a missing anchor site. The atrial model is shown in a posterior oblique view. Color coding displays the ACh concentration. The rotor trajectory is displayed by a white line. After its initiation near the RLPV the rotor drifts in a meandering fashion in direction of decreasing ACh level. Close to the border of the ACh region the drift accelerates and the rotor moves without meandering down to the posterior septal left atrium. Here it dies out by collision with a PS of opposite chirality. The action potential at one site (gray marker) near the RLPV is shown together with the computed power spectrum (FFT). CS ... coronary sinus muscle sleeve, IVC ... inferior vena cava, LAA ... left atrial appendage, LPV ... left pulmonary vein, RLPV ... right lower pulmonary vein, SVC ... superior vena cava.

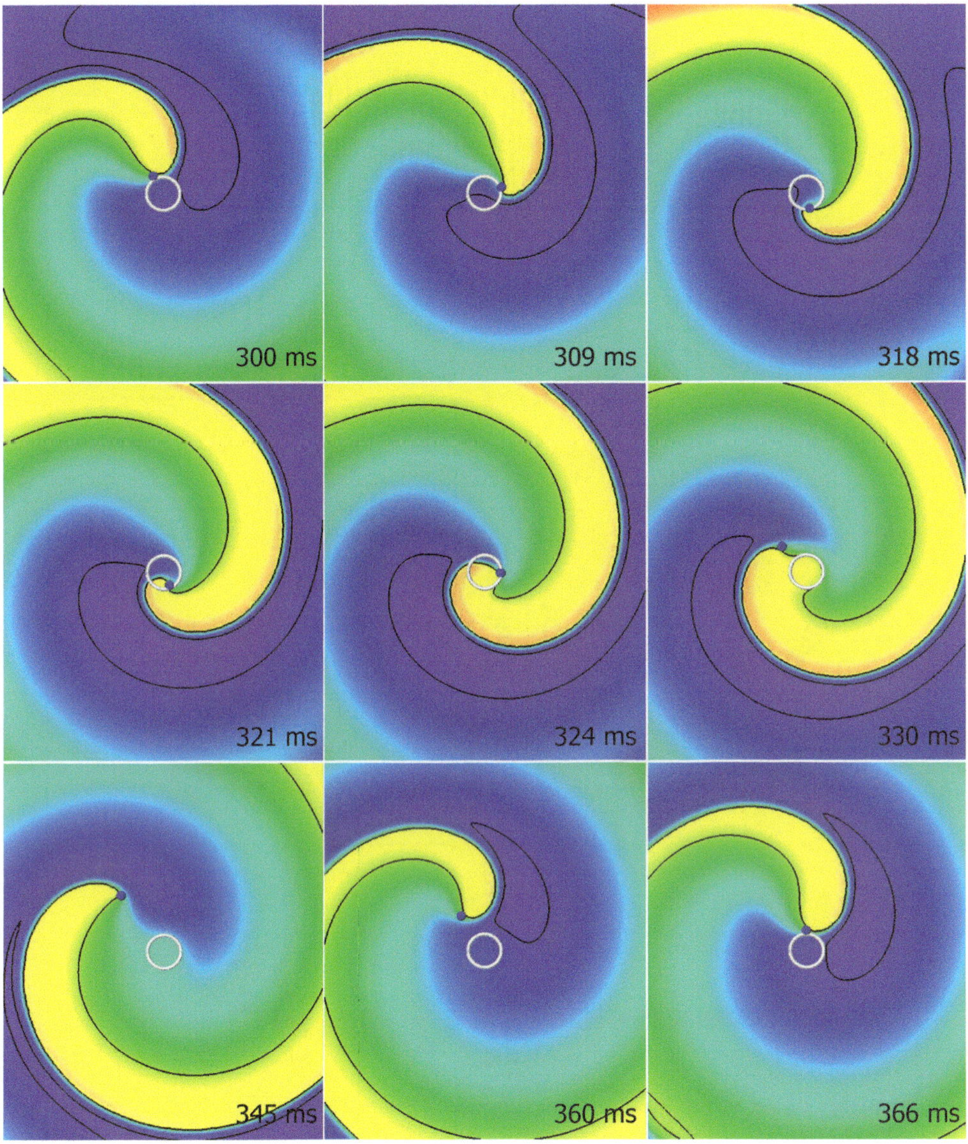

Fig. 2. One rotation of the anchored motor in the square model. Color coding depicts the action potential in the range of −80 mV (blue) to 0 mV(red). At t =300 ms the rotor (blue marker) has reached the bundle (white circle). The bundle region has not fully recovered yet and the activation front travels around its border (309 ms and 318 ms). Due to the potential gradient, pull currents are drawn from the wave front (area right from the bundle). At t =321 ms the bundle has recovered and the activation front can enter. Now the PS travels back along the bundle border as the excitable tissue is now inside the bundle (324 ms). When the PS has detached push currents increase the potential in the bundle prolonging APD (330 ms and 345 ms).

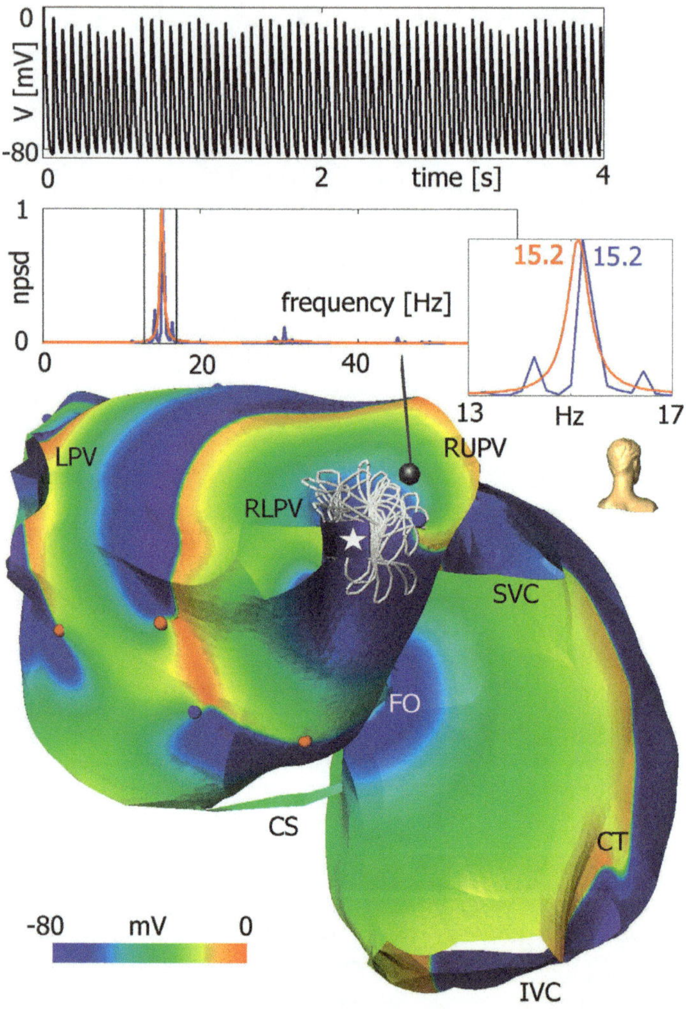

Fig. 3. Snapshot of the action potential after mother rotor anchoring. The atrial model is shown in a posterior oblique view. The mother rotor trajectory is displayed by a white line. Note meandering around the bundle insertion (white asterisk). Spherical markers represent PSs of clockwise (blue) and counter-clockwise (red) chirality. The action potential at a high frequency site (gray marker) is shown together with the power spectrum obtained by the FFT (blue) and the AR-model (red). A portion of the spectrum is zoomed for comparison.
CS ... coronary sinus muscle sleeve, CT ... crista terminalis, IVC ... inferior vena cava, FO ... fossa ovalis, LPV ... left pulmonary vein, RLPV ... right lower pulmonary vein, RUPV ... right upper pulmonary vein, SVC ... superior vena cava.

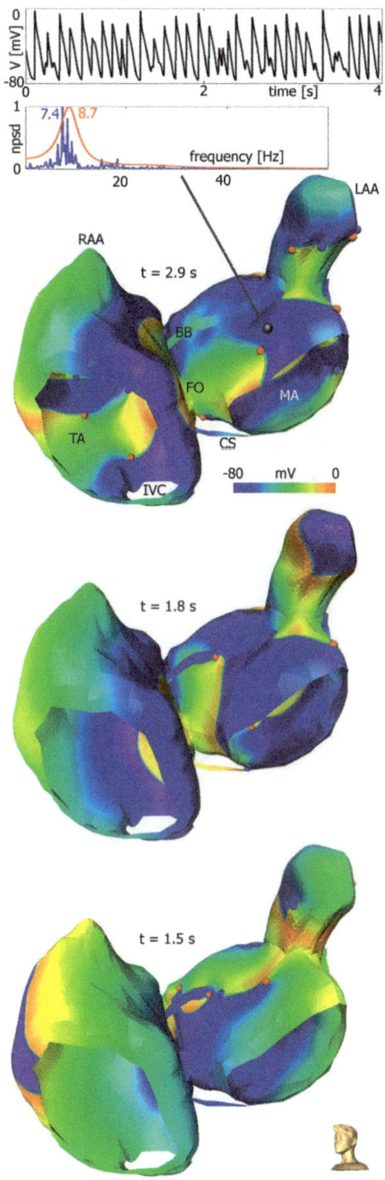

Fig. 4. Three snapshots of the action potential in a left anterior oblique view. On top the action potential in a low frequency site (gray marker) is shown together with the power spectrum. At 1.5 s a wave break can be observed at the left atrial insertion of the BB. At 1.8 s short time rotor anchoring takes place at the BB. Note that in general more PSs are on the left atrium compared to the right. Color coding and markers are the same as in Fig. 3.
BB ... Bachmann's bundle, CS ... coronary sinus muscle sleeve, FO ... fossa ovalis, IVC ... inferior vena cava, LAA ... left atrial appendage, MA ... mitral annulus, RAA ... right atrial appendage, TA ... tricuspid annulus.

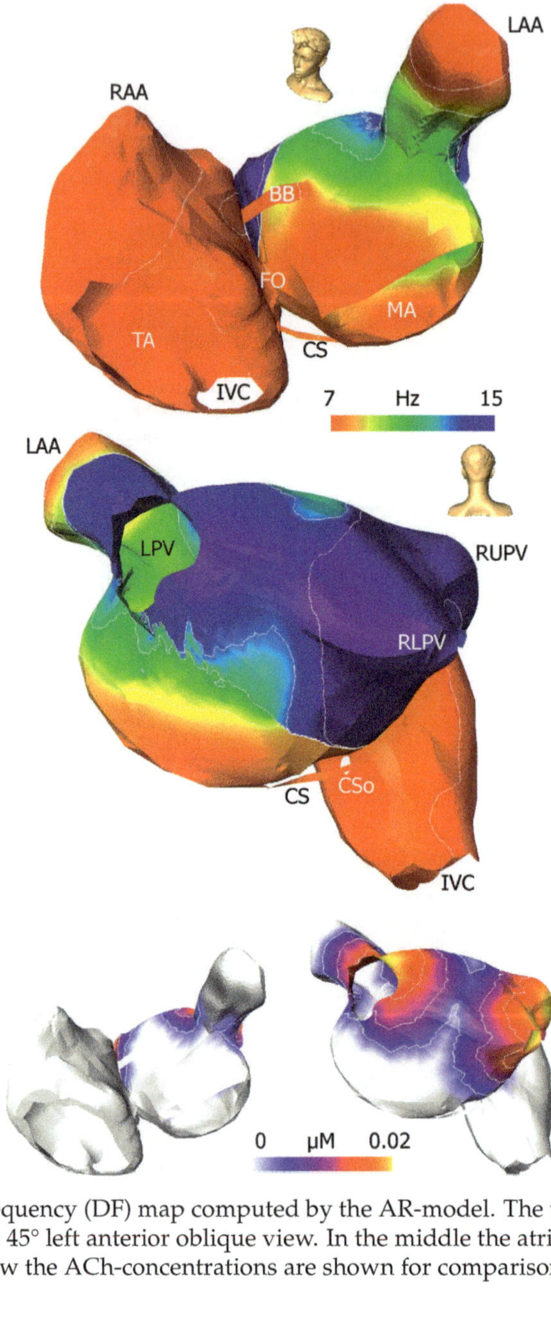

Fig. 5. Dominant frequency (DF) map computed by the AR-model. The upper panel shows the atrial model in a 45° left anterior oblique view. In the middle the atria are shown in a posterior view. Below the ACh-concentrations are shown for comparison.

6.5 Conclusions

A tissue branching (muscle sleeve, bundle, branching fibers) in a region of shortened action potential duration can serve as an anchor site for an organized activation pattern in vagotonic AF. The interplay of pull and push currents in the branching stabilizes the rotor pathway. The rotor repeatedly attaches and detaches. The locally short APD is necessary for maintaining the rotor. If APD prolongs (e.g., due to a reduced vagal tonus) the rotor can drift away from the anchor site and collide with another PS (possible spontaneous termination of AF).
Folding of the rotor trajectory and APD prolongation in the bundle (push currents) caused a modest decrease of DF at the anchor site. In our simulations the DF map was mainly influenced by the spatial distribution of acetylcholine. Thus, the DF map reflected the underlying assumed vagal activity.

7. References

Armour, J., Murphy, D., Yuan, B.-X., MacDonald, S. & Hopkins, D. (1997). Gross and microscopic anatomy of the human intrinsic cardiac nervous system, *The Anatomical Record* 247: 289–298.

Berger, T., Fischer, G., Pfeifer, B., Modre, R., Hanser, F., Th. Trieb, F. R., Stühlinger, M., Pachinger, O., Tilg, B. & Hintringer, F. (2006). Single-beat noninvasive imaging of cardiac electrophysiology (NICE) of ventricular preexcitation, *Journal of the American College of Cardiology* 48: 2045–2052.

Cappato, R., Calkins, H., Chen, S.-A., Davies, W., Iesaka, Y., Kalman, J., Kim, Y.-H., Klein, G., Packer, D. & Skanes, A. (2005). Worldwide survey on the methods, efficacy, and safety of catheter ablation for human atrial fibrillation, *Circulation* 111: 1100–1105.

Chen, J., Mandapati, R., Berenfeld, O., Skanes, A., Gray, R. & Jalife, J. (2000). Dynamics of wavelets and their role in atrial fibrillation in the isolated sheep heart, *Cardiovascular Research* 48: 220–232.

Fast, V. & Kléber, A. (1995). Cardiac tissue geometry as a determinant of unidirectional conduction block: assessment of microscopic excitation spread by optical mapping in patterned cell cultures and in a computer model, *Cardiovascular Research* 29: 697–707.

Fischer, G., Stühlinger, M., Nowak, C., Wieser, L., Tilg, B. & Hintringer, F. (2007). On computing dominant frequency from bipolar intracardiac electrogram, *IEEE Transactions on Biomedical Engineering* 54: 165–169.

Haïssaguerre, M., Jaïs, P., Shah, D., Takahashi, A., Hocini, M., Quiniou, G., Garrigue, S., Le Mouroux, A., Le Metayer, P. & Clementy, J. (1998). Spontaneous initiation of atrial fibrillation by ectopic beats originating in the pulmonary veis, *The New England Journal of Medicine* 339: 659–666.

Iyer, A. N. & Gray, R. A. (2001). An experimentalist's approach to accurate localization of phase singularities during reentry, *Annals of Biomedical Engineering* 29: 47–59.

Kneller, J., Kalifa, J., Zou, R., Zaitsev, A. V., Warren, M., Berenfeld, O., Vigmond, E. J., Leon, L. J., Nattel, S. & Jalife, J. (2005). Mechanisms of af termination by pure sodium channel blockade in an ionically-realistic mathematical model, *Circulation Research* 96: 35–47.

Kneller, J., Zou, R., Vigmond, E. J., Z.Wang, Leon, L. J. & Nattel, S. (2002). Cholinergic atrial fibrillation in a computer model of a two-dimensional sheet of canine atrial cells with realistic ionic properties, *Circulation Research* 90: e73–e87.

Kucera, J. & Rudy, Y. (2001). Mechanistic insights into very slow conduction in branching cardiac tissue: a model study, *Circulation Research* 89: 799–806.

Mandapati, R., Skanes, A., Chen, J., Berenfeld, O. & Jalife, J. (2000). Stable microreentrant sources as a mechanism of atrial fibrillation in the isolated sheep heart, *Circulation* 101: 194–199.

Nattel, S. (2002). New ideas about atrial fibrillation 50 years on, *Nature* 415: 219–226.

Ramirez, R., Nanttel, S. & Courtemanche, M. (2000). Mathematical analysis of canine atrial action potentials: rate, regional factors, and electrical remodeling, *American Journal of Physiology Heart Circulation Physiology* 279: H1767–H1785.

Rantner, L. J., Wieser, L., Stühlinger, M. C., Hintringer, F., Tilg, B. & Fischer, G. (2007). Detection of phase singularities in triangular meshes, *Methods of Information in Medicine* 46: 646–654.

Rostock, T., Rotter, M., Sanders, P., Takahashi, Y., Jaïs, P., Hocini, M., Hsu, L., Sacher, F., Clémenty, J. & Haïssaguerre, M. (2006). High-density activation mapping of fractionated electrograms in the atria of patients with paroxysmal atrial fibrillation, *Heart Rhythm* 3: 27–34.

Samie, F. H., Berenfeld, O., Anumonwo, J., Mironov, S. F., Udassi, S., Beaumont, J., Taffet, S., Pertsov, A. M. & Jalife, J. (2001). Rectification of the background potassium current – A determinant of rotor dynamics in ventricular fibrillation, *Circulation Research* 89: 1216–1223.

Sanders, P., Berenfeld, O., Hocini, M., Jaïs, P., Vaidyanathan, R., Hsu, L.-F., Garrigue, S., Takahashi, Y., Rotter, M., Sacher, F., Scavée, C., Ploutz-Snyder, R., Jalife, J. & Haïssaguerre, M. (2005). Spectral analysis identifies sites of high-frequency activity maintaining atrial fibrillation in humans, *Circulation* 112: 789–797.

Signorini, M., Magenes, G., Cerutti, S. & Arduini, D. (2003). Linear and nonlinear parameters for the analysis of fetal heart rate signal from cardiotocographic recordings, *IEEE Transactions on Biomedical Engineering* 50: 365–374.

Ten Tusscher, K. H. & Panfilov, A. V. (2002). Reentry in heterogeneous cardiac tissue described by the Luo-Rudy ventricular action potential model, *American Journal of Physiology Heart Circulation Physiology* 284: H542–H548.

Vigmond, E. J., Ruckdeschel, R. & Trayanova, N. (2001). Reentry in a morphologically realistic atrial model, *Journal of Cardiovascular Electrophysiology* 12(9): 1046–1054.

Virag, N., Jacquemet, V., Henriquez, C. S., Zozor, S., Blanc, O., Vesin, J.-M., Pruvot, E. & Kappenberger, L. (2002). Study of atrial arrhythmias in a computer model based on magnetic resonance images of human atria, *Chaos: An Interdisciplinary Journal of Nonlinear Science* 12: 754–763.

Wieser, L., Fischer, G., Nowak, C. & Tilg, B. (2007). Fibrillatory conduction in branching atrial tissue–Insight from volumetric and monolayer computer models, *Computer Methods and Programs in Biomedicine* 86: 103–111.

Wieser, L., Nowak, C., Tilg, B. & Fischer, G. (2008). Mother rotor anchoring in branching tissue with heterogeneous membrane properties, *Biomedizinische Technik* 53: 25–35.

Wieser, L., Richter, H., Plank, G., Pfeifer, B., Tilg, B., Nowak, C. & Fischer, G. (2008). A finite element formulation for atrial tissue monolayer, *Methods of Information in Medicine* 47: 131–139.

Wijffels, M., Kirchhof, C., Dorland, R. & Alessie (1995). Atrial fibrillation begets atrial fibrillation: a study in awake chronically instrumented goats, *Circulation* 92: 1954–1968.

Xie, F., Qu, Z., Garfinkel, A. & Weiss, J. (2002). Electrical refractory period restitution and spiral wave reentry in simulated cardiac tissue, *American Journal of Physiology Heart Circulation Physiology* 283: H448–H460.

4

The Thrombogenic Role of Platelets in Valvular Atrial Fibrillation

Hanan Ahmed Galal Azzam
Mansoura University, Faculty of Medicine,
Egypt

1. Introduction

Atrial fibrillation is the most common sustained cardiac arrhythmia, which is associated with a high risk of stroke and thromboembolism. The association of atrial fibrillation and valvular heart disease results in a substantial stroke and thromboembolic risk, with a 17-fold greater risk than unaffected controls (Wipf & Lipsky, 1990).
Important insights into the pathophysiology of thrombus formation (thrombogenesis) in atrial fibrillation can be made by reference to the different components of Virchow's triad for thrombogenesis, that is, abnormal blood flow, abnormal blood constituents and vessel wall abnormalities (Brotman et al., 2004).
There have been many studies which have focused on risk factors for thrombogenesis in atrial fibrillation . However, the studies exploring the presence of a hypercoagulable state in atrial fibrillation (Lip1995; Lip et al., 1995) have concentrated on various clotting factors, and markers of endothelial damage or dysfunction, rather than on platelets per se. In this chapter, we present an overview of the thrombogenic role of platelets in valvular atrial fibrillation.

2. The platelet physiology

2.1 The platelet structure

Platelets were recognized as a distinct blood element in the late 19th century (and not white blood cells) (Bizzozero, 1882). Platelets are anucleated cells arising from cytoplasmic fragmentation of megakaryocytes in the bone marrow, and have a typical diameter of ~2-3 µm. Platelets circulate in a discoid form and their average lifespan in humans is ~10 days (Hanson & Slichter, 1985). However, following activation, they undergo dramatic changes in shape and ultrastructure; the membranes become ruffled with cytoplasmic projections and the granules are centralized and discharged (Spaet, 1974; White, 2008). Normal human platelet count is ~150,000–400,000/µl, though spontaneous bleeding resulting from reduced (but functionally normal) platelets is unusual at levels >10,000/µl (Slichter, 2004).
Despite their lack of a nucleus, platelets are actively involved in a broad range of physiologic and pathologic processes. Platelets contain a variety of mediators that regulate hemostasis and thrombosis as well as a myriad of other functions including recruitment of other cells (chemotaxis), vasomotor function, cell growth, and inflammation, among others. Relevant constituents for thrombosis are present both on the cell membrane and in the cytoplasm, mainly within platelet granules. The platelet membrane, which consists of a

typical bilayer of phospholipids, contains membrane glycoproteins that interact with various ligands, either soluble ligands that activate the platelets, or fixed ligands within the vessel wall or on other cells through which the platelets adhere to these structures. One unique feature of the platelet is that its plasma membrane contains a network of numerous invaginations into the platelet interior, connected to the exterior through small pores (White et al., 1999; White & Clawson, 1980), known as the open canalicular system (OCS).

Dense granules	Nucleotides Adenine: ATP, ADP Guanine: GTP, GDP Amines Serotonin Histamine Bivalent cations
α-granules	Adhesion molecules Platelet endothelial cell adhesion molecule-1 (PECAM- 1/CD31) Fibrinogen von Willebrand factor (vWF) Thrombospondin-1 (TSP1) Vitronectin, Fibronectin Mitogenic factors Platelet-derived growth factor (PDGF) Vascular endothelial growth factor (VEGF) Transforming growth factor-ß (TGF-ß) Membrane proteins P- selectin CD40L Glycoprotein IIb/IIIa (GPIIb/IIIa, aIIbß3 integrin, CD41/CD61) Coagulation factors Fibrinogen, Plasminogen, Protein S, Kininogens Factors V, VII, XI, XIII Protease inhibitors C1 inhibitor Plasminogen activator inhibitor-1 (PAI-1) Tissue factor pathway inhibitor (TFPI) Matrix breakdown Hydrolytic enzymes MMP - 2, MMP – 9 Leucocyte recruitment Chemokines: PF4, RANTES, β- thromboglobulin, ENA-78, SDF - 1α
Lysosomes	Glycosidases Proteases Cationic proteins

Table 1. Contents of the three different granule subpopulations (α-granules, dense granules, and lysosomes) of platelets (modified from Rendu & Brohard-Bohn, 2001).

This feature imparts upon the platelet a much greater surface area than would normally be found on such a small cell. Platelets contain a second channel system, derived from megakaryocyte smooth endoplasmic reticulum, known as the dense tubular system (DTS). The DTS stores calcium and a variety of enzymes involved in platelet activation; in contrast to the OCS, the DTS does not associate with the plasma membrane (Ebbeling et al., 1992; Rendu & Brohard-Bohn, 2001). Three main populations of platelet granules (alpha granules,dense granules,lysosomes) serve as secretory vesicles, releasing components to the extracellular fluid and also serve to direct molecules to the plasma membrane in a process of exocytosis (table 1) (Rumbaut & Thiagarajan, 2010).

2.2 The platelet function

Although platelets have an important role in the normal haemostatic response, they probably contribute to several diverse processes beyond hemostasis and thrombosis, including promoting inflammatory and immune responses, maintaining vascular integrity, and contributing to wound healing (Smyth et al., 2009).

The contribution of platelets to hemostasis is different in arteries and veins. In the venous system, low-flow rates and stasis permit the accumulation of activated coagulation factors and the local generation of thrombin largely with a less prominent contribution from platelets. Venous thrombi contain platelets, but the dominant cellular component consists of trapped erythrocytes. In the arterial circulation, higher flow rates limit fibrin formation by washing out soluble clotting factors. Platelets, which work best at higher shear rates, help to form a physical barrier against further blood loss and, at the same time, provide a surface on which thrombin is generated and fibrin can accumulate (Brass, 2010).

The formation of a stable platelet plug following vascular injury is often described as occurring in three distinct stages: (1) initiation, (2) extension, and (3) stabilization (Figure 1). Initiation by collagen fibrils (within the vessel wall which become exposed to the circulation when the endothelial cell monolayer is breached, forming a complex with von Willebrand factor (VWF) and glycoprotein (GP) Ibα on the platelet surface binds to the VWF A1 domain)produces a platelet monolayer that supports the subsequent adhesion of activated platelets to each other. Extension occurs when additional platelets adhere to the initial monolayer and become activated. Thrombin, ADP, and thromboxane A_2 (TxA_2) play an important role in this step, activating platelets via cell surface receptors coupled to heterotrimeric G proteins. ADP is secreted from storage sites within platelet-dense granules. TxA_2 is synthesized from arachidonic acid released from platelet membrane phospholipids when platelets are activated.TxA_2 formation in platelets is dependent on cyclooxygenase-1(COX-1). The local generation of thrombin is facilitated by activated platelets that provide a surface on which clotting factor complexes can be assembled once phosphatidylserine has moved to the platelet surface from the inner leaflet of the plasma membrane. Intracellular signaling downstream of agonist receptors activates integrin$\alpha_{IIb}\beta_3$ (GP IIb-IIIa), making cohesive interactions between platelets (ie, aggregation) via fibrinogen possible .Stabilization refers to the later events of platelet plug formation that help to stabilize the platelet plug and prevent premature disaggregation, in part by amplifying signaling within the platelet. Examples include outside-in signaling through integrins and signaling through receptors whose ligands are located on the surface of adjacent platelets. The net result is a hemostatic plug comprised of activated platelets embedded within a cross-linked fibrin mesh, a structure stable enough to withstand the shear forces generated by flowing blood in arterial circulation (Brass, 2010).

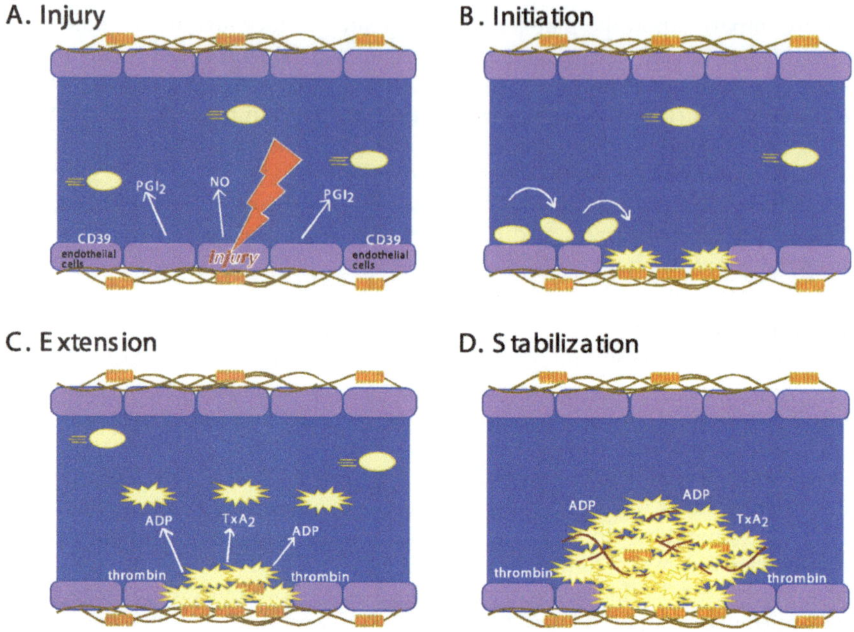

Fig. 1. Stages in platelet plug formation. A classical model. (A) Prior to vascular injury, platelet activation is suppressed by endothelial cell-derived inhibitory factors. These include prostaglandin PGI2 (prostacyclin), nitric oxide (NO), and CD39, an ADPase on the surface of endothelial cells that can hydrolyze trace amounts of ADP that might otherwise cause inappropriate platelet activation. (B) Initiation. The development of the platelet plug is initiated by thrombin and by the collagen-VWF complex, which captures and activates moving platelets. Platelets adhere and spread, forming a monolayer. (C) Extension. The platelet plug is extended as additional platelets are activated via the release or secretion of TxA2, ADP, and other platelet agonists, most of which are ligands for G protein-coupled receptors on the platelet surface. Activated platelets stick to each other via bridges formed by the binding of fibrinogen, fibrin, or VWF to activated $\alpha IIb\beta 3$. (D) Stabilization. Finally, close contacts between platelets in the growing hemostatic plug, along with a fibrin meshwork (shown in red), help to perpetuate and stabilize the platelet plug. This model is being revised as new observations (described in the text) of the behavior of individual platelets within the hemostatic plug add additional refinements (Brass, 2010 ,with permission).

3. The assessment of platelet activation

In general, the quantification of platelet abnormalities can be performed using a wide variety of measures, such as platelet volume, aggregometry (Gabassov et al., 1989), excretion of metabolites (FitzGerald et al., 1988), flow cytometry (Corash, 1990) to detect various platelet antigens, and by the measurement of increased plasma levels of platelet products, such as platelet factor 4, beta thromboglobulin (Chen &Wu, 1980; Ikeda et al.,1997) , the soluble adhesion molecule P-selectin (Blann et al., 1997),soluble CD40L(Choudhury et al.,2007) and matrix metalloproteinase-1(Martin et al.,2003) (Table 2). However, some measures (such as platelet volume) are less useful or practical. Furthermore, the choice of method may depend on the nature of the study. For example, measurement of large numbers, say, in epidemiological studies may require the use of plasma markers rather than the more specialized, time-consuming techniques such as flow cytometry(Kamath et al., 2001).

1) Platelet aggregation in response to
ADP Collagen Epinephrine Thrombin Thromboxane or arachidonic acid
(2) Measurement of platelet release products
In plasma: Beta thromboglobulin Platelet factor 4 Soluble P-selectin Soluble CD40L Matrix metalloproteinases In urine: Thromboxane
(3) Measurement of platelet surface antigens
Flowcytometry: GP IIb/IIIa P selectin (CD63) Platelet microparticles CD40L

Table 2. Assessment of platelet activation.

4. The thrombogenesis in atrial fibrillation

The association between atrial fibrillation and the risk of stroke and thromboembolism has long been recognized. Approximately one in three patients with atrial fibrillation not receiving anticoagulants will develop an ischemic stroke in their lifetime, with roughly two-thirds being cardioembolic and one-third being atherothrombotic. Cardioembolic strokes are more disabling than atherothrombotic strokes, with a higher early mortality rate (Bejot et al., 2009; Lip & Lim, 2007).

Evidence suggests that the thrombogenic tendency in atrial fibrillation is related to several underlying pathophysiological mechanisms, which can be discussed in relation to Virchow's triad for thrombogenesis (fig 2). Abnormal changes in flow are evident by stasis in the left atrium, and seen as spontaneous echocontrast. Abnormal changes in vessel walls—essentially, anatomical and structural defects—include progressive atrial dilatation, endocardial denudation, and oedematous or fibroelastic infiltration of the extracellular matrix. Additionally, abnormal changes in blood constituents are well described, and include haemostatic and platelet activation, as well as inflammation and growth factor changes (Choudhury & Lip, 2004; Watson et al., 2009). These changes result in the prothrombotic or hypercoagulable state in this arrhythmia.

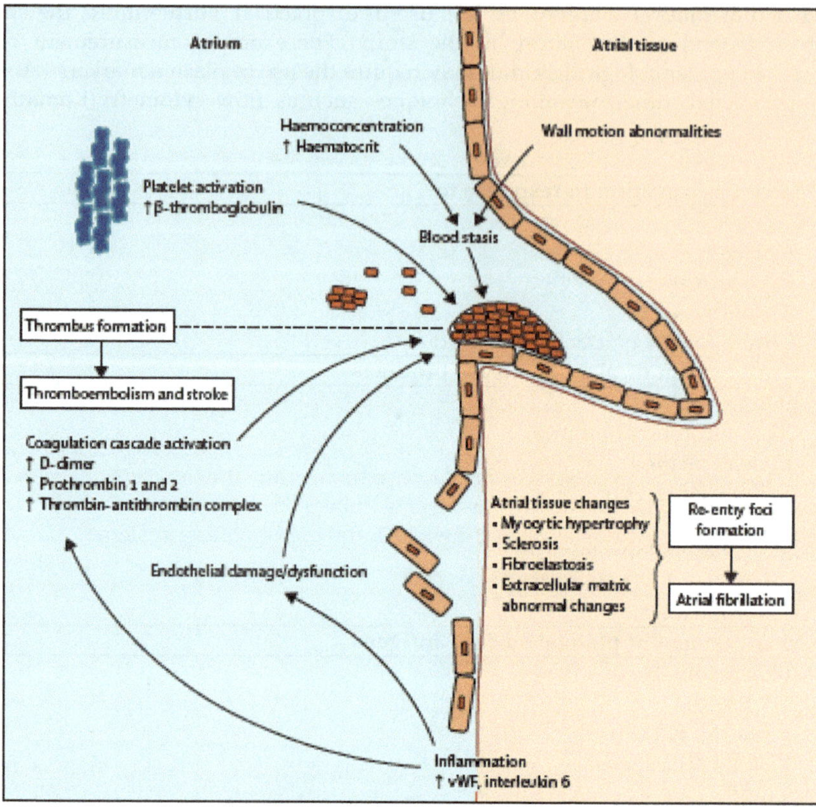

Fig. 2. Components of Virchow's triad for thrombogenesis in atrial fibrillation Abnormal changes shown in the vessel wall (eg, atrial tissue changes, endothelial damage and dysfunction), in flow (stasis—eg, in the left atrial appendage), and in blood constituents (eg, haemoconcentration, platelets, coagulation cascade activation, inflammation), all factors contribute to propensity for thrombus formation (thrombogenesis) in atrial fibrillation. vWf=von Willebrand factor (Watson et al., 2009,with permission).

An understanding of left atrial—left atrial appendage thrombogenesis may have its roots in distinguishing hemostatic and thrombotic clotting. Studies performed by Hoffman et al., 2006 offer potential mechanistic insight and their experimental findings suggest that a large volume of blood must flow over an injured surface, such as the left atrial—left atrial appendage endocardium in a person with atrial fibrillation for significant tissue factor, derived from both circulating cells and microparticles (George, 2008; Lechner & Weltermann, 2008), to accumulate in high concentrations. Furthermore, hemostasis occurs rapidly, with tissue factor of local origin determining the rate of thrombus development .The cell-based model of coagulation translates well to left atrial-left atrial appendage thrombogenesis and supports a primary role for tissue factor-based thrombin generation, with a secondary role being played by platelets .While the results of clinical trials (Connolly et al., 2006; Healey et al., 2008) and meta-analyses are consistent with this hypothesis, several biological constructs potentially provide a mechanistic platform as well.

The integrated complexity of coagulation in general and platelet-dependent thrombin generation in particular is becoming evident. One of the most interesting and clinically relevant observations over the past decade is the concomitant interdependence and independence of platelet activation and thrombin generation. The former is best considered in the context of primary hemostasis and possibly arterial thrombosis-both highly dependent on platelet activation, platelet aggregation and thrombin generation (in concentrations sufficient to provoke further platelet activation).In the latter instance, platelet subpopulations with distinct intracellular calcium signaling properties yield procoagulant domains (Munnix et al., 2007) The down regulation of platelet aIIb/b3, in turn, attenuates proaggregatory potential.

5. The role of platelets in valvular atrial fibrillation

The risk of stroke and thromboembolism is a major complication of atrial fibrillation. The risk of thrombogenesis with atrial fibrillation increases over five-fold in the presence of rheumatic heart disease, especially mitral valve stenosis. Rheumatic heart disease is observed in 15% of Western atrial fibrillation patients, but this is even a larger problem worldwide (Bejot et al., 2009). This increase in thrombogenic risk with valvular heart disease could in part explained by activation of platelets and the coagulation system.

5.1 Mitral stenosis

Platelet activation appears to play an important role in the initial step of thrombus formation in patients with rheumatic mitral stenosis (Kranidis et al., 1993). Evidence has been shown that shear stresses in turbulent flow occur as a result of stenotic valves induce platelet activation (Stein & Sabbah, 1976; Yu et al., 1978).

Many studies have demonstrated that platelet activation, evaluated by measuring the secretory substance of platelets as beta- thromboglobulin (BTG) , Platelet factor 4 (PF4) and soluble P-selection, occurs in the peripheral blood of patients with rheumatic mitral stenosis and atrial fibrillation (Chen at al., 2004; Kataoka et al., 1994; Yetkin et al., 2003).

Chen et al., 2003 demonstrated that in patients with moderate to severe mitral stenosis, increased regional left atrial platelet P-selection expression detected by flow cytometry had a significantly direct relationship with the severity of mitral stenosis. Also, they found that the fraction of peripheral venous platelets expressing P-selection in patients with chronic lone atrial fibrillation did not differ from that of healthy volunteers who were in sinus rhythm and this result provided one possible basic mechanism to clarify the ineffectiveness of aspirin in preventing thromboembolism in patients with non valvular atrial fibrillation according to previous large clinical trials (Petersen et al., 1989; The Stroke Prevention in Atrial Fibrillation Investigatiors,1993).

The role of the CD40-CD40L axis in patients with atherothrombotic diseases has generated interest as this molecule may play a pivotal link among platelets (Henn et al., 2001; Langer et al., 2005; Slupsky et al., 1998), inflammation (Anand et al., 2003; Henn et al., 2001), the endothelium (Slupsky et al., 1998; Zhou et al., 1998), coagulation (Slupsky et al., 1998; Zhou et al., 1998) and, ultimately, thrombosis. The triad of functional activity of CD40L in atherosclerotic models, high content in platelets, and mobilization during platelet thrombosis provide a readily testable hypothesis and places platelet-derived CD40L as a possible important mitigating factor in atrial fibrillation. In patients with moderate to severe mitral stenosis and atrial fibrillation, the plasma soluble CD40L levels were found to be higher than healthy controls or patients with lone atrial fibrillation (Chen et al., 2005).

Azzam & Zagloul, 2009 demonstrated that patients with rheumatic mitral stenosis and atrial fibrillation have enhanced platelet activation, assessed by elevated platelet microparticles in the plasma which have a significantly direct relationship with the severity of mitral stenosis. Platelet microparticles are generated from activated platelets and may not only be a marker of platelet activation but also a pathophysiological mediator leading to thrombosis (Niuwland & Strurk, 2002).

Correction of mitral stenosis by performing percutaneous transluminal mitral valvuloplasty (PTMV) not only confers significant beneficial haemodynamic effects but also seems to affect platelet activation. Yetkin et al., 2003 reported that soluble P-selection and BTG levels which are markers of platelet activation decreased significantly after PTMV, indicating a reduction in platelet activity. Zaki et al.,2000 also shown significant decrease in prethrombotic state 30 min. after PTMV by measuring BTG, PF4 in patients with a left atrial pressure <10mm HG after PTMV. Also, Chen et al., 2005 found that PTMV rapidly reduced platelet activity in patients with moderate-to-severe mitral stenosis, consequently rapidly reducing soluble CD40L released from platelets. On the contrary, Goldsmith et al., 2000a reported that increased levels of soluble P-selection immediately post procedure and at 24h, in association with increased venous von Willebrand factor levels at 24h after PTMV are in keeping with the increase in platelet activation and endothelial dysfunction following PTMV. These changes may contribute to the increased risk of thromboembolism following the procedure and suggest the need for adequate antiplatelet and anticoagulant therapy following PTMV. These studies therefore suggest that the degree of platelet activation corresponds inversely with the mitral valve orifice area and the more severe the mitral stenosis, the greater is the degree of platelet activation. Furthermore, damage or disease of the atrial wall, including endocrinal damage secondary to valve disease, may contribute to further thrombogenesis.

5.2 Mitral valve prolapse

Mitral valve prolapse has been linked with systemic thromboembolism, especially in young women (Barnett et al., 1980), and transient ischemic attacks or partial strokes occurring as a complication of mitral valve prolapse accounted for 40% of these cases in patients aged under 45 years .Mechanisms for this appear to be related to clot or platelet aggregates originating from the rough surface of prolapsed mitral valves or from the traumatized adjacent left atrial surface (Jeresaty, 1985). Indeed, thrombi have been found on the leaflets of patients with mitral valve prolapse who died of cerebral embolism (Lewis, 1988). There are also reports of shortened platelet survival and increased platelet coagulant activity in patients with cerebral embolism and mitral valve prolapse (Lewis, 1988).

On the other hand, recent population based and case-control studies demonstrated no increased frequency of mitral valve prolapse among patients with stroke or transient ischemic attacks, including young patients (Gilon et al., 1999; Orenica et al., 1995; Petty et al., 1994). In addition, patients with mitral valve prolapse who had strokes were similar in age to the general stroke population, and many had other risk factors for strokes, including atrial fibrillation (Gilon etal., 1999; Nishimura et al., 1985; Orenica et al., 1995). Also, some studies on the platelets have failed to demonstrate an association of platelet activation with pure mitral valve prolapse alone (Tse et al., 1997), suggesting that if the predisposition of mitral valve prolapse to thromboembolism were true, it may well operate via a mechanism other than platelet activation alone. Perhaps the severity of mitral regurgitation in mitral valve prolapse may be a factor as reported by Martini et al., 1996 who studied the platelet and coagulation activation in patients with mitral valve prolapse and suggested that mitral valve prolapse is not responsible per se for blood clotting activation, but in patients with severe mitral insufficiency an increase in thrombin generation can occur. These alterations in hemostatic system may represent a mechanism by which mitral regurgitation increases the risk of thromboembolic events in patients with mitral valve prolapse.

5.3 Mitral regurgitation

Mitral regurgitation appears to have variable effects on platelet activation and the risk of thromboembolism, which is dependent on the underlying status of the mitral valve and whether or not there is coexisting atrial fibrillation. Some studies have shown an increase in platelet activation in patients with severe mitral regurgitation (Tse et al., 1997) in association with mitral valve prolapse, when compared to patients with mitral valve prolapse and mild to moderate mitral regurgitation, which was independent of age and left atrial size. However, other studies failed to demonstrate the same effect (Martini et al., 1996), but instead report increased activation of the coagulation system and thrombin generation in these patients.

For example, Karatasakis *et al.*, 1995 showed that significant mitral regurgitation correlates with a lower incidence of spontaneous echo contrast, thrombi and embolization in patients with rheumatic mitral valve disease. Similar studies by Hwaang *et al.*, 1994 and Movsowitz *et al.*, 1993 confirmed similar findings. In patients with non-valvular atrial fibrillation, moderate to severe mitral regurgitation seems to protect against stroke especially in patients with left atrial enlargement (Nakagami et al., 1998). Also, Kranidis et al., 2000 demonstrated that mitral regurgitation has a protective effect on the development of left atrial thrombus in patients with rheumatic valve disease and atrial fibrillation .Furthermore, the presence of mitral regurgitation appears to reduce intracardiac thrombus in patients with dilated cardiomyopathy (Maze et al., 1989).

Nevertheless, there are limited data relating these clinical observations to the degree of platelet activation or thrombogenesis. However, Goldsmith *et al.*, 2000b reported an intraoperative study of patients with severe mitral regurgitation, where soluble P-selectin levels (as an index of platelet activation) were significantly lower within the left atrium compared to peripheral vein levels, indicating reduced platelet activation in association with the 'stirring' effect of the (severe) mitral regurgitation jet.

Does moderate to severe mitral regurgitation increase the risk of thromboembolism in mitral valve prolapse but paradoxically decrease the risk in rheumatic mitral valve disease and/or non-valvular atrial fibrillation? To answer this question, further studies are needed which would clarify the influence of mitral regurgitation on platelet activation in mitral valve prolapse, rheumatic mitral valve, and non-valvular atrial fibrillation.

5.4 Aortic valve disease

Haemodynamic studies have shown that diseased cardiac valves, whether stenosed or incompetent, create regions of increased turbulence and shear stresses that are large enough to damage the vascular endothelium and cellular blood elements, leading to abnormal haemorheology, platelet activation, and endothelial dysfunction (Stein & Sabbah, 1976). For example, the intensity of turbulence in patients with pure aortic stenosis may be 10 times greater than normal while the intensity of turbulence in patients with pure aortic regurgitation may be three times greater than normal (Stein & Sabbah, 1976).

Goldsmith et al., 2000c measured plasma concentrations of soluble P-selectin (a marker for platelet activation), von Willebrand factor (a marker for endothelial cell dysfunction) and fibrinogen (as an index of haemorheology and a clotting factor), in 61 patients with moderate to severe aortic valve disease in sinus rhythm, and reported that patients with aortic valve disease had higher mean plasma fibrinogen, von Willebrand factor and soluble P-selectin levels, which were not significantly different between patients with aortic stenosis or regurgitation.
Also, Prohaska et al., 2008 studied the platelet function in 660 patients considered for isolated coronary artery bypass graft (CABG) surgery, and in 421 patients considered for single aortic valve replacement (AVR). Platelet function was monitored preoperatively using the platelet function analyzer device (PFA-100), and reported that due to disturbed flow and shear exposition following an initial activation, the platelets are partially degranulated, shed microparticles, and might become involved in the pathogenesis of microvascular dysfunction and thrombotic events in patients with aortic valve disease. Furthermore , Dimitrow et al., 2009 determined markers of thrombin generation (thrombin-antithrombin complex , prothrombin fragment 1+2), platelet activation (soluble CD40 ligand , beta-thromboglobulin , P-selectin) in seventy-five patients with aortic stenosis, and reported that mean concentrations of thrombin and platelet markers were higher approximately two-fold in patients than in controls and maximal gradient as an index of turbulent flow associated with activation of coagulation and platelets.

6. The role of platelets in non- valvular atrial fibrillation

Whilst abnormalities of clotting markers are well recognized in non-valvular atrial fibrillation, abnormal platelet activation has also been reported in these patients (Lip, 1995; Yamauchi et al., 1986). However, Kamath et al., 2002 found that platelet markers (plasma beta-thromboglobulin, soluble glycoprotein V) and coagulation markers (fibrin D-dimer) were higher in atrial fibrillation compared to healthy controls with no significant abnormalities of platelet aggregation in response to standard platelet agonists, again casting doubt on the extent and significance of platelet activation in atrial fibrillation- which they have previously reviewed (Kamath et al., 2001). Choudhury et al., 2008 assessed platelet activation using 4 different aspects of platelet pathophysiology: 1) platelet surface expression of CD62P (P-selectin) and CD63 (a lysosomal glycoprotein) (by flow cytometry); 2) mean platelet volume (MPV) (by flow cytometry); 3) plasma levels of soluble P-selectin (sP-selectin, enzyme-linked immunoadsorbent assay); and 4) total amount of P-selectin per platelet (pP-selectin) ("platelet lysis" assay). They concluded that there is a degree of excess of platelet activation in atrial fibrillation compared with "healthy control subjects," but no significant difference between atrial fibrillation patients and "disease control subjects" in sinus rhythm. Platelet activation may differ according to the subtype of atrial fibrillation, but this is not in excess of the underlying comorbidities that lead to atrial fibrillation. Platelet activation in atrial fibrillation may be due to underlying cardiovascular diseases, rather than due to atrial fibrillation per se. Also, Choudhury et al., 2007 suggested that there is an excess of platelet activation in AF patients compared to healthy control subjects, as measured by sCD40L and sP-selectin levels. However, there was no excess of platelet activation in atrial fibrillation patients compared to disease control subjects. This would support the argument that platelet activation in atrial fibrillation patients is more related to the associated vascular diseases than to the arrhythmia itself. Furthermore patients with atrial fibrillation have been noted to have impaired matrix degradation, with abnormalities in matrix metalloproteinase-1 (MMP-1) and its inhibitor, tissue inhibitor of matrix metalloproteinase-1 (TIMP-1), although these again were not independently associated with the presence of atrial fibrillation on multivariate analysis (Marin et al., 2003). However, an independent relationship was noted between the MMP/TIMP system and the prothrombotic state (assessed by prothrombin fragments 1 and 2 levels). From the available data, it seems that increased interstitial fibrosis in atrial tissue is more likely due to underlying comorbidities, like hypertension, ischemic heart disease, or uncontrolled heart failure (circumstances associated with high risk to develop atrial fibrillation), rather than the presence of the arrhythmia itself.

The heart rate does not seem to be related to the extent of platelet activation in atrial fibrillation (Yamauchi et al., 1986). Therefore, heart rate control therapy itself is unlikely to offer significant benefit in terms of reducing thromboembolic risk in atrial fibrillation. Nevertheless, exercise may increase platelet activation in atrial fibrillation (Furui et al., 1987). For example, Furui et al., 1987 report an increase in platelet sensitivity to ADP aggregation and the level of beta thromboglobulin in the plasma in 20 patients with lone atrial fibrillation in comparison with age-matched controls when exercising at up to 85% of predicted maximal heart rate. However, Li Saw Hee et al., 2001 did not demonstrate any significant increase in soluble P-selectin levels amongst patients with atrial fibrillation exercised to exhaustion. One reason for the difference in findings between the studies by Furui et al., 1987 and Li Saw Hee et al., 2001 may be the choice of markers of platelet activation, and hence, different pathophysiological release mechanisms. Furthermore, there does not appear to be any significant diurnal variation in abnormal platelet activation in atrial fibrillation, as reflected by changes in soluble P-selectin levels (Li Saw Hee et al., 2000), but this may simply reflect the high thrombogenic state associated with chronic atrial fibrillation.

The extent of platelet activation in non-valvular atrial fibrillation may be related to the other features of the left atrium. For example, an enlarged left atrium and reduced left atrial appendage flow velocity has been correlated with increased platelet ctivation by (Shinohara et al., 1998). The study by Shinohara et al., 1998 reported a significant difference in platelet activation amongst patients with nonvalvular atrial fibrillation with a low left atrial appendage velocity (<40 cm. s_1) when compared to patients with a high left atrial appendage velocity _40 cm. s_1. The patients with a low atrial appendage velocity also had a significantly higher prevalence of spontaneous echo contrast and left atrial thrombus, suggesting a relationship between platelet activation and pre-embolic events if atrial fibrillation was accompanied by abnormal flow dynamics within the left atrium. Using scanning electron microscopy, we have recently demonstrated atrial endocardial cell damage, which was most commonly seen in the left atrial appendage amongst patients with mitral valve disease and atrial fibrillation (Goldsmith et al., 2000d). The interaction between activated platelets or clotting factors and the damaged endocardium may in part contribute to thrombogenesis within the left atrium.

Whether the peripheral venous levels of markers of platelet activation and thrombogenesis truly and wholly reflect left atrial levels of coagulation and platelet activation in non-valvular atrial fibrillation is not exactly clear. Li Saw Hee et al., 1999 demonstrated that there was no significant difference in the markers of platelet activation and thrombogenesis between the atria and the periphery vein amongst patients with atrial fibrillation due to mitral stenosis . Peverill et al., 1996 found that the markers of coagulation activity in similar patients were no different between the left atrium and the periphery in the absence of left atrial spontaneous echo contrast. However, levels were significantly raised in the left atrium when compared to the periphery in the presence of left atrial spontaneous echo contrast, irrespective of the underlying rhythm. Similarly, Yamamoto et al., 1995 demonstrated a significant difference in the levels of some markers of coagulation between the left atrium and the periphery, namely, thrombin-antithrombin III complex and fibrinopeptide A in patients with mitralstenosis, but failed to demonstrate the same with respect to another marker of platelet activation, namely, beta-thromboglobulin.

7. Platelet activation and thromboembolic risk in atrial fibrillation

Perhaps a continuum exists between normal platelet function, 'statistically' abnormal platelet function and overt thrombosis in patients with cardiovascular disease and stroke. Thus the abnormal platelet activation in atrial fibrillation, as summarized in the evidence above, may represent a 'pre-embolic' status in non-valvular atrial fibrillation (Pongratz et al., 1997). Indeed, platelet activation seems to occur even before the occurrence of spontaneous echo contrast in patients with atrial fibrillation (Heppell et al., 1997) and is correlated with both spontaneous echo contrast (Pongratz et al., 1997) and left atrial thrombus (Heppell et al., 1997) in atrial fibrillation.

For example, Pongratz *et al.*, 1997 demonstrated that the amount of circulating platelets expressing P-selectin was significantly higher in the patients with spontaneous echo contrast or left atrial thrombus in comparison with patients without either of these, or healthy controls. The study by Heppell *et al.*, 1997 reported that plasma levels of beta thromboglobulin were independently associated with left atrial thrombus whether or not spontaneous echo contrast was present. Studies in canine models have also demonstrated that platelet activation is significantly associated with silent cerebral infarction in atrial fibrillation (Minamino et al., 1998).

However, other clinical studies have demonstrated platelet activation in atrial fibrillation but failed to relate the former to the risk of thromboembolism. Thus, even though platelet activation appears to be significantly correlated with spontaneous echo contrast and left atrial thrombus, it does not seem to be convincingly correlated with stroke (or transient ischaemic attack) in nonvalvular atrial fibrillation. For example, the study by Gustafsson *et al.*, 1990 showed that patients with atrial fibrillation and stroke had no greater platelet activation than patients with atrial fibrillation without stroke, whilst patients with sinus rhythm and stroke had no greater platelet activation than controls in sinus rhythm without stroke; patients with non-valvular atrial fibrillation without stroke had significantly more platelet activation than individuals with stroke in sinus rhythm. Whether platelet activation contributes to stroke/transient ischaemic attack in atrial fibrillation is not clear, and whether it can be used as a predictor of risk of stroke in atrial fibrillation in addition to other parameters, such as hypertension and left ventricular dysfunction still needs to be clarified.

Thus, the available evidence suggests that thromboembolism in atrial fibrillation is probably due to enhancement of various components of the coagulation system due to stasis of blood in the inordinate and irregular atria, rather than to platelet activation per se (Nagao et al., 1995). The relative role of coagulation versus platelet activation in the pathogenesis of thrombogenesis in patients with atrial fibrillation can roughly be inferred from the results of antithrombotic drug interventions that have been tested in randomized clinical trials. Among non-vavular atrial fibrillation patients, the relative risk reduction (RRR) for stroke that is achieved with moderate intensity oral anticoagulant [international normalized ratio (INR)=2-3] compared to placebo is approximately 65%, as opposed to the 20% RRR achieved with aspirin versus placebo (Hart et al., 2007; Lip & Lim, 2007). Consistently, moderate intensity oral anticoagulant produces a RRR for stroke of 40% compared to aspirin, and of 30% compared to aspirin +clopidogrel (Hart et al., 2007). Interestingly, among medium-high risk non-valvular AF patients not eligible to make warfarin, aspirin+ clopidogrel was superior to aspirin alone for stroke prevention (Connolly et al., 2009).

Taken together, these results indicate that inhibition of coagulation remains the mainstay in preventing atrial fibrillation -related thrombogenesis. The lesser but significant role of platelets- best inhibited by a combined antiplatelet drug regimen - is presumably related to the prominent involvement of platelets in the pathogenesis of atherothrombotic (that is, non-cardiombolic) events (Lip et al., 2009).

8. Conclusion

The thrombogenic role of platelets in atrial fibrillation is clearly complex and remain partly understood. Definitive answers to the questions of whether platelet activation contribute towards stroke in atrial fibrillation or is it just an associated factor? Does a reduction in platelet activation beneficially influence thromboembolic risk in atrial fibrillation? are far from simple and compare with the somewhat equivocal benefits of antiplatelet drugs in atrial fibrillation in clinical trials. Future directions in this field should involve further clarification of the role of different aspects of platelet activation in atrial fibrillation.

9. References

Anand, SX., Viles- Gonzalez, JF., Badimon, JJ., Cavusoglu, E. & Marmur, JD. (2003). Membrane- associated CD40L and sCD40L in atherothrombotic disease. *Thromb Haemost,*Vol. 90:pp.377–84.

Azzam, H.& Zagloul, M. (2009). Elevated Platelet Microparticle Levels in Valvular Atrial Fibrillation. *Hematology*, Vol.14:pp.357-60.

Barnett, HJ.; Boughner, DR.; Taylor, DW.; Cooper, PE.; Kostuk, WJ.& Nichol, PM. (1980). Further evidence relating mitral valve prolapse to cerebral ischemic events. *N Engl J Med, Vol.*302:pp.139–44.

Bejot, Y.; Ben Salem, D.; Osseby, GV.; Couvreur, G.; Durier J.; Marie C.; Cottin Y.; Moreau T.& Giroud M. (2009). Epidemiology of ischemic stroke from atrial fibrillation in Dijon, France, from 1985 to 2006. *Neurology,* Vol.72:pp.346-53.

Bizzozero, J. (1882). Ueber einen neuen formbestandtheil des blutes und dessen rolle bei der thrombose und der blutgerinnung. *Virchows Arch Pathol Anat Physiol Klinishe Medicine,* Vol. 10: pp. 261–332.

Blann, AD.; Lip, GY.; Beevers, DG.& McCollum, CN. (1997). Soluble P-Selectin in atherosclerosis: a comparison with endothelial cell and platelet markers. *Thromb Haemost*, Vol. 77:pp.1077–80.

Brass, L. (2010). Understanding and Evaluating Platelet Function. *Hematology,Vol.1:* pp.387-96.

Brotman, DJ.; Deitcher, SR.; Lip, GY.& Martzdorff, AC. (2004). Virchow's triad revisited. *South Med J*, Vol. 97:pp. 213–14.

Chen, MC., Chang, HW., Juang, SS., Yip, HK. & Wu, CJ. (2004). Increased plasma levels of soluble P-selection in rheumatic mitral stenosis. *Chest*, Vol.126:pp.54-58.

Chen, MC.; Chang, HW.; Wu, CJ.; Yang, CH.; Hung, WC.; Yeh, KH.,& Fu, M. (2005). Percutaneous transluminal mitral valvuloplasty reduces circulating soluble CD40 ligand in rheumatic mitral stenosis. Chest, Vol.128:pp.36-41.

Chen, MC.; Wu, CJ.; Yip, HK.; Chang, HW.; Fang, CY.; Yu, TH.& Fu, M. (2003). Left atrial platelet activity with rheumatic mitral stenosis. Correlation Study of Severity and Platelet P-Selectin Expression by Flow Cytometry. *Chest*, Vol.124:pp.1663-69.

Chen, YC. & Wu, KK. (1980). A comparison of methods for the study of platelet hyperfunction in thromboembolic disorders. *Br J Haematol*, Vol.46:pp. 263–8.

Choudhury, A. & Lip, GY. (2004). Atrial fibrillation and the hypercoagulable state: from basic science to clinical practice. *Pathophysiol Haemost Thromb*, Vol.33:pp. 282–89.

Choudhury, A.; Chung, I.; Blann, AD.& Lip, GY.(2007). Platelet surface CD62P and CD63, mean platelet volume, and soluble/platelet P-selectin as indexes of platelet function in atrial fibrillation: a comparison of "healthy control subjects" and "disease control subjects" in sinus rhythm. *J Am Coll Cardiol.*, Vol.49:pp.1957-64.

Choudhury, A.; Chung, I.; Panja, N.; Patel, J. & Lip, GYH. (2008). Soluble CD40 Ligand, Platelet Surface CD40 Ligand, and Total Platelet CD40 Ligand in Atrial Fibrillation :Relationship to Soluble P-Selectin, Stroke Risk Factors, and Risk Factor Intervention, Vol.10:pp.2707-45.

Connolly, S.; Pogue, J.; Hart, R.; Pfeffer, M.; Hohnloser, S.; Chrolavicius, S.; Pfeffer, M.; Hohnloser, S.& Yusuf, S. (2006). Clopidogrel plus aspirin versus oral anticoagulation for atrial fibrillation in the Atrial fibrillation Clopidogrel Trial with Irbesartan for prevention of Vascular Events (ACTIVE W): a randomised controlled trial. *Lancet*, Vol.367:pp.1903–12.

Connolly, SJ., Pogue, J., Hart, RG., Hart, RG., Hohnloser, SH., Pfeffer, M., Chrolavicius, S. & Yusuf, S. (2009). Effect of clopidogrel added to aspirin in patients with atrial fibrillation. ACTIVE Investigatiors, *N Engl J Med*, Vol. 360:pp.2066-78.

Corash, L. (1990). Measurement of platelet activation by fluorescence activated flow cytometry. *Blood Cells*, Vol.16:pp. 97–106.

Dimitrow, PP.; Hlawaty, M.; Undas, A.; Sniezek-Maciejewska, M.; Sobień, B.; Stepień, E.& Tracz, W. (2009). Effect of aortic valve stenosis on haemostasis is independent from vascular atherosclerotic burden. *Atherosclerosis*,Jun, Vol.204:e103-8.

Ebbeling, L.; Robertson, C.; McNicol, A.& Gerrard, JM. (1992). Rapid ultrastructural changes in the dense tubular system following platelet activation. *Blood*, Vol.80: pp. 718–23.

FitzGerald, DJ.; Catella F.; Roy, L.& FitzGerald, GA. (1988): Marked platelet activation in vivo after intravenous streptokinase in patients with acute myocardial infarction. *Circulation*, Vol.77:pp. 142–50.

Furui, H.; Taniguchi, N.; Yamauchi, K.; Sotobata, I.; Saito, H.& Inagaki, H. (1987). Effects of treadmill exercise on platelet function, blood coagulability and fibrinolytic activity in patients with atrial fibrillation. *Jpn Heart J*, Vol.28:pp. 177–84.

Gabassov, VA. ; Popov, EG. ; Gavrilov, I IU. ; Pozin, EIA.& Markosian, RA. (1989). New methodical approach to the study of platelet aggregation in vitro. *Biull Eksp Biol Med*, Vol.108:pp. 437–40.

George, FD. (2008). Microparticles in vascular diseases. *Thromb Res*, Vol.122:pp.S55–59.

Gilon, D., Buonanno, FS., Joffe, MM., Leavitt, M., Marshall, JE., Kistler, JP., Levine, RA. (1999). Lack of evidence of an association between mitral-valve prolapse and stroke in young patients. N Engl J Med,Vol.341:pp.8–13.

Goldsmith, I.; Li Saw Hee, FL.; Blann, AD.& Lip, GYH. (2000a). Increased platelet activation and endothelial dysfunction in patients immediately following percutaneous balloon mitral valvuloplasty. *Clin Cardiol*,Vol. 23:pp. 587–90.

Goldsmith, I.; Blann, AD.; Patel, RL.& Lip, GYH. (2000b). Reduced indices of left atrial hypercoagulability in patients with severe mitral regurgitation. *Am J Cardiol,* Vol. 86:pp. 234–6.

Goldsmith, I.; Blann, AD.; Patel, RL.& Lip, GYH. (2000c). Plasma fibrinogen, soluble P-selectin and von Willebrand factor in aortic valve disease: evidence for abnormal haemorheology, platelet activation and endothelial dysfunction. *Heart,* Vol. 83:pp. 577–8.

Goldsmith, I.; Kumar, P.; Carter, P.; Blann, AD.; Patel, RL.& Lip, GYH. (2000d). Atrial endocardial changes in mitral valve disease: a scanning electron microscopy study. *Am Heart J,* Vol. 140:pp.777–84.

Gustafsson, C.; Blomback, M.; Britton, M.; Hamsten, A.& Svensson, J. (1990). Coagulation factors and the increased risk of stroke in Nonvalvular atrial fibrillation. *Stoke,* Vol.21:pp.47–51.

Hanson, SR. and Slichter, SJ. (1985). Platelet kinetics in patients with bone marrow hypoplasia: evidence for a fixed platelet requirement. *Blood,* Vol. 66:pp. 1105–09.

Hart, RG.; Pearce, LA.& Aguilar, MI. (2007). Meta-analysis: antithrombotic therapy to prevent stroke in patients who have nonvalvular atrial fibrillation. *Ann internal Med,* Vol. 146:pp.857-67.

Healey, JS., Hart, RG., Pogue, J., Pfeffer, MA., Hohnloser, SH., De Caterina, R., Flaker, G., Yusuf, S. & Connolly, SJ. (2008). Risks and benefits of oral anticoagulation compared with clopidogrel plus aspirin in patients with atrial fibrillation according to stroke risk: the atrial fibrillation clopidogrel trial with irbesartan for prevention of vascular events (ACTIVE-W). *Stroke,* Vol.39:pp.1482–86.

Henn, V.; Steinbach, S.; Buchner, K.; Presek, P. & Kroczek, RA. (2001). The inflammatory action of CD40 ligand (CD154) expressed on activated human platelets is temporarily limited by coexpressed CD40. *Blood,* Vol.98:pp.1047–54.

Heppell, RM.; Berkin, KE.; McLenachan, JM.& Davies, JA. (1997). Haemostatic and haemodynamic abnormalities associated with left atrial thrombosis in non rheumatic atrial fibrillation. *Heart,*Vol.77:pp. 407–11.

Hoffman, M.; Whinna, HC.& Monroe, DM. (2006). Circulating tissue factor accumulates in thrombi, but not in hemostatic plugs. *J Thromb Haemost,* Vol.4: pp.2092–93.

Hwaang, JJ.; Shyu, KG.; Hsu, KL.; Chen, JJ.; Kuan, P.& Lien, WP. (1994). Significant mitral regurgitation is protective against left atrial spontaneous echo contrast formation but not against systemic embolism. *Chest,* Vol. 106:pp. 8–12.

Ikeda, U.; Yamamoto K.& Shimada, K. (1997). Biochemical markers of coagulation activation in mitral stenosis, atrial fibrillation and cardiomyopathy. *Clin Cardiol,* Vol. 20:pp. 7–10.

Jeresaty, RM. (1985). Mitral valve prolapse. An update. *JAMA,*Vol. 254: pp.793–5.

Kamath, S.; Blann, AD.& Lip, GYH. (2001). Platelets and atrial fibrillation . *Eur Heart J,*Vol.22:pp. 2233-42.

Kamath, S.; Blann, AD.; Chin, BSP.; Lanza,F.; Aleil, LB.;Cazenave, JP.& Lip GYH (2002). A study of platelet activation in atrial fibrillation and the effect s of antithrombotic therapy. *European Heart J,* Vol.23:pp.1788-95.

Karatasakis, GT.; Gotsis, AC.& Cokkinos, DV. (1995). Influence of mitral regurgitation on left atrial thrombus and spontaneous echo contrast in patients with rheumatic mitral valve disease. *Am J Cardiol,* Vol. 76:pp.279–81.

Kataoka, H.; Yano, S.& Mikuriya, Y. (1994). Relationship of mitral valve area to hemostatic condition in rheumatic mitral stenosis. *J Cardiol,* Vol.24:pp.387-95.

Kranidis, A. ; Koulouris, S.& Anthopoulos, L. (1993). Clinical implications of left atrial spontaneous echo contrast in mitral valve disease. *J Heart Valve Dis*, Vol.2:pp. 267–72.

Kranidis, A.; Koulouris, S.; Filippatos, G.; Kappos, K.; Tsilias, K.; Karvounis, H.& Exadaktylos, N. (2000). Mitral regurgitation protects from left atrial thrombogenesis in patients with mitral valve disease and atrial fibrillation. *Pacing Clin Electrophysiol*, Vol.23 :pp.1863-6.

Langer, F.; Ingersoll, SB.; Amirkhosravi, A.; Meyer, T.; Siddiqui, FA.; Ahmad, S.; Walker, JM.; Amaya, M.; Desai, H.& Francis, JL. (2005). The role of CD40 in CD40L- and antibody-mediated platelet activation. *Thromb Haemost, VOL.*93:PP.1137–46.

Lechner, D., Weltermann, A. (2008). Circulating tissue factor exposing microparticles. *Thromb Res, Vol.*122:pp.S47–54.

Lewis, RP. (1988). Cerebral embolism in mitral valve prolapse, In: Mitral valve prolapse and mitral valve prolapse syndrome, Boudoulas H, Wooley CF,(eds) , pp.289–98, *Mount Kisco, : Future Publishing*, NY.

Li Saw Hee, FL.; Blann, AD.& Lip, GYH. (2000). A cross-sectional and diurnal study of thrombogenesis amongst subjects with chronic atrial fibrillation. *J Am Coll Cardiol*, Vol.35:pp. 1926–31.

Li Saw Hee, FL.; Blann, AD.; Gibbs, CR.; Edmunds, E.& Lip, GYH. (2001). Effect of exercise on haemostatic markers in patients with chronic atrial fibrillation. *Clin Cardiol*, in press.

Li Saw Hee, FL.; Blann, AD.; Goldmsith, I.& Lip, GY. (1999). Indexes of hypercoagulability measured in peripheral blood reflect levels in intracardiac blood in patients with atrial fibrillation secondary to mitral stenosis. *Am J Cardiol*, Vol.83:pp. 1206–9.

Lip, GY. & Lim, BS. (2007). Atrial fibrillation and stroke prevention. *Lancet Neurol*, Vol.6:pp.981-93.

Lip, GYH. (1995). Does atrial fibrillation confer a hypercoagulable state? *Lancet*, Vol. 346: pp.1313–14.

Lip, GYH.; Huber, K.; Andreotti, F.; Arnesen, H.; Airaksinen KJ; Cuisset, T.; Kirchhof, P.& Marin, F. (2009). Management of antithrombotic therapy in atrial fibrillation patients presenting with acute coronary syndrome and/or undergoing percutaneous coronary intervention/stenting. *Thromb Haemost*, Vol. 102:pp.1-15.

Lip, GYH.; Lowe, GD.; Rumley, A.& Dunn, FG. (1995). Increased markers of thrombogenesis in chronic atrial fibrillation: effects of warfarin treatment. *Br Heart J*, Vol. 73: pp.527–33.

Marin, F.; Roldan, V.; Climent, V.; Garcia, A.; Marco, P.& Lip, GYH. (2003). Is thrombogenesis in atrial fibrillation related to matrix metalloproteinase-1 and its inhibitor, TIMP-1? *Stroke*, Vol.34:pp.1181-86.

Martini, F., Zuppiroli, A., Gori, A. Chiarantini, E., Fedi, S., Prisco, D., Cellai, A,, Boddi, V., Abbate, R., Dolara, A., Gensini, G. (1996). Platelet and blood clotting Activation in patients with mitral valve prolapse. *Thromb Res*, Vol. 83:pp. 299–306.

Maze, SS.; Kotler, MN.& Parry, WR. (1998). Flow characteristics in the dilated left ventricle with thrombus: qualitative and quantitative Doppler analysis. *J Am Coll Cardiol*, Vol. 13:pp. 873–81.

Minamino, T., Kitakaze, M., Sanada, S. Asanuama, H., Kurotobi, T., Koretsune, Y., Fukunami, M., Kuzuya, T., Hok,i N. & Hori, M. (1998). Increased expression of P-selectin on platelets is a risk factor for silent cerebral infarction in patients with atrial fibrillation: role of nitric oxide. *Circulation*, Vol. 98:pp. 1721–7.

Movsowitz, C.; Movsowitz, HD.; Jacobs, LE.; Meyerowitz, CB.; Podolsky, LA.& Kotler, MN. (1993). Significant mitral regurgitation is protective against left atrial spontaneous echo contrast and thrombus as assessed by transesophageal echocardiography. *J Am Soc Echocardiography*, Vol. 6: pp.107-14.

Munnix, IC., Kuijpers, MJ., Auger, J. Thomassen, CM., Panizzi, P., van Zandvoort, MA., Rosing, J., Bock, PE., Watson, SP. & Heemskerk, JW. (2007). Segregation of platelet aggregatory and procoagulant microdomains in thrombus formation: regulation by transient integrin activation. *Arterioscler Thromb Vasc Biol*, Vol.27:pp.2484-90.

Nagao, T.; Hamamoto, M.; Kanda, A.; Tsuganesawa, T.; Ueda, M.; Kobayashi, K.; Miyazaki, T.& Terashi, A. (1995). Platelet activation is not involved in acceleration of the coagulation system in acute cardioembolic stroke with nonvalvular atrial fibrillation. *Stroke*, Vol.26:pp.1365-8.

Nakagami, H.; Yamamoto, K.; Ikeda, U.; Mitsuhashi, T.; Goto, T.& Shimada, K. (1998). Mitral regurgitation reduces the risk of stroke in patients with non rheumatic atrial fibrillation. *Am Heart J*, Vol. 136:pp.528-32.

Nishimura, RA., McGoon, MD., Shub, C., Miller FA, Jr., Ilstrup, DM. & Tajik, AJ. (1985). Echocardiographically documented mitral-valve prolapse: long-term follow-up of 237 patients. *N Engl J Med* ,Vol. 313:pp.1305-9.

Niuwland, R.& Strurk, A. (2002). Platelet derived microparticles,In: *Platelet* , Michelson AD, (ed), pp:*255 – 65, Academic Press*,c.

Orencia, AJ., Petty, GW., Khandheria, BK., Annegers, JF., Ballard, DJ., Sicks, JD., O'Fallon, WM. & Whisnant, JP.. (1995). Risk of stroke with mitral valve prolapse in population-based cohort study. *Stroke*, Vol. 26:pp.7-13.

Petersen, P.; Boysen, G.; Godtfredsen, J.; Andersen, ED.& Andersen, B. (1989). Placebo controlled, randomized trial of warfarin and aspirin for prevention of thromboembolic complications in chronic atrial fibrillation: The Copenhagen AFASAK study. *Lancet*, Vol.28:pp. 175:9.

Petty, GW.; Orencia, AJ.; Khandheria, BK.& Whisnant, JP. (1994). A population-based study of stroke in the setting of mitral valve prolapse: risk factors and infarct subtype classification. *Mayo Clin Proc*;Vol. 69:pp.632-34.

Peverill, RE.; Harper, RW.; Gelman, J.; Gan, TE.; Harris, G.& Smolich, JJ. (1996). Determinants of increased regional left atrial coagulation activity in patients with mitral stenosis. *Circulation*, Vol 94:pp.331-9.

Pongratz, G., Brandt-Pohlmann, M., Henncke, KH., Pohle, C., Zink, D., Gehlingm, G. & Bachmann, K. (1997). Platelet activation in embolic and preembolic status of patients with non rheumatic atrial fibrillation. Chest, Vol. 111: pp.929-33.

Prohaska, W.; Zittermann, A.; Lüth, JU.; Inoue, K.; Köster-Eiserfunke, W.; Baller, D.; Körfer, R.& Kleesiek, K. (2008). Prevalent platelet dysfunction in patients with aortic valve disease ,Vol.17:pp.542-7.

Rendu, F. & Brohard-Bohn, B. (2001). The platelet release reaction: granules' constituents, secretion and functions. *Platelets*, Vol. 12:pp. 261-73.

Rumbaut, RE. & Thiagarajan, P. (2010). *Platelet-Vessel Wall Interactions in Hemostasis and Thrombosis. Morgan & Claypool Life Sciences.*

Shinohara, H., Fukuda, N., Socki, T., Takeichi, N., Yui, Y., Tamura, Y. & Oki, T. (1998). Relationship between flow dynamics in the left atrium and hemostatic abnormalities in patients with nonvalvular atrial fibrillation. *Jpn Heart J*, Vol.39:pp. 721-30.

Slichter, SJ. (2004). Relationship between platelet count and bleeding risk in thrombocytopenic patients. *Transfus Med Rev*, Vol. 18:pp. 153-67.

Slupsky, JR.; Kalbas, M.; Willuweit, A.; Henn, V.; Kroczek, RA.& Müller-Berghaus, G. (1998). Activated platelets induce tissue factor expression on human umbilical vein endothelial cells by ligation of CD40. *Thromb Haemost*,Vol.80:pp.1008–14.

Smyth, SS.; Mcever, RP.; Weyrich, AS.; Morrell, C.; Hoffman, MR.; Arepally, GM.; French, PA.; Dauerman, HL. & Becker, RC. (2009). Platelet functions beyond hemostasis. *Journal of Thrombosis and Haemostasis*, Vol.7:pp. 1759–66.

Spaet, TH. (1974). *Progress in Hemostasis and Thrombosis*. Volume 2. Grune & Stratton, New York.

Stein, PD.& Sabbah, IIN. (1976). Turbulence blood flow in the ascending aorta of humans with normal and diseased aortic valves. *Circ Res*, Vol.39:pp.58-65.

The Stroke Prevention in Atrial Fibrillation Investigators (1993) . A differential effect of aspirin on prevention of stroke in atrial fibrillation. *J stroke Cerebrovase Dis*,Vol.3:pp.181-8.

Tse, HF.; Lau, CP.& Cheng, G. (1997). Relation between mitral regurgitation and platelet activation. *J Am Coll Cardiol*, Vol.30:pp. 1813–8.

Watson, T.; Shantsila, E.&Lip, GYH. (2009). Mechanisms of thrombogenesis in atrial fibrillation: Virchow's triad revisited. *Lancet*, Vol. 373:pp. 155–66.

White, JG. & Clawson, CC. (1980). The surface-connected canalicular system of blood platelets–a fenestrated membrane system. *Am J Pathol*, Vol.101:pp. 353-64.

White, JG. (2008). Electron opaque structures in human platelets: which are or are not dense bodies? *Platelets*: Vol.19: pp. 455–66.

White, JG.; Krumwiede, MD.& Escolar, G. (1999). Glycoprotein Ib is homogeneously distributed on external and internal membranes of resting platelets. *Am J Pathol*, Vol.155:pp. 2127–34.

Wipf, JE.& Lipsky, BA. (1990). Atrial fibrillation. Thromboembolic risk and indications for anticoagulation. *Arch Intern Med*, Vol. 150:pp. 1598–603.

Yamamoto, K., Ikeda, U., Seimo, Y., Mito, H., Fujikawa, H., Sekiguchi, H. & Shimada, K. (1995). Coagulation activity is increased in the left atrium of patients with Mitral Stenosis. *J Am Coll Cardiol*, Vol.25:pp. 107–12.

Yamauchi, K.; Furui, H.; Taniguchi, N.& Sotobata, I. (1986). Plasma beta-thromboglobulin and platelet factor 4 concentrations in patients with atrial fibrillation. *Jpn Heart J*, Vol. 27:pp.481–7.

Yetkin, E., Erbay, AR., Turhan, H., Ileri, M., Ayaz, S., Atak, R., Senen, K. & Cehreli, S. (2003). Decreased platelet activation and endothelial dysfunction after percutaneous mitral balloon valvuloplasty. *Int J Cardiol*, Vol. 91:pp.221-25.

Yu, SK., Latour, JG., Marchandise, B. & Bois, M. (1978). Shear stress-induced changes in platelet reactivity . *Thromb Haemost*, Vol.40:pp.551-60.

Zaki, A.; Salama, M.; El Masry, M.; Abou-Freikha, M.; Abou-Ammo, D.; Sweelum, M.; Mashhour, E.& Elhendy, A. (2000). Immediate effect of ballon valvuloplasty on hemostatic changes in mitral stenosis. Am J Cardiol, Vol.85:pp. 370-75.

Zhou, L. ; Stordeur, P. ; de Lavareille, A. ; Thielemans, K. ; Capel, P. ; Goldman, M.& Pradier, O. (1998). CD40 engagement on endothelial cells promotes tissue factor-dependent procoagulant activity. *Thromb Haemost*,Vol.79:pp.1025–28.

5

New Gene-Candidate in Atrial Fibrillation Polymorphism of β1-Adrenoreceptor Gene

Svetlana Nicoulina, Anna Chernova,
Vladimir Shulman and Pavel Shesternya
Krasnoyarsk State Medical University,
Russia

1. Introduction

Atrial fibrillation (AF) is the most common sustained cardiac arrhythmia, occuring 1-2% of the general population (European Society of Cardiology, 2010). The lifetime risk of the development of AF at age 40 years has been estimated to be approximately 1 in 4 (Lloyd-Jones et al., 2004). In most cases atrial fibrillation is secondary, i.e. caused by some cardiovascular disease. However, in minimum 1/3 of patients causes of AF are impossible to identify. In these situations idiopathic or lone AF is being the case. It is assumed that a significant number of cases of idiopathic (lone) AF is hereditary inflicted.

Significant influence of heredity on the development of AF was first stated by H. Gould in 1950. He assumed hereditary character of AF in several generations of one family, who had been under observation for 36 years. Most publications on the genealogy of AF were issued in the 1990s. They describe cases of families whose members had AF or atrial flutter. (Bertram et al., 1996; Bharati et al., 1992; Gillor et al., 1992; Girona et al., 1997; Poret et al., 1996). At the same period was published the results of observing the development of AF in two embryos during the 23rd and 25th weeks of antenatal development. Both children were born with persistent AF (Tikanoja et al., 1998).

Families, where intraventricular conduction disorders alongside with various tachyarrythmias tended to accumulate, were of special interest for the researchers. There are families described, whose members of several generations had AF and/or atrial flutter combined with block of different branches of His' bundle or atrio-ventricular heart block (Amat-y-Leon et al., 1974; Bertram et al., 1996; M.S.; Friedli, 1993).

There was point out that AF at parents increases the risk of development of atrial fibrillations in posterity. Among 2 243 relatives examined 681 (30%) had at least one parent with the registered AF (Fox et al., 1997). Priority in postulation of the AF autosomal-dominant model belongs to J. Girona. They presented two families where 20 out of 70 examined persons had paroxysmal or permanent form of AF (Girona et al., 1997).

The clinical, electrophysiological and genetic examinations were conducted in three Spanish families with AF. Genetic analysis showed that the gene responsible for the AF in these families was localized on the 10q chromosome in the area 10q22-24. Genetic typing of the patients with AF revealed the locus of the pathologic gene between D10S1694 and D10S1786. The disease is inherited with a high degree of penetrance. The authors suggest that the candidate genes for this pathology are genes of β-adrenoreceptors (ADRB1), α-adrenoreceptors (ADRA2) and genes of G-protein coupled receptor-kinase (GPRR5) as localized on the same 10 chromosome, in locus 23-26. In the families studied cardiac fibrillation was found in 21 out of 49 members. Genealogies of these families are shown in Fig. 1. One of the diseased members (II-8) died of stroke at the age of 68. Another one (III-2), who had paroxysmal cardiac fibrillation since he was 20 years old, suddenly died at the age of 36, but autopsy was not performed. Out of 19 alive family members 18 had chronic AF and 1 suffered from paroxysmal form of AF (Brugada et al., 1997).

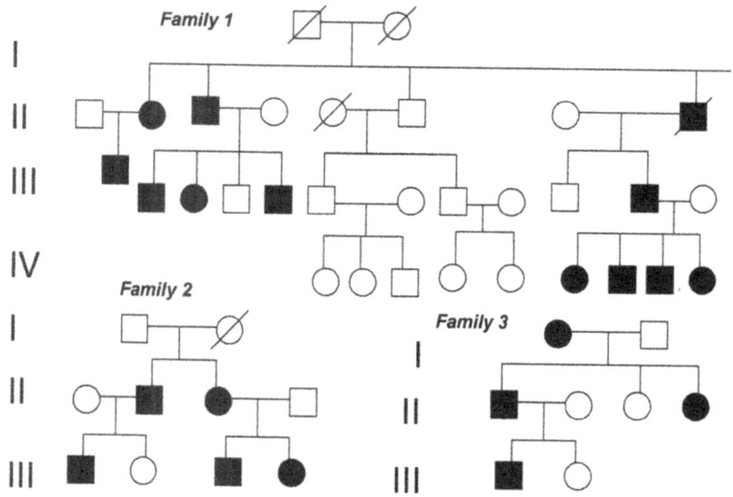

Fig. 1. Genealogy of 3 Spanish families with AF.

The hereditary AF was defined as a monogenic arrhythmia, which suggests, according to the author, that there is a possibility to correct this condition early (Roden, 2004). However, this type of rhythm disorder is characterized by genetic heterogeneity as an identical phenotypic pattern can be seen in mutations in different genetic loci. Along with the AF locus situated in the 10th chromosome, investigators mapped AF gene on a proximal long shoulder of 6q 14-16 in the interval between D6S286 and D651021 (Ellinor et al., 2004). In this particular family AF was inherited as Mendelian disease.

Finally, Chinese researchers identified 2 genes responsible for inherited AF (Yang et al., 2004). Those were the genes of myocyte potassium channels' proteins. Specifically, they reported replacement of arginine to cycteine in 27 position of gene KCNE2 on chromosome 21q22.1-22, which codes β-subunit of potassium channels. These mutations were found in 2 out of 28 examined Chinese families with inherited AF. The mutation (S140G) of gene KCNQ1 on chromosome 11p15.5, which codes α-subunit of cardiac potassium channel was identified. Occurrence of AF in these cases is caused by the fact that the function of respective potassium channels in the genes influenced by the described mutations, increases. This leads to shortening of the action potential and effective atrial refractory period. As was mentioned above, when the function of the described channels decreases, long QT syndrome occurs, thus variants LQT1 and LQT6 take place. It is also worth reminding that one of the leading phenotypic manifestations of a short QT syndrome, when the function of potassium channels increases, is paroxysmal AF. Thus, the given data of the Chinese researchers prove the suggestion that some of the familial AF variants can be classified as channels pathology (Yang et al., 2004).

There is established a relative association between inherited AF and other genetic disorders: long QT syndrome, dilation cardiomyopathy, hypertrophic cardiomyopathy, Wolff-Parkinson-White syndrome. The results of a forty-year long observation over nine generation of one family with cardiomyopathy and AF were reported in 2000. Out of 325 examined persons 106 were found to have AF (Sparks et al., 2000).

The discovery of a missense mutation (D1275N) of sodium channels gene SCN5A in patients with dilatation cardiomyopathy and of a missense mutation (replacement of arginine to histidine in 663 position) in the heavy chain of β-cardiac myosin allowed to suggest it, which caused linked inheritance of hypertrophic cardiomyopathy and AF (Gruver et al., 1999; Olson et al., 2005).

A combination of Wolff-Parkinson-White syndrome and hypertrophic cardiomyopathy caused by the pathology of PRKAG gene, which codes γ2-subunit of adenosine monophosphate - activated protein kinase was presented in 2001. The 38-44% of patients with a familial form of this syndrome had AF, as opposed to 15-20% with sporadic forms of the disease. The gene of this pathology is mapped on chromosome 7q34-36. Sequence analysis of these patients' DNA showed replacement of arginine to glutamine in position 302 (Gollob et al., 2001).

Recent years' research is aimed to find candidate genes associated with the development of AF. One of such candidate genes is a polymorphous marker of G-protein β3-subunit gene. (BNB3). Multifunctional G-protein is localized in cell membranes of cardiac hystiocytes, smooth muscular vessel cells, fibroblasts; it can be involved in the processes of cardiac muscle and vessel wall remodeling. The connection between polymorphism (deletion) of mitochondrial DNA and development of lone AF was also proved (Lai et al., 2004). In another study was discovered association of polymorphous C825T marker of BNB3 gene, which codes β-3 subunit of G-protein. As a result of genetic typing the patients fell into the following categories: C-allele homozygotes (CC genotype); heterozygotes (CT genotype) and T-allele homozygotes (TT genotype). The association between TT genotype and decreasing risk of AF was established (Schreieck et al., 2004).

The increasing of connexin 43 in AF was correlated with enlargement of the left atrium. The mutation in gene 1q21.1, which causes connexin 40 decreasing, was found out that contributes to development of aortic arch anomalies with AF (Christiansen et al., 2004).

Morphologic substrate of AF electrogenesis can be genetically determined imperfection of connective tissue development in embryogenesis, which leads to disorder in intertissue interactions and electromechanical instability. It can be proved by the work of Japanese researchers, who showed significantly frequent development of AF through experiments on transgenic mice with atrial fibrosis (Nakajima et al., 2000).

At the 21st Annual Scientific Sessions of the North American Society of Pacing and Electrophysiology (2000) there was an interesting report on the fact that myocardial "pump cuffs", which form in embryogenesis around pulmonary veins openings, are morphological substrate of ectopic activity that can cause atrial fibrillation and flutter. Myocytes in these are characterized by spontaneous electric activity, as opposed to cardiac hystiocytes of the left atrium. Clinical features of primary AF, its clinical pathogenetic forms, anatomical and electrophysiological risk factors for this pathology are not studied to a sufficient extent.

Inheritance patterns of this pathology as well as phenotypic predictors of this pathology were not studied in all the details.

2. Results

2.1 Atrial fibrillation genealogy

In relation to that, during the last five years we have examined 103 probands with the diagnosed AF and 301 members of their families (I, II, III degrees of relation) in our clinic. The probands' families were divided into groups based on the etiology of AF. Thus, we got Group 1, comprising 53 probands with idiopathic AF and 154 members of their families; Group 2 had 50 probands with secondary AF and 147 family members.

The study established the fact of family disease aggregation in the probands' families with AF. Secondary AF aggregation in the families reached 7.31% (22 diseased family members out of 301), which was significantly larger than population frequency (0.4%) of the disease (H. Kulbertus et al., 1982). In the probands' families with AF the biggest percentage of the diseased was among the family members of the first degree of relation. Specifically, the pathology in question was found at 9.86% of the examined family members within the first degree of relation and only 1.16% of the family members within the second degree of relation had it.

According to our data, among the family members of the first degree of relation, the most susceptible to atrial fibrillation are mothers (36.36%), sisters (19.44%) and fathers (16.67%) as shown in Fig.2.

Heritability of susceptibility (H^2) was defined within the framework of Falconer's model which postulates normal distribution of susceptibility in a population and among the family members of the first degree of relation. According to this model, regression coefficient of AF susceptibility was:

$$b = \frac{Xq - Xr}{a} = \frac{2{,}65 - 1{,}287}{2{,}962} = 0{,}460$$

Xq - a threshold point of susceptibility distribution in population;
Xr - a threshold point of susceptibility distribution among family members;
a – average susceptibility of the diseased in a population sample.

The values were taken from the tables - appendix to the formula of regression coefficient calculation. Heritability coefficient:

$$H^2 = \frac{b}{r} = \frac{0{,}460}{2} = 0{,}230$$

r - a relation coefficient, $r = 2$ for the family members of the first degree of relation.

Thus, heritability of AF susceptibility according to Falconer's model was 23%; the rest 77% of AF development cases are caused by the environmental factors.

To conduct the formal genetic analysis of inheritance type Weinberg's method is used for unit registration. The sick siblings in the probands' families with idiopathic AF, where this pathology was traced in several generations were used for the segregation analysis. Taking into account the results received from the sibs and probands' methods of segregation analysis for the families where probands suffer from idiopathic AF, we can assume autosomal-dominant type of this pathology inheritance.

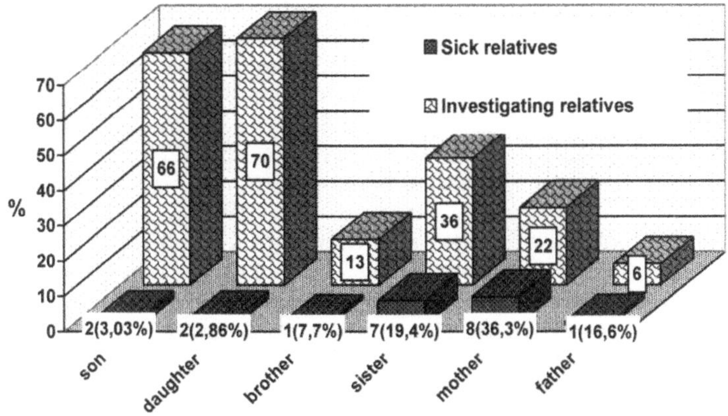

Fig. 2. Family AF aggregation in the probands' families with AF.

2.2 Family history

Proband - female, 54 years old, was examined in February, 2002. She complained about fits of unrhythmical heartbeat accompanied by dyspnea; headaches occurring after rise in blood pressure (BP). According to the anamnesis, paroxysmal atrial fibrillation was first diagnosed in 1992. The patient had several examinations in hospital. Amiodaron was administered, but treatment was not regularly. When she stops taking the medication, AF paroxysms recur, usually twice a month, mostly on exertion. Those were terminated with procainamide hydrochloride. In recent two years the blood pressure started to rise. The highest levels were 200/100 mmHg. The blood pressure did not reach with the use of ACE inhibitors. The skin was normal color and moistness. The chest was not deformed. No abnormalities in the precordial area. Apical beat was palpated on the left midclavicular line. Left heart border was dilated within the left midclavicular line. Heart sounds were clear, rhythmical, no murmur. Heart rate was 65 bpm. BP was 140/90 mmHg. No other systems' pathologies were found. In admittance, ECG showed sinus rhythm with the heart rate 65 bpm, axis = + 15°, P 0.1″, PQ 0.16″, QRS 0.08″, QT 0.38″, $R_{V5,V6}$ > R_{V4}. Conclusion: signs of the left ventricular hypertrophy. On 20jun2002 ECG showed atrial fibrillation with the ventricular heart rate 100-135 bpm. We revealed hardening of aorta and aortic valve cusps, slight symmetric left ventricular hypertrophy (interventricular septum – 1.1 cm; left ventricle posterior wall – 1.2 cm) by echo. The left atrium size was normal (2.8 cm). Left ventricular ejection fraction (LVEF) was normal. Diagnosis: Idiopathic heart rhythm disorder: paroxysmal atrial fibrillation type. Concomitant disease: Arterial hypertension.

Proband's mother, 75 years old, with complains about unrhythmical heart beat; shortness of breath on slight exertion, sometimes at rest, which worsens in the lying position; heaviness in the right hypochondrium; swollen ankles, constricting retrosternal pain on exertion (walking about 500 m on the level road). Those were stopped by taking nitroglycerine. Further complains include seeing little dots when the BP rises; weakness and dizziness. According to the anamnesis, chronic AF was first diagnosed 17 years ago. Before becoming chronic, paroxysms had been recurring for 10 years. At the age of 60 angina pectoris symptoms started to reveal, the BP began to rise. Maximal BP levels were 220/115 mmHg. Around the same time clinical picture of heart failure was observed. The treatment included cardiac glycosides, β-blockers, ACE inhibitors, diuretics, antithrombotic. The skin was pale, dry. Chest was not deformed. No abnormalities in the precordial area. Apex beat was palpated at 1 cm to the outside of the left midclavicular line. Left heart border was dilated up to the 1 cm from the left midclavicular line. Heart sounds were muffled, arrhythmical, systolic murmur was heard on the aorta and Botkin-Erb point. Heart rate was 100 bpm; BP was 150/85 mmHg. Respiration was rough, no crackles with breathing rate 20 per minute. Palpatory tenderness in the right hypochondrium. Percussion findings showed the lower end of the liver to be below the edge of the costal margin. Pastosity of the knees was noticed. ECG showed rhythm of atrial fibrillation with the ventricular rate 85-130 bpm, axis =0°, QRS 0.08″, QT 0.36″, $R_{V5,V6} > R_{V4}$. Signs of the left ventricle hypertrophy were seen. Echo data revealed aorta and aortic valve cusps hardening; severe left ventricle hypertrophic (interventricular septum 1.4 cm, left ventricle back wall is 1.5 cm). The left atrium was dilated (4.6 cm). LVEF was slightly reduced (52%, by Teicholz). Diagnosis: Idiopathic heart rhythm disorder: chronic atrial fibrillation type. Concomitant disease: Arterial hypertension. Coronary heart disease. Angina pectoris.

Proband's son, 17 years old, complained about stabbing pains in the cardiac apex. Irregularities in the cardiac performances were not subjectively noticed. According to the anamnesis, during last 5 years ECG records showed frequent ventricular premature beats. The patient s regularly taking β-adrenergic blockers with no positive antiarrhythmical effect. The skin was slightly hyperemic, of normal moistness, red dermographism. Chest was not deformed. No abnormalities in the precordial area. Apex beat was palpated at 1 cm to the inside of the left midclavicular line. Heart borders were within normal ranges. Heart sounds were clear, arrhythmical, no murmur. Heart rate was 70 bpm, (with frequent extrasystole). BP was 130/85 mmHg. No other systems' pathologies were found. ECG showed sinus rhythm with the heart rate 80 bpm, axis = + 40 °, P 0,06″, PQ 0,16″, QRS 0,08″. QT 0,34″. Conclusion: Frequent ventricular extrasystole, trigeminy. Bicycle ergometry registered frequent ventricular premature beats at rest; the number of premature beats did not reduce at exertion. Echo did not reveal any pathology. Transesophageal left atrium stimulation results: Wenckebach point - 176 per minute, sinus node recovery time (SNRT) - 1050 msec, corrected sinus node recovery time (SNRTc) - 250 msec. Ultrafrequent stimulation with a short volley of stimuli provoked a paroxysm of atrial fibrillation with the ventricular rate 79-120 bpm. Frequent ventricular premature beats were also registered. Diagnosis: Idiopathic heart rhythm disorder: type of frequent ventricular premature beats and paroxysmal atrial fibrillation.

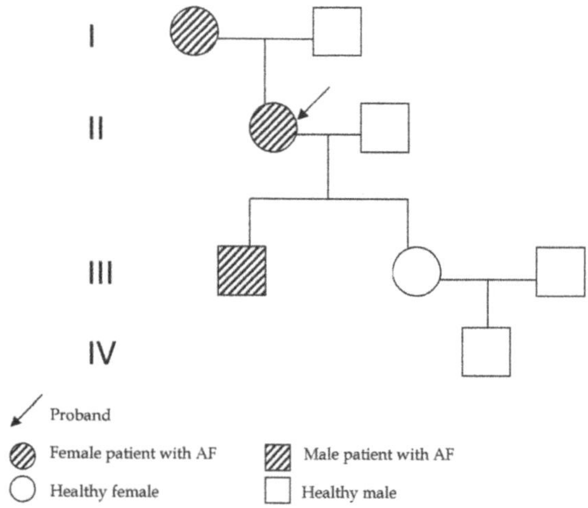

Fig. 3. Genealogy of the family with atrial fibrillation.

Proband's daughter, 35 years old, with complains about stabbing pains in the cardiac apex, feeling of incomplete inhalation, dizziness. The patient can not indicate for sure when the above mentioned symptoms appeared. According to the patient, their possible causes were physical and emotional overstrain. Taking sedatives given positive effect. No irregularities in the cardiac performance were revealed. The skin was normal tone and moistness. Chest was not deformed. No abnormalities in the precordial area. Apex beat was palpated at 1 cm to the inside of the left midclavicular line. Heart borders were within normal ranges. Heart sounds were clear, rhythmical, no murmur. Heart rate was 65 bpm. BP was 120/80 mmHg. No other systems' pathologies were found. ECG showed a sinus rhythm with the heart rate 64 bpm, axis = + 30°, P 0.08″, PQ 0.16″, QRS 0.08″, QT 0.36″. Echo did not reveal any abnormalities. Bicycle ergometry revealed no cardiac rhythm disorders. Exertion tolerance is high. No hypertension syndrome. Holter ECG-monitoring registered a sinus rhythm with normal variability. No cardiac rhythm disorders were found during the examination period. Proband's grandson, 13 years old, did not any complains. Cardiac rhythm disorder had never occurred. According to the anamnesis, patient had some minor respiratory diseases and chickenpox. The examination did not reveal any abnormalities. ECG showed a sinus rhythm with the heart rate 76 bpm, axis = + 40 °, P 0.06″, PQ 0.16″, QRS 0.06″, QT 0.34″. Echo revealed first degree mitral valve prolapse (mitral valve cusps sagging up to 4 mm).

2.3 New gene-candidate of atrial fibrillation

We evaluated β1-adrenoreceptor candidate gene polymorphism in the patients with lone and secondary AF. Genetic study has been performed using DNA extracted from peripheral blood leukocytes (Smith, 1990). Amplification was achieved with PCR. Genetic tests were performed in 30 patients of the 1st group (lone AF) and 25 their healthy relatives; and in 30 patients of the 2nd group (secondary AF) and 44 their healthy relatives. Besides, 198 patients, who did not have any signs of cardiovascular diseases, were genetically typed (control group).

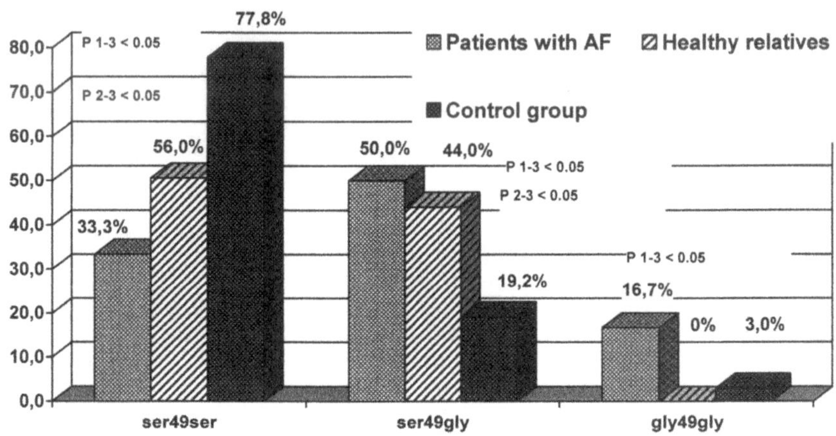

Fig. 4. Polymorphism of β1 – adrenoreceptors gene among patients with lone AF.

According to own data, probands and their relatives with lone AF had significantly prevailing heterozygous genotype of β1-adrenoreceptors (Ser49 Glu) in comparison with the control group: 15 probands (50%) and 11 relatives (44%) in comparison with 38 (19.2%) of the control group. The 1st group probands also showed domination on the rare allele

(Glu49Glu) in comparison with the control group: 5 (16.7%) and 6 (3.2%) respectively. However, the described genotype was found in none of the healthy relatives of the 1st group probands (Fig.4).
The 2nd group patients also demonstrated a significant domination of a heterozygous allele (Ser49Glu): 14 (46.7%) in comparison with the control group 38 (19.2%). However, the genotype in question was not significantly predominant in these patients' relatives in comparison with the control group. Frequency of genotype Glu49Glu occurrence in the patients with secondary AF and their relatives was not significantly different from that of the control group (Fig.5).

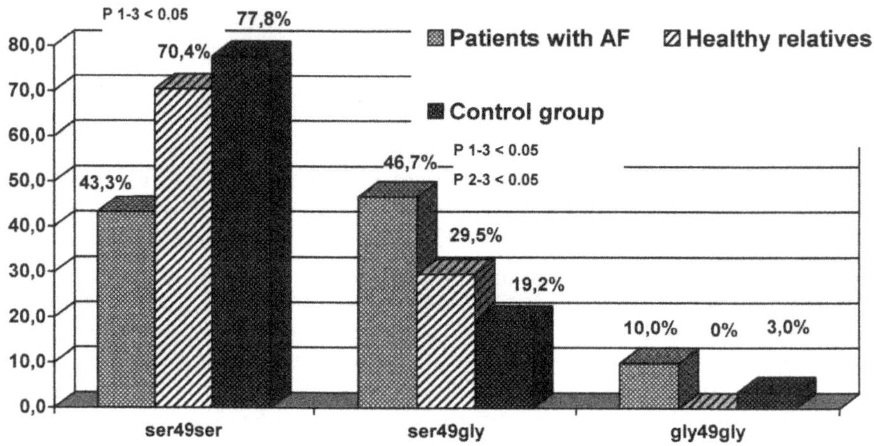

Fig. 5. Polymorphism of β1-adrenoreceptors gene in patients with secondary atrial fibrillation.

Taking everything presented above into account, heterozygous variant of the genotype of β1-adrenoreceptors gene Ser49Glu can be considered one of the genetic predictors of both lone and secondary AF. Genotype Ser49Glu can also serve as a predictor of lone AF. Relatives of those probands with the lone AF and Ser49Glu genotype are under the risk of developing this pathology.

3. Conclusion

On the whole, analysis of our own data and the data presented in literature shows that AF can be caused by hereditary predisposition. The most obvious manifestation of hereditary predisposition is in the patients with lone AF. Hereditary AF is often associated with other cardiovascular diseases (primary cardiomyopathy, Wolff-Parkinson-White syndrome, long- and short QT syndromes etc.). In some cases hereditary AF is a monogenic disease. However, as seen in many cases, AF is caused by a particular combination of certain genes' polymorphism (candidate genes). Our study of polymorphism of β1-adrenoreceptors gene in the patients with lone and secondary AF can assist in solution of one of the aspects of this problem. It is also beyond all doubt that further search for candidate genes causing both lone and secondary AF remains urgent. This search's findings can contribute greatly to the prevention of one of the most common and dangerous arrhythmias. As genetic are gradually incorporated into routine clinical practice, classification system may facilitate individualized AF therapy based on pharmacogenomic principles (Roberts & Gollob, 2010).

4. Acknowledgment

We would like to thank Mikhail Voevoda, Vladimir Maksimov and staff of the Research Institute of Therapy, Novosibirsk, Russia for help with genetic testing and their continued support and assistance in our studies.

5. References

Amat-y-Leon, F., Racki, A. & Denes, P. (1974). Familial atrial dysrhythmia with A-V block. Intracellular microelectrode, clinical electrophysiologic, and morphologic observations. *Circulation*, Vol.50, No. 6, pp.1097-1104.

Bertram, H., Paul, T. & Beyer, F. (1996). Familial idiopathic atrial fibrillation with bradyarrhythmia. *European Journal of Pediatrics*, Vol.155, No. 1, pp.7-10.

Bharati, S., Surawicz. B. & Vidaillet, H. (1992). Familial congenital sinus rhythm anomalies: clinical and pathological correlations. *Pacing and Clinical Electrophysiology*, Vol.15, No. 11, pp.1720-1729.

Brugada, R., Tapscott, T. & Czernusczewicz, G. (1997). Identification of a genetic locus for familial atrial fibrillation. *New England Journal of Medicine*, Vol. 336, pp. 905-911.

Chen, Y., Xu, S. & Bendahhou, S. (2003). KCNQ1 Gain-of-Function Mutation in Familial Atrial Fibrillation. *Science*, Vol.299, No. 5604, pp. 251-254.

Christiansen, J., Dyck J. & Elyas B. (2004). Chromosome 1q21.1 contiguous gene deletion is associated with congenital heart disease. *Circulation Research*, Vol. 94, No. 11, pp. 1429-1435.

Das, S., Makino, S. & Melman Y. (2009). Mutation in the S3 segment of KCNQ1 results in familial lone atrial fibrillation. *Heart Rhythm*, Vol.6, No. 8, pp. 1146-1153.

Ellinor, P., Moore, R. & Patton, K. (2004). Mutations in the long QT gene, KCNQ1, are an uncommon cause of atrial fibrillation. *Heart*, Vol. 90, pp. 1487-1488.

Friedli, B. (1993). Arrhythmias in the adolescent and adult with a congenital heart defect. *Schweizerische medizinische Wochenschrift*, Vol.123, No. 43, pp. 2065-2071.

Fox, C.S., Parise, H., D'Agostino, R.B. (2004). Parental atrial fibrillation as a risk factor for atrial fibrillation in offspring. *Journal of the American Medical Association*, 291, pp.2851–5. 278.

Gillor, A., Korsch, E. (1992). Familial manifestation of idiopathic atrial flutter. *Monatsschrift Kinderheilkunde*, Vol.140, No. 1, pp. 47-50.

Girona, J., Domingo. A. & Albert, D. (1997). Familial auricular fibrillation. *Revista Española de Cardiología*, Vol. 50, pp. 548-551.

Gollob, M., Green, M. &Tang A. (2001). Identification of a gene responsible for familial Wolff-Parkinson-White syndrome. *New England Journal of Medicine*, Vol. 344, No. 24, pp.1823-1831.

Gould, L., Reddy, V. & Becher, H. (1978). The sick sinus syndrome. *Journal of electrocardiology*, Vol.11, No.1, pp.11-14.

Gruver, E., Fatkin, D. & Dodds G. (1999). Familial hypertrophic cardiomyopathy and atrial fibrillation caused by Arg663His beta-cardiac myosin heavy chain mutation. *American Journal of Cardiology*, Vol. 83, No. 12A, pp.13-18.

Guidelines for the the management of atrial fibrillation. (2010). The Task Force for the Management of Atrial Fibrillation of the European Society of Cardiology (ESC). *European Heart Journal*, Vol. 31, No.19, pp. 2369-2429.

Lai, L., Su, M. & Yeh, H. (2002). Association of the human minK gene 38G allele with atrial fibrillation: evidence of possible genetic control on the pathogenesis of atrial fibrillation. *American Heart Journal,* Vol. 144, No. 3, pp. 485-490.

Lloyd-Jones, D., Wang, T. & Leip, E. (2004). Lifetime risk for development of atrial fibrillation: the Framingham Heart study. *Circulation,* Vol. 110, pp. 1042-1046.

Nakajima, H. Nakajima, H.O. & Salcher O. (2000) Atrial but not ventricular fibrosis in mice expressing a mutant transforming growth factor-b1 transgene in the heart. *Circulation Research,* 86, 571–579.

Olson, T., Michels, V. & Thibodeau, S. (1998). Actin mutations in dilated cardiomyopathy, a heritable form of heart failure. *Science,* Vol. 280, pp.750-752.

Olson, T., Michels, V. & Ballew, J. (2005). Sodium channel mutations and susceptibility to heart failure and atrial fibrillation. *Journal of the American Medical Association,* Vol. 293, No. 4, pp. 491-493.

Poret, P., Mabo, P., & Deplace, C. (1996). Is isolated atrial fibrillation genetically determined? Apropos of a familial history. *Archives des maladies du coeur et des vaisseaux,* Vol. 89, pp. 1197-1203.

Roberts, J., Gollob, M. (2010). Impact of Genetic Discoveries on the Clasification of Lone Atrial Fibrillation. *Journal of the American College of Cardiology,* Vol. 55, pp. 705-712.

Roden, D. (2004). Human genomics and its impact on arrhythmias. *Trends in cardiovascular medicine,* Vol.14, No. 3, pp. 112-116.

Schreieck, J., Dostal, S. & Von Beckerath, N. (2004). C825T polymorphism of the G-protein beta3 subunit gene and atrial fibrillation: association of the TT genotype with a reduced risk for atrial fibrillation. *American Heart Journal,* Vol.148, No 3, pp. 545-550.

Sparks, E.A., Graber, H. & Boudoulas, H. (2000). Atrial myopathy and atrial fibrillation: phenotypes in heritable cardiac conduction and myocardial disease. *European Heart Journal,* Suppl K, pp.78-90.

Tikanoja, T., Kirkinen P. & Nikolajev K. (1998). Familial atrial fibrillation witl fetal onset. *Heart,* Vol.79, p. 637-641.

Yan, H., Chen, J. & Zhu, J. (2004). Expression of connexin in atrium of patients with atrial fibrillation and its signal transduction pathway. *Zhonghua Yi Xue Za Zhi,* Vol. 84, No. 3, pp. 209-213.

Yang, H., Xia, M. & Jin, Q. (2004). Identification of a KCNE2 - gain of function mutation in patients with familial atrial fibrillation. *American Journal of Pathology,* Vol.165, No 3, pp. 1010-1032.

Part 2

Mapping and Detection

6

Current Status and Future of Cardiac Mapping in Atrial Fibrillation

Doosang Kim[1] and Hyuk Ahn[2]
[1]*Seoul Veterans Hospital,*
[2]*Seoul National University,*
Korea

1. Introduction

AF is a major concern in general population worldwide. Every year, 3 million suffer from AF related stroke, 1.5 million die from AF related stroke within a year, and 1 million are severely disabled by AF related stroke. Only 1% of AF patients underwent a treatment such as ablation or AF surgery. 99% remain as they are or prophylactic anticoagulation medication only. The reason why is due to the limitation in diagnostic mapping and ablation treatment. Incomplete, vague and fragmented maps give us incomplete AF information, and lead to incomplete cure chance. Standard 12-lead ECG, which composed of 6 bipolar Einthoven limb leads and 6 unipolar Wilson pre-cordial leads, are used for more than 100 years giving us the information about rhythm, electric axis, activation sequence, and repolarization pattern. However, the F wave information of standard ECG signals during AF has limitation that only a few signals are available to show whether AF or not, or little information of source or location of its origin. The exact location of source origin and propagation route or pattern of reentry is too difficult to be elucidated by conventional low-sensitive ECG method due to its very weak signal amplitude of F-wave. Therefore, in order to manage AF successfully, we should get detailed information of AF activity in atrium using a high sensitive mapping methodology. Accurate mapping is the essential to successful treatment of arrhythmia. Endocardial mapping techniques for AF are now well developed and its accuracy reached high to treat AF effectively, however, they demand invasiveness, moderate costs and selection of patients. They are not suitable for mass screening to general population yet. Non-invasive mapping for AF is still far from bed-side due to its insufficient information of AF, not enough to detect F wave and to make a sufficient map to treat AF. According to the recently updated worldwide survey on AF ablation by Cappato *et al.* [1] in 2010, anti-arrhythmic drug-off success rate and overall success rate are 75% and 83% for paroxysmal AF, 65% and 75% for persistent AF, and 63% and 72% for long-standing persistent AF. Major complications were reported 4.5% from catheter ablation for AF. They reported that CARTO-guided left atrial circumferential ablation (48% of all treated patients) and Lasso-guided ostial electric disconnection (27% of all treated patients) were the most commonly used techniques for AF treatment. To improve the success rate, exact cardiac mapping of AF is essential.

In this chapter, we described several topics of cardiac map, such as history, importance, composition, classification, basic principle, clinically available maps, and my study work, Magnetocardiography Action Potential Activity mapping for AF and future frontiers.

2. History of cardiac activation mapping

Cardiac activity is an electro-physiologic phenomenon including time course and wave propagation distribution of excitatory process of the myocardium. To understand this complicated phenomenon, we need the isolated beating heart model. It began with the basic investigation of Oskar Langendorff who developed a method for investigation of the isolated heart (Langendorff, 1895). In 1950s, Dick Durrer, cardiologist and Henk van der Tweel, physist opened the Amsterdam era of cardiac activation study. They developed instruments to reveal the excitation of heart with ECG. They reported the monumental ventricular wall excitation in 2D and 3D results from dog heart [2-5]. After success of dog heart model, in 1970, with informed consent of family members, human isolated hearts were obtained from individuals who had died, within 30 minutes after death. Thru the isolated Langendorff human heart perfusion apparatus, the hearts were perfused with an oxygenated, heparinized, modified Tyrode solution, with washed bovine erythrocytes, and resumed beating spontaneous sinus rhythm for periods ranging from 4 to 6 hours. During the activity, electrical activity of the heart was recorded from epicardial activity by hand-held electrodes and intramural activity by needle electrodes using 14-channel Ampex tape recorder with 870 terminals. They reported the 2D and 3D isochronic representation of atrial activation of an isolated normal human heart at first (fig.1) [6].

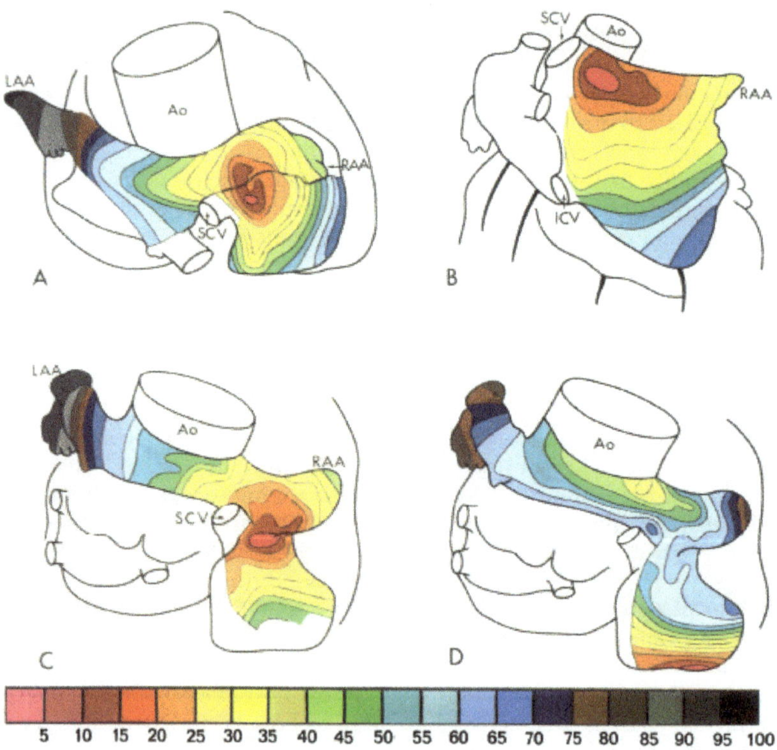

Fig. 1. Isochronic representation of the normal human atrial activation from isolated Langendorff human heart perfusion apparatus made by Durrer et al. at first. Reprinted with permission from Ref. 6

First atrial epicardial excitation mapping in atrial arrhythmia (atrial flutter) was performed during open heart surgery in a patient with atrial arrhythmia (atrial flutter) and rheumatic mitral and aortic valve disease was reported in 1971 by Wellens *et al.* [7]. They made the inferred propagation map from the atrial excitation (Fig.2).

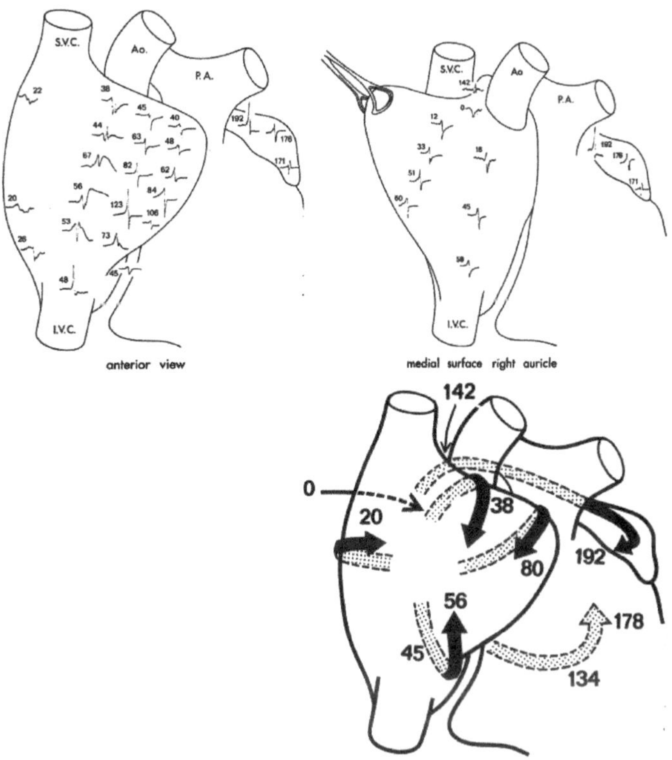

Fig. 2. Atrial epicardial excitation recordings and suggested spread in a patient having atrial flutter at first. Reprinted with permission from Ref. 7

Another important breakthrough is the development of pulse generator or stimulator, made by engineer Leo Schoo *et al.* with reproducible high accuracy [8]. It helps to be possible to map by placing catheters at different sites in the hearts.

In the early 1960s, the term "body surface mapping" was coined by Taccardi B *et al.* Multiple unipolar or bipolar leads were recorded from the body surface in dogs [9] and in humans [10] to display and analyze the complexity of potential distribution on maps. Next important work of body surface mapping is ECGI which have been studied by Rudy Y *et al.* for several decades.

Endocardial contact mapping under fluoroscopic control is the most widely applied current technique for diagnostic electrophysiology study. It involves recordings of electric signals at multiple sites of the heart, such as high right atrium, coronary sinus, left atrium via septal puncture, right ventricular apex and His bundle area using bi/quadri/multi-polar catheters. With the increase in complexity of catheter technology and modern computerized mapping technique, the classical endocardial electrogram recording via a few positioned catheters appeared old-fashioned more and more.

New mapping technologies are under development actively. CARTO, CARTO Merge (Biosense-Webster, Baldwin Park, CA, USA), Real-time Position Management (RPM) (Cardiac Pathways-Boston Scientific EP Medsystems, Sunnyvale, CA, USA), NavX (St. Jude Medical, Inc., St. Paul, MN, USA), Ensite 3000 (St. Jude Medical, Inc., St. Paul, MN, USA) hane been introduced recently and used actively worldwide now. We describe these new mapping technologies in detail at this chapter.

3. Body surface potential mapping (BSPM)

Isopotential body surface maps are used to provide a complete picture of the effects of the currents from the heart on the body surface. The potential distributions are represented by contour lines of equal potential, and each distribution is displayed instant throughout activation or recovery, or both. Since Body surface mapping was introduced, its role has been proved in the field of ischemia detection, accessory pathway localization, Brugada syndrome, long QT syndrome, and idiopathic VT and reentrant VT analysis, which have abnormalities of relatively big enough signal, QRS activity, ventricular activation to be detected easily. However, for AF, very weak signal, F wave activity is too small to be used as a definite diagnostic solution by BSPM. Body surface potential mapping of atrial events was first described by SippensGroenewegen *et al.* in characterizing P waves during ectopic atrial activation [11] and during atrial flutter [12] in 1998. This system uses many leads, more than 12 lead-standard ECG. BSPM records simultaneously all signals from all leads, not sequential acquisition of endocardial signals from contact-based conventional endocardial mapping. Therefore, BSPM results in real-time characterizing and localizing the pattern and propagation route of AF. Guillem *et al.* reports 40+16 leads systems in 16 AF patients with 2,048 Hz sampling rate, 1 μV resolution, and 500 Hz bandwidth (fig.3) [13]. Using 240-seconds recordings, wavefront propagation maps were classified according to the different patterns; I (single wavefront), II (single wavefront with wave breakages and splitting) or III (multiple simultaneous wavefronts). This classification showed to be highly reproducible over 4 minutes, and these results give us new insights of varing AF characteristics, from simple pattern to very chaotic ones.

Similar AF pattern analysis was also made by Kornings *et al.* using epicardial contact mapping electrode, and this will be described later in the part of "epicardial contact mapping" of this chapter.

In spite of limited usefulness, non-invasive cardiac mapping, such as BSPM, has unique necessity for (i) screening people with genetic predisposition or altered myocardial substrate for risk of life-threatening arrhythmias, in order to take prophylactic measures; (ii) specific diagnosis of the arrhythmia mechanism to determine the most suitable intervention; (iii) determination of cardiac location for optimal localized intervention (such as ablation, pacing, targeted drug delivery or targeted gene transfer); (iv) evaluation of efficacy and guidance of therapy over time; (v) studying the mechanisms and properties of cardiac arrhythmias in human, where the electrophysiological substrate is quite different from experimental animal models used thus far for this purpose [14]. Although these procedures are of interest, their clinical utilities have not been established yet.

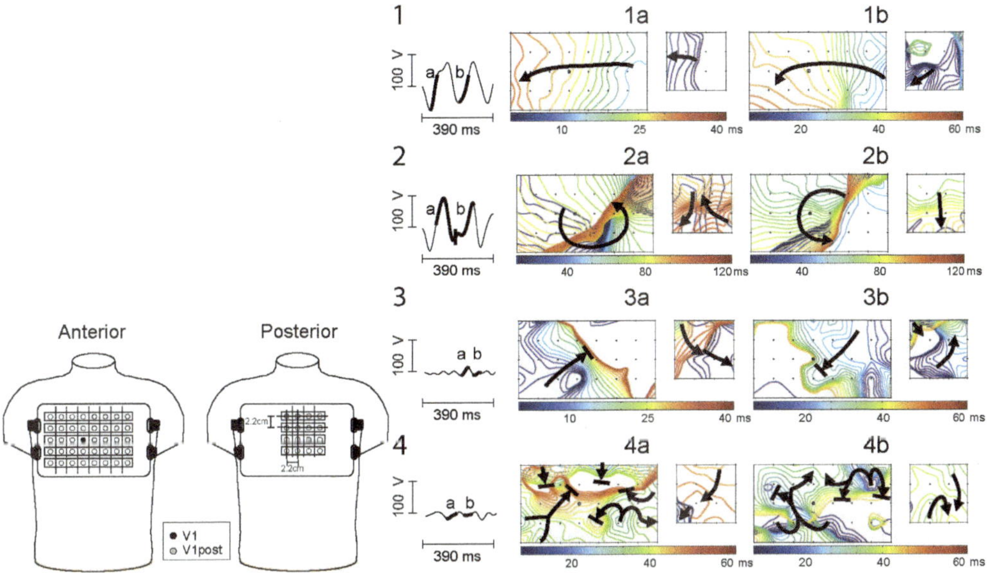

Fig. 3. Body surface potential mapping (BSPM) is a non-invasive simultaneous mapping. (a) Left panel; Arrangement of the electrodes and belt used for their attachment to the patient. A total of 56 ECG leads were placed on the chest over the atria on the front (n=40) and on the back (n=16). (b) Right panel; Wavefront propagation maps of three dominant activation patterns were shown in AF patients; single wavefront (1), single wavefront with wave breakages and splitting (2 and 3), and multiple simultaneous wavefronts (4). Fine figures by courtesy of Prof. MS Guillem and Reprinted with permission from Ref. 13

4. Electrocardiographic Imaging (ECGI)

ECGI combines alleged established technologies, BSPM and CT in a unique fashion to generate noninvasive images of cardiac electrical activity. Rudy Y *et al.* provided ECGI applications in normal heart, heart with a conduction disorder, focal activation initiated by right or left ventricular pacing, and atrial flutter, successfully using a multi-electrode vest records 224 body-surface electrograms [14]. Electrical potentials and isochrones are reconstructed on the heart's surface using geometrical information from computed tomography (CT) and a mathematical algorithm. Left panel of Fig.4 shows the ECGI application procedures briefly. A 224-electrode vest strapped to the patient's torso and connected to a multichannel mapping system measured body surface potential (a), and then the patient underwent a thoracic CT scan (b). The CT images provided epicardial surface geometry and vest-electrode positions (c). The potential and geometry data were processed through ECGI software (CADIS) (f). Through this process, ECGI isochrones map and epicardial surface potential map were constructed (g). Right panel of Fig.4 shows the normal atrial isochrone map (a) and atrial flutter isochrones map (b) having the reentrant circuit beginning from isthmus, entering septum, emerging from Bachman bundle and propagating down RAFW (right atrial free wall) to reenter isthmus again. Wang *et al.* reported the successful ECGI isochrones map in scar-related atypical atrial flutter with a high spatial and temporal resolution [15].

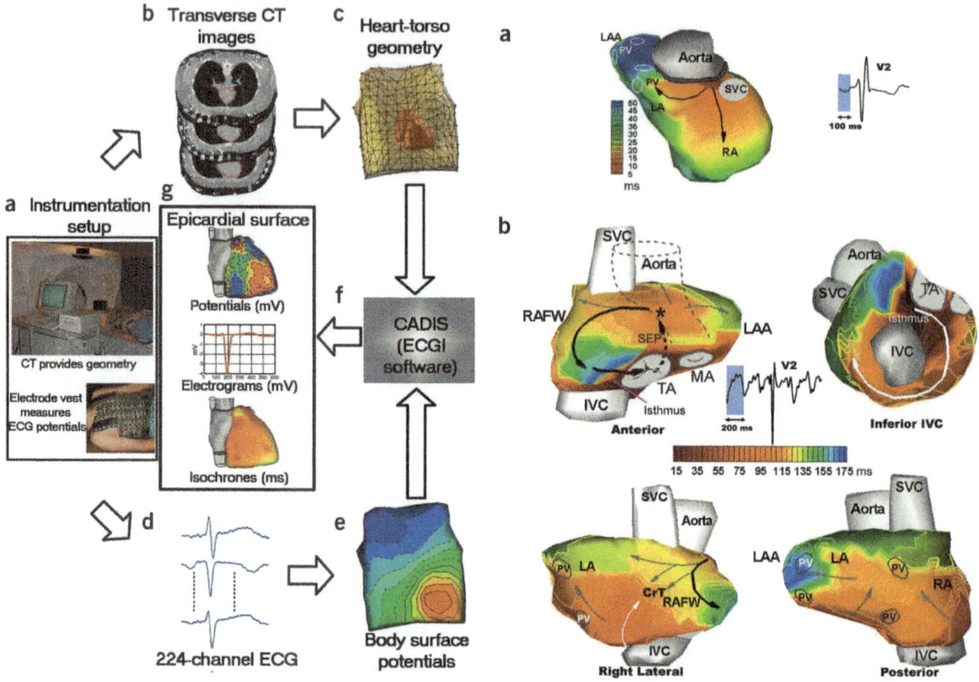

Fig. 4. ECGI application procedure (Left panel) and atrial activation ECGI map (Right panel) in nomal conduction (a) and atrial flutter (b). In Left panel, a 224-electrode vest strapped to the patient's torso and connected to a multichannel mapping system measured body surface potential (a), and then the patient underwent a thoracic CT scan (b). The CT images provided epicardial surface geometry and vest-electrode positions (c). The potential and geometry data were processed through ECGI software (CADIS) (f). Through this process, ECGI isochrones map and epicardial surface potential map were constructed (g). In Right panel, the normal atrial isochrone map (a) and atrial flutter isochrones map (b) having the reentrant circuit beginning from isthmus, entering septum, emerging from Bachman bundle and propagating down RAFW (right atrial free wall) to reenter isthmus again. ECGI is a non-invasive simultaneous BSPM mapping, not sequential invasive endocardial contact mapping. Reprinted with permission from Ref. 14

ECGI has higher results in resolution than BSPM, which located pacing sites to within 7mm in RV and 11mm in LV. It results in clinical benefit to explore source origin during troublesome catheter work.

Recently, Patient-specific volume conductor modeling with magnetic resonance imaging was reported by Pfeiter *et al.* in 2008 [16]. They used 1.5 Tesla cine MRI images, and makes volume conductor model using (i) segmentation, (ii) extraction process of chest, lung, and blood mass, (iii) myocardial reconstruction, and (iv) volume conductor integration. And using 62 channel Mark-8 system (Biosemi V.O.F.), body surface potential map is acquired and defines by Wilson-Central-terminal (WCT) with 2048 Hz sampling rate, and band-filtered with a lower and upper edge frequency of 0.3 and 400 Hz, respectively, so the AC resolution of them was $500nVit^{-1}$ (16 bits per channel) (Fig.5). This method gives a fast and accurate insight to us non-invasively. Still, it is remained not at clinic but at experimental circumstances.

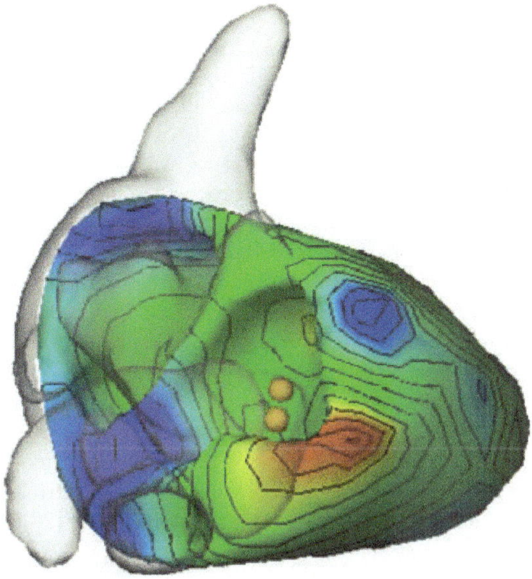

Fig. 5. Patient-specific volume conductor model using 62 channel body surface potential and MR image integration shows activation time estimation having accessory pathway in WPW syndrome patient. This is first personalized simultaneous BSPM with MR mapping. Reprinted with permission from Ref. 16

5. Electrophysiologic endocardial contact mapping

Catheter or surgical ablation has evolved to be the treatment of choice in patients with a broad spectrum of cardiac tachy-arrhythmias including atrial fibrillation. The most important requirement for successful ablation is the exact mapping of arrhythmia, focal or reentrant, and identification of target sites during the electro-physiologic study. Conventional classic mapping needs on fluoroscopy, marked x-ray hazard during procedure, and leads to low spatial resolution and inaccurate navigation to a target. Classical endocardial contact mapping techniques basically depend on electrical information from endocardial contact electrodes and on anatomic information from fluoroscopic endocardial contour images. Activation sequence mapping, pace mapping and entrainment mapping are the classical methods of contact catheter mapping. Activation sequence mapping uses the timing of electrograms from roving catheter during arrhythmia with a timing of a reference signal to identify early signal or propagation of activation. It is useful to detect focal arrhythmias, such as focal atrial tachycardia or RVOT tachycardia. Pace mapping is helpful for source identification of reproducible arrhythmia by pacing at source origin with similar cycle length. Entrainment mapping is used to confirm macro-reentrant circuit having an excitable gap. These classical mapping methods are moderate x-ray hazard, time-consuming, technically difficult, not completely reproducible, and most of all, not suitable for hemodynamically unstable patients or transient arrhythmias with short duration. To overcome these weak points, several technical advances have been made since 1997 [17].

5.1 CARTO mapping

CARTO (Biosense Webster, Diamond Bar, CA, USA) is a non-fluoroscopic electro-anatomical real-time high-resolution most-widely used 3D mapping system composing with magnetic field sensor tip catheter on the magnetic field emitter pad, which was introduced in 1996 at first [18]. Nowadays, CARTO-guided left atrial circumferential ablation (48% of all AF treatment patients) is the most commonly used techniques in AF treatment and drug-off success rate is 70%, overall success rate 80% according to the recent worldwide survey [1]. The sensing of magnetic field by location sensor enables the exact location of the tip with high accuracy, 1mm. Fig.6 shows the basic mechanism of CARTO to localize the tip location [19]. A tiny location sensor is embedded in the catheter tip consisting of three miniaturized coils that is tracked by the CARTO system. The locator pad placed beneath the patient table generates 3 ultra-low magnetic fields to identify the location and orientation of the sensor. The mapping catheter and reference patch are plugged into the junction box and signals are sent over to the electrophysiology recording systems. ECG signals and location information are sent to a data acquisition and display system that analyzes the signals, determines location of catheter tip, and generates maps using the previously collected anatomical and electro-physiologic data. The accuracy of CARTO was tested in vitro and in vivo studies and reported highly reproducible and accurate with 1mm error range [20].

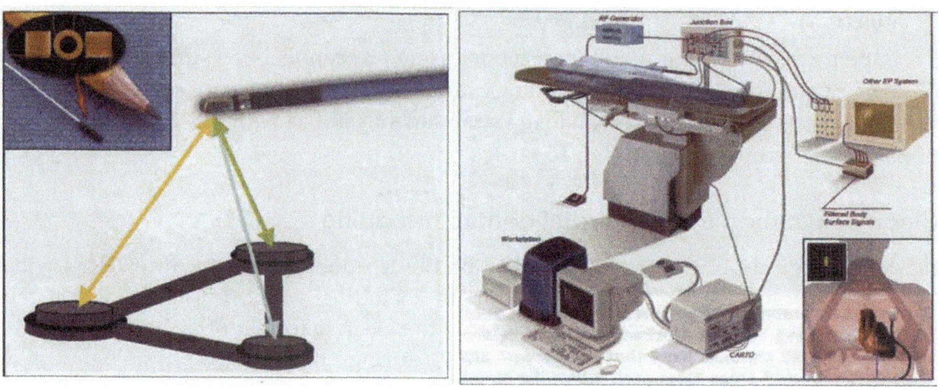

Fig. 6. Basic mechanism and typical setup of the CARTO electro-anatomical mapping system (a) A tiny location sensor is embedded in the catheter tip consisting of three miniaturized coils that is tracked by the CARTO system. The locator pad placed beneath the patient table generates 3 ultra-low magnetic fields to identify the location and orientation of the sensor. (b) Typical setup of the CARTO electro-anatomical mapping system in the electro-physiology laboratory. Fine figures by courtesy of and Reproduced with permission of the Anatolian Journal for Cardiology/AVES Publishing, from Copyright 2002, *Firat Duru.* Ref. 16

CARTO is a very useful tool in mapping for sustained atrial tachycardias, macroreentrant atrial arrhythmias after surgical correction of congenital heart disease, and ventricular tachycardia of post myocardial infarction or other structural heart disease, and useful in isthmus dependent atrial flutter and idiopathic ventricular tachycardia. Basically the CARTO system makes map by contact-based sequential acquisition of endocardial signals, for construction of 3D electro-anatomical maps, it takes 30 minutes or more, very time consuming. Therefore, if the arrhythmia is not sustained or has varying cycle lengths, or in the patient who is hemodynamically not well tolerated, or unstable catheter location during intra-cardiac activation and patient movement, CARTO sequential mapping is not possible or inaccurate, requiring the reconstruction of a whole new map. CARTO XP improves some these drawbacks. The other limitations of CARTO include that it is mostly applied to single target chamber only per one trial, and it is impossible to obtain information from the epicardial activity. Risk to patient from invasiveness during procedure, higher costs and limited reusability of this system is another hurdle to prevent widely distribution.

5.2 CARTO Merge mapping

CARTO Merge (Biosense Webster, Diamond Bar, CA, USA) is a recently developed fusion system of 3D CT or MR images with an electro-anatomic map. Fig. 7 shows the differences between CARTO and CARTO Merge systems for right atrium [21].

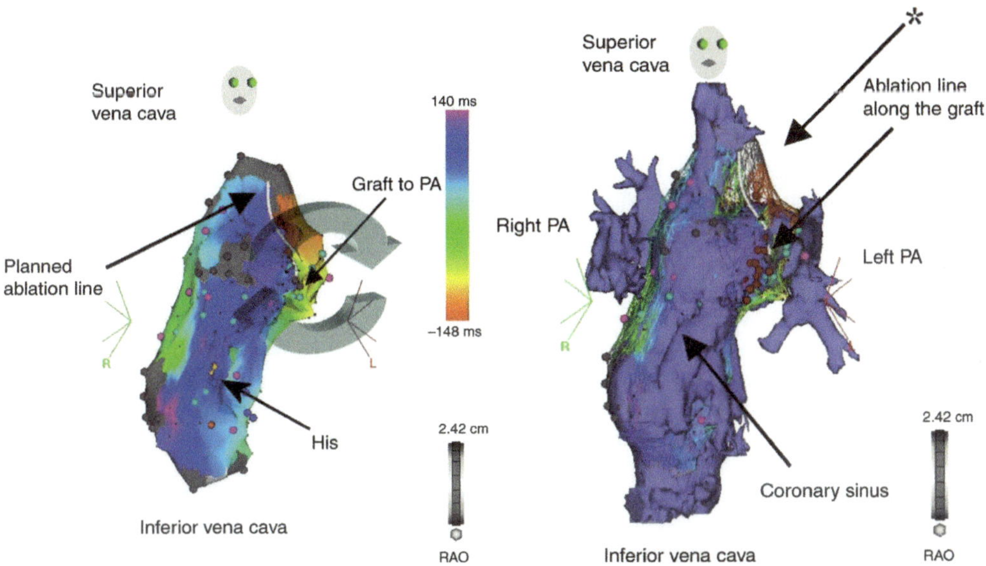

Fig. 7. CARTO (Left) and CARTO Merge (Right) map in right anterior oblique view of right atrium from postoperative Fontan operation patient. In CARTO Merge, CT based anatomy (blue) and underlying map (mesh) show the detailed anatomy of right atrium with coronary sinus, connected pulmonary arteries and its branches from postoperative Fontan patient. CARTO and CARTO Merge are sequential endocardial contact mapping. Reprinted with permission from Ref. 21

In CARTO Merge, the high-resolution anatomical information from contrast enhanced 64-slice cardiac computed tomography (CT) was reconstructed and the heart chambers were segmented and implemented in the new electro-anatomical mapping system.

However, roving magnetic tip catheter mapping is basically a sequential, beat-by-beat approach, which demands stable rhythm and fixed reference point, and may have possible error from ferromagnetic noise. Multiple factors create discrepancies between electro-anatomic maps and merged, preacquired computed tomographic images. The accuracy of the integrated 3D geometry is highly dependent on image quality and on the merge process. Errors may develop from changes in cardiac chamber volume or rhythm occurring between the time of 3D anatomic image acquisition and electro-anatomic mapping in EP lab. Gating of image acquisition to the cardiac cycle and respiratory phase may affect rendered volumes. Usually volume image acquisitions were gated at 80% of the R-R interval for atrial and at 0% of the R-R interval (R wave) for ventricular imaging during the end-expiratory phase.

5.3 NavX mapping

Next to CARTO, the NavX (Endocardial Solutions, Inc., St. Paul, MN, USA) is the 2nd widely used 3D non-fluoroscopic mapping system using transthoracic low-power electrical currents to enable localization of endocardial electrode catheters, which was published in 1999 [22]. NavX has advantages in multiple endocardial catheter real-time visualization with a respiratory compensation algorithm. The other advantage is the effect on radiation exposure reduction. NavX is significantly higher than others in x-ray hazard reduction, median fluoroscopy time is 13 min conventionally, 6 min with CARTO, 4 min with NavX [23]. NavX system measures the local voltage on every standard intra-cardiac electrode and calculates the electrode position in 3D space. Additionally, it labels any individual electrode of each catheter. The ability to visualize and label electrodes on both the circular mapping and the ablation catheters may offer a great benefit in ablation procedures. NavX is built on the principles of LocaLisa. It creates 3D images of the catheters, based on a low-current electrical field of 350 μA at a frequency of 5.68 kHz, generated by three pairs of nominally orthogonal skin patches in X, Y, and Z axes. The measured voltage and impedance sensed by these catheter electrodes are proportional to the distance of the electrode from the patches, thus allowing calculation of the location of the catheter in 3D space. The potentials are defined with respect to a reference electrode, which is a surface electrode or an internal fixed electrode such as a coronary sinus catheter electrode that presents the origin of the coordinate system. After impedance calibration, the position in space of each electrode can be determined for a wide range of patient body masses (34-115 kg) with the accuracy of 0.6 mm. To control variations related to the cardiac cycle, acquisition is gated to any selected electrogram to need. Compensation for respiratory movements is also conducted, the respiratory motion artifact is measured and subtracted from the measurement or roving electrode position. Using this, 3D geometry reconstruction of heart chambers is performed to guide treatment. However, 3D atrial reconstruction using NavX system is not fully reliable yet. In spite of all, NavX enables a significant reduction in fluoroscopy time and total procedure duration compared with the conventional- fluoroscopy-based approach. By using the Penta-array catheter each with 4 electrodes, sequential acquisition of the contact electrogram activity obtained as the penta-array catheter is swept up, therefore rapid activation mapping can be performed as Fig.8 [24].

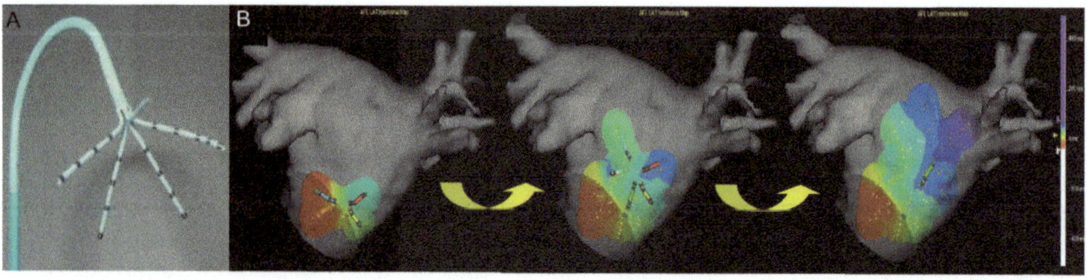

Fig. 8. Penta-array catheter (A) having each 4 electrodes and sequential swept up contact mapping are displayed (B). NavX system is basically sequential endocardial contact mapping. Reprinted with permission from Ref. 24

5.4 Real-time Position Management mapping

Another new mapping system is Real-time Position Management (RPM) (Cardiac Pathways-Boston Scientific EP Medsystems, Sunnyvale, CA, USA) system that was first described by de Groot *et al.* in 2000 [25]. RPM uses ultrasound to measure the distance between the reference ultrasound transducer and catheters. Two reference catheters and one mapping catheter were introduced by either arterial or venous approach. Ultrasound ranging technique is used to (i) construct a 3D representation of catheters including electrodes and transducers, anatomic structures, and ablation sites and (ii) display real-time movement of the tip and shaft of the catheters. As a non-fluoroscopic map-guide system, RPM, cooled RF ablation was tested in animal experience [26]. RPM system has advantages over CARTO or NavX system regarding stable catheter position that is minimally influenced by body, cardiac, respiratory movement, and sweating, and also no need for skin electrodes or patches. However, one major disadvantage is that the RPM system requires a special catheter, a mapping catheter and two reference catheters equipped with ultrasound transducers which limited steerability of the mapping catheter, and dislocation of the reference catheters due to roving catheter manipulation.

5.5 Clinical Implication

We described briefly several mapping systems having current clinical usage. New technical advance in mapping system results in new treatment concept and clinical success. Substrate CFAE mapping in AF, activation/propagation mapping in atrial tachycardia/atrial flutter, and voltage mapping in scar-related atrial tachycardias are the current useful examples of 3D electro-anatomical mapping systems. From the data acquisition of single mapping system, several maps are generated such as activation map, propagation map, voltage map, frequency map and geometric map. Activation map describes the dispersion of activation times in the mapped region. Propagation map is a dynamic graphic representation of the activation wavefront throughout the cardiac cycle. Voltage map is a graphic representation of the peak-to-peak voltage of the local electrograms recorded. Frequency map is a graphic representation of the frequency spectra, such as dominant frequency (DF) or complex fractionated atrial electrogram (CFAE), of the local electrogram recorded. Geometric map present graphic representation of the mapped anatomy.

Substrate mapping is benefit to treat AF by substrate modification. In 1959, Moe and Abildskov hypothesized that AF is due to multiple randomly propagating reentry waves in the atrium, suggesting that functional reentry is the mechanism underlying fibrillation [27]. Wijffels *et al.* confirmed that AF was shown to require at least 6 to 8 circulating reentrant wavefronts [28]. Maintenance of AF depends on a critical atrial mass on conduction velocity and refractory periods in the atrial tissue to support functional reentry. Since Cox *et al.* reported the higher success rate in AF treatment using surgical Maze procedure [29-30], substrate modification is accepted as a new target for AF treatment and substrate mapping is recently accepted as very important one. The Cox-Maze procedure incorporates 4 lesion sets and involves; (i) encirclement of the Pulmonary Veins, (ii) a lesion joining the circumferential PV lesion to the mitral annulus with amputation of the left atrial appendages, (iii) a circumferential lesion in the Coronary Sinus, and (iv) ablation of the right atrium. However, Maze procedure remains complex and is associated with a significant increase in cardiopulmonary bypass time, morbidity, and mortality.

Although the exact mechanisms of AF treatment by linear lesion set like surgical Maze procedure still remains not completely elucidated yet, (i) reduction of excitable LA myocardial mass may be account for these success. Besides mass reduction, (ii) attenuation of vagal innervations, (iii) abolition of non-PV foci, especially related with ligament of

Marshall, and (iv) elimination of anchor circuits confined to LA-PV region are the reason of importance of substrate mapping [31].

Two different parameters were used to display the substrate mapping, one is voltage and the other is frequency. In frequency, complex fractionated atrial electrogram (CFAE) is the parameter indicated for the fractionation of atrial activity, and dominant frequency (DF) is the largest peak frequency of the atrial activity spectrum. Fig.9 shows the comparison of the CFAE map and DF map in same AF patients. [32].

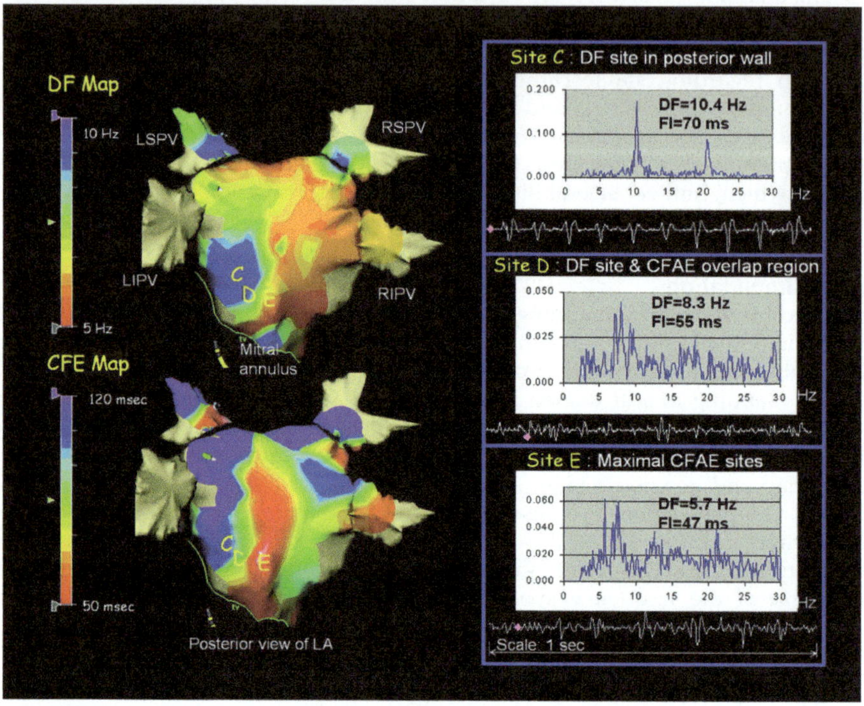

Fig. 9. Comparison of the regional distribution of the DF map (upper) and CFAE map (lower) using NavX sequential mapping system in same AF patients. The intracardiac bipolar electrogram and corresponding frequency spectra during AF are shown in right panels. The most fractionated areas (shortest FI, site E) in the LA low posterior wall are in the periphery of the high-frequency sites of AF (highest DF site, site C) near the lateral mitral isthmus. CFAE ablation did not terminate AF; however, linear ablation in the lateral mitral annulus crossing the highest DF site successfully terminated AF. Reprinted with permission from Ref. 32

Nademanee *et al.* reported that CFAE map-guided left atrial (LA) ablation terminated sustained AF in 95% of patients, resulting in excellent clinical outcomes (1 year AF-free rate, 91%) and improved mortality rates [33]. However, the electro-physiologic mechanism of CFAE has not been clearly elucidated yet. CFAE regions are predominantly located at the septum, roof, and LA appendage (LAA) with low voltage surrounded by a high voltage area and low conduction velocity in patients with AF. CFAE cycle length was longer, and % area of CFAE was smaller in patients with an enlarged LA or low-voltage LA [34]. High plasma concentrations of TGF-beta and TIMP-1 had lower LA voltage and greater LA volume significantly in non-valvular AF patients [35].

RF ablation of atrial flutter, focal atrial tachycardia, AV nodal reentry tachycardia, and scar-related (incisional) atrial reentrant tachycardia under activation/propagation mapping using CARTO or NavX are accepted as clinical success. Especially, incisional atrial tachycardias in patients following surgery for congenital heart disease having complex structural abnormalities were treated by catheter ablation [36]. Electroanatomical activation 3D map allowed a rapid distinction between focal and reentrant mechanisms and visualization of the activation wavefronts along anatomical and surgically created barriers, such as reentrant tachycardia propagating through the tricuspid annulus-vena cava inferior isthmus or along peri-atriotomy loops. Target sites in complex congenital heart disease patients are often slow-conducting narrow isthmus bordered by areas of scar tissue [37] and voltage criteria have been developed by areas of scar tissue by De Groot et al. [38]. Voltage-based scar-related delineation in patients with congenital heart disease is the good example of 3D electroanatomic mapping which has clinical impact.

In spite of many clinical advantages, endocardial contact mapping has several weak points to be solved, (i) detection source problem, alteration or interference of magnetic field or ultrasound, (ii) contact issues, missing or noise signals from contact problems, (iii) motion artifact from reference point, cardiac cycle, respiration movement, (iv) un-mappable arrhythmia, (v) sequential fragmented map, not simultaneous single snapshot map, (vi) fractionated electrograms not to trace whole propagation of each F wave, and (vii) position error during image registration. However, in spite of several weak points, these endocardial contact maps provide us valuable insights into the mechanism of arrhythmias and enhanced understanding of substrate -EP relationships.

6. Non-contact endocardial mapping

The most important drawback of contact mapping is the error from the missing or noisy signal due to poor contact problem. So, some electrograms were deleted when artifacts or poor contact were observed. To overcome this problem, noncontact concept was introduced in 1987 by Taccardi B *et al.* in which intra-cavitary potentials were measured from olive-shape probe electrodes introduced through the LV apex of animal heart [39]. 64 Multi-electrode array (MEA) (EnSite Array, St. Jude Medical, St. Paul, MN, USA) is very rapid, 3360 virtual electrogram complete map generation on a single beat, relatively accurate, and usable even in hemodynamically unstable or non-sustained VT patients. However, this system has limitations in (i) distance problem, between catheter and tissue, decreased accuracy more than 34mm apart from tissue, (ii) signal-to-noise ratio problem, (iii) chamber size dependent, and (iv) virtual electrogram not real one, (v) inadequate substrate mapping and (vi) the associated moderate costs.

Recently, an ultrasound-based 3D imaging modality, CARTO-based 3D ultrasound image system (Biosense Webster Inc., USA) has been developed to minimize merge process error [34]. The axial CT images were transferred to the electro-anatomic mapping system equipped with CARTO Merge image integration software (Biosense Webster). The surface reconstruction of the RA with superior vena cava, left arium, pulmonary veins, right ventricle, and left ventricle were segmented from each chamber volume. An electro-anatomic location sensor was incorporated into the IntraCardiac Echocardiography (ICE) catheter tip to allow the establishment of (i) tip location in 3D space, (ii) tip direction, and

(iii) the origin and direction of the 2D ICE sector image. Three second segments of 2D ultrasound images were acquired during ECG gating to a coronary sinus atrial electrogram for atrial imaging, and ECG gating to the R wave of V1-3 electrogram for ventricular imaging. This system was not automatically gated to respiration, so the images were acquired in late expiration phase (79%). Point-to-point component interpolation from a family of the chamber contour data makes the complete volume rendering and 3D geometry. They reported the point-source error of 3D ultrasound-derived geometries was 2.1mm for atrial and 2.4mm for ventricular sites, and significantly less than CARTO Merge CT images, 3.3mm for atria and 4.8mm for ventricle. Fig.10 shows 3D ultrasound geometry creation [40].

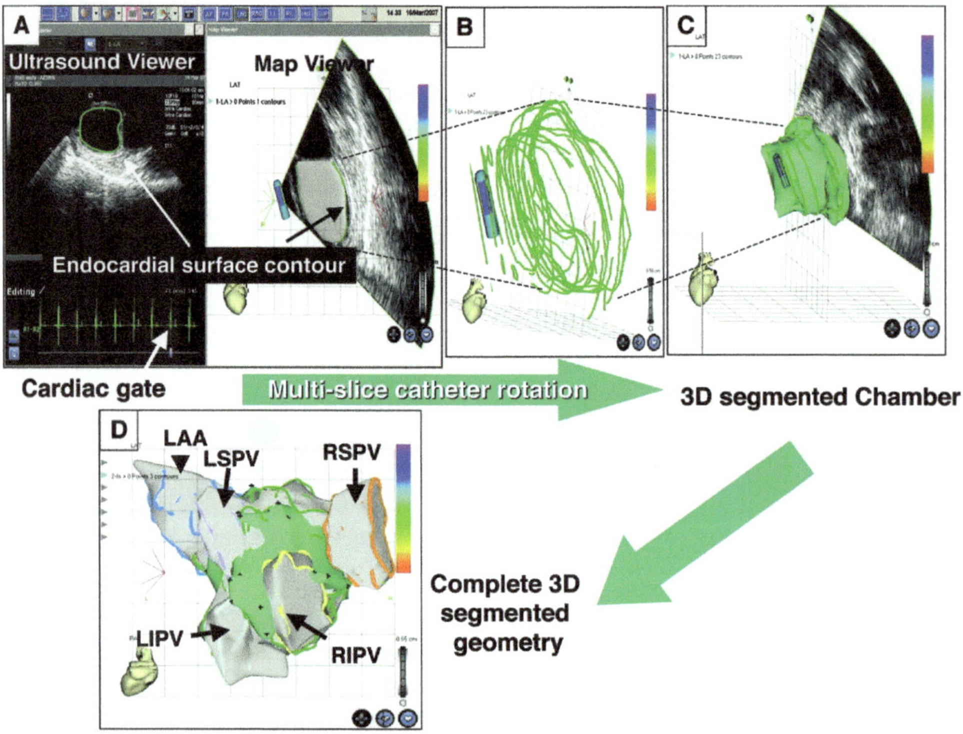

Fig. 10. CARTO-based 3D ultrasound geometry creation. A) 2D ICE view of the LA with endocardial perimeter (left) and simultaneously rendered endocardial contour (right). B) Collated multiple LA perimeters created with multiple catheter rotations. C) Overall segmented volume using point-to-point component interpolation. D) Complete LA and PV geometry created from individual volume components. LA indicates left atrium; LAA, left atrial appendage; PV, pulmonary vein; RS, right superior; RI, right inferior; LS, left superior; and LI, left inferior. It took some time to make several contours for each chamber. This is an invasive non-contact endocardial sequential mapping. Reprinted with permission from Ref. 40

In canine experimental model, a 3D ultrasound-derived geometry was created by 51 contours for RA, 22 contours for SVC, 22 contours for LA, 7 contours for PV and 8 contours for LAA. So, the total rendering time was 23 minutes for RA and 26 minutes for LA. The limitations of this 3D US derived images are (i) error from respiratory cycle, (ii) poorer resolution than CT imaging, (iii) error from acoustic shadowing or incomplete penetration of ultrasound, (iv) not fully contact images.

7. Epicardial contact mapping

Unlike the invasive endocardial sequential mappings such as CARTO, NavX, MEA, etc, Body surface potential mapping (BSPM) or ECGI gives us non-invasive simultaneous electrical information, but their resolution is limited due to relatively weak signal intensities from F-wave of AF. Epicardial contact mapping helps to show exact propagation route of F-wave. 256-channel 3-dimensional dynamic mapping system with intra-operative epicardial patch electrodes was used [42]. Successful results were reported, but it is useful only during the operation, so it is still invasive, useless for preoperative exam or follow-up, and it does not show normal activity under physiological conditions, such as closed chest, no anesthesia, presence of neural inputs, mechanical loading, and normal perfusion in intact human subjects. Epicardial electrode system has also limitation to detect any conduction via

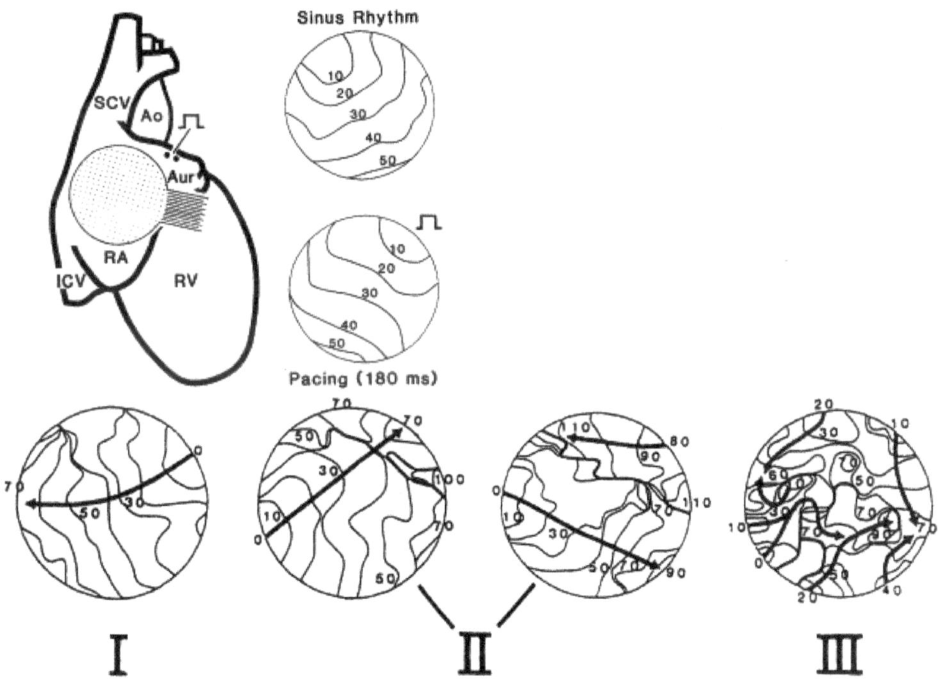

Fig. 11. Using 244-lead epicardial electrode mapping systems (upper), three different AF types were classified along mapping results (lower) in RA free wall of AF patients, such as single uniformly propagating waves (I), single non-uniformly conducting waves or two wavelets (II) and three or more wavelets associated with multiple areas of slow conduction and arcs of conduction block (III). This invasive epicardial contact mapping is simultaneous mapping to show the different pattern of AF complexity. Reprinted with permission from Ref. 42

inter-atrial septum and coronary sinus musculature. However, epicardial contact mapping gives us some clue of AF characteristics to understand their pathophysiology of different propagation pattern like previously described report by Guillem *et al.* [13]. Konings *et al.* reported three different types of AF according to the F-wave propagation pattern using 244-lead epicardial mapping electrode system in RA free wall (Fig.11). They classified AF as the degree of complexity of atrial activation during fibrillation, (i) single broad wave fronts propagating without significant conduction delay, exhibiting only short arcs of conduction block or small areas of slow conduction not disturbing the main course of propagation, (ii) single waves associated with a considerable amount of conduction block and/or slow conduction or the presence of two wavelets, and (iii) three or more wavelets associated with areas of slow conduction (<10 cm/s) and multiple arcs of conduction block [42].

Patients with a left atrial (LA) thrombus are accepted as a known contraindication for endocardial mapping and procedure. In this circumstance, hybrid epicardial and endocardial mapping and ablation technique would be possible [43]. Mapping catheter is inserted into pericardial space via a subxyphoid approach. Although this new approach resulted in a successful outcome for LA thrombi patient, the risk of complications such as hemo-pericardium, phrenic nerve injury, great vessel injury, coronary artery damage or pericarditis should also be considered before procedure.

8. Magnetocardiographic action potential activity mapping

Magnetocardiographic action potential activity mapping is a new experimental non-invasive non-contact high-sensitive simultaneous 3D mapping system for AF using superconducting quantum interface device and CT image co-registration. It is very rapid to register signals like an ECG, but very sensitive enough to analyze F-wave for source localization sufficiently, having many channels, more than 64 channels simultaneously, and shows results easily to physician as a 3D map. Its feasibility were reported in 2007 at first [44], and we introduce it for understanding including basic concept, history, main differences between ECG and MCG, its resolution, source localization, CT co-registration, clinical application, MCG studies at rhythm disorders, *etc.* in this chapter.

8.1 Biomagnetism

The movement of charged ions such as Na, K, and Ca across cell membranes generates electrical potentials on body surface which can be detected by electrographic mapping methods such as ECG. The same ion fluxes also generate electrical currents, which in turn give rise to magnetic fields. These magnetic fields can be registered outside the body, and measurement of the biomagnetic fields generated by the electrical activity of the human body is termed *biomagnetism*. The magnetic field strength is quantified with field density, whose unit is the Tesla (T). The magnetic fields of the body are so weak, for example, the magnetic field of the heart is < 100 picotesla (1 pT = 10^{-12} T) and that of the brain is femtotesla (1 fT = 10^{-15} T) (the earth's magnetic field is 10^{-4} T), so therefore some kind of shielding from external magnetic fields and high sensitive device are usually necessary. Biomagnetic measurements have been performed on several organs, besides the heart with electrical activity including the brain (magneto-encephalogram, MEG), eye (magneto-oculogram, MOG) and peripheral nerves (magneto-neurogram, MNG). MEG is currently used world-wide and studied actively to localize brain lesion such as epileptic focus, and gives higher information than EEG.

8.2 History of MCG

Magnetocardiography(MCG) is a technique to register the extracorporeal magnetic field of the heart which is generated by the same currents as the ECG. First MCG signals were registered in 1963 using a set of two copper coils and no external shielding by Baule *et al.* [45]. In 1967, MCG measurement was performed in a magnetically shielded room to cancel out the effects of external magnetic fields such as the earth's magnetic field and that of urban traffic [46]. A significant step forward was the invention and implementation of the superconducting quantum interference device (SQUID) in liquid helium at 4.2 °K (-269 °C) at 1970 by Cohen *et al.* [47]. During the next two decades, MCGs were registered with single channel device, and mappings were performed by placing the sensor at several locations over the thorax and measuring signals from one location at a time. First normal MCG patterns based on such mapping systems was reported in 1978 by Saarinen *et al.* [48]. In the 1990's, multi-channel devices have emerged, allowing simultaneous recording of the magnetic signals over large precordial areas by Van Leeuwen *et al.* [49-50]. Today, MCG measurements can be performed with highly sensitive second-order SQUID gradiometers sensors in low-cost aluminium magnetically shielded rooms, resulting in high sensitivities, and with a modern multi-channel device, MCG registration can be performed in a few minutes, rendering the method suitable for clinical patient measurements.

8.3 Main differences between MCG and ECG

MCG has morphological features similar to the P-wave, QRS complex, and T- and U- waves of the ECG and the temporal relationships between them are generally the same [48]. The main difference between spatial ECG and MCG patterns is the spatial angle of 90° between them, an essential feature of the MCG and ECG maps [51]. ECG and MCG are sensitive to different configurations of the source current: body surface potential measurements reflect the flux of the primary current distribution whereas the magnetic measurements are associated with the curl of the same source [52]. Therefore, certain source configurations can be undetectable in one measurement but visible in the other. A radial dipole in a sphere produces no magnetic signal outside the volume conductor, on the other hand, a vortex type current, curl current, a loop current would be undetectable in ECG measurements, but generates a measurable magnetic field. Almost all MCG studies are based on measurement of the magnetic field component perpendicular (radial or Z-component) to the anterior chest (Bz). MCG is thus most sensitive to currents tangential to the chest surface, whereas especially chest leads of ECG are more sensitive to radial currents. MCG is more sensitive to the terminal phase of the depolarization when the activation wavefront occurs in a more tangential direction than at the initial part [53]. ECG (the isointegral BSPM maps) shows abnormalities mainly during the depolarization period, whereas in MCG, better discrimination results from use of the abnormalities in the repolarization period [54]. MCG is also not affected by conductivity variations caused by the lungs, pericardial effusion, muscles, and skin, unlike ECG [51]. In MCG, there are no potentials generated by the skin-electrode interference needing to be filtered out, it does not require skin-electrode contact, which is prone to noise, as in body surface ECG. MCG is totally non-invasive and even non-contact device.

8.4 Temporal and spatial resolution of MCG

Bioelectric and biomagnetic studies offer functional information about electrically active organs, such as the heart and the brain, which is difficult to obtain by other imaging techniques. For example, MRI, computed tomography (CT) and X-ray imaging mainly provide only static anatomical information with relatively good spatial resolution. The alternative functional imaging methods, such as perfusion-MRI, PET, and SPECT, involve the use of intravenous enhancing markers to produce knowledge about metabolic process. In addition, the time resolution of perfusion-MRI, PET and SPECT is only around one second and the spatial resolution is only around a few centimeters. As with ECG signals, the MCG signals of the heart are obtained relatively good within millisecond time resolution.

In spite of higher temporal resolution of MCG, spatial resolution of MCG has a few measurable error ranges. In a phantom study by Fenici et al in 1998 [55], the accuracies of MCG dipole localizations were investigated by using a non-magnetic stimulation catheter, and the average MCG localization accuracy was 2-7 mm, while Body Surface Potential Mapping was 4-10 mm [56]. MCG localization accuracy is dependent to the signal-to-noise ratio (SNR) of MCG. With the SNR between 5 and 10, the average localization error was found to be 9 ± 8 mm, while for the SNR between 30 and 40, and for the goodness of fit between 99.5 % and 100 %, the average error reduced to 3.2 ± 0.3 mm. Therefore, the high SNR is essential to have a good spatial resolution. These previous resolution were originated from the QRS study. In atrial F wave localization, the F wave localization error is larger than QRS wave, because of its small size and irregularly irregular pattern. To minimize the atrial F wave localization error, co-registration with MDCT and MCG signals is essential.

8.5 Source localization

In source localization studies, the *forward problem* has to be solved first, i.e. one has to calculate the electrical potential or the magnetic field, generated by the current sources in the heart, on and outside of the body, respectively. In the *inverse problem*, the current source is determined from the MCG and BSPM measurements. However, even with a complete knowledge of the electromagnetic field outside of the source region, the inverse problem cannot be uniquely solved because the same field distribution can be produced by infinitely many current source configurations. Therefore, restrictive assumptions about the current sources are needed. The conventional way is to use equivalent source models for describing the actual currents. The parameters of the source model can then be determined from the measured data, e.g., in a least-squares sense. In addition to the current source, the media surrounding it needs to be modeled. The volume conductor models used in cardio-magnetic source imaging studies are usually referred to as *torso models*. For atrial F wave source localization, **separative Surface Potential Activation Beamformer** (sSPAB) is introduced by Kim *et al.* [44].

Minimum variance beamformer (MVB) is a well-known spatial filtering technique explaining the covariance matrix of measured fields and the technique is proper to deal with rhythmic oscillation fields like F-waves in atrial arrhythmia because the covariance matrix of the measured signal contains spatiotemporal information. However, the MVB has two intrinsic drawbacks: First, the result is not robust to the source dipole orientation although the technique has originally been developed for Equivalent current dipole (ECD) source model - a collective excitation of pyramidal cells on the brain cortex can be well approximated by the ECD source. Because the dipole orientation estimation prior to calculating the source power at the position is crucial to obtain a good result with MVB, the estimation should be done very carefully. Moreover, in a heart as opposed to a brain, the ECD is not a good model describing heart current sources. Second, MVB is unable to separate one source from the others for correlated multi-sources, especially for successively activating sources just like the myocardial current sources. Separative Surface Potential Activation Beamformer (sSPAB) is an effective dynamic source localization technique for electrical reentrant excitation of myocardium from AF. sSPAB technique is based on Minimum varience beamformer (MVB), but it circumvent the drawbacks of MVB mentioned previously by adopting Equivalent double layer (EDL) model rather than Equivalent current dipole (ECD) and by using higher order statistics of measured signals.

Current dipole sources are not suitable for explaining the reentrant excitation feature appearing on the myocardium. Instead of Equivalent current dipole (ECD), this surface source model based on the Equivalent double layer (EDL) model is utilizing the fact that all the primary current sources in a heart can be described by epicardial transmembrane action potential on the closed surface enclosing the heart. With the Boundary element model (BEM) - conductor model considering the effect of the volume current, it confines the dependent variables to the action potentials on the Boundary element model (BEM) heart surface. The estimated sSPAB power is corresponding to each other the source activity on the heart tissue. Therefore, it is no need to estimate the orientation of current dipole at the vertexes. The lead fields are calculated by a multi-surface Boundary element model (BEM) consists of heart, lung and torso. The source potentials are located only on the heart surface using sSPAB technique [44].

By using the Independent component analysis (ICA), the F-wave was separated from the other activations such as ventricular excitation, and also the feature in a time sequence. Generally, Minimum varience beamformer (MVB) uses a covariance matrix of measured signals obtained by multi-channel detectors, which means that Minimum varience beamformer (MVB) separate sources with the second order statistics (e.g. according to the magnitude of variance). The second order statistics are not enough to separate an MCG signal into the characteristic components such as P-wave, QRS complex, and T-wave. Therefore, higher order statistics of the measured signals are required. Separative Surface Potential Activation Beamformer (sSPAB) adopts the JADE algorithm using the 4th order cumulants of the measured data. The moving dipole forms a magnetic field trace at each sensor position as it moves along a route. The measured magnetic field can be separated into several independent waveforms by Independent component analysis (ICA) with a degree of freedom in permutation.

Fig.12 shows some examples of Activity map of action potential (AMAP) as application results of separative Surface Potential Activation Beamformer (sSPAB) for clinical use of source localization. Fig. 12 (a) and (b) are AMAPs for patients having dimished F-wave and coarse F-wave respectively. Patient 1 is a 61 years-old male diabetes with rheumatic valvular heart disease. He suffered from severe mitral stenosis (mitral valve area is 0.68 cm^2) and he has calcified Aortic valve leaflet with leaflet fusion of Rt coronary cusp and noncoronary cusp. He has large LA (size 67 mm) and long-standing persistent AF. High amplitude activity of action potential can be observed around the inferior part of right atrial surface. Patient 2 is a 57 years-old male with rheumatic valvular heart disease showing severe mitral regurgitation. It is due to A1 and A3 prolapse of mitral valve leaflet. His LA size is 67 mm big and his rhythm is long-standing persistent AF. He shows coarse F-wave in MCG, the excitation is very strong and expanded to the ventricle so that we could guess it transferring an atrial flutter.

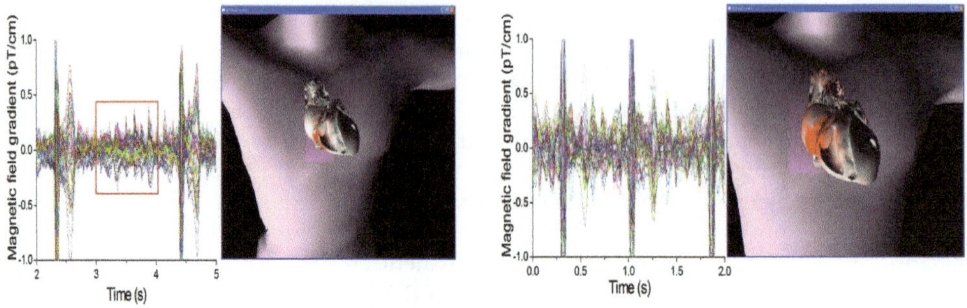

Fig. 12. Activity map of the action potential (AMAP) examples produced by sSPAB method. Red color implies high activity amplitude on the atrial myocardial surface. (a) Patient I: diminished F-wave and high activity on the inferior of Right atrium. (b) Patient II: coarse F-wave and activity on the RAA expanded to ventricle.

8.6 Clinical application of MCG

MCG has been used for many cardiac disorders. MCG can detect exercise-induced myocardial ischemia in heterogeneous CAD patient population with several ST-segment and T-wave parameters as well as ST amplitude, and spatial evaluation of ischemia-induced post-exercise T-wave changes may be useful in localization of the ischemic myocardial region [57]. MCG can detect patients with LV hypertrophy [58] and quantify its degree in patients with increased LV mass [59]. In patients with acute chest pain and without ST-segment elevation (Non-STEMI), MCG predicted CAD with a 97.8% probability and excluded CAD with an 84.8% probability, superior to ECG, Troponin I and Echocardiography [60].

Fetal MCG recordings are another important application of magnetic measurements to detect the heart rate of the fetus and even some cardiac abnormalities throughout the course of pregnancy [61], because the ECG signal of a fetus decreases after the 25th week of gestation and becomes practically undetectable due to vernix caseosa, an insulating layer covering the fetus, while the MCG signal increases [62]. After the 30th week, the ECG signal increases again together with the MCG signal [63].

8.7 MCG studies at rhythm disorders

MCG has proven accurate in localization of accessory pathways causing pre-excitation in Wolff-Parkinson-White syndrome [64], as well as in localization of the tachycardia points of origin [65] and premature ventricular ectopic complexes [66]. MCG have been superior to signal-averaged ECG in indicating a propensity toward life-threatening arrhythmias and magnetocardiographic intra-QRS fragmentation [67] and QT dispersion have identified post-MI patients prone to ventricular arrhythmias [68], the former being independent of the extent of LV dysfunction. All of this study targets for rhythm disorders are the relatively big signal component, QRS complex. Atrial F wave is very weak and small, so hard to detect and analyze, that is the reason why it prevents the study of atrial rhythm disorders using MCG. To overcome this hurdle of sensitivity, top-notched DROS SQUID 64 channel MCG system and software is used to detect atrial F wave easily.

8.8 MCG recording and data processing

MCG signals were recorded at supine position with about 5 minutes (30 to 60 seconds a session, several sessions) recording time under the MCG dewar. The MCG system utilizes double relaxation oscillation Superconducting Quantum Interference Device sensors [69-70]. The average noise spectral density of the whole system in a magnetic shielded room is 10 fT/√Hz @ 1 Hz and 5 fT/√Hz @ 100 Hz. The KRISS MCG has 64 planar first-order SQUID gradiometers, which measure the tangential components of the cardiomagnetic fields. Measuring tangential field components is effective to obtain the overall heart information with a relatively small area of sensor distributions, that is, feasible to detect deeply-located sources like an electrical activity caused by the atrial excitation [71]. In this system, the tri-polar magnetic field map patterns were changed into ordinary dipolar field maps by using the minimum norm estimate [72]. The typical recording time is 30 to 60 seconds and the subjects are in their supine position under the MCG dewar. In Root mean square (RMS) peak ratio, supine position gives lesser P than T in ratio, however the real size of amplitude of P wave is 1.5 fold larger in supine. Therefore, the signal of P wave is well detected in supine position from MCG (Fig.13). [71].

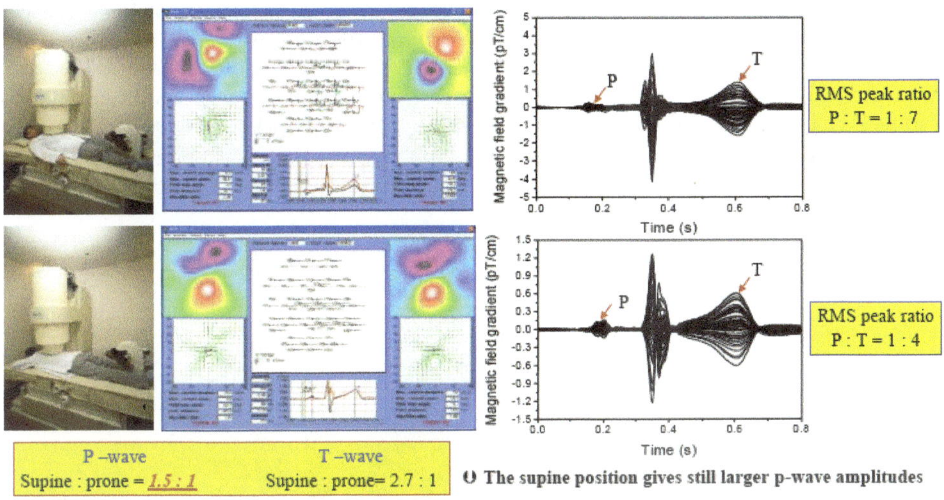

Fig. 13. Comparison of supine versus prone position for adequate MCG signal register. Modified reprinted with permission from Ref. 71

The MCG data of all subjects were analyzed by the application software KRISSMCG64 (Biomagnetism Research Center, Korea Research Institute of Standards and Science, Daejeon, KOREA). The signal processing software provides automatic digital filtering, synthetic gradiometer formation, and baseline correction for the acquired records. To analyze atrial F-wave in atrial surface, F-wave were separated from other components such as P, QRS, and T-wave component in a time sequence using Minimum variance beamformer (MVB) localization combined Independent component analysis (ICA), which separate successfully waveforms of moving current dipoles.

8.9 Generation of CT geometry for 3D heart modeling

In order to make an exact conductor model and to combine anatomical information with MCG results, Computed tomogram (CT) images were recorded previously for the individual patients. The generation procedure of geometric heart modeling is as follows: (i) Heart image preparation from computed tomography having several landmarks for co-registration with MCG, (ii) Characteristic line data extraction of the heart shape from CT images, (iii) Surface constructions from the extracted line data. This modeling is achieved by computer aided Non-Uniform Rational B-Spline (NURBS) procedure. It uses the absolute coordinate data as the reading coordinates, creates ASCII file, interpolate NURBS curve creation, generates curve by modification and optimization, and finally gives NURBS surface creation for modeling.

By the co-registration process between MCG and CT, the volumetric conductor models were established. The conductor model explains the volume current effect in calculation of forward problems with the Boundary element model, which results in a more accurate localization than in case of using a simple conductor model such as a horizontally layered model.

8.10 Propagation path tracing (Inferred route) from AMAPs

From the Activity map of action potential (AMAP) using separative Surface Potential Activation Beamformer (sSPAB) and Independent component analysis (ICA), the propagation route of the atrial activity were inferred as a MCG map. Fig. 14 shows the process for inferring an atrial excitation route originating the F-wave. The AMAP examples by using sSPAB for AF demonstrated in other patient, 70 years-old male who had severe mitral stenosis (MVA 0.67 cm^2) due to severe calcified MV leaflet, large LA (size 60 mm) and chronic AF. The measurement and analysis were shown in Fig. 14. As expected, the F-wave

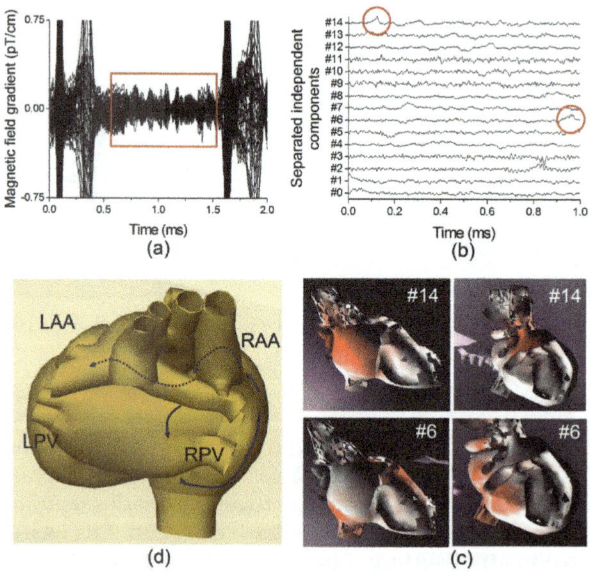

Fig. 14. The process for inferring propagation route as a MCG map. (a) Atrial fibrillation time traces recorded by using an MCG. The R-and T-waves were chopped for their relatively large amplitudes. (b) The separated independent components of the f-waves. The time window is corresponding to the red box in the Fig (a). (c) The activity maps of the action potential found by using sSPAB; the upper row is corresponding to the #14 waveform (early excitation) in Fig. (b), and the bottom row is corresponding to the #6 waveform (later excitation), respectively. The red color implies the active change in the action potential for each corresponding waveform. (d) The inferred propagation trace of the atrial excitation. LAA, left atrial appendage; RAA, right atrial appendage; LPV, left pulmonary vein; RPV, Right pulmonary vein. Reprinted with permission from Ref. 44

caused by AF is relatively small compared to R- and T-peaks. The oscillatory behavior of F-wave between the previous T-wave and the next R-waves can be observed in the multi-channel MCG record (fig. 14(a)). Using the ICA process in the sSPAB, we can separate the independent components of the F-waves and each the waveform can be marked visually time by time (fig. 14(b)). In Fig. 14(c), the Activity maps of the action potential were found by using sSPAB; the upper row is corresponding to the #14 waveform (early excitation) in Fig. 14(b), and the bottom row is corresponding to the #6 waveform (later excitation), respectively. The left panels are seen from the right lateral side of the subject and the right panels are seen from the right posterior position of the subject. The red color on the myocardium implies the active change in the action potential for each corresponding waveform. From the AMAPs at the two sequential time instants, we can infer the propagation trace of the atrial excitation. The expected propagation route was drawn in Fig. 14(d) [44].

8.11 Reproducibility test of MCG AMAP source localization

To confirm whether AF source localization by my methods is reproducible or not, MCG data sets of twelve AF patients were analyzed. From each MCG data set, seven records were collected randomly with same time interval, like as around 1 sec, 10 sec, 20 sec, 30 sec, 40 sec, 50 sec and 60 sec records from the 60 seconds MCG data, and around 1 sec, 5 sec, 10 sec,

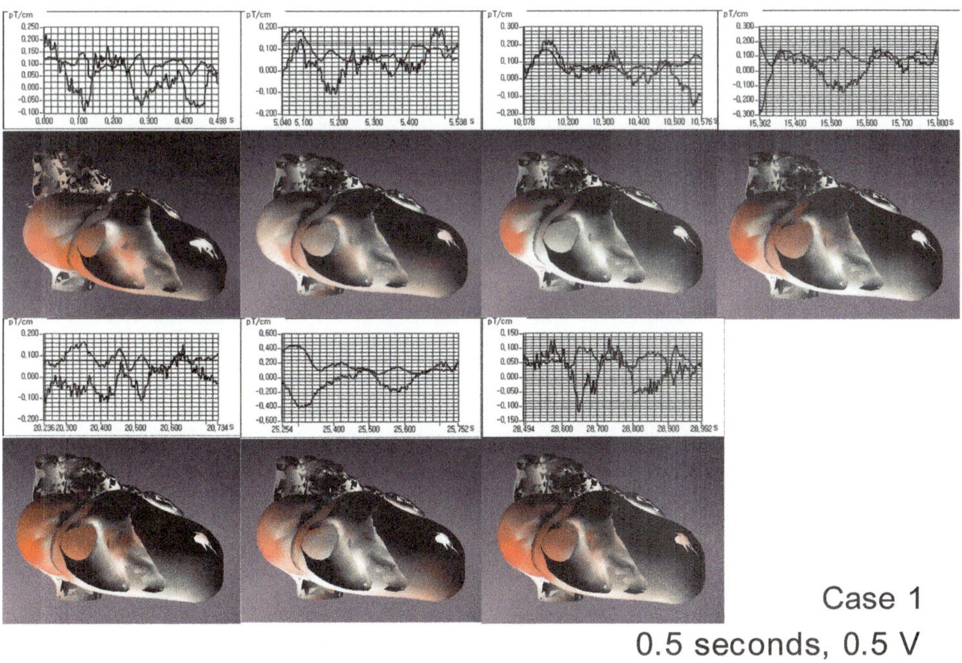

Fig. 15. Reproducibility test result of AF source localization using MCG, ICA, and sSPAB methods. Seven F wave records from different time period with 5 seconds interval shows very irregular F wave, however, their source localization results is similar each other in activity and location. Due to the irregularity of F wave characteristics, they are not completely identical in the time, activity intensity and dispersion.

15 sec, 20 sec, 25 sec, 30 sec records from the 30 seconds MCG data. Each record is 0.5 second-long and moved a little to acquire only F wave without QRS and T wave. Each record is used to make 3D AF source localization through baseline correction filtering without averaging, raw data analysis and 3D Equivalent double layer (EDL) localization method in sSPAB algorithm of KRISSMCG64 application software. The relative locations of AF source are similar between them, but some different in activity strength and in detailed location each other so, not completely identical in all (Fig. 15). However, the relative reproducibility is more than 5 of 7. The reason why they show no completely identical result is might be originated from the irregularity of F wave. AMAP source localization could not acquire identical acquisition of F wave in time, activity intensity, and dispersion. However, the F wave source is localized within near location with variant activity.

8.12 MCG map-guided minimal AF surgery

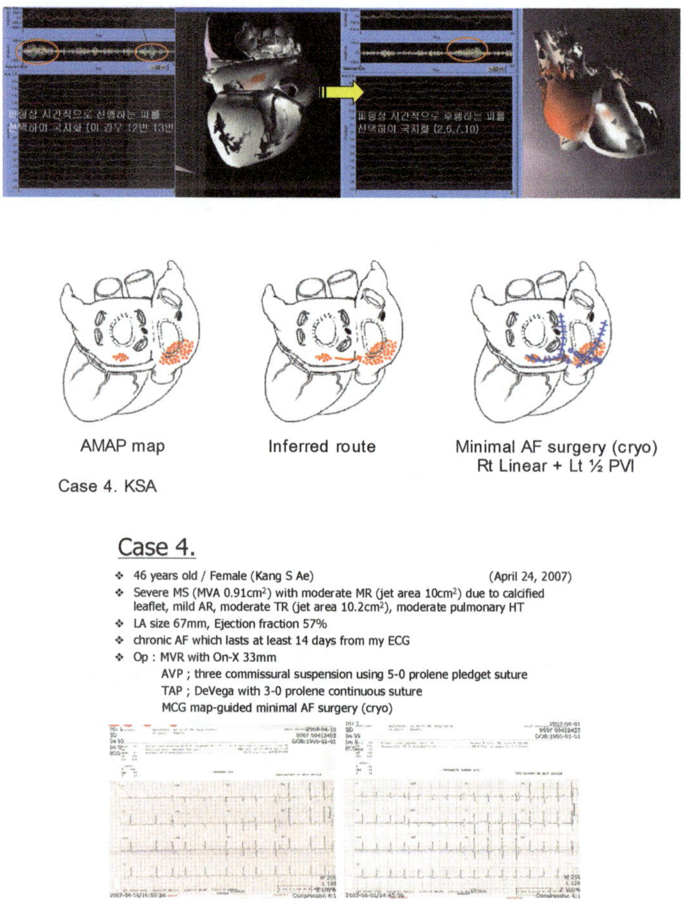

Fig. 16. Example of successful MCG map-guided minimal AF surgery. (a) Sequential 3D source localization (upper) and schematic view of AMAP map, inferred route and minimal AF surgery (lower) (b) Case summery and ECG results, pre and postoperative status.

After making the MCG map for AF, AF ablation operation method were planned, such as location and length of incision or cryo-ablation, and other combined procedures according to the patient's disease status; atrium size, valve incompetence, coronary artery stenosis, etc. Under the institutional ethical review board's approval, using MCG map, 8 cases of MCG map-guided minimal AF surgery were conducted successfully. 46 years-old female patient case is shown at fig. 16. There are no sick sinus syndrome, no permanent pacemaker insertion, 100% sinus conversion at immediate postoperative time and 5 of 7 reached sinus rhythm successfully with drug-off.

9. Conclusions

The proposed separative Surface potential activation beamformer (sSPAB) visualized successfully the Activity map of action potential (AMAP) corresponding to the F-wave in the Magnetocardiography (MCG) records of a patient with AF. In addition, a prompt visualization of the electrical excitation of the myocardium is crucial for a clinical application of the MCG. By confining the source power calculation of the sSPAB to the coordinates on the endocardial and epicardial surfaces, the AMAP could be obtained on the heart boundary in a very short time, a couple of minutes. The obtained F-waves show periodic oscillatory behaviors. By using the sSPAB, the F-wave was separated from the other activations and localized the position of a reentry circuit corresponding to the F-wave. By separating the F-wave time-by-time and visualizing the AMAP for each time-separated waveform, the propagation trace of the AF was able to be inferred.

From the reproducibility test of source localization using Equivalent double layer 3D method, the result is very similar to each other in different seven records. Map-guided AF surgery facilitates less-extensive procedures and has an ultimate benefit to patient. Smaller incision, simple minimal procedure, reduced postoperative bleeding, shortened cardiopulmonary bypass time, etc could be the advantages of map-guided surgery. MCG is a totally noninvasive and even non-contact method for analyzing AF. The visualization of the myocardial current distribution corresponding to the reentrant excitation would be a great help for planning the AF surgery and the follow-up examination. However, more technical development in sensitivity of MCG system and image processing solution are required for more accurate source localization and propagation.

10. Future experimental mappings

Ideal future mapping methods should offer (i) high sensitivity to detect very small targets, (ii) high spatio-temporal resolution to localize precisely and follow a propagation route in real-time, (iii) noninvasiveness to allow repeat exam, (iv) personalized anatomical information, (v) feasibility in clinical application, (vi) minimal adverse effects including radiation hazard. To fulfill these goals, many experimental studies are conducted. Novel mapping and imaging technologies such as cardiac MRI, MR spectroscopy, diffused optical spectroscopy, optical imaging, cardiac coherence tomography is under development for clinical use.

Optical mapping, cardiac electrical activity mapping using fluorescence imaging techniques provides unprecedented details of cardiac electrical activity at high spatial and temporal resolution and optical recordings of action potentials with signals similar to the shape and time course of action potentials recorded with intracellular microelectrodes. It can image electrical activity at sufficiently fast rates to map rapid activation of cardiac tissue during reentry, and provide detailed maps of repolarization sequences. Experimental studies using high-resolution optical mapping of impulse propagation during AF in the isolated sheep heart demonstrate that acetylcholine (Ach) dose-dependent reentrant sources in the left atrium can drive the fibrillatory activity throughout both atria. Using phase representation of the local impulse kinetics, Berenfeld *et al.* [73-74] establish that rotors can arise from unidirectional blocks of propagation at functional obstacles. Further spatiotemporal tracking of the wavebreak sites identifies a functional isthmus in the wake of such an obstacle whose minimal width supporting a figure-of-eight reentry substance is about 4 mm. In the absence of Ach, increasing the intra-atrial pressure revealed a consistent increase in the frequency and dominance of activation in an area between the atrium and a pulmonary vein with the appearance of intermittent reentrant activity there. From the development of molecular biology and genetics, channelopathy, disease of structure and function of cardiac ion channel, results in atrial tachyarrhythmias. The role of mapping in channelopathies is important subjects such as in Brugada syndrome, long-QT syndrome, idiopathic VF, etc. To overcome the limitation of current morphological and functional imaging technique, molecular cardiovascular imaging with SPECT and PET will be facilitated, which directly and noninvasively visualize molecular pathways in normal and diseased condition in vivo.

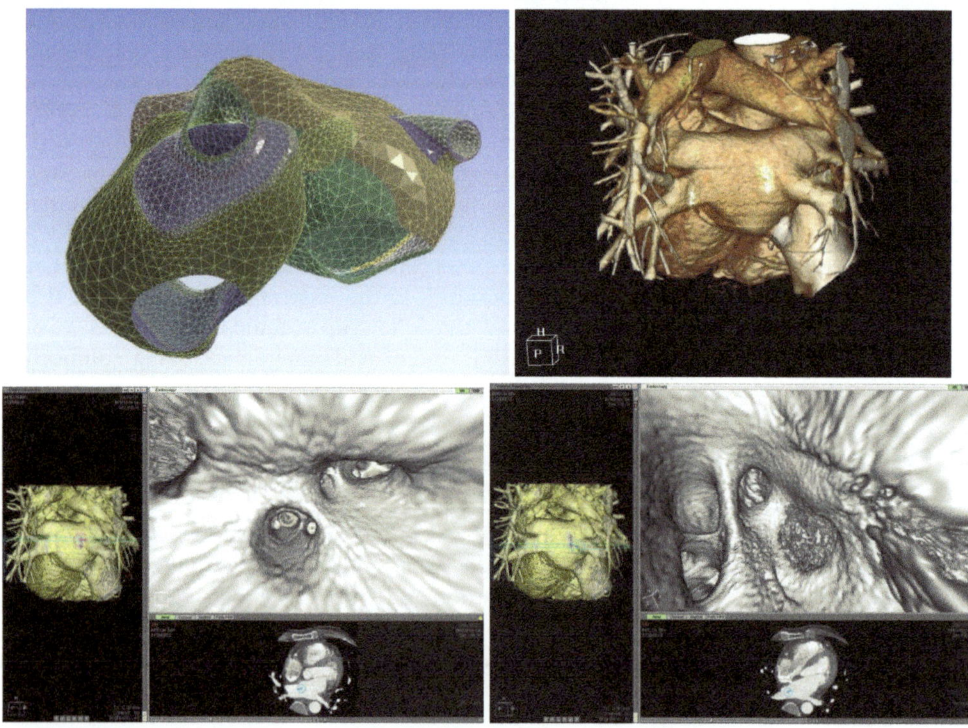

Fig. 17. Future advancement in mapping including (upper left) personalized 3D atrial modeling, (upper right) detailed anatomy information including PA, LAA, etc, (lower) detailed endoscopic view. Courtesy from Prof. Eun-Bo Shim and Whal Lee.

The role of mapping will be expanded in the fields of early detection of disease, risk evaluation, treatment guidance and outcome accessment. In technical viewpoint of mapping in AF, (i) personalized 3D atrial modeling, (ii) detailed anatomy information including PA, LAA, etc, (iii) detailed endoscopic view, (iv) real-time processing map, and (v) 4D cine-MR based map should be made near future (Fig.17).

11. References

[1] Cappato R, Calkins H, Chen SA, Davies W, Iesaka Y, Kalman J, Kim YH, Klein G, Natale A, Packer D, Skanes A, Ambrogi F, Biganzoli E. Updated worldwide survey on the methods, efficacy, and safety of catheter ablation for human atrial fibrillation. Circ Arrhythm Electrophysiol 2010; 3:32-38.

[2] Durrer D, van der Tweel LH. Spread of activation in the left ventricular wall of the dog. I. *Amer Heart J* 1953; 46:683-91.

[3] Durrer D, van der Tweel LH. Spread of activation in the left ventricular wall of the dog. II. *Amer Heart J* 1954; 47:192-203.

[4] Durrer D, van der Tweel LH, Blickman JR. Spread of activation in the left ventricular wall of the dog. III. *Amer Heart J* 1954; 48:13-35.

[5] Durrer D, van der Tweel LH, Berreklouw S, van der Wey LP. Spread of activation in the left ventricular wall of the dog. IV. *Amer Heart J* 1955; 50:860-82.

[6] Durrer D, van Dam R Th, Freud GE, Janse MJ, Meijler FL, Arzbaecher RC. Total excitation of the isolated human heart. *Circulation* 1970; 41:899-912.

[7] Wellens HJ, Janse MJ, van Dem RT, Durrer D. Epicardial excitation of the atria in a patient with atrial flutter. British Heart J 1971; 33:233-237.

[8] Durrer D, Schoo LM, Schuilenburg RM, Wellens HJJ. The role of premature beats in the initiation and the termination of supraventricular tachycardia in the Wolff-Parkinson_White syndrome. *Circulation* 1967; 36:644-62.

[9] Taccardi B. Distribution of heart potentials on dog's thoracic surface. Circ Res 1962; 11:862-69.

[10] Taccardi B. Distribution of heart potentials on the thoracic surface of normal human subjects. Circ Res 1963; 12:341-52.

[11] SippensGroenewegen A, Roithinger FX, Peeters HA, Linnenbank AC, van Hemel NM, Steiner PR, *et al.* Body surface mapping of atrial arrhythmias: Atlas of paced P wave integral maps to localize the focal origin of right atrial tachycardia. *J Electrocardiol* 1998; 31(Suppl):85-91.

[12] SippensGroenewegen A, Lesh MD, Roithinger FX, Ellis WS, Steiner PR, Saxon LA, Lee RJ, Scheinman MM. Body surface mapping of counterclockwise and clockwise typical atrial flutter: A comparative analysis with endocardial activation sequence mapping. *J Am Coll Cardiol* 2000; 35:1276-1287.

[13] Guillem MS, Climent AM, Castells F, Husser D, Millet J, Arya A, Piorkowski C, Bollmann A. Noninvasive mapping of human atrial fibrillation. *J Cardiovasc Electrophysiol* 2008; 1-7.

[14] Ramanathan C, Ghanem RN, Jia P, Ryu K, Rudy Y. Noninvasive electrocardiographic imaging for cardiac electrophysiology and arrhythmia. *Nat Med* 2004 April; 10(4):422-28.

[15] Wang Y, Schuessler RB, Damiano RJ, Woodard PK, Rudy Y. Noninvasive electrocardiographic imaging (ECGI) of scar-related atypical atrial flutter. Heart Rhythm 2007; 4(12):1565-67.
[16] Pfeifer B, Hanser F, Seger M, Fischer G, Modre-Osprian R, Tilg B. Patient-specific volume conductor modeling for non-invasive imaging of cardiac electrophysiology. The Open Medical Informatics J 2008; 2:32-41.
[17] Gepstein L, hayam G, Ben HS. A novel method for non-fluoroscopic catheter-based electroanatomical mapping of the heart: in vitro and in vivo accuracy results. *Circulation* 1997; 95:1611-22.
[18] Ben-Haim SA, Osadchy D, Schuster I et al. Nonfluoroscopic, in vivo navigation and mapping technology. *Nat Med* 1996; 2:1393-95.
[19] Firat Duru. CARTO Three-Dimensional Non-Fluoroscopic Electroanatomic Mapping for Catheter Ablation of Arrhythmias: A Useful Tool or an Expensive Toy for the Electrophysiologist? Anadolu Kardiyol Derg 2002; 4:330-7.
[20] Gepstein L, Hayam G, Ben-Haim SA. A novel method for nonfluoroscopic catheter-based electroanatomical mapping of the heart. In vitro and in vivo accuracy results. Circulation 1997; 21:1268-78.
[21] Pflaumer A, Deisenhofer I, Hausleiter J, Zrenner B. Mapping and ablation of atypical flutter in congenital heart disease with a novel three-dimensional mapping system (CARTO Merge). Europace 2006; 8:138-139.
[22] Wittkampf F, Wever E, Derksen R et al. LocaLisa: new technique for real-time 3-dimensional localization of regular intracardiac electrodes. *Circulation* 1999; 99:1312-17.
[23] Early MJ, Showkathali R, Alzetani M et al. Radiofrequency ablation of arrhythmias guided by nonfluoroscopic catheter location: a prospective randomized trial. *Eur heart J* 2006; 27:1223-29.
[24] Patel AM, d'Avila A, Neuzil P, Kim SJ, Mela T, Singh JP, Ruskin JN, Reddy VY. Atrial tachycardia after ablation of persistent atrial fibrillation. Circ Arrhythmia Electrophysiol. 2008; 1:14-22.
[25] De Groot NM, Bootsma M, van der Velde ET, Schalij MJ. Three-dimensional catheter positioning during radiofequency ablation in patients: first application of a real-time position management system. *J Cardiovasc Electrophysiol* 2000;11:1183-92.
[26] Watanabe I, Min N, Okumura Y, Ohkubo K, Kofune M, Ashino S, Nagashima K, Nakai T, Kasamaki Y, Hirayama A. Temperature-controlled cooled-tip radiofrequency linear ablation of the atria guided by a realtime position management system. Int Heart J 2011; 52:50-55.
[27] Moe GK, Abildskov JA. Atrial fibrillation as a self-sustaining arrhythmia independent of focal discharge. Am Heart J 1959; 58:59-70.
[28] Wijffels MC, Kirchof CJ, Dorland R, Allessie MA. Atrial fibrillation begets atrial fibrillation. A study in awake chronically instrumented goats. Circ 1995; 92:1954-68.
[29] Cox JL, Boineau JP, Schuessler RB, Jaquiss RD, Lappas DG. Modification of the maze procedure for atrial flutter and atrial fibrillation. I. Rationale and surgical results. J Thorac Cardiovasc Surg 1995; 110:473-84.

[30] Cox JL, Jaquiss RD, Schuessler RB, Boineau JP. Modification of the maze procedure for atrial flutter and atrial fibrillation. II. Surgical technique of the maze III procedure. J Thorac Cardiovasc Surg 1995; 110:485-95.

[31] Willems S, Klemm H, Rostock T, Brandstrup B, Ventura R, Steven D, Risius T, Lutomsky B, Meinertz T. Substrate modification combined with pulmonary vein isolation improves outcome of catheter ablation in patients with persistent atrial fibrillation: a prospective randomized comparison. Eur Heart J 2006; 27:2871-78.

[32] Lin YJ, Tai CT, Kao T, Chang SL, Lo LW, Tuan TC, Udyavar AR, Wongcharoen W, Hu YF, Tso HW, Tsai WC, Chang CJ, Ueng KC, Higa S, Chen SA. Spatiotemporal organization of the left atrial substrate after circumferential pulmonary vein isolation of atrial fibrillation. Circ Arrhythmia Electrophysiol. 2009; 2:233-241.

[33] Nademanee K, McKenzie J, Kosar E, Schwab M, Sunsaneewitayakul B, Vasavakul T et al. A new approach for catheter ablation of atrial fibrillation: mapping of the electrophysiologic substrate. J Am Coll Cardiol 2004;43:2044-53.

[34] Park JH, Park SW, Kim JY, Kim SK, Jeoung B, Lee MH, Hwang C, Kim YH, Kim SS, Pak HN. Characteristics of complex fractionated atrial electrogram in the electroanatomically remodeled left atrium of patients with atrial fibrillation. Circ J 2010; 74:1557-63.

[35] Kim SK, Park JH, Kim JY, Choi JI, Joung B, Lee MH, Kim SS, Kim YH, Pak HN. High plasma concentrations of transforming growth factor-beta and tissue inhibitor of metalloproteinase-1. Circ J 2011; 75:557-564.

[36] Reithmann C, Hoffmann E, Dorwarth U, Remp T, Steinbeck G. Electroanatomical mapping for visualization of atrial activation in patients with incisional atrial tachycardias. Eur Heart J 2001; 22:237-246.

[37] Nakagawa H, Shah N, Matsudaira K et al. Characterization of reentrant circuit in macroreentrant right atrial tachycardia after surgical repair of congenital heart disease: isolated channels between scars allow "focal" ablation. Circ 2001; 103:699-709.

[38] De Groot NMS, Kuijper AFM, Blom NA et al. 3-D distribution of bipolar atrial electrogram voltages in patients with congenital heart disease. Pacing Clin Electrophysiol. 2001; 24:1334-42.

[39] Taccardi B, Arisi G, Macchi E, Baruffi S, Spaggiari S. A new intracavitary probe for detecting the site of origin of ectopic ventricular beats during one cardiac cycle. *Circulation* 1987;75:272-81.

[40] Okumura Y, Henz BD, Johnson SB, Bunch TJ, O'Brien CJ, Hodge DO, Altman A, Govari A, Packer DL. Three-dimensional ultrasound for image-guided mapping and intervention: methods, quantitative validation, and clinical feasibility of a novel multimodality image mapping system. Circ Arrhythm Electrophysiol 2008; 1:110-119.

[41] Nitta T, Ohmori H, Sakamoto S, Miyagi Y, Kanno S, Shimizu K. Map-guided surgery for atrial fibrillation. J Thorac Cardiovasc Surg 2005;129:291-9.

[42] Konings KTS, Kirchhof CJHJ, Smeets JRLM, Wellens HJJ, Penn OC, Allessie MA. High-density mapping of electrically-induced atrial fibrillation in humans. *Circulation* 1994; 89:1665-1680.

[43] Choi JI, Pak HN, Kim YH. Hybrid epicardial and endocardial catheter ablation in a patient with atrial fibrillation and suspicious left atrial thrombus. Circ J 2009; 73:384-87.

[44] Doosang Kim, Kiwoong Kim, Yong-Ho Lee, Hyuk Ahn. Detection of atrial arrhythmia in superconducting quantum interference device magnetocardiography; preliminary result of a totally-noninvasive localization method for atrial current mapping. Interact CardioVasc Thorac Surg 2007;6:274-279.

[45] Baule G, McFee R. Detection of magnetic field of the heart. Am Heart J 1963;66:95-96.

[46] Cohen D. Magnetic fields around the torso: production by electrical activity of the human heart. Science 1967;156:652-54.

[47] Cohen D, Edelsack EA, Zimmermann JE. Magnetocardiograms taken inside a shielded room with a superconducting point-contact magnetometer. Appl Phys Lett 1970;16:278-280.

[48] Saarinen M et al. The normal magnetocardiogram: I Morphology. Ann Clin Res 1978;10(suppl21):1-43.

[49] Van Leeuwen P et al. A 67-channel biomagnetometer designed for cardiology and other applications. In: Yoshimoto T et al. eds. Recent Advances in Biomagnetism. Tohoku University Pres, Sendai 1999:89-92.

[50] Montonen J et al. Magnetocardiographic functional imaging studies in Biomag laboratory. In: Aine C et al. eds. Biomag96, Proceedings of the 10th international conference on biomagnetism. Springer, New York 2000:494-497.

[51] Maniewski R, Katila T, Poutanen T, Siltanen P, Varpula T, Wikswo JP Jr. Magnetic measurements of cardiac mechanical activity. IEEE Trans Biomed Eng 1988;35(9):662-70.

[52] Plonsey R. Capability and limitations of electrocardiography and magnetocardiography. IEEE 1972;19:239-244.

[53] Nousiainen JJO Lekkala JO, Malmivuo JAV. Comparative study of the normal vector magnetocardiogram and vector electrocardiogram. J Electrocardiol 1986; 19:275-290.

[54] Lant J et al. Complementary nature of electrocardiographic and magnetocardiographic data in patients with ischemic heart disease. J Electrocardiol 1990;23:315-322.

[55] Fenici R et al. Nonfluoroscopic localization of an amagnetic catheter in a realistic torso phantom by magnetocardiographic and body surface potential mapping. Pacing Clin Electrophysiol 1998;21:2485-2491.

[56] Pesola K et al. Bioelectromagnetic localization of a pacing catheter in the heart. Phys Med Biol 1999a;44:2565-2578.

[57] Hanninen H, Takala P, Korhonen P, Oikarinen L, Makijarvi M, Nenonen J, Katila T, Toivonen L. Features of ST segment and T-wave in exercise-induced myocardial ischemia evaluated with multichannel magnetocardiography. Ann Med 2002;34(2); 120-9.

[58] Fujino K, Sumi M, Saito K, Murakami M, Hiquchi T, Nakaya Y, Mori H. Magnetocardiograms of patients with left ventricular overloading recorded with a second-derivatives SQUID gradiometer. J Electrocardiol 1984; 17(3):219-28.

[59] Karvonen M, Oikarinen L, Takala P, Kaartinen M, Rossinen J, Hanninen H, Montonen J, Nenonen J, Makijarvi M, Keto P, Toivonen L, Nieminen MS, Katila T. Magnetocardiographic indices of left ventricular hypertrophy. J Hypertens 2002;20(11):2285-92.

[60] Park JW, Jung F. Qualitative and quantitative description of myocardial ischemia by means of magnetocardiography. Biomed Technik 2004; 49:267-73.

[61] Kariniemi V, Ahopelto J, Karp PJ, Katila TE. The fetal magnetocardiogram J Perinat Med 1974;2(3):214-6.

[62] Hamada H et al. Prenatal diagnosis of long QT syndrome using fetal magnetocardiography. Prenat Diagn 1999;19:677-680.

[63] Oostendorp TF, van Oosterom A. Modeling the fetal magnetocardiogram. Clin Phys Physiol Meas 1991;12(suppl.A):15-18.

[64] Makijarvi M et al. Localization of accessory pathways in Wolff-Parkinson_White syndrome by high-resolution magnetocardiographic mapping. J Electrocardiol 1992;25:143-155.

[65] Moshage W et al. Evaluation of the non-invasive localization accuracy of the cardiac arrhythmias attainable by multichannel magnetocardiography (MCG). Int J Cardiac Imaging 1996;12:47-59.

[66] Oeff M et al. Magnetocardiographic localization of the origin of ventricular ectopic beats. Pacing Clin Electrophysiol 1994;17:517-522.

[67] Korhonen P, Montonen J, Makijarvi M, Katila T, Nieminen MS, Toivonen L. Late fields of the magnetocardiographic QRS complex as indicators of propensity to sustained ventricular tachycardia after myocardial infarction. J Cardiovasc Electrophysiol 2000;11(4):413-20.

[68] Oikarinen L et al. Postmyocardial infarction patients susceptible to ventricular tachycardia show increased T wave dispersion independent of delayed ventricular conduction. J Cardiovasc Electrophysiol 2001;12:1115-1120.

[69] Lee YH, Kwon H, Kim JM, Park YK, Park JC. Double relaxation oscillation SQUID with high flux-to-voltage transfer and its application to a biomagnetic multichannel system. J Korean Phys Soc 1998; 32(4):600.

[70] Kim K, Lee YH, Kwon H, Kim JM, Kim IS, Park YK. Optimal sensor distribution for measuring the tangential field components in MCG. Neurol Clin Neurophysiol 2004; 1:60.

[71] Kim K, Kwon H, Kim KD, Lee YH, Kim JM, Kim IS, Lim HK, Park YK, Kim D, Lim SP. Detection of Rapid Atrial Arrhythmias in SQUID Magnetocardiography. Progress in Superconductivity 2005; 7(1): 28-35.

[72] Numminen J, Ahlfors S, Ilmoniemi R, Montonen J, Neonen J. Transformation of multichannel magnetocardiographic signals to standard grid form. IEEE Trans Biomed Eng. 1995; 42(1):72-8.

[73] Jalife J, Berenfeld O, Mansour M. Mother rotors and fibrillatory conduction: a mechanism of atrial fibrillation. Cardiovasc Res 2002;54:204-16.

[74] Berenfeld O, Mandapati R, Dixit S, et al. Spatially distributed dominant excitation frequencies reveal hidden organization in atrial fibrillation in the Langendorff perfused sheep heart. J Cardiovasc Electrophysiol 2000;11:869-79.

7

Digital Signal Processing and Artificial Intelligence Methods for Intracardial Signal Complexity Evaluation

Vaclav Kremen and Lenka Lhotska
Department of Cybernetics, Faculty of Electrical Engineering, Czech Technical University in Prague
Czech Republic

1. Introduction

Advances in catheter ablation therapy have led to a widespread increase in its use in management of arrhythmias. The high success rates and low complication rates of this technique have revolutionized treatment of such conditions as Wolff-Parkinson-White syndrome, AV nodal reentrant tachycardia, and atrial tachycardia. More recently, catheter ablation has become a useful alternative to medical therapy in patients with atrial flutter and AF. Because these arrhythmias are among the most common seen in clinical practice and can at times be difficult to manage pharmacologically, primary care physicians need to be aware of new developments in treatment in order to offer an alternative to pharmacological therapy when it is contraindicated, ineffective, or poorly tolerated (Kosinski et al., 1998).
Since the milestone publication more than a decade ago by Haissaguerre et al (Haissaguerre et al., 2003) describing the role of ectopic foci within the pulmonary veins (PV), much progress has been achieved in the field of (potentially) curative ablation of atrial fibrillation. It is possible that the multiple linear lesions (ie, a mitral isthmus line, roofline) in addition to pulmonary vein isolation effectively modify AF substrate skin to a surgical Maze procedure. However, treating all chronic AF patients with an identical approach has one glaring weakness: Not all chronic AF patients are the same. Subjecting every patient to the same ablation set is not logical and likely results in many unnecessary lesions. The search for a new approach to identify target areas for AF ablation resulted in 2 new strategies in latest years: mapping of high-dominant-frequency areas and mapping of areas with stable complex fractionated atrial electrograms (CFAEs) (Nademanee, 2007). Mapping of CFAE as target sites for AF ablation has shown great promise (Nademanee et al., 2004). Nademanee et al. (Nademanee et al., 2004) concluded that CFAE areas represent critical sites for AF perpetuation and can serve as target sites for AF ablation (Kottkamp & Hindricks, 2007). Other works that showed new quantification measures of A-EGM during AF used morphological features of the atrial waves (Faes & Ravelli, 2007) in contrast to previously proposed measures to describe A-EGMs. In a recent study Scherr et al. (Scherr et al., 2007) showed the first use of an algorithm for automatic search of CFAEs and A-EGM complexity description in A-EGMs recorded during AF mapping procedures.
Nademanee et al. (Nademanee et al., 2004) sought to investigate the electrophysiological substrate and referred in their publication introduction to the work of Allessie's group. In

a landmark publication, Konings et al. (Konings et al., 1997) described high-density mapping of electrically induced AF in patients with Wolff-Parkinson-White syndrome undergoing surgery using a spoon-shaped electrode with 244 unipolar electrodes. In that study, the right atrium was investigated and was found to be activated by one or multiple wavelets propagating in different directions. Three types of right atrial activation during AF were identified. From type I to type III, the frequency and irregularity of AF increased, and the incidence of continuous electrical activity and reentry became higher (Konings et al., 1994). Electrogram morphology was found to be an indicator for collision of wavefronts (short double potentials), conduction block (long double potentials), and pivoting points or slow conduction (fragmented potentials) (Konings et al., 1997) and (Kottkamp & Hindricks, 2007). Unfortunately, mapping of high-dominant-frequency areas has been shown not to be effective in chronic AF patients (Sanders et al., 2005). On the other hand, mapping of CFAE as target sites for AF ablation has shown great promise (Nademanee et al., 2004). This approach is based on observations of several recent mapping studies in human AF. During sustained AF, CFAEs often are recorded in specific areas of the atria and exhibit surprisingly remarkable temporal and spatial stability (Nademanee et al., 2004) and (Jais et al., 1996) Nademanee et al. concluded (Nademanee et al., 2004) that CFAE areas represent critical sites for AF perpetuation and can serve as target sites for AF ablation (Kottkamp & Hindricks, 2007).
However, currently used algorithms still have some settings that need to be set up manually, so that execution of the algorithms are not fully automatic and it needs to be tested under a range of conditions. New stable algorithms for automatic evaluation of fibrillation electrograms are thus not only of scientific interest but can also provide a proper basis for selecting the most appropriate AF treatment (Kottkamp & Hindricks, 2007; Scherr et al., 2007).
In 2007 and 2008 we developed a background methodology and techniques to extract more A-EGM features that are based on several possible information dimensions (degree of freedom) of the A-EGM signal, for example entropy, DF and CFAEs based features, as well as time and frequency domain analysis features. We introduced the unique wavelet transform based algorithm for searching fractionated segments (FSs) in A-EGM signal, sequentially followed by extraction algorithms that allow to mine the information of level of fractionation of the signal (A-EGM signal complexity) based on local electrical activity, which is automatically found by this algorithm (Křemen & Lhotská, 2007b). We described and tested more than 40 features, and based on several selection criteria we selected the most important 15 features that entered the sequential steps of features evaluation and A-EGM complexity classification/evaluation (Křemen & Lhotská, 2008). The major and methodological part of this work is presented here to uncover these new possibilities of artificial intelligence and signal processing of A-EGM for broader spectrum of electrophysiologists and cardiologists or scientists who are interested in this field of AF treatments.

2. Defining A-EGM classes of fractionation

First of all, we would like to make clear what kind of measurements and A-EGM signals we had at our disposal and we used for the analysis. All atrial bipolar electrograms used in this work were collected during left-atrial endocardial mapping using 4-mm irrigated-tip ablation catheter (NaviStar, Biosense-Webster) in 12 patients (9 males and 3 females, aged 56 ± 8 years) with persistent AF. The A-EGMs acquired before the ablation procedure were band-pass filtered ($30 - 400$ Hz) and sampled at frequency of 977 Hz by CardioLab 7000 (Prucka Inc.). Continuous recording from mapping catheter was exported in digital format, and subsequently split into 1500 ms segments exhibiting good endocardial contact, stable signal pattern, and reasonable signal-to-noise ratio. A-EGM signals were stored and analyzed later in off-line regime manually by the experts.

All A-EGM signals preselected by the expert using the above described procedure were ready to be ranked by other experts into classes of fractionation (CF), which would reflect the level of fractionation of each individual A-EGM signal in dataset. This ranking was used in the study in next steps of A-EGM signal preprocessing, description (defining measures of A-EGM) and classification (see sections 3, 4, and 5).

Although the degree of fractionation of the A-EGM signals in the dataset, and also in reality, was assumed to be naturally continuous, a discrete set of CF was chosen for the purposes of study to be used by experts as ranking options. This was decided due to impossibility to classify signals by experts in smoother scale (the experts classified A-EGMs simply by looking at signal in time domain). From the same reason the ranking options were set up to four degree sets of classes of fractionation (four CF) for the purposes of the study. The four CF enabled to get a uniform dataset of A-EGMs with significant number of samples in each class, so that such dataset could be used in next steps in data processing, A-EGMs description and classification to get desirable statistical significance of results of experiments. These four CF were set up as ranking options for experts:

1. Organized activity – high percentage of organized signal activity in current signal (above 90 %).
2. Mild degree of fractionation – approximatelly same level of organized and disorganized activity of the signal.
3. Intermediate degree of fractionation – high percentage of disorganized activity of the signal (above 50%).
4. High degree of fractionation – disorganized A-EGM signal (highly fractionated).

Three independent experts were asked to assign each A-EGM signal in the dataset to one of four optional CF. The ranking was done manually by simply displaying an individual A-EGM signal from the dataset, looking at it in time domain (simulation of real-time mapping procedure) and assigning the signal to a considered CF. Custom written software developed for this purpose was programmed in software Matlab v.7 and it was used by each expert. The experts had the same information and condition to classify signals, which are commonly used during AF mapping procedure. They used A-EGM signal displayed on the screen followed bottom with ECG signal, captured from the same time as partial A-EGM signal, having possibility to switch between $I, aVF, V1, CS1.2, CS3.4, ABL1.2, ABL3.4$ and $Stim$ inputs. The only difference from current clinical practice was no time pressure as during real-time mapping procedure and experts had enough time to evaluate or reevaluate individual A-EGMs.

After the experts ranked a displayed A-EGM signal, they switched to next one in the dataset. They could go through all ranked signals after they performed individual ranking and they had possibility to change the ranking for partial A-EGMs to make corrections at any time of ranking procedure. No specific criteria for signal assessment (e.g. dominant frequency or percentage of continuous electrical activity) were given. The experts were just asked to classify the A-EGMs by their subjective judgment according to how the ablation at particular site would be valuable for atrial debulking. The examples of the A-EGMs assigned by experts to class $1-4$ are shown in Figure 1.

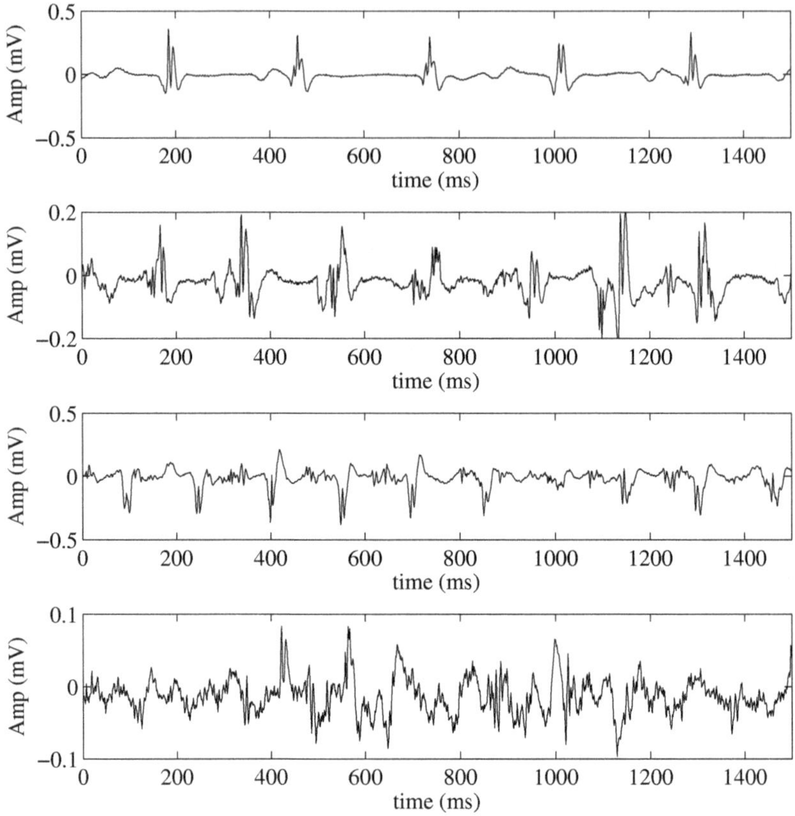

Fig. 1. Four complex fractionated atrial electrograms are shown. These are representatives of each CF used in the study. From the top to bottom:
1 – organized atrial activity,
2 – mild,
3 – intermediate,
4 – high degree of fractionation.

3. A-EGM signal preprocessing

Signal preprocessing plays a very important role for further A-EGM signal analysis and classification of level of fractionation of a given A-EGM signal. In this section the main problem which normally arises in signal processing task is described, namely signal denoising. The filtering methods will be presented as part of wavelet framework. Other filtering approaches, such as classical and adaptive filters (AR, ARMAX models (Gustafsson, 2000) etc.) were also tested and can be used for filtering of A-EGM, but for the presented tasks of A-EGM preprocessing and further features extraction the best results were achieved by wavelet filtering methods. In this section, attention is focused on the application of wavelet transform and filters. A concrete denoising of A-EGM signal will be demonstrated.

Fundamental viewpoints of wavelet transform merely for terminology and notation conventions are presented as a background of the A-EGM preprocessing used during this application. More detailed information on this topic can be found in (Burrus, 1997; Daubechies, 1992).

3.1 Wavelet transform

The classical Fourier transform (FT) is not suitable if the signal has time varying frequency, i.e. the signal is non-stationary. This means that the FT tells whether a certain frequency component exists or not. This information is independent on where in time this component appears. It is possible to analyze any signal by using an alternative approach called wavelet transform (WT). WT analyzes the signal at different frequencies with different resolutions. WT is designed to give good time resolution and poor frequency resolution at high frequencies and good frequency resolution and poor time resolution at low frequencies (Novak, 2003). This approach makes sense especially when the signal at hand has high frequency components for short durations and low frequency components for long durations, which is the case in most biological signals, mainly EEG, EMG, ECG and also A-EGM. One example of the wavelet analysis of A-EGM of CF 1 is shown in Figure 2.

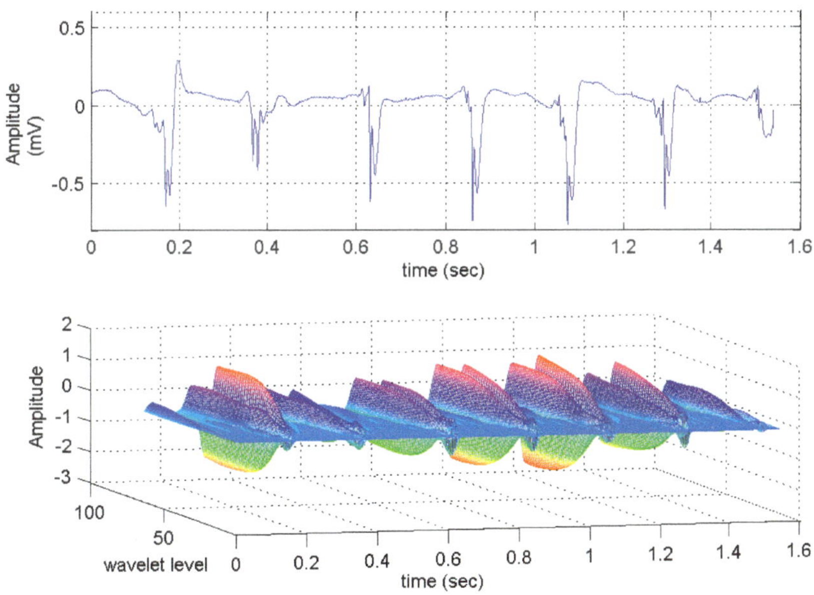

Fig. 2. Example of continuous Wavelet Transform (CWT) for A-EGM signal, which was ranked by three independent experts into class 1 – organized atrial activity. The A-EGM signal to be decomposed by CWT is shown at the top. Corresponding wavelet coefficients are depicted at the bottom.

3.2 Finalized A-EGM wavelet filter

In the described approach we used filtering (de-noising) of A-EGM signals performed using wavelet transform filter based on multilevel signal decomposition and thresholding of detailed coefficients (Mallat, 1999) described bellow. We found optimal filter setup by particle swarm optimization procedure (Křemen et al., 2007). The Coiflet of order four mother wavelet (MW) was used to decompose signal into 5 levels (Daubechies, 1992). Detail coefficients were thresholded by soft-thresholding (Donoho, 1995) with these settings of thresholds (level 1 (WT_{L1}) to level 5 (WT_{L5})): $0.02, 0.04, 0.008, 0.008, 0.008$. Reconstruction of the filtered signal was computed by wavelet reconstruction based on the original approximation coefficients and the modified detail coefficients of levels from 1 to 5.
Figure 3(a) shows a wavelet decomposition of A-EGM signal at 5 levels using Coiflet mother wavelet. From the Figure 3(a) subfigures a_1 and a_2 it is obvious that the main noise is focused in level 1 and 2 that corresponds to optimal filter thresholds setup found by optimization procedure (thresholds $WT_{L1} = 0.02$ and $WT_{L2} = 0.04$) (Křemen et al., 2007). Figure 3(b) shows the progression of described de-nosing procedure using optimal filter setup found by optimization procedure (Křemen et al., 2007). The optimal thresholds setup is used and depicted together with detailed coefficients before and after thresholding. The filtered signal shows the effectiveness of the filter that can be seen by watching the signal (Figure 4) or by comparing residuals in Figure 5.
Unfortunately, although using strong optimization particle swarm optimization procedure, some useful information for A-EGM classification was probably discarded during filtering process. This can be seen in analysis of residuals in Figure 5. The autocorrelation diagram of filtering residuals still shows some patterns, that are slightly correlated. It is obvious that these parts of the filtered signal are about tenth of amplitude of original signal in this partial example of the A-EGM signal which we are using here in this chapter for demostration of filtering. But although we used and tested more filtering approaches (classical filters, adaptive filters, wavelet filters) and strong optimization procedure, this effect of the filter could not be probably avoided. We concluded that the method outperformed the classical approaches as median or elliptic filters and that also after visual inspection the obtained results looked very clean which can be seen in Figure 4. This figure finally shows the example of original and filtered A-EGM signal to demonstrate the filtering efficacy in relation to visual aspects only.

4. A-EGM signal description - finding attributes

4.1 Basic concepts of feature construction

Before any modelling and classification of the signal takes place, a data representation must be chosen. In this chapter data is represented by a fixed number of features which can be binary, categorical or continuous. Feature is synonymous of input variable or attribute[1]. Finding a good data representation is very domain specific and related to available measurements. In A-EGM signal processing task, the "raw" data is represented by the matrix of A-EGM signals of 1.5 s length resampled at 1 kHz (section 2) and the extracted features (measures of A-EGM signal) that will be described in this section. That is, a set of variables of A-EGM signal that

[1] It is sometimes necessary to make the distinction between "raw" input variables and "features" or "measures" of signal that are variables constructed from the original input variables. Original input variables are in that case time series of amplitudes of the signal or other representation of this time domain signal (for example frequency spectrum of the A-EGM or wavelet representation of A-EGM). We will make it clear when this distinction is necessary.

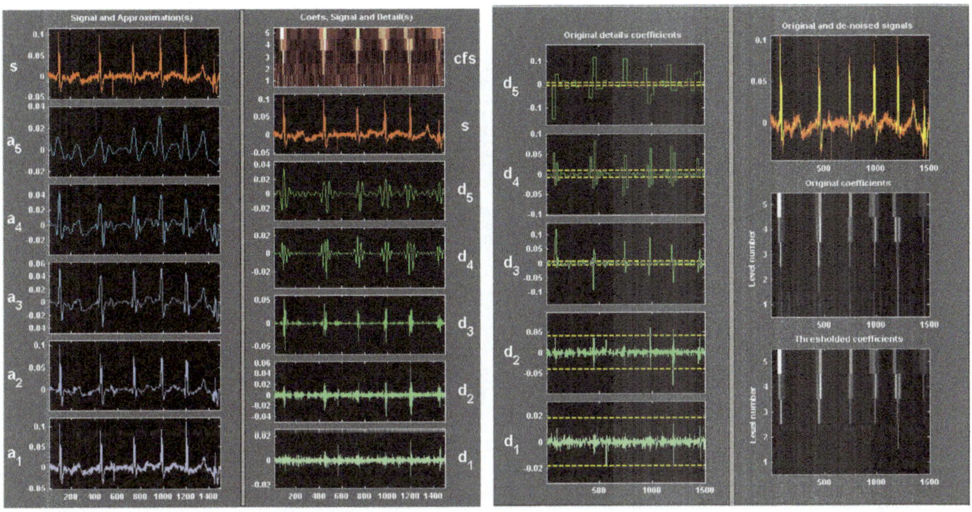

(a) Wavelet decomposition of A-EGM signal of CF 1.

(b) Wavelet denoising of A-EGM signal of CF 1

Fig. 3. (a) Wavelet decomposition of A-EGM signal, ranked by experts into CF 1. Decomposition at 5 levels was used performed with Coiflet of order four mother wavelet. Approximations and details are shown. From approximations and details of level 1 and 2 it is obvious that the main noise is focused in level 1 and 2, which corresponds to filter thresholds setup.
(b) Wavelet denoising of the same A-EGM signal shown on (a). The original signal is depicted in red and the filtered signal in yellow color. Decomposition at 5 levels was used and performed with Coiflet of order four mother wavelet. Thresholding of the detailed coefficients at 5 levels was performed to de-noise the signal. Dashed yellow lines show the values of individual optimal thresholds at all levels.

enable to categorize the A-EGM complexity (continually or to discrete classes of fractionation $1-4$).

4.2 Measurement of intervals between discrete peaks

The extraction of this A-EGM feature (measure) is based on an algorithm that works in time domain and calculates index of fractionation of A-EGM as a mean of the intervals between discrete peaks of A-EGMs (Figure 6), which are detected using input parameters of the algorithm: peak-to-peak sensitivity, signal width and refractory period. Input parameters of this algorithm were found by exhaustive search ($10x10$ validation) using measured dataset of A-EGM. The finally used optimal settings of the algorithm are: sensitivity = 0.2 mV, signal width = 8 ms, refractory period = 14 ms. The feature is refereed to as MIDP in the chapter. This algorithm was first introduced by (Křemen et al., 2008).

4.3 Features based on description of local activation waves found automatically in A-EGM

These algorithms for A-EGM features extraction were developed in frame of this new methodology of A-EGM processing we introduce here. It enables to describe A-EGM

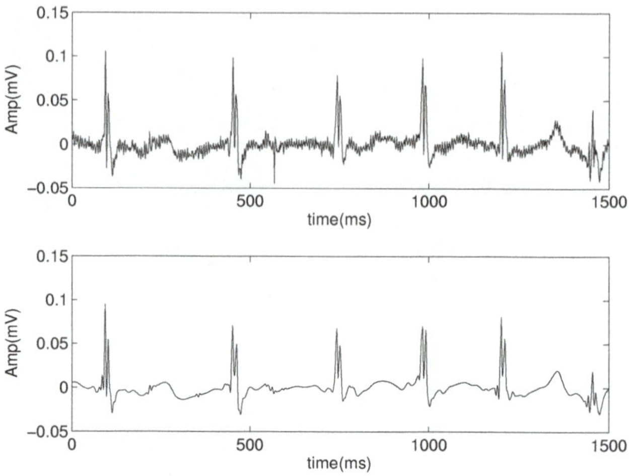

Fig. 4. The original (top) and filtered (bottom) A-EGM signal of CF 1. The filtering was performed by described wavelet filter.

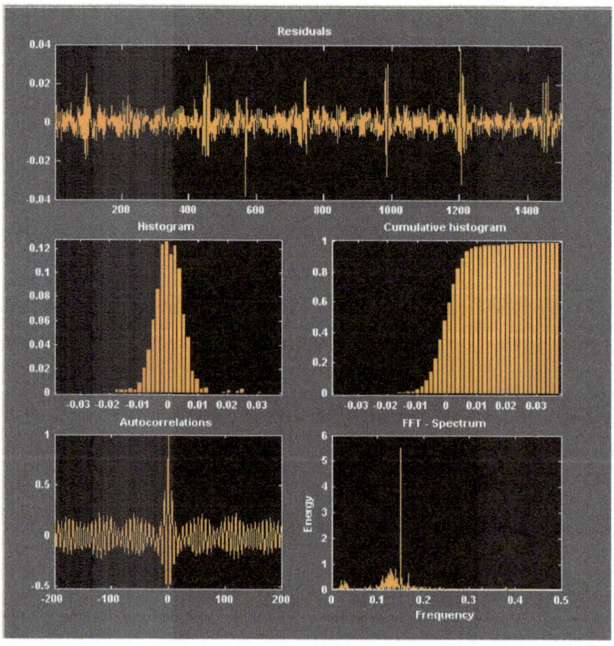

Fig. 5. The analysis of residuals after wavelet denoising procedure using described filter for A-EGM signal of CF 1. The residuals and autocorrelation diagrams show that some information about segments of local activation in A-EGM was filtered out with noise even in the best found "optimal" filter setup.

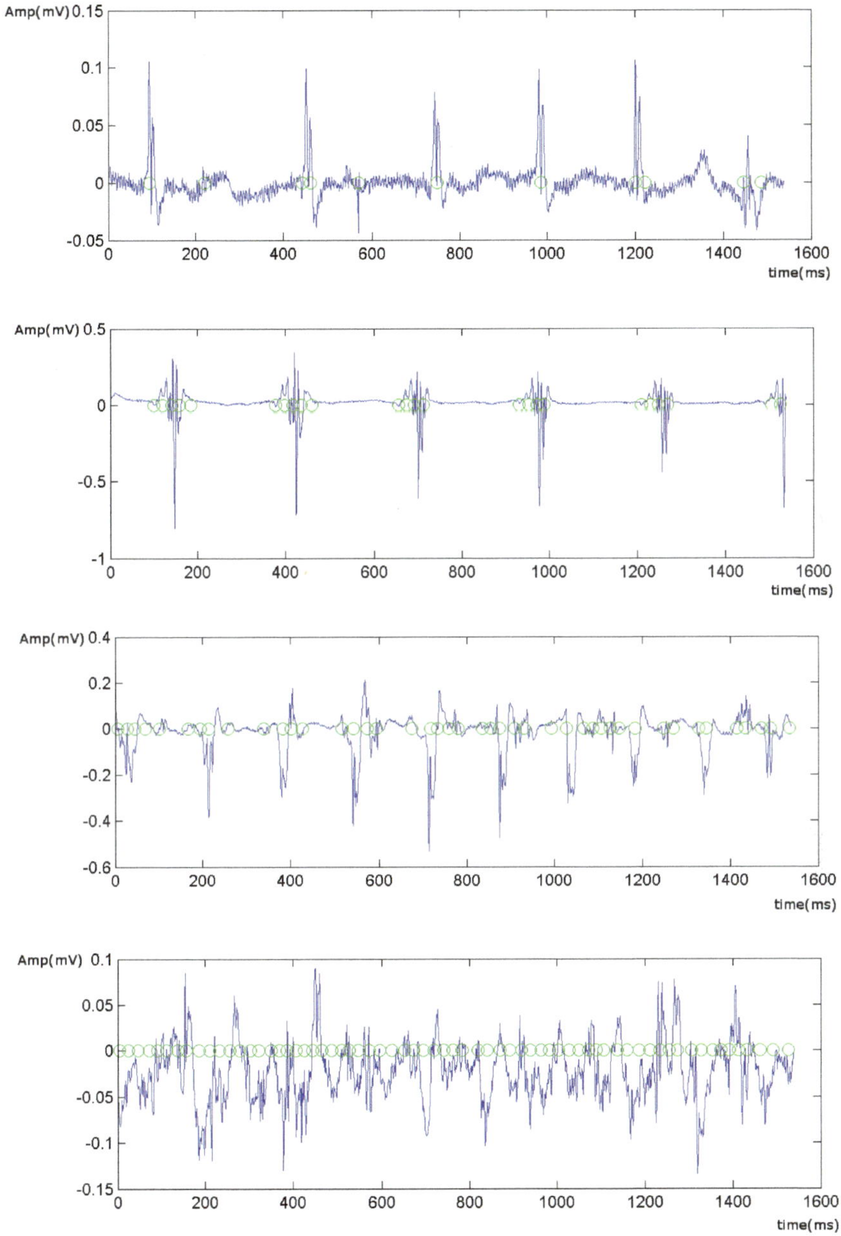

Fig. 6. The A-EGM representatives of each defined CF from cleared dataset are shown (from class 1 to class 4 from the top to bottom). Green circles show found discrete peaks of the signal defined by sensitivity 0.02 mV, signal width 8 ms and refractory period 14 ms in each A-EGM.

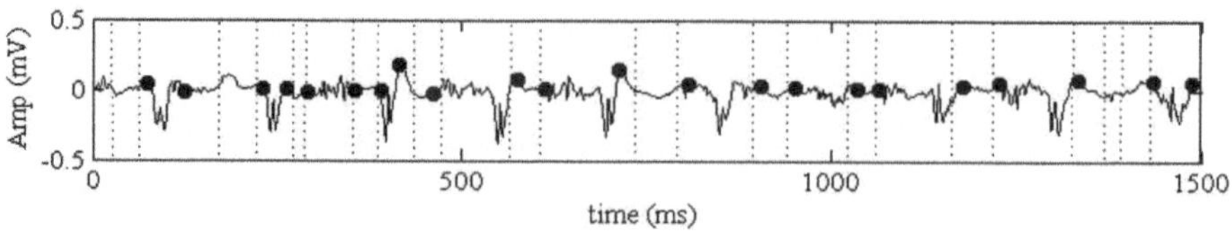

Fig. 7. Original A-EGM signal recorded during AF mapping procedure of persistent AF captured in left atria. Experts' ranking of the signal was into CF 3. Black dots denote the beginnings and the ends of FSs marked manually by expert to made a gold standard for comparison and optimizing of FSs searching algorithms. Dashed lines denote the beginnings and the ends of FSs found automatically by WTA.

complexity in a new way. The algorithms perform several automatic signal preprocessing steps. Based on this preprocessing, the algorithms then automatically search for areas of the A-EGM signal, where local electrical activity is found (areas of interest – fractionated segments (FSs), see Figure 7), also described by Faes et al. as local activation waves (LAWs) (Faes et al., 2007) and (Faes & Ravelli, 2007). Several features of A-EGM are then defined based on automatic FSs description. The features are therefore derived from the characteristics of the automatically observed FSs or LAWs.

Algorithm for automatic searching FSs

Fist we describe the algorithm for automatic searching FSs and then derived extraction of defined A-EGM measures. The problem of searching FSs is similar to problems of adaptive segmentation of the signal. The aim is to find the best algorithm that searches automatically (without need of a supervisor) for local electrical activity in the A-EGM signal to find FSs in that signal (Figure 7). We tried to approach the A-EGM signal in time domain only and also tried to find other adaptive segmentation methods suitable for this task, but the results were significantly worse than the results produced by the novel algorithm (Křemen & Lhotská, 2007b; 2008) that used a wavelet decomposition. We introduce this algorithm here very briefly. The algorithm searched for segments with local electrical activity (FSs) within A-EGMs (Figure 8a). The denoised signal (Figure 8b) was decomposed by discrete wavelet transform multilevel decomposition into 5 levels using the Coiflet wavelet of order 4. The detailed coefficients of the signal were reconstructed at level 3 (L_3). L_3 was normalized to its maximum absolute value (Figure 8c) and thresholded at 0.014 (A_T) (Figure 8d). All parts of the signal with non-zero absolute amplitude were set to arbitrary value of 1 denoting primary FSs (Figure 8e). Secondary FSs were defined as all nests of adjacent primary FSs with intersegment space < 5 ms (T_T). The individual steps of the algorithm are shown in Figure 8. The parameters of this algorithm (type of mother wavelet, decomposition level L_3, thresholds A_T, and T_T) were found by particle swarm optimization technique (Křemen & Lhotská, 2007a). The individual steps of the algorithm are thoroughly shown in (Křemen & Lhotská, 2007b) and (Křemen & Lhotská, 2008). The algorithm is refereed to as WTA (wavelet transform algorithm) here.

New A-EGM measures defined

We designed this WTA as the basic preprocessing algorithm that serves to automatically search through measured A-EGM signal to find FSs in that signal. Based on these found

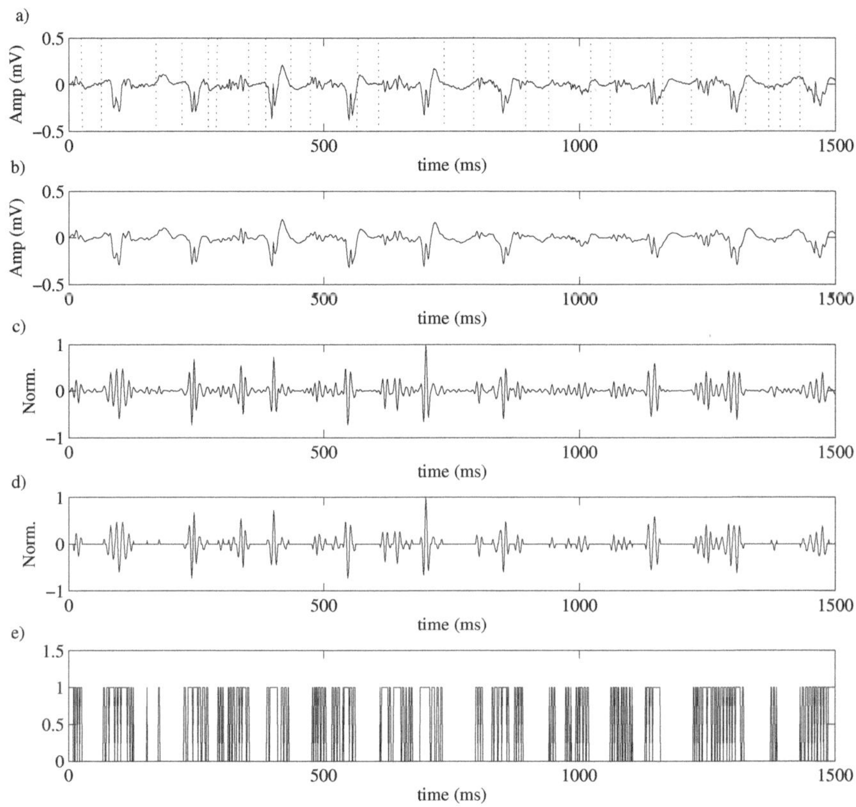

Fig. 8. a) De-noised A-EGM signal, assigned by three experts to class 3 is filtered by proposed wavelet filtering algorithm (b). The filtered signal entered the algorithm to find the individual FSs in that signal. c) Level 3 of the detailed coefficients of the discrete wavelet transform normalized with respect to its absolute maximal value. This signal was used to identify the individual FSs of the original A-EGM signal. d) The signal from c) thresholded by threshold value 0.014. e) The individual signal peaks (primary FSs) are marked by value 1. The peaks show areas of interest, where local electrical activity is visible. These peaks are joined/merged by threshold 5 ms to form areas of individual FSs (secondary FSs). The beginnings and ends of the automatically observed FSs are marked by dashed lines.

FSs we can define then several statistically dependent or independent features of A-EGM. We describe these individual features here briefly. To introduce these features we often use the statistical measures that are commonly known. We also tested other statistical measures, such as weighted mean etc., but they did not give such good results in A-EGM classification, therefore we did not introduce them here.

Number of fractionated segments

We defined a feature FS as a number of fractionated segments found by WTA in particular A-EGM signal in the dataset.

Statistical description of inflexion points in FSs

Number of Inflection Points calculated in automatically found FSs in A-EGM was defined as the new feature IPFS. We also defined four new features based on statistical analysis of IPFS in current one A-EGM signal:

- **MINIPFS** – Minimum of Inflection Points in found FSs in a particular A-EGM signal.
- **MAXIPFS** – Maximum of Inflection Points in found FSs in a particular A-EGM signal.
- **MIPFS** – Arithmetical Mean value of Inflection Points added together in automatically found FSs and calculated as $\bar{x} = 1/N \cdot \sum_{i=1}^{N} x_i$, where x_i is a number of inflection points in one FS number i, and N is total number of FS in particular A-EGM.
- **SDIPFS** – We used Standard Deviation of Inflection Points added together in automatically found FSs and calculated as $\sigma = \sqrt{1/N \cdot \sum_{i=1}^{N} (x_i - \bar{x})^2}$, where x_i is a number of inflection points in one FS number i, and N is total number of FS in particular A-EGM.

Statistical description of Zero level crossing points in FSs

Number of Zero level crossing points (the points where the signal changes the sign or the polarity) calculated in automatically found FSs in A-EGM was used as the new feature ZCPFS. We defined four new features based on statistical analysis of ZCPFS in current one A-EGM signal:

- **MAXZCPFS** – Maximum of Zero level Crossing Points in found FSs.
- **MINZCPFS** – Minimum of Zero level Crossing Points in found FSs.
- **MZCPFS** – Arithmetical Mean value of Zero level Crossing Points added together in automatically found FSs and calculated as $\bar{x} = 1/N \cdot \sum_{i=1}^{N} x_i$, where x_i is a number of inflection points in one FS number i, and N is total number of FS in particular A-EGM.
- **SDZCPFS** – We used Standard Deviation of Zero level Crossing Points added together in automatically found FSs and calculated as $\sigma = \sqrt{1/N \cdot \sum_{i=1}^{N} (x_i - \bar{x})^2}$, where x_i is a number of inflection points in one FS number i, and N is total number of FS in particular A-EGM.

Statistical description of inter-segment distance of FSs

The new feature was defined and calculated as total length of all inter-segment distances in particular A-EGM and refereed to as TDFS. We defined two new features based on statistical analysis of inter-segment distance of automatically found FSs in A-EGM signal:

- **MDFS** – Arithmetical Mean value of inter-segment distance of automatically found FSs calculated as $\bar{x} = 1/N \cdot \sum_{i=1}^{N} x_i$, where x_i is the inter-segment distance i of two corresponding FSs, and N is total number of inter-segment distances found automatically in particular A-EGM.
- **SDDFS** – We used Standard Deviation of inter-segment distance of automatically found FSs calculated as $\sigma = \sqrt{1/N \cdot \sum_{i=1}^{N} (x_i - \bar{x})^2}$, where x_i is the inter-segment distance i of two corresponding FSs, and N is total number of inter-segment distances found automatically in particular A-EGM.

Statistical description of width of FSs

This new feature was defined as sum of width of all FSs found in particular A-EGM, refereed to as TWFS. We also defined four new features based on statistical analysis of the widths of automatically found FSs in A-EGM signal:

- **MINWFS** – Minimal width of found FSs in particular A-EGM signal.
- **MAXWFS** – Maximal width of found FSs in particular A-EGM signal.
- **MWFS** – Arithmetical Mean value of widths of automatically found FSs calculated as $\bar{x} = 1/N \cdot \sum_{i=1}^{N} x_i$, where x_i is the width of one FS i, and N is total number of FSs found automatically in particular A-EGM.
- **SDWFS** – We used Standard Deviation of widths of automatically found FSs calculated as $\sigma = \sqrt{1/N \cdot \sum_{i=1}^{N} (x_i - \bar{x})^2}$, where x_i is the width of one FS i, and N is total number of FSs found automatically in particular A-EGM.

Statistical description of maxima of amplitude in FSs

Three new features were defined based on statistical analysis of maxima of amplitudes in automatically found FSs in A-EGM signal:

- **MAXAFS** – Maximal absolute value of Amplitude in found FSs in particular A-EGM signal.
- **MAFS** – Arithmetical Mean value of maximal absolute value of Amplitude in automatically found FSs calculated as $\bar{x} = 1/N \cdot \sum_{i=1}^{N} x_i$, where x_i is the maximal absolute value of amplitude in one FS number i, and N is total number of FSs found automatically in particular A-EGM.
- **SDAFS** – We used Standard Deviation of maximal absolute value of Amplitude in automatically found FSs calculated as $\sigma = \sqrt{1/N \cdot \sum_{i=1}^{N} (x_i - \bar{x})^2}$, where x_i is the maximal absolute value of amplitude in one FS number i, and N is total number of FSs found automatically in particular A-EGM.

Mean interval of peaks found in FSs

We used the features described in Section 4.2 and calculated the same features only for automatically found fractionated segments. We therefore acquired four new features:

1. **MIDPFS** – Mean of the Intervals between Discrete Peaks of A-EGM in found FSs.
2. **FIDPFS** – Mean of Intervals between Discrete Peaks using filtered A-EGM signals and in found FSs.

3. **NIDPFS** – Mean of Intervals between Discrete Peaks using normalized A-EGM signals and in found FSs.
4. **FNIDPFS** – Mean of Intervals between Discrete Peaks using filtered and normalized A-EGM signals and in found FSs.

Joining features MIDP & FIP & IPFS

We aggregated two features MIDP and IPFS into one MIDP&IPFS feature using simple formula: MIDP&IPFS = $\sqrt{MIDP^2 + IPFS^2}$, and next two features FIP and IPFS into new feature FID&IPFS by adding: FIP&IPFS = FIP + IPFS.

Measurement of morphological regularity and similarity of FSs

As showed by Faes et al., a morphological variations of the consecutive atrial depolarization waves (FSs or LAWs) can be described by an automated algorithm (Faes et al., 2007) and (Faes & Ravelli, 2007). Faes et al. also showed that atrial activity has a repetitive characteristics and regularity of present LAWs during organized atrial rhythms (flutter or type I AF) and on the contrary, highly disorganized electrograms showing fragmented LAWs with complex morphology contain more dissimilar LAWs, thus leading to zero the probability to find similar depolarizations (Faes & Ravelli, 2007). The algorithms describing the morphological similarity thus could play an important role to describe A-EGM complexity. We suggested and implemented a simple algorithm, which automatically describes the morphological similarity of automatically found FSs in individual A-EGM from used datasets.
The WTA algorithm was first used to find the FSs in currently processed A-EGM. Let's consider A-EGM signal $\mathbf{x}$ of length N, where $\mathbf{x} = [x_1, x_2, ...x_N]$. The FSs found by WTA in A-EGM signal $\mathbf{x}$ can be written as $\mathbf{y}$, where $\mathbf{y} = [\mathbf{y}_1, \mathbf{y}_2, ...\mathbf{y}_m]$, where m is the number of found FSs. We performed the estimate of cross-correlation of $\mathbf{x}$, and all vectors in $\mathbf{y}$. One cross-correlation of $\mathbf{x}$ and $\mathbf{y}_i$, where $i \in (1, m)$ was defined as:

$$\widehat{\mathbf{R}}_{xy_i}(m) = \begin{cases} \sum_{n=0}^{N-m-1} x_{n+m} y_{i_n}^* & m \geq 0 \\ \widehat{\mathbf{R}}_{xy_i}^*(-m) & m < 0 \end{cases} \tag{1}$$

If length of $\mathbf{y}_i$ was less than N, the vector $\mathbf{y}_i$ was zero padded to number of samples N.
The sequence $\widehat{\mathbf{R}}_{xy_i}$ was then normalized with respect to its absolute maxima, therefore normalized cross-correlation of $\mathbf{x}$ and $\mathbf{y}_i$ was calculated as: $\widehat{\mathbf{R}}'_{xy_i} = \widehat{\mathbf{R}}_{xy_i} / max|\widehat{\mathbf{R}}_{xy_i}|$. Thresholding of $\widehat{\mathbf{R}}'_{xy_i}$ was used to found the segments, where the higher correlation of $\mathbf{x}$ and $\mathbf{y}_i$ is present. Threshold $\delta = 0.7$ was find by particle swarm optimization procedure (Křemen & Lhotská, 2007a) to set to zero the segments of $\widehat{\mathbf{R}}'_{xy_i}$ with less correlated $\mathbf{x}$ and $\mathbf{y}_i$:

$$\widehat{\mathbf{R}}'_{xy_i}(m) = \begin{cases} \widehat{\mathbf{R}}'_{xy_i}(m) & \delta \geq 0.7 \\ 0 & \delta < 0.7 \end{cases} \tag{2}$$

The correlation peaks were found in $\widehat{\mathbf{R}}_{xy_i}(m)$ and determined as a index of morphological similarity ρ.
The performance of the algorithm could be adjusted by using more sophisticated approach that could be object of separate investigation (e.g. using of time warping methods etc.), but we are not describing it here in the chapter.

5. A-EGM signal classification

To determine the generalization ability of a model one would need to measure the average risk for the set of all possible data objects. In real life applications it is not feasible, so we estimated the risk using a test set. When doing this we should be aware of the danger of testing models on a single test set (for example resulting from a rigid partition of the set of all available data to the training and test parts). Model selection based on testing trained models on a single test set does not get rid of the danger of overfitting. A more accurate estimation of the empirical risk can be obtained with K-fold cross-validation (Guyon et al., 2006). In this technique we split the set of available data into n parts and perform n training and test processes (each time the test set is one of the parts and the training set consists of the rest of the data). The average test risk can be a good estimate of real generalization ability of the tested algorithm, especially when the whole cross-validation is performed several times (each time with different data split) and n is appropriately chosen. To get a good estimate of generalization ability of a learning machine, it is important to analyse not only the average test error, but also its variance, which can be seen as a measure of stability.

We found out, that comparison of the 10-fold cross-validation error is not stable enough to decide, which configuration of the classifier is better. Therefore we used 10 fold 10 cross-validation setup and calculated classification errors in each step of 10 fold 10 cross-validation for each classifier. A mean value of the classification error was calculated from these errors in 10 fold cross-validation and was taken as representation of the classification results for partial classifier. The comparison of the classifiers was done using these mean errors.

Group of Adaptive Model Evolution

Group of Adaptive Models Evolution (GAME) (Kordík, 2005) proceeds from the Group Model Data Handling (GMDH) theory (Ivakhnenko, 1971). GMDH was designed to automatically generate model of the system in the form of polynomial equations. An example of inductive model created by GAME algorithm is depicted in the Figure 9. Similarly to Multi-Layered Perceptron (MLP) neural networks, GAME units (neurons) are connected in a feedforward network (model). The structure of the model is evolved by special niching genetic algorithm, layer by layer. Parameters of the model (coefficients of units' transfer functions) are optimized independently (Kordík et al., 2007). Model can be composed of units of different transfer function type (e.g sigmoid, polynomial, sine, linear, exponential, rational, etc). Units with transfer function performing well on given data set survive the evolution process and form the model. Often, units of several different types survive in one model, making it hybrid.

Here in the chapter, we using GAME models as predictors (continuous output variable) and also as classifiers (four output classes). The evolutionary design of the GAME algorithm makes this possible without need to change the learning strategy. For classification purposes, the GAME model consists mainly of units with sigmoid transfer function and for regression, polynomial, linear or exponential units are often selected to fit the input-output relationship.

Data analysis

The character of the used data set, particularly the uncertain boundary of middle classes excludes the possibility to classify into 10 classes of fractionation with reasonable error. Even for classification into four classes, we got perfect (95%) accuracy for class 1 and 4 only, the accuracy for other two classes was bad (around 65%). Reflecting these preliminary experiments we projected the data into two dimensions (using (Drchal et al., 2007)) and found

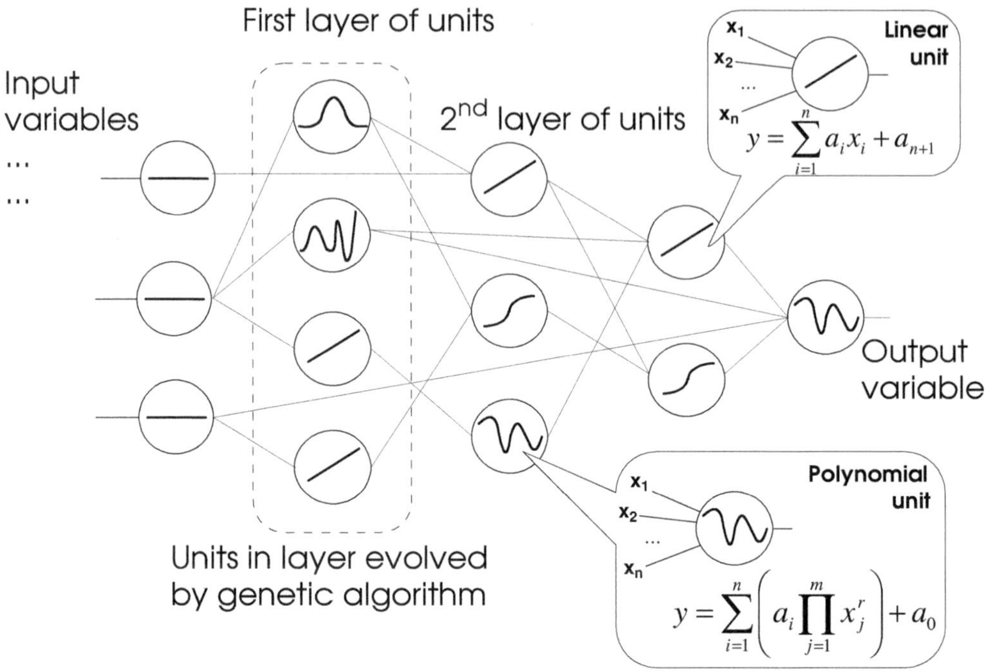

Fig. 9. The structure of the GAME model is evolved layer by layer using special genetic algorithm. While training a unit, selected optimization method adjusts coefficients $(a_1, ..., a_n)$ in the transfer function of the unit.

boundaries better separating the data vectors. We prepared two versions of the data set. The first was A-EGM-regression data set, where the output was continuous number taken from raw dataset (not using CF classified by experts). The second was A-EGM-classification data set with three output classes: (1 – organized atrial activity; 2 – intermediate; 3 – high degree of fractionation), where for class one the average one particular A-EGM signal classification (ACF - average class of fractionation) by three experts was below 1.9, for class two the ACF in $\langle 1.9, 3 \rangle$ interval and for the class three the ACF was above 3.

Results of GAME approach

At first, we studied the regression performance of GAME models produced by different configurations of the algorithm. The target variable was the average A-EGM signal ranking by three experts (the A-EGM-regression data set). We found out, and it is also apparent in the box-plot charts, that comparison of the 10 fold cross validation error is not stable enough to decide, which configuration is better. Therefore we repeated the 10 fold cross validation ten times, each time with different fold splitting. For each box plot it was necessary to generate and validate hundred models.

For all experiments we used three default configurations of the GAME algorithm available in FAKE GAME environment (*The FAKE GAME environment for the automatic knowledge extraction*, 2008). The *std* configuration uses just subset of units (those with implemented analytic gradient for faster optimization). It evolves 15 units for 30 epochs in each layer. The *quick*

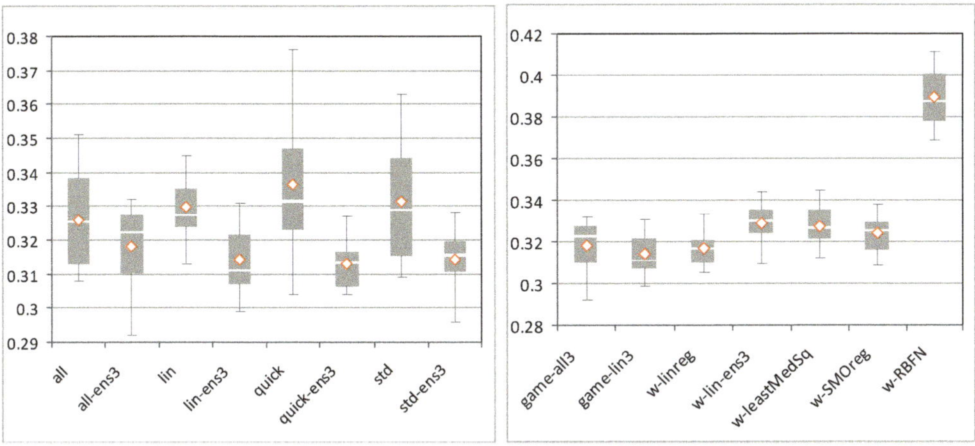

Fig. 10. The comparison of RMS cross validation errors for several configuration of the GAME engine (left). Selected GAME models compared with models generated in WEKA environment (right).

configuration is the same as *std* except that it does not use the niching genetic algorithm (just 15 units in the initial population). The *linear* configuration restricts type of units that can be used to linear transfer function units. The *all* configuration is the same as *std* configuration, in addition it uses all units available in the FAKE GAME environment. This configuration is more computationally expensive, because it also optimizes complex units such as BPNetwork containing standard MLP neural network with the back-propagation of error (Mandischer, 2002).

The GAME algorithm also allows to generate ensemble of models (Brown, 2004; Hansen & Salamon, 1990). Ensemble configurations contain digit (number of models) in their name.

The Figure 10 shows that the regression of the ACF output is not a very difficult task. All basic GAME configurations performed similarly (left chart) and ensembling of three models further improved their accuracy. The ensemble of three linear models performed best in average, but the difference from $all - ens3$ configuration is not statistically significant.

In WEKA data mining environment, *LinearRegression* with embedded feature selection algorithm was the best performing algorithm. Ensembling (bagging) did not improved results of generated model, quite the contrary. The Radial Basis Function Network (RBFN) failed to deliver satisfactory results in spite of experiments with its optimal setting (number of clusters).

Secondly, our experiments were performed on the A-EGM-classification data set. The methodology remained the same as for regression data. Additionally we tested classification performance of 5 models ensembles. Figure 11 left shows that the classes are not linearly separable – *linear* configuration generates poor classifiers and ensembling does not help. Combining models in case of all other configurations improves the accuracy. For *all* configuration the dispersion of cross validation errors is quite high. The problem is in the configuration of the genetic algorithm – with 15 individuals in the population some "potentially useful" types of units do not have chance to be instantiated. Ensembling models generated by this configuration improves their accuracy significantly.

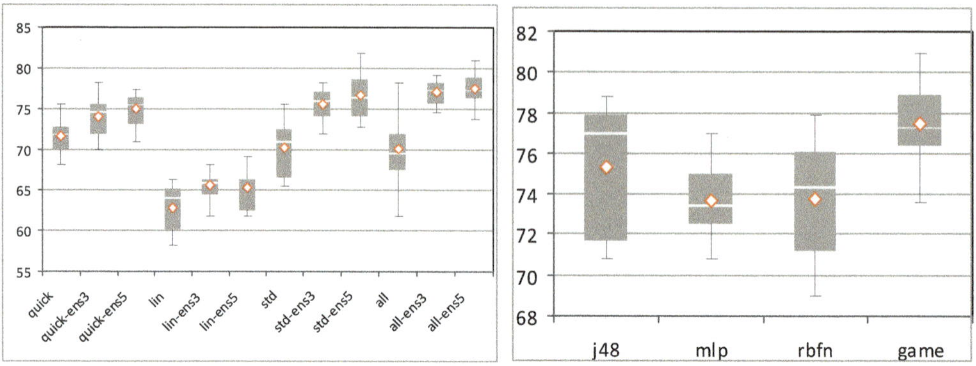

Fig. 11. Classification accuracy in percent for several GAME configurations (left) and comparison with Weka classifiers (right).

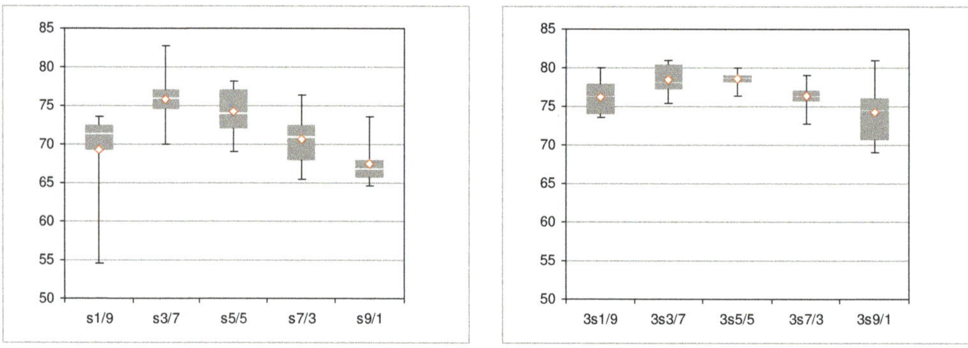

Fig. 12. Classification performance for different ratios of training/validation data split. Left – results for single game models generated by *std* configuration. Right – results for GAME ensemble ($std - ens3$).

Comparison with WEKA classifiers (Figure 11 right) shows that GAME ensemble significantly outperforms Decision Trees (j48), MultiLayered Perceptron (mlp) and Radial Basis Function network (rbfn) implemented in WEKA data mining environment.

The last experiment (Figure 12) showed that the best split of the training and validation data set is $\frac{40\%}{60\%}$ (training data are used by optimization method to adjust parameters of GAME units transfer functions, whereas from validation part, the fitness of units is computed).

Implicitly, and in all previous experiments, training and validation data set was divided $\frac{70\%}{30\%}$ in the GAME algorithm. Changing the implicit setting to $\frac{40\%}{60\%}$ however involves additional experiments on different data sets.

Conclusion of GAME approach classification

Our results showed, that extracted features for CFAEs bear significant information allowing us to classify signals into three classes of fractionation with 80% accuracy for ACF and raw dataset. That is good result with respect to 60% of consistent assignments into four

CF performed by three independent experts. For this data set, the GAME algorithm outperformed well established methods in both classification and regression accuracy. What is even more important, both winning configurations were identical $all - ens$.

6. Discussion and conclusion

Described methodology of the signal processing allowed us to construct several systems that can effectively work with the A-EGM signal in real-time. Figure 13 shows the whole signal path from its recording by catheter touching the endocardial tissue, through the robust wavelet based filtering method, feature extraction and selection phase towards the regression or classification. The result of regression or classification can be then used as a number (color shade) to be mapped into real electro-anatomical maps during the ablation of AF.

In the era of catheter ablation of AF, the initial attempts to describe A-EGMs during AF were predominantly based on frequency-domain analysis of atrial signals (Sanders et al., 2005), (Lazar et al., 2004) and (Lin et al., 2006). Wave morphology similarity approach was alternatively investigated (Ravelli et al., 2005). The pitfalls of spectral mapping have been recently recognized (Ng et al., 2006) and (Ng et al., 2007). Besides technical difficulties, it soon became clear that not only dominant frequency (DF) but also the level of fractionation is clinically important descriptor of local atrial signal (Nademanee et al., 2004) and (Takahashi et al., 2008). Both characteristics are often concordant. Sites with highly fractionated A-EGMs almost fully encompass the sites with high DF but not always vice versa. For that reason, algorithms implemented in commercially available mapping systems were designed for detection of CFAEs rather than high DF (Scherr et al., 2007) and (Verma et al., 2008). These time-domain algorithms require specific input parameters being more flexible but, on the other hand, operator-dependent. In addition, relatively simple mathematical definition of fractionation in those algorithms suggests that more sophisticated analytical methods may provide better performance in CFAEs detection.

Our study showed for the first time that wavelet-based approach to the description of endocardial A-EGMs during AF offers fractionation indexes and classifiers which tightly correlate with the expert classification and have reasonable power to detect highly fractionated A-EGMs. To our best knowledge this is also the first study that utilized atrial signal database and expert ranking to validate automated software algorithm for the quantification of A-EGMs fractionation.

Previous reports on the automated detection of CFAEs showed also promising agreement between CFAEs detection performed automatically and by investigators. In the study by Verma et. al (Verma et al., 2008), the overall agreement between algorithm-labeled (defined as mean cycle length $<$ 120 ms) and investigator-labeled CFAEs sites was 86% for two independent investigators combined. In the study by Wu et. al (Wu et al., 2008), 82.5% of effective sites with significant AF cycle length prolongation after ablation were judged retrospectively as CFAEs sites (defined as shortest cycle interval between $60 - 120$ ms) (Křemen et al., 2008).

Number of A-EGMs in experimental dataset was limited and representative A-EGMs were preselected based on quality from vast amount of data obtained during left-atrial mapping. This could have introduced a bias towards our algorithms. It should be emphasized, however, that fractionation analysis even under "real world conditions" requires much more diligent approach compared to conventional voltage or activation mapping and that higher standards for A-EGM quality are prerequisite for meaningful results. In contrast to DF assessment, stable endocardial contact is crucial for valid fractionation analysis. Consequently, preselection of

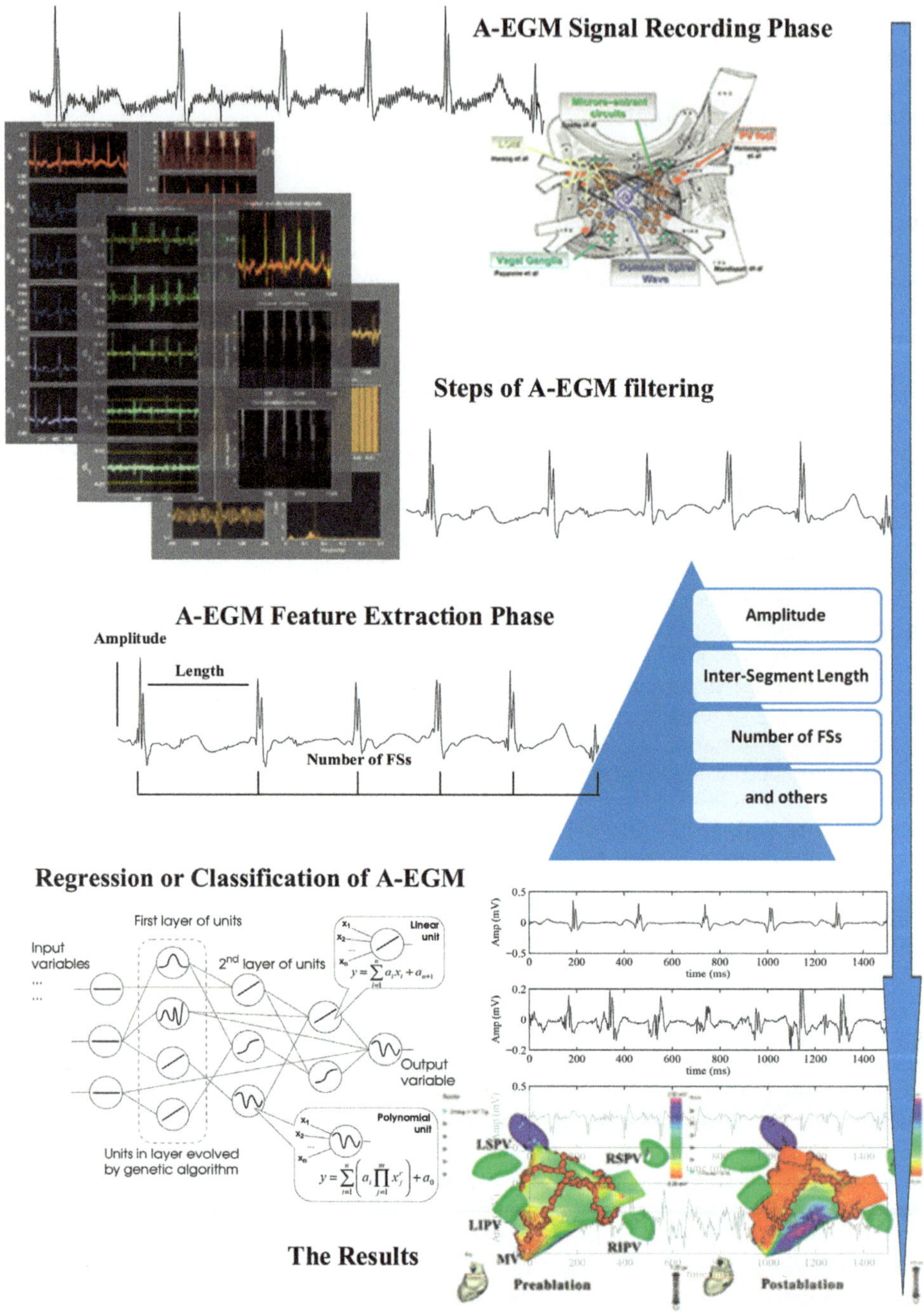

Fig. 13. Schema of described methodology of A-EGM processing and evaluation.

A-EGMs, according to our opinion, is fully appropriate for pilot testing of a new algorithms even if these algorithms are designed quite robustly in order to ensure good performance also for signals with less than optimum signal-to-noise ratio (Křemen et al., 2008).

Some objections may be raised to mere four categories used for expert ranking of A-EGMs. Optimal classification should have been performed in a continuous scale reflecting inherent features of fractionation. However, such classification is difficult to achieve in reasonable time span because of within-expert "drift" in evaluation of consecutive A-EGMs which requires many additional re-evaluation steps. We circumvented this problem by averaging the classification by 3 experts to obtain semi-continuous scale of fractionation (Křemen et al., 2008).

Because of temporal variation in appearance of A-EGMs during AF at some sites, it was shown that the signal assessment requires recording duration > 5 seconds to obtain reproducible fractionation measures Lin et al. (2008) and Stiles et al. (2008). In our study, we used only 1.5 s A-EGMs. This approach seems to be fully adequate because only A-EGMs with stable activation pattern within this period were selected. Assuming that dominant cycle length during AF is usually < 200 ms, the A-EGM duration of 1.5 s covers at least $7-8$ signal pattern repetitions which ensures sufficient statistical stability. Temporal alterations of A-EGMs are certainly problematic issue during real-time fractionation mapping but the results of our validation study were not clearly affected by this phenomenon (Křemen et al., 2008).

Our algorithm is fully automatic and does not need any initial settings by the operator like voltage criteria required in CFAEs software of commercially available mapping systems (Scherr et al., 2007) and (Verma et al., 2008) which might be particularly sensitive to background noise and dispersion of voltages at different sites within mapped atrium. Parameter settings in our algorithms were manifold cross-validated using random split of experimental dataset into training and testing subsets. Because correlation between fractionation index and expert classification was chosen as one of the test criterion (instead of CFAEs detection), general performance of algorithms within the whole range of A-EGMs fractionation was confirmed. For all these reasons and because of robust preprocessing steps, the algorithms will hopefully perform well in larger independent sample of A-EGMs with the identical parameter settings. However, this should be a subject of subsequent investigation as well as the definition of cut-off value of indexes of fractionation or classifiers setup for CFAEs detection.

Ablation of CFAEs as adjutant target sites appears to increase success rate of ablation for persistent AF and improves short-term outcome of AF patients as shown in numerous clinical studies. Feasibility of real-time automated detection of CFAEs was investigated, but only in two of studies this feature was directly used for ablation (Verma et al., 2008) and (Porter et al., 2008). So far, any information is missing on the utility of automated assessment of CFAE compared to investigator-based detection in directing the ablation procedure.

7. Acknowledgement

This work was supported by the research projects $\#MSM$ 6840770012 "Interdisciplinary Biomedical Engineering Research II" from Ministry of Education, Youth and Sports of the Czech Republic and post doctoral research project by Czech Science Foundation GACR $\#P103/11/P106$.

8. References

Brown, G. (2004). *Diversity in Neural Network Ensembles*, PhD thesis, The University of Birmingham, School of Computer Science, Birmingham B15 2TT, United Kingdom.

Burrus, S. (1997). *Introduction to Wavelets and Wavelet Transforms.*, Prentice Hall.

Daubechies, I. (1992). *Ten lectures on wavelets.*

Donoho, D. (1995). De-noising by soft-thresholding, *IEEE Transactions on Information Theory* 41(3): 613–627.

Drchal, J., Kordík, P. & Šnorek, M. (2007). Dataset Visualization Based on a Simulation of Intermolecular Forces, *IWIM 2007 - International Workshop on Inductive Modelling*, Vol. 1, Czech Technical University in Prague, Praha, pp. 246–253.
URL: *http://cig.felk.cvut.cz*

Faes, L., Nollo, G., Antolini, R., Gaita, F. & Ravelli, F. (2007). A method for quantifying atrial fibrillation organization based on wave morphology similarity, *IEEE Trans Biomed Eng.* 49: 1504–1513.

Faes, L. & Ravelli, F. (2007). A morphology-based approach to the evaluation of atrial fibrillation organization, *IEEE Eng Med Biol Mag.* 26(4): 59–67.

Gustafsson, F. (2000). *Adaptive Filtering and Change Detection*, John Wiley & Sons, Ltd.

Guyon, I., Gunn, S., Nikravesh, M. & Zadeh, L. (2006). *Feature Extraction, Foundations and Applications*, Physica-Verlag, Springer.

Haissaguerre, M., Jais, P., Shah, D., Takahashi, A., Hocini, M., G, Q., Garrigue, S., Le Mouroux, A., Le Metayer, P. & Clementy, J. (2003). Spontaneous initiation of af by ectopic beats originating in the pulmonary veins, *N Engl J Med* 339: 659–666.

Hansen, L. & Salamon, P. (1990). Neural network ensembles, *IEEE Trans. Pattern Anal. Machine Intelligence* 12(10): 993–1001.

Ivakhnenko, A. G. (1971). Polynomial theory of complex systems, *IEEE Transactions on Systems, Man, and Cybernetics* SMC-1(1): 364–378.

Jais, P., Haissaguerre, M., Shah, D., Chouairi, S. & Clementy, J. (1996). Regional disparities of endocardial atrial activation in paroxysmal atrial fibrillation, *Pacing Clin Electrophysiol.* pp. 1998–2003.

Konings, K., Kirchhof, C., Smeets, J., Wellens, H., Penn, O. & Allessie, M. (1994). High-density mapping of electrically induced atrial fibrillation in humans, *Circulation* 89: 1665–1680.

Konings, K., Smeets, J., Penn, O., Wellens, H. & Allessie, M. (1997). Configuration of unipolar atrial electrograms during electrically induced atrial fibrillation in humans, *Circulation* 95: 1231–1241.

Kordík, P. (2005). Game - group of adaptive models evolution, *Technical Report DCSE-DTP-2005-07*, Czech Technical University in Prague, FEE, CTU Prague, Czech Republic.

Kordík, P., Kovářík, O. & Šnorek, M. (2007). OPTIMIZATION OF MODELS: LOOKING FOR THE BEST STRATEGY, *Proceedings of the 6th EUROSIM Congress on Modelling and Simulation*, Vol. 2, ARGESIM, Vienna, pp. 314–320.
URL: *http://neuron.felk.cvut.cz/ kordikp/iw/eurosim07.pdf*

Kosinski, D., Grubb, P., Wolfe, A. & Mayhew, H. (1998). Catheter ablation for atrial flutter and fibrillation an effective alternative to medical therapy, *POSTGRADUATE MEDICINE* 103.

Kottkamp, H. & Hindricks, G. (2007). Complex fractionated atrial electrograms in atrial fibrillation: A promising target for ablation, but why, when and how?, *Heart Rhythm* pp. 1021–1023.

Křemen, V. & Lhotská, L. (2007a). Automatic Search of Individual Signal Complexes in Complex Fractionated Atrial Electrograms Using Wavelet Transform, *8th International Workshop on Mathematical Methods in Scattering Theory and Biomedical Engineering - book of abstracts*, University of Ioannina, Crete, p. 37.

Křemen, V. & Lhotská, L. (2007b). Novel approach to search for individual signal complexes in complex fractionated atrial electrograms using wavelet transform, *6th International Special Topic Conference on ITAB - Proceedings*, IEEE, Piscataway, pp. 83–86.

Křemen, V. & Lhotská, L. (2008). Evaluation of Novel Algorithm for Search of Signal Complexes to Describe Complex Fractionated Atrial Electrogram, *Biosignals 2008 - II.*, Vol. 2, INSTICC Press, Setúbal, pp. 416–419.

Křemen, V., Lhotská, L., Čihák, R., Vančura, V., Kautzner, J. & Wichterle, D. (2008). A new approach to automated assessment of endocardial electrograms fractionation in human left atrium during atrial fibrillation., *Physiol. Measurement* .

Křemen, V., Lhotská, L. & Macaš, M. (2007). Using PSO Algorithm to Optimize Parameters of Time-Domain Method for Complex Fractionated Atrial Electrograms Evaluation , *8th International Workshop on Mathematical Methods in Scattering Theory and Biomedical Engineering - book of abstracts*, University of Ioannina, Crete, p. 36.

Lazar, S., Dixit, S., Marchlinski, F., Callans, D. & Gerstenfeld, E. (2004). Presence of left-to-right atrial frequency gradient in paroxysmal but not persistent atrial fibrillation in humans, *Circulation* 110: 3181–3186.

Lin, Y., Tai, C., Kao, T., Chang, S., Wongcharoen, W., Lo, L., Tuan, T., Udyavar, A., Chen, Y., Higa, S., Ueng, K. & Chen, S. (2008). Consistency of complex fractionated atrial electrograms during atrial fibrillation, *Heart Rhythm* 5: 406–12.

Lin, Y., Tai, C., Kao, T., Tso, H., Higa, S., Tsao, H., Chang, S., Hsieh, M. & Chen, S. (2006). Frequency analysis in different types of paroxysmal atrial fibrillation, *J. Am. Coll. Cardiol.* 47: 1401–1407.

Mallat, S. (1999). *A Wavelet tour of Signal Processing. 2. edition*, Academic Press.

Mandischer, M. (2002). A comparison of evolution strategies and backpropagation for neural network training, *Neurocomputing* (42): 87–117.

Nademanee, K. (2007). Trials and travails of electrogram-guided ablation of chronic atrial fibrillation, *Circulation* 115: 2592–2594.

Nademanee, K., McKenzie, J., Kosar, E., Schwab, M., Sunsaneewitayakul, B., Vasavakul, T., Khunnawat, C. & Ngarmukos, T. (2004). A new approach for catheter ablation of atrial fibrillation: mapping of the electrophysiologic substrate, *J Am Coll Cardiol* 43: 2044–53.

Ng, J., Gold, J. & Goldberger, J. (2007). Understanding and interpreting dominant frequency analysis of af electrograms, *Journal of Cardiovascular Electrophysiology* pp. 680–685.

Ng, J., Kadish, A. & Goldberger, J. (2006). Effect of electrogram characteristics on the relationship of dominant frequency to atrial activation rate in atrial fibrillation, *Heart Rhythm* pp. 1295–1305.

Novak, D. (2003). *Electrocardiogram Signal Processing using Hidden Markov Models*, PhD thesis, Czech Technical University in Prague, Faculty of Electrical Engineering, Technicka 2, 166 27 Prague 6, Czech Republic.

Porter, M., Spear, W., Akar, J., Helms, R., Brysiewicz, N., Santucci, P. & Wilber, D. (2008). Prospective study of atrial fibrillation termination during ablation guided by automated detection of fractionated electrograms., *J. Cardiovasc. Electrophysiol.* . [May 5; electronic publication ahead of print].

Ravelli, F., Faes, L., Sandrini, L., Gaita, F., Antolini, R., Scaglione, M. & Nollo, G. (2005). Wave similarity mapping shows the spatiotemporal distribution of fibrillatory wave complexity in the human right atrium during paroxysmal and chronic atrial fibrillation, *J. Cardiovasc. Electrophysiol.* 16: 1071–1076.

Sanders, P., Berenfeld, O., Hocini, M., Jais, P., Vaidyanathan, R., Hsu, L., Garrigue, S., Takahashi, Y., Rotter, M., Sacher, F., Scavee, C., Ploutz-Snyder, R., Jalife, J. & Haissguerre, M. (2005). Spectral analysis identifies sites of high frequency activity maintaining atrial fibrillation in humans, *Circulation* 112: 789–797.

Scherr, D., Dalal, D., Cheema, A., Cheng, A., Henrikson, C., Spragg, D., Marine, J., Berger, R., Calkins, H. & Dong, J. (2007). Automated detection and characterization of complex fractionated atrial electrograms in human left atrium during atrial fibrillation, *Heart Rhythm* 4: 1013–1020.

Stiles, M., Brooks, A., John, B., Shashidhar, Wilson, L., Kuklik, P., Dimitri, H., Lau, D., Roberts-Thomson, R., Mackenzie, L., Willoughby, S., Young, G. & Sanders, P. (2008). The effect of electrogram duration on quantification of complex fractionated atrial electrograms and dominant frequency, *J. Cardiovasc. Electrophysiol.* 19: 252–258.

Takahashi, Y., OŃeill, M., Hocini, M., Dubois, R., Matsuo, S., Knecht, S., Mahapatra, S., Lim, K., Jais, P., Jonsson, A., Sacher, F., Sanders, P., Rostock, T., Bordachar, P., Clementy, J., Klein, G. & Haissaguerre, M. (2008). Characterization of electrograms associated with termination of chronic atrial fibrillation by catheter ablation., *J. Am. Coll. Cardiol.* 51: 1003–1010.

The FAKE GAME environment for the automatic knowledge extraction (2008). available online at: http://www.sourceforge.net/projects/fakegame.

Verma, A., Novak, P., Macle, L., Whaley, B., Beardsall, M., Wulffhart, Z. & Khaykin, Y. (2008). A prospective multicenter evaluation of ablating complex fractionated electrograms (CFEs) during atrial fibrillation (AF) identified by an automated mapping algorithm: acute effects on AF and efficacy as an adjuvant strategy, *Heart Rhythm* 5: 198–205.

Wu, J., Estner, H., Luik, A., Ucer, E., Reents, T., Pflaumer, A., Zrenner, B., Hessling, G. & Deisenhofer, I. (2008). Automatic 3D mapping of complex fractionated atrial electrograms (CFAE) in patients with paroxysmal and persistent atrial fibrillation., *J. Cardiovasc. Electrophysiol.* . [March 28; electronic publication ahead of print].

8

Automatic Detection of Paroxysmal Atrial Fibrillation

Redmond B. Shouldice, Conor Heneghan and Philip de Chazal
BiancaMed, NovaUCD, Belfield Innovation Park, Ireland

1. Introduction

The purpose of this chapter is to provide a tutorial level introduction to (a) the physiology and clinical background of paroxysmal (intermittent) atrial fibrillation (PAF), and (b) methods for detection of patterns consistent with AF using electrocardiogram (ECG) processing. The document assumes that the reader is familiar with basic signal processing concepts, but assumes no prior knowledge of AF or pattern classification. A practical implementation of an automatic AF detector is presented; a supervised linear discriminant classifier is used to estimate the likelihood of a block of inter-heartbeat intervals being PAF, with accuracies of 92%, 94%, 100% and 100% when the method was used to process the publically available Physionet (Goldberger et al., 2000) signal databases MITDB, AFDB, NSRDB and NSR2DB respectively.

2. Clinical background: Atrial fibrillation

2.1 Physiology, prevalence and health consequences

Atrial fibrillation (AF) is the most commonly found sustained cardiac arrhythmia in clinical practice, and has serious associated mortality and morbidity (Benjamin et al., 1998). For example, about 15% of strokes occur in people with atrial fibrillation, so AF is a significant risk factor for stroke. The prevalence of AF increases with age and is slightly more common in men than in women. The prevalence of AF is 0.5% for the group aged 50 to 59 years and rises to 8.8% in the group aged 80 to 89 years (Kannel et al., 1982). 1-2% of the population suffer from AF at present, and the number of affected individuals is expected to double or triple within the next two to three decades both in Europe and in the USA; in addition, the presence of AF is associated with a marked reduction in everyday functioning and quality of life (Kirchhof et al., 2009).

AF is where the heart's atria quiver instead of beating in a coordinated fashion, reducing effectiveness as a pump, and potentially causing clots to form if blood pools within the atria. Disorganized continuous atrial activity (giving rise to ECG "fibrillatory" waves) may give rise to irregular ventricular rate, visible as "irregularly irregular" variations in the RR ECG interval.

2.2 Clinical implications of automatic detection of PAF

The major hazard of AF is stroke. Frequent episodes of PAF can be captured by 24 hour Holter; however, if episodes are rare or asymptomatic, then long term Holter ECG or ECG

event recorders can help. For instance, Roche et al. (2002) note that in patients still complaining of palpitations after one negative 24-hour Holter, numerous, prolonged, and often asymptomatic episodes of PAF can be revealed by long-term automatic event recorders.
It has been shown that trans-telephonic ECG monitoring can increase the detection rate of PAF in stroke and transient ischaemic attack patients whose 24-hour Holter result was negative (Gaillard et al., 2010). Short duration monitoring (24-72hr Holter) identifies new AF in only about 5% of patients post stroke. In contrast, longer monitoring (e.g., 4 or 7-day event loop recorder) detected new atrial fibrillation/flutter in 5.7%-7.7% of consecutive patients in 2 studies (Liao et al., 2007).

2.3 Diagnostic techniques for PAF

Cardiac event recorders have been shown to have a higher diagnostic yield in patients with intermittent symptoms such as palpitations or dizziness. Since paroxysmal AF may often be the underlying cause of some of these symptoms, event recorders are widely used to document PAF. However, a limitation of patient triggered recorders is that AF may be asymptomatic or occur whilst the patient is sleeping. There may also be inconsistent use of a manual trigger by the elderly. Therefore, the newest generation of AF recorders incorporate auto-trigger features, which will automatically record ECG strips, when certain parameters are recognized - for example, physician defined thresholds of bradycardia or tachycardia.
Accordingly, there is interest in algorithms for the automated recognition of AF in event recorders. As a result, automated methods of detecting these intermittent episodes have been explored. An episode-based classification system which removes the QRS complex is described by Stridh et al. (2001). Other techniques analyse RR interval dynamics to determine AF episodes; for instance the following authors (Dash et al., 2009; Hong-Wei et al., 2009; Lombardi et al., 2004; Maier et al. 2001 & Tateno & Glass, 2001) apply a mixture of time and frequency analysis techniques to RR intervals.
A smart system based on temporal features of RR intervals (Shouldice et al., 2004; Shouldice et al., 2007) for the classification of ECG blocks that contain AF is presented in this chapter.

3. Methods

This section discusses

1. PAF detection block based system
2. Mapping of expert annotations to a quantized signal suitable for the development of a block based system
3. Performance measures
4. Detailed discussion of linear discriminant analysis and an example.

3.1 Classification

A common task in medicine is to distinguish two groups of measurements or subjects. For example, one may wish to identify all people with a particular disease by combining results from blood tests, physical measurements, and symptoms. Such a task is called classification, and is typically the job of the human expert in the system. It is useful to automate the process of classification, particularly where large quantities of data or large numbers of subjects are required. For example, the FDA has recently approved a system (AutoPap from NeoPath) which analyses Pap smears automatically and returns a classification of positive, negative, or indeterminate.

The design of such automated systems has been, and continues to be an area of active research, particularly with increases in computational speed and the increasing use of information technology in medicine.

There are a large number of approaches for developing automated classification systems. Among the most popular are techniques based on discriminant analysis (linear and quadratic), k-means cluster analysis, neural networks, fuzzy logic, and support vector machines. The algorithm outlined here for detection of blocks consistent with PAF uses linear discriminant analysis (LDA), operating on a block by block based measure.

3.2 Block based system

A number of methods exist for processing real time data and then performing classification. For instance, in the case of a PAF classifier, one could analyze incoming QRS detections on a beat by beat basis and make some decision at a particular QRS point based on a small number of previous QRS points. However, in practice some form of windowing (perhaps incorporating many QRS points) is desirable to combat the effect of dropped or erroneous QRS detections, e.g., so as not to be unduly influenced by a profound change due to electromyographic artifact.

The algorithm outlined here uses the concept of per block processing. This involves buffering a certain length of ECG signal and associated QRS detection points and then making a classification decision; in other words, fixed length sequences of ECG beats are inspected. The output classification decision, whether it be PAF, NONPAF or undetermined (i.e. when no QRS points are available due to noise) provides a trigger to store the associated ECG signal to flash memory or not.

A block based system, for instance using non overlapping blocks containing 100 QRS detections, requires that an expert label be appended to each block for performance estimation purposes. This step involves the quantization of the expert annotations (e.g. such annotations might be at the start of a period of atrial fibrillation or at the return to normal sinus rhythm) to the block length. The original expert annotations are also stored on a per beat basis; this step facilitates the estimation of "beat based" performance measures.

Fig. 1 illustrates the segmentation of an expert signal into 5 non overlapping blocks. In this case, a block is tagged as PAF if at least half of the block (i.e. 50 beats) was determined by the expert to be PAF.

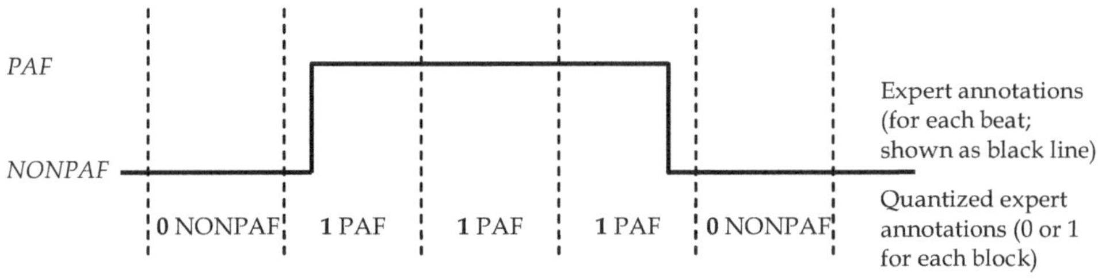

Fig. 1. The quantized expert signal (0 or 1 annotations, perhaps at half the block length) provide the quantized training information (reference) to compare with classifier output. Thus, block performance measures can be calculated from TP, TN, FP, FN figures. However, it should be noted that the inherent quantization will limit the upper bound of performance measures such as 'episode', 'duration' and on a 'beat' basis.

These expert annotations are then available for comparison with the classifier output and thus to generate performance figures. The training process involves the choice of certain characteristics (features) that describe how PAF-like behaviour manifests itself in the block of RR intervals (derived from the difference of the block QRS points). The actual features used in the BiancaMed system are discussed in Section 4; however, it may be useful at this point to inspect a flowchart indicating the main steps involved in the training and testing of the block system used (see Fig. 2).
One can also consider an improvement of the block based system whereby an overlap is introduced. As an example, for a 100 beat block system, an extreme case of overlapping is where each block is used to classify a single middle beat. The block is then shifted by one beat and another classification is performed. Obviously, this is a rather computationally expensive method of classifying on a per beat basis, although it does remove the possible quantization error of the expert signals. A system utilizing somewhat less overlap (say 50% overlap or a shift of 50 beats when a 100 beat block is considered) can be used to trade computational complexity for possible quantization error.
At this stage, it is useful to consider how the power of diagnostic tests can be assessed. Some of the most favoured measures used by clinicians are sensitivity and specificity. These can be explained by reference to Table 1. For a two-class problem, there is an associated table with four cells. There are two rows representing 'true' atrial fibrillation and 'false' non-AF (i.e. all other rhythms).

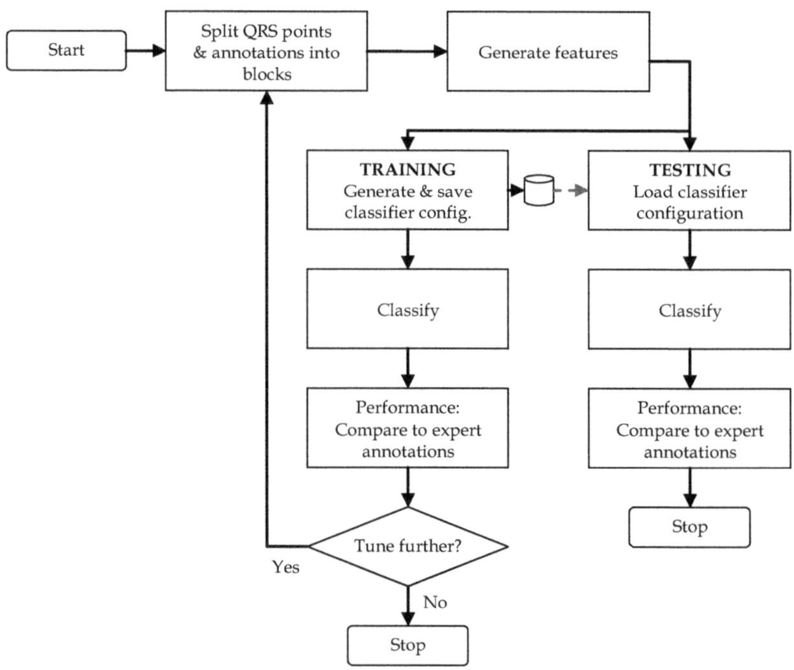

Fig. 2. Main steps involved in both the training and testing of a block based classification system utilizing expert annotations.

There are also two columns representing the assignment of each beat by the test. Note that in the case of a 100 beat block system, a 'PAF' classification leads to all of those 100 beats being tagged as 'PAF'. Those beats that have been tagged as PAF by a human expert and are subsequently classified as PAF by the algorithm, are called 'true positive' (TP). Beats that are known to be PAF, but which the test classified as control are labelled as 'false negative' (FN). Beats which are NONPAF, but which the test flags as PAF are labelled 'false positive' (FP). Finally, beats which contain rhythms other than PAF, and which the test correctly labels as NONPAF are called 'true negative' (TN).

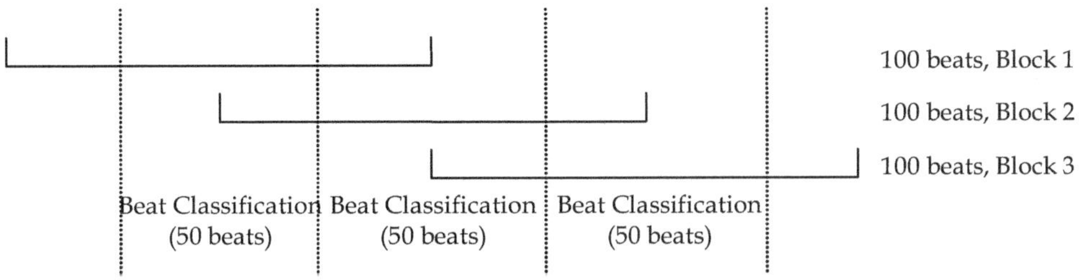

Fig. 3. If 50% overlap is used, each 100 beat block provides a classification of the middle 50 beats. Note: the start and end 50 beat segments should be padded or trimmed.

The sensitivity (*Se*) of a test is then defined as the percentage of PAF beats which are identified as PAF. The specificity (*Sp*) of the test is defined as the percentage of NONPAF beats which are identified (classified) as NONPAF. These may be expressed as

$$Se = \frac{TP}{TP + FN} \qquad Sp = \frac{TN}{TN + FP} \tag{1}$$

Note that it makes no sense to give either figure in isolation. Any diagnostic test can be made to have 100% sensitivity (by simply labelling everyone as having the disease), but such a test would have zero specificity, and would be of no practical benefit.

		EXPERT ANNOTATION	
		PAF	*NONPAF*
TEST RESULT	*PAF*	TRUE POSITIVE (TP)	FALSE POSITIVE (FP)
	NONPAF	FALSE NEGATIVE (FN)	TRUE NEGATIVE (TN)

Table 1. Definition of terms used in calculating sensitivity, specificity, positive predictive value, and negative predictive value.

Related measures are the Positive Predictive Value (*PPV*) and the Negative Predictive Value (*NPV*). These are defined respectively as the percentage of PAF-classified beats, which are expert tagged as PAF, and NONPAF-classified beats, which are actually NONPAF. The associated equations are

$$PPV = \frac{TP}{TP + FP} \qquad NPV = \frac{TN}{TN + FN} \tag{2}$$

Finally, the accuracy is given as the overall percentage of correctly classified beats

$$ACC = \frac{TP + TN}{TP + TN + FP + FN} \tag{3}$$

In the context of auto-detection of AF using a device with a limited amount of flash memory, the classifier design must balance the need to keep the number of false positive (*FP*) detections as low as possible to avoid exhausting the ECG storage memory while remaining sufficiently sensitive (i.e. keep the number of *FN* detections small) so as to capture real PAF beats.

3.3 Alternative performance measures

As can be seen from the previous section, beat based performance measures can be generated from quantized blocks (e.g. containing 100 beats) of data. However, such measures do not give any indication of how many actual episodes (events) of PAF are captured (i.e. each PAF event can vary widely in length). Jager et al. (1991) propose alternative event based performance measures based on episode and duration, for the evaluation of transient ST elevation detectors. An episode measure is designed to provide information on how well episodes (rather than beats) are captured; a duration measure describes how reliably duration is captured. As an example, such episode and duration performance figures are available for the King of Hearts AF monitor.

Jager et al. (1991) note that there are four possible outcomes in which a detector is presented with an input with is either an event or non event - FP, FN, TP and TN (as per the beat measures). However, they note that in some detectors the concept of a non event cannot be counted (e.g., stating that a subject had four "non-events" of PAF during a nights sleep does not really mean much!) and thus the false negative (FN) figure is undefined. Therefore, they concentrate on obtaining sensitivity (Se, the fraction of events which are detected) and positive predictivity (PPV, the fraction of detections which are events). Furthermore, they provide two different methods of aggregating performance figures to account for the possibly small number of events in each subject dataset. The average statistics give each subject equal weighting; in contrast, the gross statistics give each event or detection equal weighting.

3.3.1 Episode measures

An episode of PAF is deemed to have been successfully detected (a "match") if the period of overlap between the expert annotated signal and predicted signal (i.e., the classifier output) is greater than 50% or when the period of overlap contains the extrema. Of course, the original expert annotations were at a higher resolution (arbitrarily chosen as 1 annotation per sec or 1 Hz based on the per-second expert markings) than the 30 sec quantized sequences. Therefore, the quantized classifier output must be upsampled for calculation of episode and duration measures; as an example, an output of 00010 will become a train of 90 'zeros' followed by 30 'ones' followed by 30 'zeros'.

An episode based sensitivity measure (*ESe*) is an estimate of the likelihood of detecting a PAF episode where *STP* is the number of matching PAF episodes, *FN* is the number of non matching episodes and (*STP*+*FN*) is the total number of episodes. For this measure, a "match" occurs when an expert annotated episode is overlapped by at least 50% of the predicted PAF signal. The defining reference annotations are based on the human expert markings and the detector signal is the quantized classifier output, upsampled to the same rate as the expert signal. The episode positive predictivity (*EPP*) is defined based on *PTP* (capturing the number of matching episodes) and *FP* (the number of non matching episodes). For this measure, a "match" occurs when a predicted episode is overlapped by at least 50% of the expert annotated PAF signal. N.B., this is the reverse of the case for a match when determining STP. These measures are calculated using

$$ESe = \frac{STP}{STP + FN} \quad EPP = \frac{PTP}{PTP + FP} \tag{4}$$

3.3.2 Duration measures

The total duration of PAF correctly detected can be calculated as follows. The duration sensitivity (*DSe*) and duration positive predictivity (*DPP*) may be calculated using

$$DSe = \frac{\sum D \cap R}{\sum R} \quad DPP = \frac{\sum D \cap R}{\sum S} \tag{5}$$

where $\sum R$ represents the total time of expert determined PAF and $\sum D$ represents the total time of PAF determined by the predictor. $\sum D \cap R$ is the overlap (common region or intersection) between expert and predictor, calculated using a logical AND operation. In general, these duration performance figures might be expected to be broadly similar to the per beat figures.

3.4 Supervised classification using training data

When using a linear discriminant classifier (LDA), one must first derive the covariance matrix and class mean vectors (this is discussed in more detail in a later section). In general, this requires us to have access to a set of data whose class membership is known - i.e., access to expert annotated data. Such a set of data is called a "training set", and the overall approach is called "supervised learning" since the classifier is given some known outputs to begin with. As an aside, it is noted that there is much interest in unsupervised training where the classifier has no knowledge about the class memberships of any data, or perhaps a minimal set of knowledge such as the total number of classes present in the data. However, this more general class of classifier is not considered in this document.

One caveat with using supervised training of a classifier is that the classifier can become "over-trained"; that is it will assign a lot of importance to patterns which arose in the training data through chance alone. As an extreme example, given enough parameters one can draw an arbitrarily complex boundary region between the two classes of data in the training data which will achieve 100% accuracy in identifying class membership. This is shown in Fig. 4 (left) where a complex decision boundary between the two classes using 20 training data vectors is shown. It would appear that the test has 100% performance in all parameters. However, when it is tested on additional data (Fig. 4 (right)), it is clear that in fact the test makes a lot of errors. Therefore, in general one should be cautious in assessing the performance of a classifier on training data alone, since this will tend to bias the results upwards.

A better methodology is to develop the diagnostic test using available training data, and then assess its performance on an independent (test) set, which was never used in the design or training of the classifier. Ideally, the training data and the test data should both be sufficiently large to well represent the general population statistics (where population refers to the subjects likely to be classified using the test, not necessarily the general population). In the system outlined in this document, the population of interest will be subjects with suspected PAF episodes. The values of class mean vectors, and covariance matrices supplied by the authors represent the pool of training data that has currently been well characterized. These values can be altered as the test data set grows, or to deal with specific sub-populations with different statistical distributions.

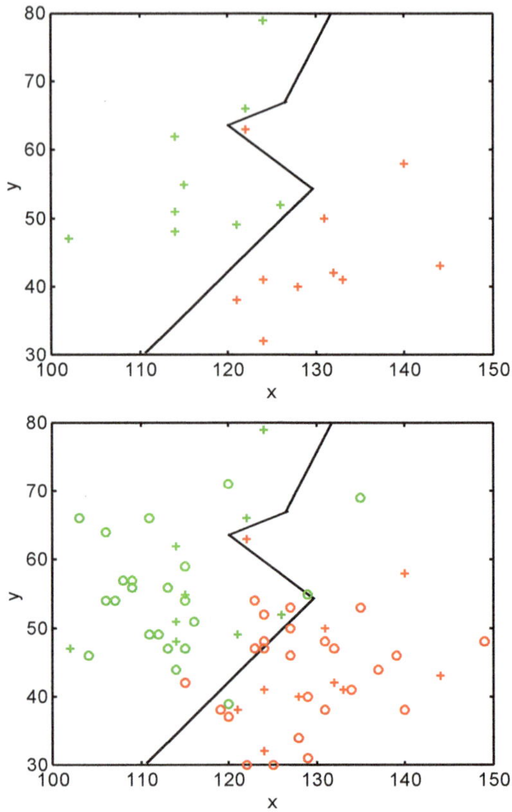

Fig. 4. A relatively complex decision rule to separate two classes with 100% accuracy (upper). Classification performance of the complex decision rule when independent data is tested. The decision rule which produced 100% accuracy for the training data now produces a significant number of errors (lower). This is an example of overtraining.

3.5 Example: Pattern recognition using discriminant analysis

Imagine one is devising a test to identify people with a (hypothetical) disease called "bilurosis". The clinical measurements from each subject consist of two blood measurements: the number of red blood cells (RBC) per unit volume (denoted as x in the following discussion) and the number of lymphocytes per unit volume (denoted as y in the following discussion). For convenience, it will be assumed that there are an equal number (n=40) of control subjects and subjects with the disease. However, in practice this is not likely to be the case. Table 2 gives a truncated view of the measured values from our experimental test. The task is to find an automated means of discriminating control subjects and disease subjects.

In an ideal world, one might hope to make a single measurement that would correctly distinguish the two groups. Initially, one might consider the information offered by the x and y measurements individually. Fig. 5 shows the individual histograms of the x and y variables. This histogram reveals that the distributions of x and y differ for the control and disease subjects, which implies that they are useful diagnostic measurements.

CONTROL SUBJECTS		DISEASE SUBJECTS	
RBC (x)	**LBC (y)**	**RBC (x)**	**LBC (y)**
114	51	128	40
126	52	144	43
...	...	...	...
111.4 (9.8)	**54.4 (9.0)**	**128.4 (7.2)**	**42.1 (9.1)**

Table 2. Data values used for Example 1 (note - these have been truncated at two rows for display here). The values in the last row are mean and standard deviation.

The histograms can allow one to devise a simple diagnostic test. For instance, it may be noted that the mean x value (111.4) in the control subjects is lower than that of the disease subjects (128.4). Therefore it is possible to make a decision rule that everyone with x values lower than or equal to 120 is a control subject. However, if the x value alone is used as a means of diagnosis, it is noted that 6 control subjects have values greater than this, and 4 disease subjects have lower values, so these subjects would be wrongly classified.
The corresponding performance table for the test (x>120 is disease) in Table 3. The following performance figures are derived:

Sensitivity	90%	Specificity	85%
PPV	85.7%	NPV	84.5%
Accuracy 87.5%			

		REALITY	
		DISEASE	*CONTROL*
TEST RESULT	*DISEASE*	36	6
	CONTROL	4	34

Table 3. Values of TP, FP, FN, and TN for the simple decision rule x>120

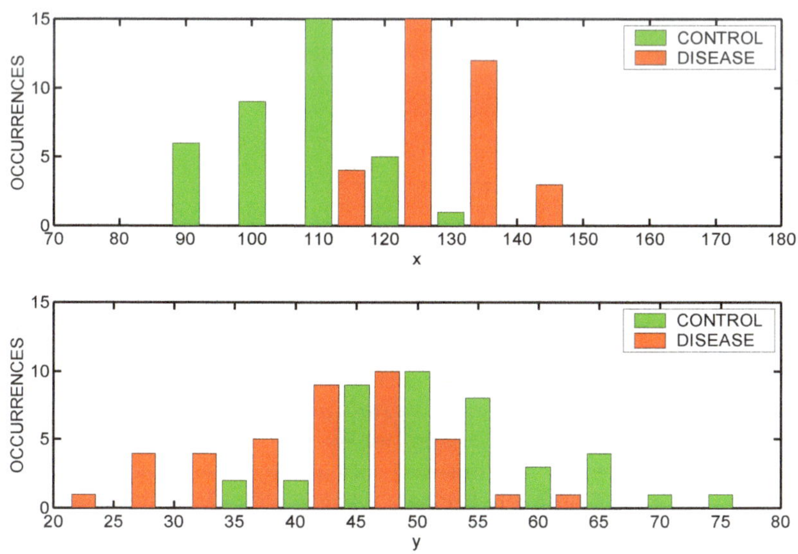

Fig. 5. Histograms of the x and y values for the data contained in Table 2.

It is not hard to see that the exact performance figures of a test are highly dependent on the exact decision rule used. For example, if the decision rule was changed to "x>114 is disease", then every disease subject would be classified as having the disease, but unfortunately 19 control subjects would also be classed as having the disease. In such a case, the performance figures would be:

Sensitivity	100%	Specificity	52.5%
PPV	67.8%	NPV	100%
Accuracy	76.3%		

An ideal diagnostic test would have all of these values equal to 100%. Intuitively, one might suspect that a better diagnostic test would be obtained if information from both the x and y measurements was used. One means of devising such a test is linear discriminant analysis.
The concept of LDA is easy to understand. Fig. 6 shows a scatter plot of the measured x and y data for the control and disease classes. It is easy to see that the two classes fall into two clusters that are well separated. The one-parameter decision rule attempts to find these two clusters by drawing horizontal and vertical decision lines; a better cluster division can be obtained by drawing more general lines of the form $y=mx+c$ as shown in the diagram.
Linear discriminant analysis answers the question of how to find the parameters of the line (or more generally, a hyperplane in n-dimensions). It is referred to as linear since the decision rules it produces will be based on linear combinations of the measured variables.

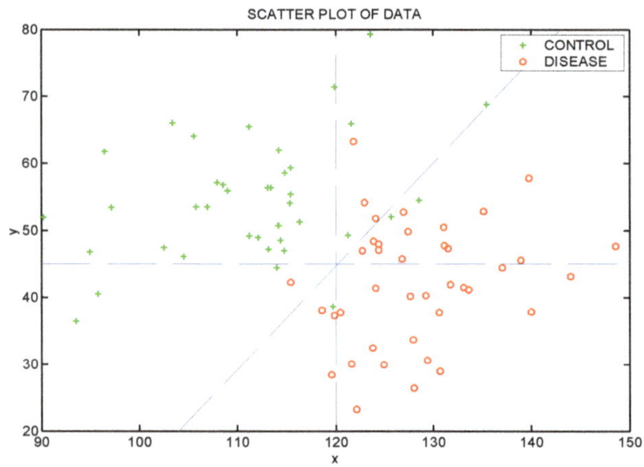

Fig. 6. Scatter plot of the x and y data used in Example 1.

A general derivation of the theory of linear discriminant analysis is beyond the scope of this chapter, but an approach will be used here based on work by Fisher (Fisher, 1936).
Conceptually, one wishes to find a line (or more generally a plane or hyperplane) which optimally separates the two classes of data. This is equivalent to finding the direction of projection onto a line, such that the projected values are well separated.
This is perhaps best explained pictorially, as seen in Fig. 7. In this figure, the two dimensional data points x=(x,y) are projected onto a line. Their value on the line is called their discriminant value. These discriminant values will have their own histograms/ probability density functions (sketched as green [or light grey] and red [or dark grey] pdfs on the discriminant line) for each class. The best choice of projection direction will separate out the two discriminant histograms to the maximum extent possible.

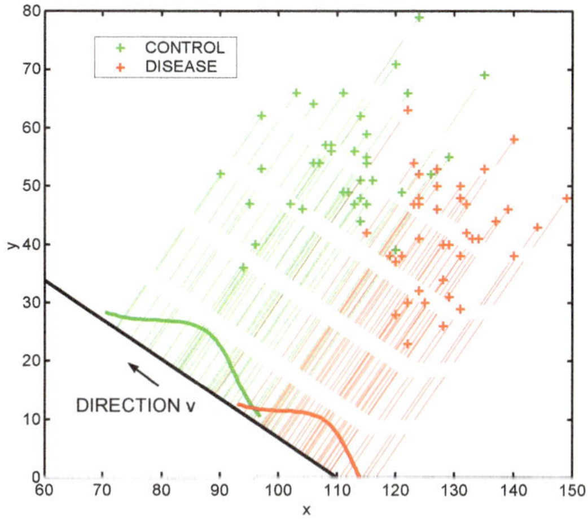

Fig. 7. Projection of the data used in Example 1 onto a vector of direction v, in order to produce a discriminant value for each data point.

This discriminant value will take on a range of (scalar) values, so the decision rule will be based on comparing the discriminant value against this threshold. A reasonable threshold is the discriminant value produced by the point which is equidistant between the two class mean vectors:

$$\frac{(\mu_A + \mu_B)}{2} \tag{6}$$

Therefore, the final decision rule to classify an arbitrary data vector x will be described by

$$(\mu_A - \mu_B)^T \Sigma^{-1} x \underset{\text{choose classB}}{\overset{\text{choose classA}}{\gtrless}} \frac{(\mu_A - \mu_B)^T \Sigma^{-1} (\mu_A + \mu_B)}{2} \tag{7}$$

If equality is achieved, the test is indeterminate.

One can apply this LDA rule to all 80 data points in the set to produce the following table of results:

		REALITY	
		DISEASE	*CONTROL*
TEST RESULT	*DISEASE*	37	4
	CONTROL	3	36

Table 4. Values of TP, FP, FN, and TN for the LDA rule in Eq. (7)

The corresponding performance values are:

Sensitivity	92.5%	Specificity	90%
PPV	90.2%	NPV	92.3%
Accuracy	91.25%		

These figures are an improvement over the single feature classifiers considered previously. The LDA decision rule described is termed Fisher's approach. An alternative derivation of a LDA classifier can be obtained using Bayes's rule. It uses the same assumptions about features being normally distributed, and having a common covariance matrix.
It yields a set of discriminant values q_k, one for each class, as follows:

$$q_k = \boldsymbol{\mu}_k{}^{\mathrm{T}}\boldsymbol{\Sigma}^{-1}\mathbf{x} - \tfrac{1}{2}\boldsymbol{\mu}_k{}^{\mathrm{T}}\boldsymbol{\Sigma}^{-1}\boldsymbol{\mu}_k + \log(\pi_k) \qquad (8)$$

where π_k is the prior probability of class k. In this case, the class with the highest discriminant value is chosen as the output class.

3.6 Modifications to linear discriminant analysis

The classification rule given above does not account for any knowledge one may have about the likely distribution of the classes prior to conducting the test (known as *the prior probabilities*). It is not unreasonable that knowledge of these distributions can be used to help the classifier (i.e., if 99% of people undergoing the test are normal, and one wishes the specificity to be good, then it may make sense to move the threshold for the discriminant value closer to the normal class). In other words, moving the discriminant value towards the normal class will result in higher specificity and lower sensitivity. As a specific example, in the above test one might set the prior probabilities of the two possible outcomes (denoted as π_A and π_B) of the test to 0.5, as based on the data available, there are equal numbers of control and disease subjects.
Alternatively, one may know from other experience that approximately 5% of the general population has the hypothetical disease "bilurosis" and hence set the prior probability of the disease outcome to 0.05 and of a normal outcome to 0.95. Knowledge or estimates of the prior probabilities, therefore, can be used to modify the discrimination rule as follows:

$$(\boldsymbol{\mu}_{\mathrm{A}} - \boldsymbol{\mu}_{\mathrm{B}})^{\mathrm{T}}\boldsymbol{\Sigma}^{-1}\mathbf{x} \quad \overset{\text{choose class A}}{\underset{\text{choose class B}}{\gtrless}} \quad \frac{(\boldsymbol{\mu}_{\mathrm{A}} - \boldsymbol{\mu}_{\mathrm{B}})^{\mathrm{T}}\boldsymbol{\Sigma}^{-1}(\boldsymbol{\mu}_{\mathrm{A}} + \boldsymbol{\mu}_{\mathrm{B}})}{2} - \log\left(\frac{\pi_B}{1-\pi_B}\right) \qquad (9)$$

Note that $\pi_A = 1 - \pi_B$. Finally, since the discriminant value is not simply a hard decision ("yes" vs. "no"), but rather a number, it may be used to estimate the confidence of the decision. Alternatively, this can be thought of as the *posterior probability* of a test vector belonging to a specific class.
A Bayesian formulation of the linear discriminant analysis test allows a convenient means to capture the confidence of our decision. It can be shown that the posterior probability of a test vector being in class k is given by

$$P_k = \frac{\exp(q_k)}{\sum_k \exp(q_k)} \qquad (10)$$

where q_k is its corresponding discriminant value for membership in set k. If any of the P_ks are close to one, then the classifier is very confident in assigning it to class k.

3.7 Techniques for improving classification performance – conversion to gaussianity

An important assumption in the derivation of a linear discriminant classifier is that the features have a Gaussian (normal) distribution. In other words, if the feature is x, then the probability density function (pdf) of x is given by

$$p_x(x) = \frac{1}{\sqrt{2\pi\sigma^2}} \exp\left(\frac{-(x-\mu)^2}{2\sigma^2} \right) \tag{11}$$

This is an assumption that is often violated by features which have useful classification information, and will lead to reduced performance of the classifier. For example, one feature which is used by the BiancaMed PAF detection system is based on the range of spread in a block of RR intervals. The resulting histogram can be more closely made to approximate a normal distribution by the application of the square root transformation.

Other transformations that are commonly used are the log transformation or the cube root. Features which are likely to be non-Gaussian include power measurements, envelope measurements, and counts (e.g., counting the number of premature ventricular contractions within a window).

4. Implementation

4.1 Block based PAF detector

Atrial fibrillation is known to be capable of causing ventricular depolarization timing changes (filtering action of the AV node) that can give rise to an irregularly irregular RR interval (difference between successive QRS complexes). As such, it is this type of RR behavior that is desirable to discriminate using suitable temporal features.

A block diagram showing input, preprocessing, feature generation, classification and output for a block based detector is provided in Fig. 8.

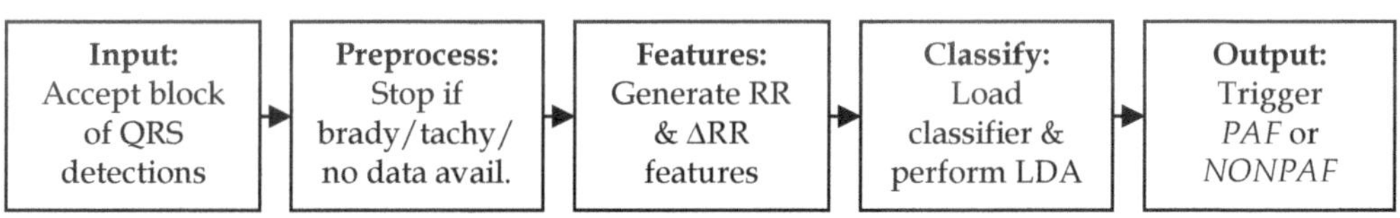

Fig. 8. Block based classification system

4.2 Deriving features using the RR series

The discussion in Section 3.4 on linear discriminant analysis describes how to derive a linear classifier from a set of features extracted from the data. The real key to a successful diagnostic test, however, is in identifying features which provide classification information. This is an art rather than a science, and in general features are found through a combination of a systematic approach and experience of the classifier designer. There are some techniques for finding optimal subsets of features, but in general it is the job of the researcher to seek out the most likely candidate features.

A first step towards selecting features for the final classifier was the formation of class-dependent histograms of each feature (a selection of these are shown in Fig. 9). Inspection of the histograms allowed features that had well separated means and approximately Gaussian distribution to be chosen.

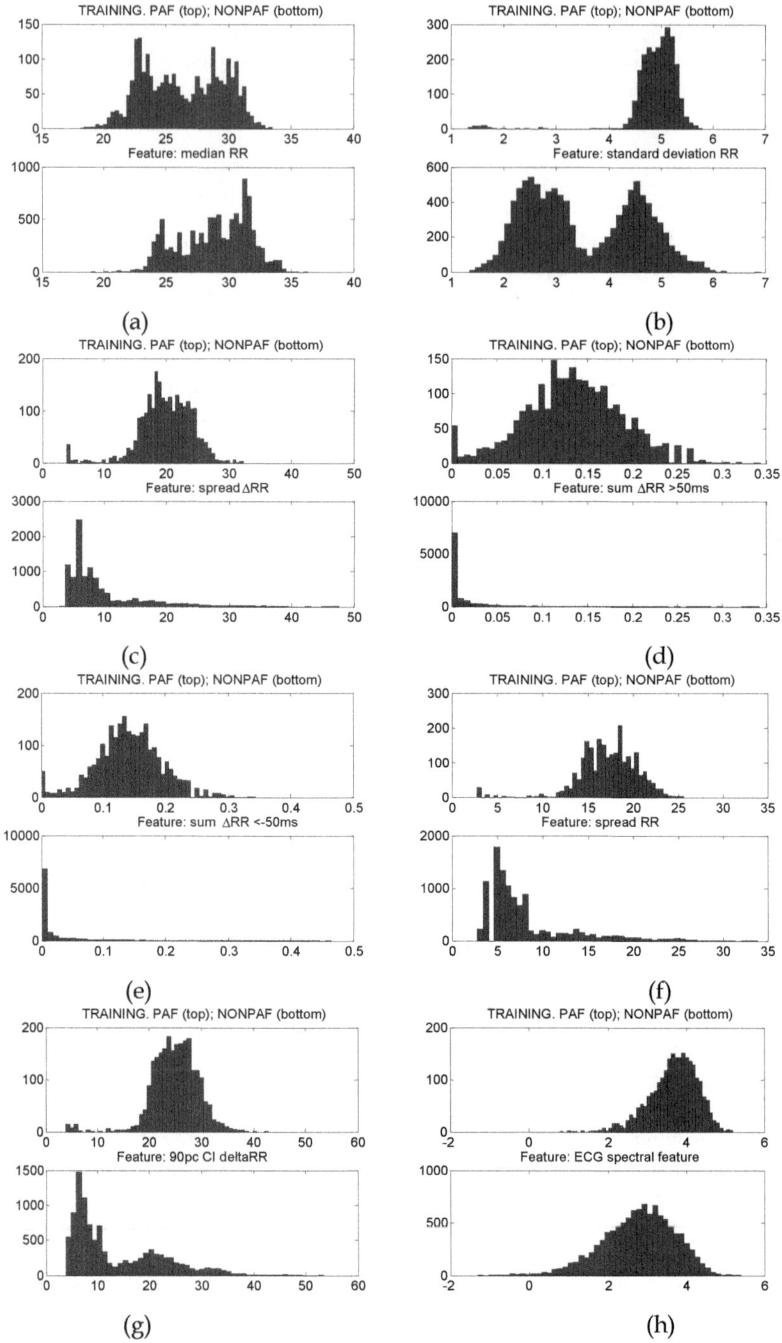

Fig. 9. Histograms of candidate features from training set.

Some features of RR and ΔRR (i.e., delta or difference between successive RR intervals) considered were:

- Mean (Huang et al., 1998; Lombardi et al., 2004)
- Root Mean Square (RMS)
- Median
- Standard deviation (Capucci et al., 1992)
- Interquartile range
- Other quantile ranges
- First 4 serial correlation coefficients (de Chazal & Heneghan, 2001)
- Power spectral density estimates (Bettoni et al., 2002; Herweg et al., 1998)
- PNN50, %NN >50 ms different that previous interval (Maier et al., 2001)
- PNN50a, %NN >50 ms longer than previous interval
- PNN50b, %NN >50ms shorter than previous interval
- Skewness
- Kurtosis
- Allan factor
- Approximate entropy

Note that power spectral (frequency based) features were excluded from the final feature set due to extra computational complexity. Also, in the case of multiple features that measure similar basic characteristics of the signal (e.g. trimmed mean, median and mean are all measures of central tendency) only one feature was chosen. The bimodal distribution of the log standard deviation of RR intervals (NONPAF) in Fig. 9(b) makes a Gaussian fit difficult. It should be noted that features which ignore extreme values (whether high or low) are likely to be more robust in a Holter based system where a certain level of QRS misdetection is possible. After analysis of the features, five were chosen that provide an insight into the spread, central tendency and count of thresholded differences.

A first preprocessing step prior to calculating ECG features is to verify that the sequence of QRS detections is within certain bounds. For instance, if the block beats per minute (bpm) value is greater than a particular threshold (suggesting tachycardia) or below a certain threshold (suggesting bradycardia), then the brady/tachy function should already have been activated; thus, it does not make sense to go through the classification process.

The RR interval series is used to generate the classification features. Since the classification is performed on 100 beat blocks, this number of QRS detections must be buffered along with the associated ECG signal. Features are generated independently for each of the blocks, whether overlapping or not.

The time-domain features were calculated as follows. The QRS intervals series, denoted by $QRS[n]$, and assuming n intervals contained within each block, the RR ($RR[n-1]$) and difference in RR ($\Delta RR[n-2]$) series were generated.

Subsequently, the following time domain measures were calculated for each block:

1. Trimmed mean (i.e. deletion of outliers) of $RR[n-1]$ at 10%.
2. Spread in $\Delta RR[n-2]$ from 5% to 95%.
3. Spread in $RR[n-1]$ from 5% to 95%.
4. Sum of $\Delta RR[n-2]$values greater than 50 ms (scaled to operating sampling rate) divided by the total number of $\Delta RR[n-2]$ values within the block, i.e. (n-2). Upper bound set to twice the trimmed mean of $RR[n-1]$.
5. Sum of $\Delta RR[n-2]$values less than –50 ms (scaled to operating sampling rate) divided by the total number of $\Delta RR[n-2]$ values within the block, i.e. (n-2). Upper bound set to twice the trimmed mean of $RR[n-1]$.

Transformations were applied to these features where appropriate. It should be noted that each of the five features operates on a subset of the block RR sequence; therefore, they might be expected to be quite robust to outlying (and perhaps erroneous) values.

4.3 Training and test data

The classifier parameters used in the block detector must first be generated. This is achieved using supervised learning on available annotated data, specifically a "training" subset. A separate "test" (i.e., independent and withheld) subset is kept separately from the "training" data; these "test" data are then used for performance validation.

The class mean vectors were calculated using

$$\boldsymbol{\mu}_{\mathbf{A}} = \frac{1}{N_A}\sum_{k=1}^{N_A} \mathbf{x}_{\mathbf{k},\mathbf{A}} \qquad \boldsymbol{\mu}_B = \frac{1}{N_B}\sum_{k=1}^{N_A} \mathbf{x}_{\mathbf{k},B} \tag{12}$$

where A denotes the normal class, B is the PAF class, N_A is the number of training vectors in class A, and $\mathbf{x}_{\mathbf{k,A}}$ is the kth vector from Class A. The common covariance matrix was calculated using

$$\Sigma = \frac{1}{N_A + N_B - 2}\left(\sum_{k=1}^{N_A}\left(\mathbf{x}_{\mathbf{k,A}} - \boldsymbol{\mu}_{\mathbf{A}}\right)^T\left(\mathbf{x}_{\mathbf{k,A}} - \boldsymbol{\mu}_{\mathbf{A}}\right) + \sum_{k=1}^{N_B}\left(\mathbf{x}_{\mathbf{k,B}} - \boldsymbol{\mu}_{\mathbf{B}}\right)^T\left(\mathbf{x}_{\mathbf{k,B}} - \boldsymbol{\mu}_{\mathbf{B}}\right)\right) \tag{13}$$

Using the calculated values of $\boldsymbol{\mu}_K, \Sigma$, an incoming feature $\mathbf{x}$ may be classified by calculating the discriminant value:

$$q = \left(\boldsymbol{\mu}_B - \boldsymbol{\mu}_A\right)^{\mathrm{T}} \boldsymbol{\Sigma}^{-1}\mathbf{x} - \tfrac{1}{2}\left(\boldsymbol{\mu}_B - \boldsymbol{\mu}_A\right)^{\mathrm{T}} \boldsymbol{\Sigma}^{-1}\left(\boldsymbol{\mu}_B + \boldsymbol{\mu}_A\right) + \log\left(\frac{\pi_B}{1 - \pi_B}\right) \tag{14}$$

and posterior probabilities for class membership calculated using

$$P_A = 1 - P_B$$
$$P_B = \frac{\exp(y)}{1 + \exp(y)}$$

The databases available for the training and testing of the algorithm are available online through the Physionet resource (Goldberger et al., 2000). These databases, containing expert annotated atrial fibrillation segments, are as follows:

1. **Database AFDB** is the MIT-BIH Atrial Fibrillation Database and includes 25 long-term ECG recordings of human subjects with atrial fibrillation (mostly paroxysmal). Of these datasets, 2 have no original ECG signal for validation with the QRS detector.
2. **Database MITDB** is the MIT-BIH Arrhythmia Database contains 48 half-hour excerpts of two-channel ambulatory ECG recordings, obtained from 47 subjects. 8 of the datasets contain periods of atrial fibrillation.
3. **Database NSRDB** is the MIT-BIH Normal Sinus Rhythm Database. This database includes 18 long-term ECG recordings of subjects. Subjects included in this database were found to have had no significant arrhythmias; they include 5 men, aged 26 to 45, and 13 women, aged 20 to 50.

4. **Database NSR2DB** is the Normal Sinus Rhythm RR Interval Database. This database includes beat annotation files for 54 long-term ECG recordings of subjects in normal sinus rhythm (30 men, aged 28.5 to 76, and 24 women, aged 58 to 73).

A PAF episode was defined to begin at either an atrial fibrillation "AFIB" or atrial flutter "AFL" annotation. Any other rhythm annotation was a non-event (i.e. NONPAF). An assumption is made here that the target hardware for the PAF classification samples ECG at 128 Hz. Due to the fact that the Physionet databases were sampled at greater than the desired sampling rate (Fs) of 128 Hz, the initial classifier development was performed by dividing the supplied database QRS detections by their respective Fs values, multiplying by 128, rounding to the nearest integer, and then scaling to milliseconds. This is an attempt to provide a rough simulation of the increased sampling (but not quantization) error that is expected in hardware. For more realistic "real world" performance estimates, it is intended that the ECG data available as part of the Physionet datasets be resampled and quantized to the expected input values and then run through the target hardware's QRS detector. This step should serve to highlight the influence (if any) of QRS misdetections/lead dropout on classification performance.

The 25 AFDB datasets were used to select the classifier features. This was achieved by using leave-one-out cross fold validation to provide a measure of generalized error and then tuning features to maximize accuracy. The leave-one-out cross-validation scheme works as follows: one subject's data is withheld and classifier parameters are obtained by using all the other available training data. The classification performance of the resulting classifier can then be estimated on the one withheld set. Overall estimated classification performance can then be obtained by averaging the results over all possible withheld sets.

When the (empirically determined) 5 features (as listed previously) were determined, the final classifier parameters were stored based on all of the AFDB datasets. Testing can then be performed on the same database, although some bias is to be expected. The other three databases, MITDB, NSRDB and NSR2DB represent independent test data.

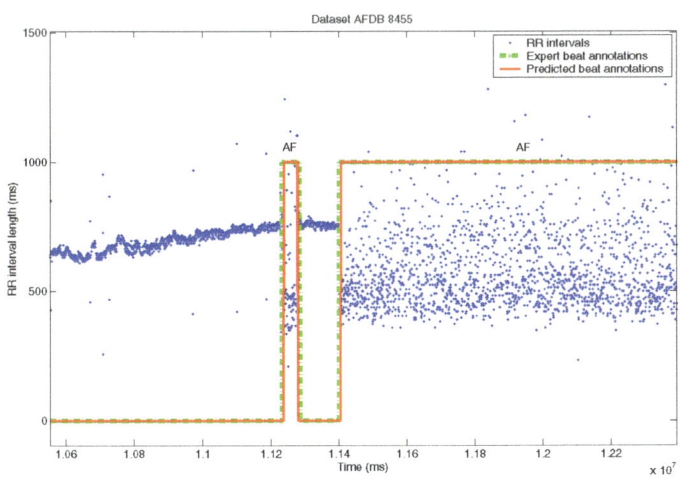

Fig. 10. BiancaMed algorithm processes multiple measures from the RR series and accurately predicts PAF events. This record excerpt is part of the AFDB.

5. Test results: Performance of the system

The classifier parameters saved during the training process were then used to classify each of the withheld test datasets from MITDB (48 records, 8 with AF), NSRDB (18 records) and NSR2DB (54 records). ROC plots of the performance on the AFDB and MITDB are presented in Fig. 11.

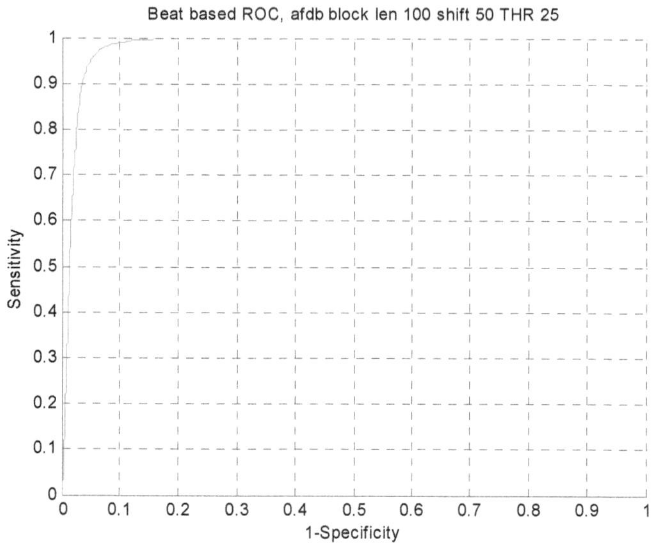

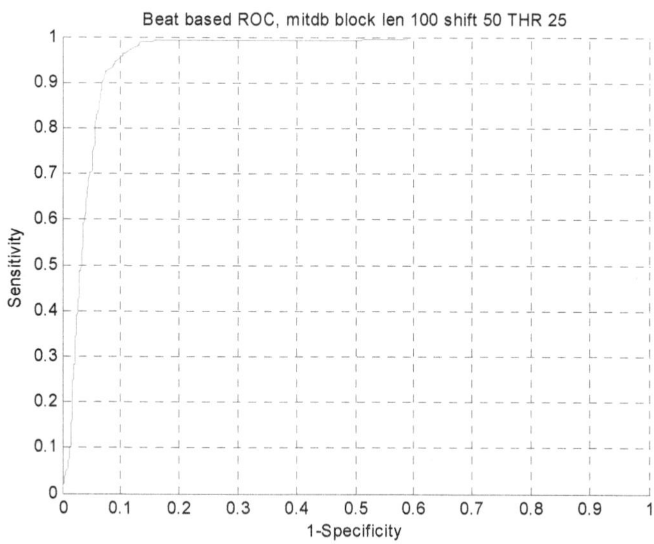

Fig. 11. Receiver operating characteristics: AFDB (left) and MITDB (right) on a per beat basis

Database	Aggregation	ESe	EPP	DSe	DPP
MITDB	Gross	81	72	74	54
	Average	88	70	81	55
AFDB	Gross	81	54	75	59
	Average	79	78	80	71

Table 5. Published 'King of Hearts Express AF' (c.f. 'Physician's Operation Manual') database test results including all events (all figures are percentages)

Database	Beat Se	Beat Sp	Beat Acc
MITDB	88	94	93
AFDB	94	97	96* estimated

Table 6. Published 'Tateno and Glass' database test results (beat basis)

Database	Aggregation	ESe	EPP	DSe	DPP
MITDB	Gross	81	90	93	89
	Average	88	88	86	87
AFDB	Gross	71	80	92	95
	Average	76	67	83	80

Table 7. BiancaMed system, 100 beat epochs with 50% overlap, episode and duration figures (compared to expert beat annotations) tested on subjects with AF episodes (i.e. all AFDB records and 8 MITDB records).

An alternate method of measuring the performance is on a beat-by-beat basis. These measures allow the determination of the expected number of false triggers on recordings free of AF such as the NSRDB, NSR2DB and those records with other arrhythmias in MITDB). Table 8 shows results for the system processing epochs containing 100 beats.

Database	Beat Se	Beat Sp	Beat Acc
MITDB	93	92	92
AFDB	92	96	94
NSRDB	--	100*	100
NSR2DB	--	100**	100

[*=1,600 FP beats out of total 1,582,715 beats; **=10,150 FP beats out of total 5,258,870 beats]

Table 8. BiancaMed system, 100 beat epochs with 50% overlap, beat figures (compared to expert beat annotations). All database records analyzed.

6. Conclusion

On a beat-by-beat basis the systems boasts high sensitivity and specificity on the MITDB (arrhythmia) and AFDB (atrial fibrillation) datasets as well as a low false trigger rate on the normal sinus rhythm records in NSRDB and NSR2DB.

As can be seen from the gross and average sensitivity and positive predictivity figures the PAF detector described in this chapter does, on average, perform well at discriminating patterns consistent with atrial fibrillation in the withheld test set.

However, it must be noted that other rhythms (whether they be arrhythmias or arising during periods that would be classed as "normal") that give rise to irregular RR interval times may also trigger the detector. Runs of ventricular premature contractions (PVCs) can cause false triggering. In addition, if the QRS detector incorrectly detects noise/artifact or T waves as QRS complexes, the false impression of "irregularly irregular" RR intervals may cause the algorithm to incorrectly trigger.

The BiancaMed PAF classification system is competitive with the published 'King of Hearts' episode and duration figures. On a beat-by-beat basis (Table 5.3) the systems boasts high sensitivity and specificity on the MITDB (arrhythmia) and AFDB (atrial fibrillation) datasets as well as a low false trigger rate on the normal sinus rhythm records in NSRDB and NSR2DB.

The episode, duration, and block accuracies of the system indicate that it performs very well in detecting PAF, and also at achieving a low false detection rate in normal subjects. As the method described only relies on inter-heartbeat intervals and low complexity time-domain features it is well suited to power-dependent applications such as ECG event recorders. It is also suited to other sensors of heart-rate, such as photoplethysmogram and ballistocardiogram.

The system outlined in this chapter has clear clinical relevance as an enabler for long term automatic capture of rare or asymptomatic paroxysmal atrial fibrillation events which might otherwise be missed by short Holter recordings or manual event recorders.

7. References

Benjamin, E.J.; Wolf, P.A.; D'Agostino, R.B.; Silbershatz, H.; Kannel, W.B. & Levy, D. (1998). Impact of atrial fibrillation on the risk of death. *Circulation*, Vol.98, No.10, pp. 946–952.

Bettoni, M. & Zimmermann, M. (2002). Autonomic tone variations before the onset of paroxysmal atrial fibrillation. *Circulation*. Vol.105, No.23, pp.2753-9.

Capucci, A.; Santarelli, A.; Boriani, G. & Magnani, B. (1992). Atrial premature beats coupling interval determines lone paroxysmal atrial fibrillation onset. *Int J Cardiol*. Vol. 36, No.1, pp.87-93.

Dash, S.; Chon, K.H.; Lu, S. & Raeder, E.A. (2009). Automatic Real Time Detection of Atrial Fibrillation. *Annals of Biomedical Engineering*. Vol.37, No.9, pp.1701-1709.

de Chazal, P. & Heneghan, C. (2001). Automated Assessment of Atrial Fibrillation, *Computers in Cardiology*, Vol.28, pp.117-120.

Fisher, R. (1936). The use of multiple measurements in taxonomic problems. *Annals of Eugenics*, Vol.7, pp.179–88.

Gaillard, N.; Deltour, S. et al. (2010). Detection of paroxysmal atrial fibrillation with transtelephonic EKG in TIA or stroke patients. *Neurology*. Vol.74, No.21, pp.1666-70.

Goldberger, A.L.; Amaral, L.A.N.; Glass, L.; Hausdorff, J.M.; Ivanov, P.Ch.; Mark, R.G.; Mietus, J.E.; Moody, G.B.; Peng, C.K. & Stanley, H.E. (2000). PhysioBank,

PhysioToolkit, and PhysioNet: Components of a New Research Resource for Complex Physiologic Signals. *Circulation.* Vol.101,No.23,pp.e215-e220.

Herweg, B.; Dalal, P.; Nagy, B. & Schweitzer, P. (1998). Power spectral analysis of heart period variability of preceding sinus rhythm before initiation of paroxysmal atrial fibrillation. *Am J Cardiol.* Vol.82, No.7, pp.869-74.

Huang, J.L.; Wen, Z.C.; Lee, W.L.; Chang, M.S. & Chen, S.A. (1998). Changes of autonomic tone before the onset of paroxysmal atrial fibrillation. *Int J Cardiol.* Vol.66, No.3, pp.275-83.

Jager, F.; Moody, G.B.; Taddei, A. & Mark, R.G. (1991). Performance measures for algorithms to detect transient ischemic ST segment changes. *Computers in Cardiology,* Los Alamitos. pp.369–372.

Kannel, W.B.; Abbott, R.D.; Savage, D.D.; McNamara, P.M. (1982) Epidemiologic features of chronic atrial fibrillation: the Framingham study. *N Engl J Med.* Vol.306,pp.1018-22.

Kirchhof, P.; Bax, J. et al. (2009). Early and comprehensive management of atrial fibrillation: proceedings from the 2nd AFNET/EHRA consensus conference on atrial fibrillation entitled 'research perspectives in atrial fibrillation'. *Europace.* Vol.11, No.7, pp.860-85.

Liao, J.; Khalid, Z.; Scallan, C.; Morillo, C. & O'Donnell, M. (2007). Noninvasive cardiac monitoring for detecting paroxysmal atrial fibrillation or flutter after acute ischemic stroke: a systematic review. *Stroke.* Vol.38,No.11,pp.2935-40.

Lombardi, F.; Tarricone, D.; Tundo, F.; Colombo, F.; Belletti, S. & Fiorentini, C. (2004). Autonomic nervous system and paroxysmal atrial fibrillation: a study based on the analysis of RR interval changes before, during and after paroxysmal atrial fibrillation. *Eur Heart J.* Vol.25,No.14,pp.:1242-8.

Hong-Wei, L.; Ying, S.; Min, L.; Pi-Ding, L. & Zheng, Z. (2009). A probability density function method for detecting atrial fibrillation using R–R intervals. *Medical Engineering & Physics.* Vol.31,No,1,pp.116-23.

Maier, C.; Bauch, M. & Dickhaus, H. (2001). Screening and prediction of paroxysmal atrial fibrillation by analysis of heart rate variability parameters. *Computers in Cardiology.* Vol 28,pp.129-32.

Roche, F.; Gaspoz, J.M.; Da Costa, A.; Isaaz, K.; et. Al (2002). Frequent and prolonged asymptomatic episodes of paroxysmal atrial fibrillation revealed by automatic long-term event recorders in patients with a negative 24-hour Holter. *Pacing Clin Electrophysiol.* Vol.25, No.11,pp.1587-93.

Shouldice, R.B.; O'Brien, L.M.; O'Brien, C.; de Chazal, P.; Gozal, D. & Heneghan, C. (2004). Detection of obstructive sleep apnea in pediatric subjects using surface lead electrocardiogram features. *Sleep.* Vol.27,No.4,pp.784-92.

Shouldice, R.B.; Heneghan, C. & de Chazal, P. (2007). Automated detection of paroxysmal atrial fibrillation from inter-heartbeat intervals. *Conf Proc IEEE Eng Med Biol Soc.* 2007, pp.686-9.

Stridh, M. & Sornmo, L. (2001). Spatiotemporal QRST cancellation techniques for analysis of atrial fibrillation. *IEEE Trans on Biomed Eng,* Vol.48, pp.105-111.

Tateno, K. & Glass, L. (2001). Automatic detection of atrial fibrillation using the coefficient of variation and density histograms of RR and deltaRR intervals. *Med Biol Eng Comput.*, Vol.139; pp.664-71.

Part 3

Remodeling and Predictors

9

Novel Index for Determining the Development of Electrophysiological and Structural Atrial Remodeling in Patient with Atrial Fibrillation

Toshiya Kurotobi
Division of Cardiac Rhythm Management, Shiroyama Hospital,
Department of Advanced Cardiovascular Therapeutics,
Osaka University Graduate School of Medicine,
Japan

1. Introduction

The development of atrial remodeling process could contribute to the structural and electrophysiological changes in pulmonary veins (PVs) and atrium; which could promote local conduction abnormalities and cause an increased the arrhythmogenecity resulting in atrial fibrillation (AF) persistency. The efficacy of treatment strategy to restore sinus rhythm such as catheter ablation (CA) might be quite decreased in such cases with advanced atrial remodeling, therefore it is crucial to know the information associating with atrial electrical and structural remodeling for promoting AF.

In this study, we attempted to determine the novel factors relating the process of structural and electrophysiological remodeling in patients with AF in the inflammatory and anatomical views.

2. Novel index as increased inflammation determining the development of atrial remodeling

2.1 Backgrounds

The causes and pathogenesis of AF recurrences are multifactorial and are related to technical factors and a multitude of clinical factors; some studies have explored the possible role of inflammatory mechanisms in the pathogenesis of AF. The C-reactive protein (CRP) is a sensitive maker for reflecting a local or systemic inflammatory response, and some clinical studies also support the association of an elevated CRP level and an increase in AF episodes. In this study, we examined the association between a pre-existent inflammatory response and the recurrence of AF after CA, and clarified the clinical and electrophysiolocgical factors related to the CRP elevation.

2.2 Method

2.2.1 Study population

The study population consisted of 257 consecutive patients with drug-refractory episodes of AF who underwent radiofrequency catheter ablation. The patients' mean age was 61 years,

187 (73%) were male, and 77 (30%) had persistent AF defined as recurrent episodes of AF lasting more than 3 months. The exclusion criteria was as follows, 1; a left atrial diameter (LAD) of more than 55mm, 2; significant valvular disease requiring surgery, 3; an ejection fraction of less than 40%, and 4; hypertrophic obstructive cardiomyopathy. All antiarrhythmic agents (AAAs) were generally discontinued for at least 3 days before the CA. Vaugham-Williams Class I (Ia 47.9%, Ic 60.7%) AAAs was prior medicated in 80.9%, class II was 15.2%, class III was 10.5%, and class IV was 12.5%.

2.2.2 Electrophysiological study and catheter ablation

Transesophageal echocardiography was performed to exclude any left atrial (LA) thrombi. A 10-pole or 20-polar diagnostic catheter was positioned in the CS for pacing and recording. A 20-pole catheter was located in the right atrium to cover the area around the tricuspid annulus or superior vena cava (SVC). The LA and PVs were accessed by a transseptal approach. We introduced 3 steerable catheters including two spiral curve catheters into the left atrium through a single transseptal puncture site. The PVs were mapped with a circumferential 10-pole or 20-pole catheter (IBI, Irvine, CA, USA). The surface ECG and intracardiac electrograms filtered between 30 to 500 Hz were recorded simultaneously with a polygraph (DUO EP Laboratory; Bard Electrophysiology, Lowell, MA, USA). A single bolus of 150 IU/kg of heparin was administered after the transseptal puncture and repeated to maintain an activated clotting time of >300 seconds.

We initially performed a PV isolation procedure by using a double circular mapping technique during an isopreterenol administration (1-2 μg/min). We confirmed the success of the electrical PV isolation by monitoring the circumferential electrical isolation at the antrum level: approximately 1 cm from the ostium of both the right and left PVs. The complete disappearance of the potentials from all 4 PVs was confirmed in all patients. In case of burst-inducible AF after the PV isolation procedure, an additional roof line was created. Then, additional RF energy applications were appropriately applied for any mitral isthmus, induced atrial tachycardia circuits and complex fractionated electrical activity. If the arrhythmogenic foci were suspected to have originated from a non-PV area, they were located by searching with a roving catheter.

Radiofrequency (RF) energy was delivered for 30 to 60 seconds at each site using an 8mm tip catheter (Japan Life Line Co., Ltd., Fantasista, Tokyo, Japan). The RF energy was delivered with the power limited to 35 W. The temperature was limited to 55°C.

2.2.3 CRP measurement

The assessment of the CRP level was assessed by a high sensitive radio-immunoassay one day before the CA procedure. The CRP level was classified into 4 quartile levels (Quartile 1; <0.02 mg/dl, Quartile 2; 0.03-0.07 mg/dl, Quartile 3; 0.08-0.27 mg/dl, and Quartile 4; 0.28< mg/dl).

2.2.4 The evaluation of cardiac parameters

We measured the end-systolic LA diameter and the left ventricular parameters with 2D-echocardiography. LA volume and PV diameter was measured by integrating the volume traced in each slice of the 64-slice-MDCT scan (Philips Medicals Systems) one day before the CA.

2.2.5 Follow-up

All patients were discharged to home 3 days after the CA procedure and were seen in our hospital at 1-2 month intervals. The in-hospital AF episodes were carefully monitored for at least 2 days after the CA, and the AF episodes after discharge were adequately assessed by the patients' complaints, 12 lead ECG and 24 hour Holter ECG recordings. AF recurrence was defined as the occurrence of atrial tachyarrhythmias after a 2 month blanking period following the CA procedure. AAAs were given for 3 to 6 months to the patients with long-lasting persistent AF or to those with paroxysmal AF and easily induced residual AF. Following that, the AAAs were withdrawn and the AF episodes were further assessed without AAAs.

2.3 Result

2.3.1 CRP level relating clinical, structural, electrophysiological findings

Table 1 shows the association between the CRP quartiles and clinical characteristics. In clinical characteristics, the age, prevalence of structural heart disease, prevalence of hypertension, and number of prior anti-arrhythmic agents were significantly increased when the CRP level was elevated.

	Quartile 1 <0.02 (N=65)	Quartile 2 0.03-0.07 (N=64)	Quartile 3 0.08-0.27 (N=64)	Quartile 4 0.28< (N=64)	p value
Age (y.o)	59±11	62±10	61±10	64±10	0.026
Male (%)	74	71	75	71	0.95
SHD(%)	32	43	29	69	0.001
HT(%)	33	37	44	51	0.27
AF duration(y)	4.8	5.8	6.5	5.7	0.33
Persistent AF	36	21	35	27	0.21
Co-AFL(%)	25	29	34	30	0.77
# of AAAs	1.6	2.1	1.7	2.1	0.035

SHD; structural heart disease, HT; hypertension, Co-AFL; coexistent atrial flutter,
# of AAAs; number of anti-arrhythmic agents

Table 1. Patient characteristics and CRP quartiles

Table 2 shows the association among the CRP quintiles and structural, electrophysiological, procedural findings. In structural findings, the left atrial diameter was significantly increased for an elevated CRP level, and the LA volume also tended to be increased with a CRP elevation. IN electrophysiological findings, arrrhythmogenisity from PVs were significantly decreased when the CRP level was increased. However, the atrial substrate after PV delineation to maintain AF were highly observed when the CRP level was elevated.

	Quartile 1 <0.02 (N=65)	Quartile 2 0.03-0.07 (N=64)	Quartile 3 0.08-0.27 (N=64)	Quartile 4 0.28< (N=64)	p value
Structural findings					
LA diameter, (mm)					
(A-P)	35.1±5.5	35.6±5.6	36.5±5.5	38.1±5.5	0.001
(S-L)	38.1±6.6	39.3±5.8	40.0±7.4	40.0±6.9	0.25
(MV-PV)	53.7±8.3	52.2±8.8	54.0±9.0	51.7±8.3	0.46
LA volume, (cm3)	76.8±42	86.8±34	91.4±34	94.4±40	0.14
PV diameter, (mm)					
(LSPV)	19.1±2.8	18.3±2.5	18.5±3.5	19.3±3.7	0.76
(LIPV)	16.0±3.0	6.4±2.5	16.2±2.5	15.9±2.2	0.80
(RSPV)	19.1±3.4	18.4±3.1	19.0±2.9	18.4±2.4	0.66
(RIPV)	16.6±3.2	16.4±2.8	16.0±2.7	6.5±2.3	0.78
LVEF, %	64.3±12	65.1±12	64.7±8.3	59.5±13.2	0.08
Electrophysiological findings					
(Triggered AF)					
AF triggered by AFC (%)	75	71	68	61	0.38
AF triggered from PVs (%)	67	65	56	55	0.04
AFC from PVs (%)	93	90	84	0.19	
(Burst inducible AF)					
Pacing induced AF (%)	63	56	62	72	0.40
Pacing induced AT (%)	54	59	70	76	0.04
Residual inducible AF (%)	8	19	9	36	0.004
Procedural findings					
(Additional CA strategy)					
Roof line creation (%)	67	71	83	74	0.22
Mitral isthmus line (%)	22	33	32	26	0.60
SVC isolation (%)	25	15	13	16	0.41

LA; left atrium, A-P; anterior-posterior. S-L; septal-lateral, MV-PV; mitral valve-upper pulmonary vein AFC; arrhythmogenic foci, AT; atrial tachycardia, CA; cathter ablation,

Table 2. Structural, electrophysiological and procedural findings and CRP quartiles

2.3.2 CRP level and clinical course

Figure 1 represents the relation between the AF occurrence after the CA and the CRP quartiles. AF occurrence after CA was significantly higher when the CRP level was elevated (quintile 1; 11%, quintile 2; 13%, quintile 3; 20%, and quintile 4; 30% $p<0.001$).

The univariate analysis revealed that the CRP quartile, left atrial diameter, persistent AF, AF duration (m), number of prior AAAs, mitral isthmus line and superior vena cava isolation were significant factors for an AF recurrence. The multivariate analysis revealed that the CRP quartile [Odds ratio (95% CI); 2.06 (1.02-4.22)] was an independent factor to AF recurrences, as well as, the left atrial diameter [1.31(1.12-1.52)] and persistent AF[1.09(1.01-1.19)].

Figure 2 represents the effects of statins on the AF recurrence. The use of statins was significantly associated with a decreased incidence of an AF recurrence (7% vs. 19%, $p<0.05$), whereas the use of ACE or AII antagonists was not significantly associated with an AF recurrence (16% vs. 16%, $p<0.05$).

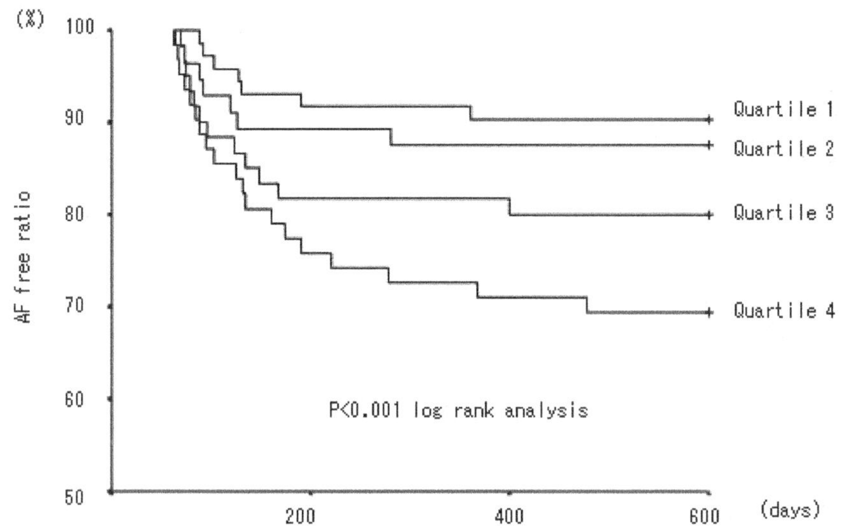

Fig. 1. The relation between the AF occurrence after the CA and the CRP quartiles.

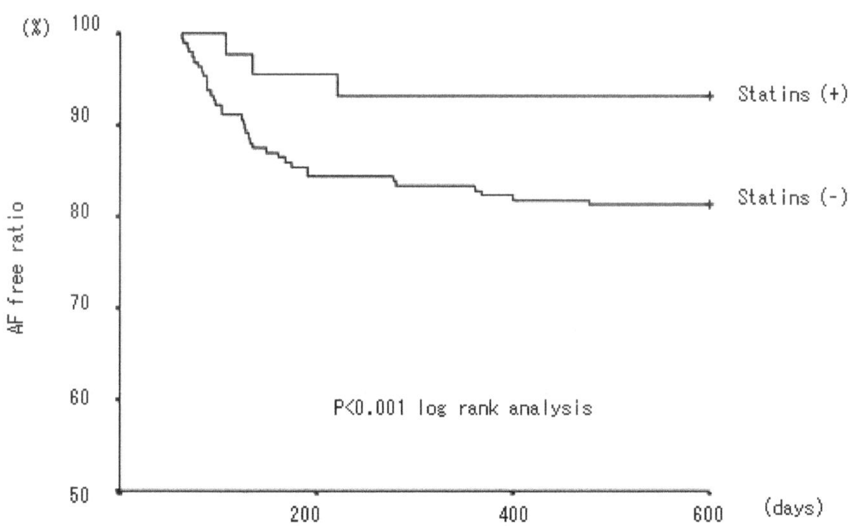

Fig. 2. The statin use and the AF occurrence after the CA.

2.3.3 The comparison of parameter and outcome between paroxysmal and persistent AF

CRP level (0.18±0.26 vs. 0.33±0.89 mg/dl, $p=0.042$) and left atrial diameter (35.1±5.4 vs. 38.9±5.2, $p<0.001$) were significantly lower in patients with paroxysmal than persistent AF. As procedural findings, the additional roof line creation (64% vs. 95%, $p<0.001$) and mitral isthmus line creation (13% vs. 37%, $p=0.038$) were significantly lower in patients with paroxysmal than persistent AF. The residual burst pacing inducible AF at the end of CA was significantly lower in patients with paroxysmal than persistent AF (14% vs. 36%, p<0.001). Figure 3 demonstrated the comparison of AF recurrence between paroxysmal and persistent AF. AF recurrence was significantly lower in patients with paroxysmal than persistent AF (15 % vs. 24%, p<0.01), although several clinical bias relating to structural remodeling were included between both groups.

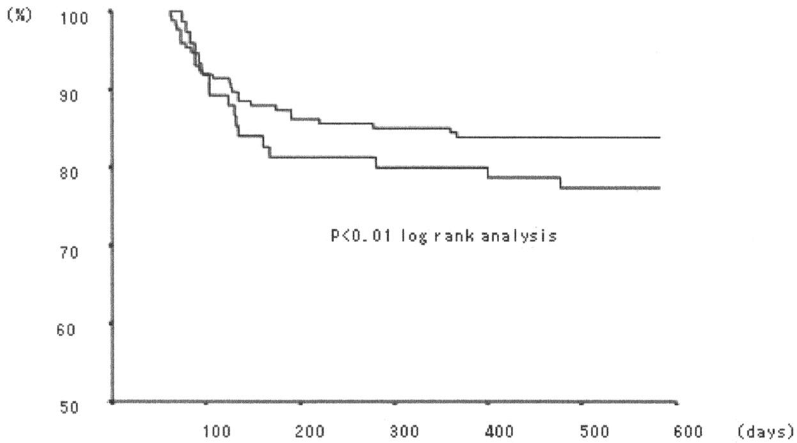

Fig. 3. The comparison of AF recurrence between paroxysmal and persistent AF.

2.4 Discussion

2.4.1 Epidemiological significance of inflammation on AF

Epidemiological studies have demonstrated that during an inflammatory response the CRP level is significantly higher in AF patients than in non-AF patients, and the increased CRP level is an independent contributing factor for the future development of an AF occurrence (Chung et al. 2001). The concept that inflammation contributes to at least some types of AF is supported by the frequent occurrence of AF after cardiac surgery (Bruins et al. 1997), a genetic study (Gaudino et al. 2003), and the association of AF with pericarditis (Spodick 1976). In particular, AF occurrences were highly observed in 5 to 70% of patients after cardiac surgery (Hogue et al. 1999); which may explain the clinically significant impact of the inflammatory response on AF occurrences, whereas hemodynamic intolerance and neuro-hormonal factors may also basically be associated with the development of AF by promoting the atrial functional and anatomical remodeling process.

2.4.2 Inflammation and the AF occurrence after CA

It has been reported that the electrical reconnection of isolated PV potentials might mainly be related to the AF occurrence after CA in patients with paroxysmal AF (Cappato et al. 2003). However, a PV electrical isolation strategy alone for patients with an enlarged atrium or persistent AF might be quite limited. It is now recognized that the development of AF leads to electrical and structural changes within the atria that perpetuate the atrial tachyarrhythmia. Shortening of the atrial refractory period and prolongation of the atrial conductivity as the result of a remodeled atrium could allow for the promotion and maintenance of multiple wavelet-re-entry circuits. The structural changes, including left atrial dilatation, further increase the fibrotic process with deposition of increased amounts of connective tissue, and promote the inconsistency and prolongation of the atrial conduction which leads to maintaining the perpetuation of AF. Previous studies have shown that AF recurrence after CA is significantly higher in patients with inducible AF after the PV isolation than in those without AF (Wright et al. 2008), and a younger age, smaller left atrial diameter(Van Gelder et al. 1991), and shorter duration of AF(Wijffels et al. 1995) are predictors of sinus rhythm maintenance. The results of those studies suggest that many of the AF recurrences are thought to be secondary to electrical and structural remodeling. In this study, the increased CRP level was significantly associated with an advanced age and structural heart disease with a significant relationship to a high AF inducibility after the PV isolation during the CA. Thus, these findings indicate that an increased CRP level might be a useful marker for the atrial remodeling process which would promote the future development of AF after the CA.

2.4.3 The mechanism of AF occurrence caused by inflammation

The precise mechanism for the increased circulating CRP level in AF is uncertain, but might reflect the active participation of CRP in the local inflammatory response within the atrial myocardium. In this study, AF recurrence was clearly associated with increased CRP levels even after the adjustment for confounding factors; which implies that the CRP may have a direct linkage to the AF occurrence, and not only be a secondary marker for atrial remodeling. Historical evidence to support a direct association between AF and inflammation can be extracted from the frequent association of AF to inflammatory conditions of the heart, such as myocarditis and pericarditis. Transient AF episodes were frequently observed after open heart surgery, and the results of the atrial biopsies taken from patients in AF have demonstrated evidence of inflammatory infiltration within the atrial tissue (Frustaci et al. 1997). The CRP could possibly bind to the membranes of the myocardial cells in inflamed tissues, and release an activating complement, leading to tissue damage. Data from ischemic heart disease also supporting the deposits of CRP, have also been demonstrated on immunohistochemical staining, in the vascular wall of active atherosclerotic plaques, where it is co-localized with the complement complex (Lagrand et al. 1997). Moreover, CRP has been shown to act as an opsonin and may participate in the clearance of apoptotic myocyte loss (Mevorach 2000). Myocyte loss is typically accompanied by replacement fibrosis. Thus, that local inflammatory response in the atrium may also be a part of the structural remodeling process associated with an increased occurrence of AF.

2.4.4 Anti-inflammatory agents for preventing AF occurrences

Recently studies have shown that the use of anti-inflammatory agents is associated with a decreased incidence of AF. The capacity of statins to reduce inflammation, CRP levels and oxidative stress is well-established (Strandberg et al. 1999) (Plenge et al. 2002). In a retrospective study, statins decreased the recurrence after successful external cardioversion of persistent lone AF (Siu et al. 2003); in a prospective analysis, statins protected against atrial fibrillation in patients with stable coronary artery disease (Young-Xu et al. 2003). The use of statins has recently been related to a 3-fold decrease in the odds of AF after noncardiac thoracic surgery (Amar et al. 2005), and has a lower incidence of AF (Marin et al. 2006) or other cardiac arrhythmias (Dotani et al. 2000) after coronary artery bypass surgery.

Pretreatment with statins, which significantly reduces the inflammatory cytokines and prevents the adhesion between the inflammatory cells and endocardium, is likely to facilitate the prevention of inflammatory mediated AF episodes.
There is evidence suggesting an association between AF and an enhanced renin angiotensin system activity. Experimental studies have revealed that angiotensin II possesses several pro-inflammatory properties which is the key mediatory factor in the inflammatory cascade (Healey et al. 2005). Further, angiotensin II exhibits a growth-enhancing effect on cardiac myocytes as well as on vascular smooth muscle cells and fibroblasts, thus resulting in the remodeling and fibrosis of the atria that could serve as a potential arrhythmogenic substrate for the development of AF. ACE-Is or angiotensin II antagonists have been shown to decrease the inflammatory response. (Brull, Sanders et al. 2002) (Hernandez-Presa et al. 1997), and prevent the development of myocardial fibrosis related to the electrical and structural remodeling process (Nakashima, Kumagai et al. 2000) (Fortuno et al. 1998) (Lopez et al. 2001).
In the data from this study, the patients with a pre-statin treatment experienced a significant decrease in AF episodes after the CA, however the patients with a pre-ACE-I or AII antagonist treatment did not experience that beneficial effect. The patients medicated with statins tended to include younger patients, whereas those medicated with ACE-Is or AII antagonists tended to include older patients with hypertension or a reduced ventricular function; which may have modified the results of the analysis of our data.
Recent clinical studies have demonstrated that the CRP level is transiently elevated after CA (Marcus et al. 2008), and that the short-term AF episodes were transiently increased (Oral et al. 2002). These reports also suggested that the increased inflammatory response from the CA procedure may increase the following transient occurrences of AF. Pretreatment with statins significantly improved the short-term outcome within 3 days, and not only the long-term outcome after the CA in this study; which may be expected to facilitate a reduction in the AF occurrences after CA and improve the symptoms due to tachyarrhythmias with the avoidance of any unnecessary second CA procedures. Further studies are required to examine the beneficial effect of anti-inflammatory agents on improving the short and long term outcome after CA.

3. Novel index as left atrial roof shape determining the development of atrial remodeling

3.1 Backgrounds

The preexistent morphology of the PVs could modify their arrhythmogenicity (Lin et al. 2000; Lee et al. 2005; Pak et al. 2006). The development of the remodeling process could contribute to the structural and electrophysiological changes in the PVs and atrium; which could promote local conduction abnormalities and cause an increased PV/non-PV arrhythmogenecity resulting in AF persistency (Lee et al. 2005) (Wijffels et al. 1995) (Hoit et al. 1998) (Chen et al. 2002) (Johnson et al. 1986). This evidence supports the observation that the morphological findings of the PVs and atrium may include a crucial role of helping to identify the characteristics of their pre-existing arrhythmogenicity (Kurotobi et al. 2011). However, there is a methodological limitation of the PVs and atrium in order to evaluate the morphological characteristics in a quantitative manner because of their own unique, variable and asymmetrical features.
The part of the left atrial (LA) roof which consists of the upper wall of the left atrium and upper PVs, incorporating the LA, was described as the LA roof silhouette, and could easily be visualized by pulmonary angiography or CT imaging. The morphological findings of the PVs and atrium may include a crucial role of helping to identify the characteristics for the

electrical and structural remodelling. In this study, we examined the hypothesis that the LA roof shape could be used as a novel predictor in patients with AF to allow us to determine the characteristics of the PVs, atrial arrhythmogenicity and substrate for promoting AF.

3.2 Methods

3.2.1 Study population

The study population consisted of 153 consecutive patients with drug-refractory episodes of AF who underwent radiofrequency catheter ablation (CA). The patients' mean age was 62 years, 122 (80%) were male, and 58 (38%) had persistent AF defined as recurrent episodes of AF lasting more than 3 months. The exclusion criteria was same as CRP study.

3.2.2 Electrophysiological study and catheter ablation

Electrophysiological study and ablation procedure was same as CRP study, and had already stated in the section of 2.2.2.

3.2.3 The induction and detection of the arrhythmogenic foci

The induction of arrhythmogenic foci was performed according to our previously reported paper (Kurotobi, Iwakura et al.). In brief, spontaneous arrhythmogenic foci in both atria were induced and carefully mapped before and after the PV isolation procedure using an intravenous infusion of high dose isoproterenol (ISP) of up to 20 μg/min without any sedation. If AF persisted or spontaneously occurred under the ISP, we attempted to cardiovert the AF up to 3 times. To detect the location of the arrhythmogenic foci, we simultaneously used five multipolar catheters to record the electrograms from the PVs and outside the PVs to search for any arrhythmogenic foci. A 20-pole catheter (2 mm inter-electrode spacing) covered the area from the SVC to the crista terminalis, coronary sinus, and ostium of the left PVs. A roving catheter was located at the right superior PV ostium. During the ablation procedure, the ISP administration was maintained at 1-2 μg/min. At the end of the procedure, the same induction maneuvers as in the initial protocol (up to 20 μg/min) were repeated. Arrhythmogenic foci were defined as direct AF triggers or spontaneous reproducible atrial premature beats with coupling intervals of < 350ms or frequent repetitive firings.

3.2.4 The evaluation of left atrial volume

We measured the end-systolic LA diameter and left ventricular parameters with 2D-echocardiography. The LA volume and PV diameter were measured by integrating the volume traced in each slice of the 64-slice-MDCT scan (Philips Medicals Systems) during several days prior to the CA. To enhance the cardiac cavity, contrast medium was injected at a flow-rate of 2.5 mL/s through an antecubital vein using an injector. The LA volume was measured by integrating the volume traced in each slice of the CT scan from the level of the mitral annulus to the roof of the left atrium with commercially available software (EP planner, Philips Medical Systems, Haifa, Israel). Each slice was automatically traced with digital markers to exclude the PVs and LA appendage at their ostial level. The LA appendage was excluded from the volumetric analysis.

3.2.5 The assessment of the LA roof shape

According to the PVs and LA dominant level, we classified the LA roof shape into a deep V shape (group A; Possible PV dominant type), shallow V shape (group B) and flat-coved shape (group C; Possible LA dominant type) using both PVs cine angiography (Figure 4). Cine angiography was performed by spontaneous contrast medium injection from the long sheath located at the upper right and left PVs. The shape of LA roof was determined by using antero-posterior projection, and was assessed by an upper angle between the right and left side LA wall silhouette. Deep V shape (A) was defined an less than 140°, shallow, V shape (B) was 140°-180°, and flat-coved shape was more than 180°(C).

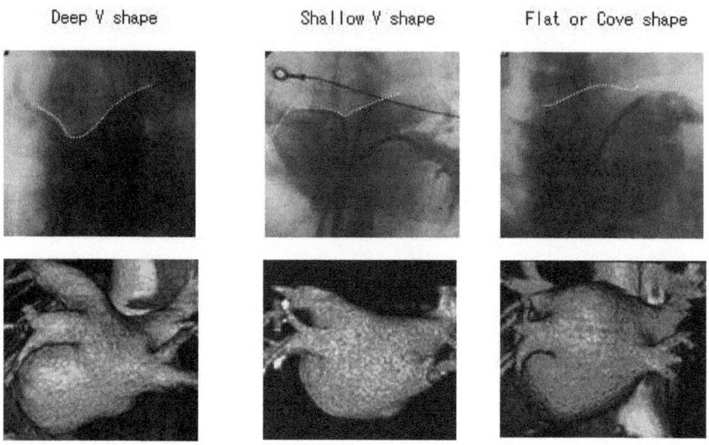

Fig. 4. Classification of roof shape.

3.3 Results

3.3.1 Patient characteristics and roof shape

The comparison of the patient characteristics among group A, B and C are shown in Table 3. Group A was observed in 35 patients (23%), B in 76 (50%), and C in 42 patients (27%). There were no significant differences in the mean age, mean AF duration, or clinical coexistence of atrial flutter, among the 3 groups. As the LA roof silhouette became flat, the number of prior of AAD's (A; 2.1±0.9 vs. B; 1.7±1.4 vs. C; 1.2±0.8, p=0.003) significantly decreased, and the prevalence of structural heart disease (A; 19% vs. B; 40% vs. C; 68%, p=0.002) and persistent AF (A; 26% vs. B; 35% vs. C; 52%, p=0.014) significantly increased.

	d-V (n=35)	s-V (n=76)	F-C (n=42)	p value
Age (years)	64.7±6.9	61.4±11.3	62.6±8.7	0.40
Male (%)	83	75	86	0. 69
SHD (%)	19	40	68	0.002
Hypertension (%)	30	24	46	0.10
AF period (m)	63.8	67.1	67.0	0.83
Per-AF	26	35	52	0.014
The duration of pe-AF	14.3	22.7	37.8	0.108
Co-AFL(%)	27	26	39	0.42
# of AAD	2.1±0.9	1.7±1.4	1.2±0.8	0.003

SHD; structural heart disease, Co-AFL; coexistent atrial flutter, AAD; anti-arrhythmic drug per-AF; persistent AF

Table 3. Clinical background and roof shape

3.3.2 Relationship among the LA roof shapes and electrophysiological and structural findings

The electrophysiological and structural findings of each roof shape group are shown in Table 4.

As the LA roof silhouette became flat, the incidence of AF arising from the PVs (A; 70% vs. B; 57% vs.C; 40%, p=0.003), AF from the upper PVs (A; 63% vs. B; 41% vs. C; 38%, p=0.046) and from arrhythmogenic foci including reproducible premature beats (A; 94% vs. B; 84% vs. C; 76%, p=0.033) significantly decreased. On the other hand, the incidence of AF arising from non-PV sites (A; 6% vs. B; 13% vs. C; 22%, p=0.041) and from arrhythmogenic foci from non-PV sites (A; 26% vs. B; 46% vs. C; 54%, p=0.016) significantly increased as the LA roof silhouette became flat. A multivariate analysis demonstrated that the deep V shape was an independent contributing factor to AF triggers from PV [Odds ratio (95% CI); 2.94 (1.27-6.80), p=0.012]. As the LA roof silhouette became flat, the incidence of pacing inducible AF just after the PV isolation (A; 51% vs. B; 65% vs. C; 79%, p=0.001) and at the end of the CA (A; 12% vs. B; 24% vs. C; 36%, p=0.016) significantly increased.

The LA diameter (A-P; 33.1±2.8 mm for A vs. 37.4±5.6mm for B vs. 40.2±6.3mm for C, p<0.001;. S-L; 36.1±5.8 mm for A vs. 39.4±6.6 mm for B vs. 43.2±6.8 mm for C, p<0.001; MV-PV; 48.2±6.0 mm for A vs. 55.3±8.7 mm for B vs. 58.4±7.6 mm for C, p<0.001.) and entire LA volume (A; 69.5±24.1 ml vs. B; 85.2±34.9ml vs. C; 105.7±45.4, p<0.001) became significantly larger, as the LA silhouette became flat. The PV diameter of each PV and left ventricular ejection fraction did not differ between the three roof shape groups.

	deep V (n=35)	shallow V (n=76)	flat or cove (n=42)	p value
Electrophysiological findings				
Trigger inducible AF (%)				
AF from 4PVs	70	57	40	0.003
AF from upper PVs	63	41	38	0.046
AF from non-PV sites	6	13	22	0.041
AFCs from 4PVs	94	84	76	0.033
AFCs from upper PVs	90	76	64	0.02
AFCs from non-PV sites	26	46	54	0.016
# of AF foci from PVs	0.86	0.76	0.80	0.82
# of all AF foci	2.03	1.93	2.29	0.28
Pacing inducible AF (%)				
Just after PVI	51	65	79	0.001
At the end of the CA	12	24	36	0.016
Structural findings				
Left atrial diameter, (mm)				
(A-P)	33.1±2.8	37.4±5.6	40.2±6.3	0.001
(S-L)	36.1±5.8	39.4±6.6	43.2±6.8	0.001
(MV-PV)	48.2±6.0	55.3±8.7	58.4±7.6	0.001
LA volume, cm^3	69.5±24.1	85.2±34.9	105.7±45.4	0.001
PV diameter (mm)				
(LSPV)	18.5±2.8	19.0±2.9	19.5±4.8	0.19
(LIPV)	15.3±2.4	15.8±2.2	15.5±3.2	0.74
(RSPV)	18.6±2.6	19±3.2	19.3±3.7	0.32
(RIPV)	15.8±2.2	15.9±2.6	15.7±2.9	0.83
LVEF, %	66.1±8.6	63.3±13.7	59.7±13.1	0.08

PVs; pulmonary veins, PVI; pulmonary vein isolation, CA; catheter ablation procedure
AF; atrial fibrillation, AFCs; arrhythmigenic foci,
AFCs include reproducible atrial premature beats as the possible AF trigger.

Table 4. Relation between the LA roof shapes and electrophysiological and strictural findings

3.3.3 Clinical outcome

An in-hospital recurrence was observed in 28/152 (18%) patients, and a long-term AF recurrence was observed in 29/152 (19%) patients. The mean follow-up period after the CA was 567 days (360-1065 days). The AADs were used were administrated after the CA in 30% of the patients (persistent; 47%, paroxysmal; 23%). The ratio of additional LA roof line (A; 64% vs. B; 84% vs. C; 88%, $p<0.05$), and mitral isthmus line (A; 14% vs. B; 22% vs. C; 34%, $p<0.05$) during CA were significantly highly required as the LA silhouette became flat, whereas the AF recurrence was not significantly different among three groups (A; 18% vs. B; 18% vs. C; 23%, n.s.) .

3.4 Discussion

3.4.1 LA roof shape and PV/LA dominancy

From the embryological view, the PV trunks are shown to derive from a common vessel, which becomes absorbed within the LA from superior-posterior direction. This incorporation transforms the branches of this common PV into separately inserting individual 4 PV trunks, first into the right and left PV trunks and subsequently into the superior and inferior trunks (DeRuiter et al. 1995) (Neill 1956) (Yamane et al. 2008). Anatomical PV structure could be caused by either anomalous branching of the common PV or by the variable absorption level of the common PV into the LA, therefore the incorporation level could mainly determine the LA roof shape according to the PV/LA dominancy level. When the common PV was incorporated into LA with a greater dominancy PVs, the silhouette of LA roof could be expressed by the upper wall of superior PVs; which the roof shape may be expressing as a V. On the other side, that was incorporated into LA with a less dominancy PVs, the silhouette of LA roof could be mainly expressed by the existent upper LA wall; which the LA roof may tend to be a flat shape.

In this study, an enlarged LA volume has a significant association with flat or coved LA roof shape. The development of the atrial structural remodeling process may also change the LA roof shape. Vertical LA enlargement could modify LA roof shape and sometimes overlap the PV silhouette as a component of LA roof, because the location of PVs is strictly stick to right and left lungs. Horizontal LA enlargement may promote the development of flat LA roof. Moreover, the advancement of cardiac rotation as a result of aging or hypertensive change; which is possibly related to atrial remodeling process, may also change the LA roof silhouette.

3.4.2 LA roof shape and PV arrhythmogenicity

AF is mainly initiated by PV triggers (Haissaguerre et al. 1998), and a rapidly firing source located within the PVs could be responsible for initiating, and in some cases, maintaining arrhythmias in patients with AF. The mechanism underlying such rapid discharges from PVs, including enhanced automaticity or triggered activity mechanisms may be involved in the initiation of AF (Patterson et al. 2005). In this study, AF triggers from PVs were highly observed in the patients with a deep V LA roof shape and PV dominancy. A previous paper reported that AF tended to originate from larger pulmonary veins (PVs) (Yamane et al. 2002). Especially in the superior PVs, the enlargement may often be consistent with the site of the arrhythmogenic PVs (Lin et al. 2000). PV enlargement caused by the stretch mechanism may increase the PV's automaticity and/or triggered activity to initiate AF (Satoh and Zipes 1996). However, there was no significant relation between the LA roof shape and PV diameter in this study. These findings may imply the novelty and independence of the LA roof shape as an index of the PV's arrhythmogenicity, as compared with the prior reports which discussed the PV features.

3.4.3 LA roof shape and non PV arrhythmogenicity

Non-PV foci could arise from the superior vena cava, left atrial posterior free wall, crista terminalis, ostium of the coronary sinus, inter atrial septum, or Marshall bundle (Hwang, Wu et al. 2000) (Chen et al. 1999) with an incidence of those ranging from 3.2 to 47% (Lin et al. 2003) (Mangrum et al. 2002) (Schmitt et al. 2002). The predominant non-PV triggering sites have a slow diastolic depolarization that enhances spontaneous depolarization (Chen et al. 2002), and the triggered activity of the non-PV triggers could also be involved in the onset and perpetuation of AF..

Because triggered activity is likely to occur in the presence of underlying disease such as cardiomyopathy (Boyden et al. 1984), the development of the atrial remodeling process may enhance the triggered activity of non PV lesions. A previous study reported that multiple PV arrhythmogenic foci may be associated with an older age, longer AF duration, and larger atrial all triggers (Lee et al. 2005), and persistent AF is more frequently triggered by foci from the LA side of the LA–PV junction than is paroxysmal AF(Pak et al. 2006). These findings could explain why the flat and cove LA roof as a result of advanced atrial remodeling increased the non PV arrhythmogenisity in this study.

3.4.4 The significance of LA roof shape as ablation strategy

It is now recognized that the development of AF leads to electrical and structural changes within the atria that perpetuate the atrial tachyarrhythmia. The structural changes, including the enlarged LA, further promote the inconsistency and prolongation of the atrial conduction which leads to maintaining the perpetuation of AF. In this study, the incidence of pacing inducible AF just after PV isolation and at the end of the CA significantly increased, as the LA roof silhouette became flat. A previous paper reported that AF recurrence after CA was significantly higher in patients with inducible AF after the PV isolation than in those without AF (Wright et al. 2008), therefore that evidence indicates the importance of a flat or coved LA roof shape as a reflection of any latent AF substrate in the atrium. And also, the development of the atrial remodeling process could enhance the triggered activity of non-PV lesions(Lee et al. 2005) (Boyden et al. 1984). In this study, non-PV foci were significantly more often observed in patients with a flat-coved LA roof shape.

P V isolation is the cornerstone of the treatment especially in patients with paroxysmal AF, however the PV electrical isolation strategy alone in patients with a remodeled atrium might be quite limited. Many of the AF recurrences are thought to be secondary to electrical and structural remodeling (Wijffels et al. 1995) (Van Gelder et al. 1991). Thus, a further additional extensive intervention following the PV isolation might be required to improve the outcome of the CA in patients with a flat-coved LA roof, whereas only a PV isolation strategy could lead to a favorable outcome in patients with a deep V LA roof.

4. Conclusion

Pre-exsistent CRP level and the shape of the LA roof shape as novel factors allowed us to understand the structural and the electrophysiological information of the pulmonary vein and atrium. This information is useful for determining the appropriate strategy for the CA of AF.

5. Ackonowledgements

There were no relationships with the industry or conflicts to disclose in this study.

6. References

Amar, D. (2005). "Statin use is associated with a reduction in atrial fibrillation after noncardiac thoracic surgery independent of C-reactive protein." Chest 128(5): 3421-7. ISSN 0012-3692

Boyden, P. A. (1984). "Mechanisms for atrial arrhythmias associated with cardiomyopathy: a study of feline hearts with primary myocardial disease." Circulation 69(5): 1036-47. ISSN 0009-7322

Bruins, P. et al. (1997). "Activation of the complement system during and after cardiopulmonary bypass surgery: postsurgery activation involves C-reactive protein and is associated with postoperative arrhythmia." Circulation 96(10): 3542-8. ISSN 0009-7322

Brull, D. J. (2002). "Impact of angiotensin converting enzyme inhibition on post-coronary artery bypass interleukin 6 release." Heart 87(3): 252-5. ISSN 1468-201X

Cappato, R. (2003). "Prospective assessment of late conduction recurrence across radiofrequency lesions producing electrical disconnection at the pulmonary vein ostium in patients with atrial fibrillation." Circulation 108(13): 1599-604. ISSN 1524-4539

Chen, S. A. (1999). "Right atrial focal atrial fibrillation: electrophysiologic characteristics and radiofrequency catheter ablation." J Cardiovasc Electrophysiol 10(3): 328-35. ISSN 1524-4539

Chen, Y. J. (2002). "Electrophysiology and arrhythmogenic activity of single cardiomyocytes from canine superior vena cava." Circulation 105(22): 2679-85. ISSN 1524-4539

Chung, M. K. (2001). "C-reactive protein elevation in patients with atrial arrhythmias: inflammatory mechanisms and persistence of atrial fibrillation." Circulation 104(24): 2886-91. ISSN 1524-4539

DeRuiter, M. C. (1995). "In normal development pulmonary veins are connected to the sinus venosus segment in the left atrium." Anat Rec 243(1): 84-92. ISSN 0003-276X

Dotani, M. I. et al. (2000). "Effect of preoperative statin therapy and cardiac outcomes after coronary artery bypass grafting." Am J Cardiol 86(10): 1128-30, A6. ISSN 0002-9149

Fortuno, M. A. (1998). "Overexpression of Bax protein and enhanced apoptosis in the left ventricle of spontaneously hypertensive rats: effects of AT1 blockade with losartan." Hypertension 32(2): 280-6. ISSN 0194-911X

Frustaci, A. (1997). "Histological substrate of atrial biopsies in patients with lone atrial fibrillation." Circulation 96(4): 1180-4. ISSN 0009-7322

Gaudino, M. (2003). "The -174G/C interleukin-6 polymorphism influences postoperative interleukin-6 levels and postoperative atrial fibrillation. Is atrial fibrillation an inflammatory complication?" Circulation 108 Suppl 1: II195-9. ISSN 1524-4539

Haissaguerre, M. (2000). "Electrophysiological end point for catheter ablation of atrial fibrillation initiated from multiple pulmonary venous foci." Circulation 101(12): 1409-17. ISSN 1524-4539

Haissaguerre, M. (1998). "Spontaneous initiation of atrial fibrillation by ectopic beats originating in the pulmonary veins." N Engl J Med 339(10): 659-66. ISSN 0028-4793

Healey, J. S. (2005). "Prevention of atrial fibrillation with angiotensin-converting enzyme inhibitors and angiotensin receptor blockers: a meta-analysis." J Am Coll Cardiol 45(11): 1832-9. ISSN 0735-1097

Hernandez-Presa, M. (1997). "Angiotensin-converting enzyme inhibition prevents arterial nuclear factor-kappa B activation, monocyte chemoattractant protein-1 expression, and macrophage infiltration in a rabbit model of early accelerated atherosclerosis." Circulation 95(6): 1532-41. ISSN 0009-7322

Hogue, C. W. (1999). "Risk factors for early or delayed stroke after cardiac surgery." Circulation 100(6): 642-7. ISSN 1524-4539

Hoit, B. D. (1998). "Left atrial systolic and diastolic function accompanying chronic rapid pacing-induced atrial failure." Am J Physiol 275(1 Pt 2): H183-9. ISSN 0002-9513

Hwang, C. (2000). "Vein of marshall cannulation for the analysis of electrical activity in patients with focal atrial fibrillation." Circulation 101(13): 1503-5. ISSN

Johnson, N. (1986). "Characteristics of initiation and termination of catecholamine-induced triggered activity in atrial fibers of the coronary sinus." Circulation 74(5): 1168-79. ISSN 0009-7322

Kurotobi, T. (2010) "Multiple arrhythmogenic foci associated with the development of perpetuation of atrial fibrillation." Circ Arrhythm Electrophysiol 3(1): 39-45. ISSN 1941-3084

Kurotobi, T. (2011) "The significance of the shape of the left atrial roof as a novel index for determining the electrophysiological and structural characteristics in patients with atrial fibrillation" Europace 13 (6): 803-8 ISSN1532-2092

Lagrand, W. K. (1997). "C-reactive protein colocalizes with complement in human hearts during acute myocardial infarction." Circulation 95(1): 97-103. ISSN 0009-7322

Lee, S. H. (2005). "Predictors of non-pulmonary vein ectopic beats initiating paroxysmal atrial fibrillation: implication for catheter ablation." J Am Coll Cardiol 46(6): 1054-9. ISSN 1558-3597

Lin, W. S. (2000). "Pulmonary vein morphology in patients with paroxysmal atrial fibrillation initiated by ectopic beats originating from the pulmonary veins: implications for catheter ablation." Circulation 101(11): 1274-81. ISSN 1524-4539

Lin, W. S. (2003). "Catheter ablation of paroxysmal atrial fibrillation initiated by non-pulmonary vein ectopy." Circulation 107(25): 3176-83. ISSN

Lopez, B. (2001). "Usefulness of serum carboxy-terminal propeptide of procollagen type I in assessment of the cardioreparative ability of antihypertensive treatment in hypertensive patients." Circulation 104(3): 286-91.ISSN 1524-4539

Mangrum, J. M. (2002). "Intracardiac echocardiography-guided, anatomically based radiofrequency ablation of focal atrial fibrillation originating from pulmonary veins." J Am Coll Cardiol 39(12): 1964-72. ISSN

Marcus, G. M. (2008). "Markers of inflammation before and after curative ablation of atrial flutter." Heart Rhythm 5(2): 215-21. ISSN 1547-5271

Marin, F. (2006). "Statins and postoperative risk of atrial fibrillation following coronary artery bypass grafting." Am J Cardiol 97(1): 55-60. ISSN 0002-9149

Mevorach, D. (2000). "Opsonization of apoptotic cells. Implications for uptake and autoimmunity." Ann N Y Acad Sci 926: 226-35. ISSN 0077-8923

Nakashima, H. (2000). "Angiotensin II antagonist prevents electrical remodeling in atrial fibrillation." Circulation 101(22): 2612-7. ISSN 1524-4539

Neill, C. A. (1956). "Development of the pulmonary veins; with reference to the embryology of anomalies of pulmonary venous return." Pediatrics 18(6): 880-7. ISSN 0031-4005

Oral, H. (2002). "Clinical significance of early recurrences of atrial fibrillation after pulmonary vein isolation." J Am Coll Cardiol 40(1): 100-4. ISSN 0735-1097

Pak, H. N. (2006). "Electroanatomic characteristics of atrial premature beats triggering atrial fibrillation in patients with persistent versus paroxysmal atrial fibrillation." J Cardiovasc Electrophysiol 17(8): 818-24. ISSN 1045-3873

Patterson, E. (2005). "Triggered firing in pulmonary veins initiated by in vitro autonomic nerve stimulation." Heart Rhythm 2(6): 624-31. ISSN 1547-5271

Plenge, J. K. (2002). "Simvastatin lowers C-reactive protein within 14 days: an effect independent of low-density lipoprotein cholesterol reduction." Circulation 106(12): 1447-52. ISSN 1524-4539

Satoh, T. and D. P. Zipes (1996). "Unequal atrial stretch in dogs increases dispersion of refractoriness conducive to developing atrial fibrillation." J Cardiovasc Electrophysiol 7(9): 833-42. ISSN 0009-7330

Schmitt, C. (2002). "Biatrial multisite mapping of atrial premature complexes triggering onset of atrial fibrillation." Am J Cardiol 89(12): 1381-7. ISSN

Siu, C. W., C. P. Lau, et al. (2003). "Prevention of atrial fibrillation recurrence by statin therapy in patients with lone atrial fibrillation after successful cardioversion." Am J Cardiol 92(11): 1343-5. ISSN 0002-9149

Spodick, D. H. (1976). "Arrhythmias during acute pericarditis. A prospective study of 100 consecutive cases." JAMA 235(1): 39-41. ISSN 0098-7484

Strandberg, T. E. (1999). "Effect of statins on C-reactive protein in patients with coronary artery disease." Lancet 353(9147): 118-9. ISSN 0140-6736

Van Gelder, I. C. (1991). "Prediction of uneventful cardioversion and maintenance of sinus rhythm from direct-current electrical cardioversion of chronic atrial fibrillation and flutter." Am J Cardiol 68(1): 41-6. ISSN 0002-9149

Wijffels, M. C. (1995). "Atrial fibrillation begets atrial fibrillation. A study in awake chronically instrumented goats." Circulation 92(7): 1954-68. ISSN 0009-7322

Wright, M. (2008). "State of the art: catheter ablation of atrial fibrillation." J Cardiovasc Electrophysiol 19(6): 583-92. ISSN 1540-8167

Yamane, T. (2008). "Prevalence, morphological and electrophysiological characteristics of confluent inferior pulmonary veins in patients with atrial fibrillation." Circ J 72(8): 1285-90. ISSN 1346-9843

Yamane, T. (2002). "Dilatation as a marker of pulmonary veins initiating atrial fibrillation." J Interv Card Electrophysiol 6(3): 245-9. ISSN 1383-875X

Young-Xu, Y. (2003). "Usefulness of statin drugs in protecting against atrial fibrillation in patients with coronary artery disease." Am J Cardiol 92(12): 1379-83. ISSN 0002-9149

10

Brain Natriuretic Peptide and the Risk of Cardiovascular Events and Death in Patients with Atrial Fibrillation

Keizo Tsuchida[1] and Kazuhiko Tanabe[2]
[1]*Tsuchida Clinic of Internal Medicine and Cardiology,*
[2]*Tanabe Clinic,*
Japan

1. Introduction

Brain natriuretic peptide (BNP) is a hormone that is secreted by the heart, especially from the ventricle (Sudoh et al., 1988; Yasue et al., 1994). The plasma BNP concentrations (BNP levels) are correlated positively with the left ventricular end-diastolic pressure and negatively with the left ventricular ejection fraction (Yoshimura et al., 1993; Maeda et al., 1998), so BNP levels should be measured to evaluate left ventricular function. BNP levels have proved to be good markers of congestive heart failure. In addition, BNP levels are useful in screening test for left ventricular dysfunction and also heart disease.

Some studies have shown that BNP levels have a prognostic value of mortality and morbidity in patients with chronic heart failure (Maeda et al., 2000; Anand et al., 2003), in general populations (Wang et al., 2004) and in clinical practice (Tsuchida & Tanabe, 2008). However, the prognostic value of BNP levels in patients with atrial fibrillation (AF) is not well known. This study investigated the relations of BNP levels to cardiovascular events and death in patients with AF.

Hohnloser et al. suggested that warfarin therapy was needed in patients with paroxysmal AF similarly as in those with sustained AF (Hohnloser et al., 2007). Another report showed that, if sinus rhythm was maintained with antiarrhythmic therapy, the prognosis of the patients with paroxsmal AF for ischemic stroke was better than those with permanent AF (Komatsu et al., 2004). We examined the necessity of warfarin therapy in patients with paroxysmal AF as in those with chronic AF.

Furthermore, $CHADS_2$ score is known to be very useful to decide the indication of warfarin therapy in patients with AF (Gage et al., 2001). The patients with $CHADS_2$ score of 2 or more are recommended to take warfarin therapy, those with $CHADS_2$ score of 1 to take Warfarin or antiplatelet drugs, and those with $CHADS_2$ score of 0 need not any take warfarin. We investigated the usefulness of BNP as an aid in $CHADS_2$ score to decide the indication of warfarin therapy in patients with $CHADS_2$ score of 0 or 1.

2. Subjects and methods

2.1 Subjects

This study included 371 consecutive outpatients with AF in the Tsuchida Clinic of Internal Medicine and Cardiology (23-93 years with an average age of 69.5±10.8 years; 205 men and

166 women; 231 paroxysmal AF and 140 chronic AF), whose BNP levels were measured to evaluate left ventricular function from 1999 to 2002. The patients were treated according to the relevant guidelines and followed up until 31 December 2006. The mean follow-up period was 5.4years (max: 7.5 years). Diagnosis was based on history, physical examination, laboratory findings, chest X-rays, electrocardiograms and echocardiograms. Paroxysmal AF was defined as AF that terminated spontaneously within 7 days after onset. Chronic AF was defined clinically when defibrillation of paroxysmal AF was unsuccessful (permanent AF) or AF was continuously observed for more than 6 months (persistent AF).

2.2 Methods

BNP levels were measured by the immunoradiometric assay method using a Shionoria BNP assay kit (Shionogi, Osaka, Japan) for the one-point blood sample taken in a sitting position. Some studies of patients with heart failure (Latini et al., 2004; Tsutamoto et al., 1997) showed that BNP levels of more than about 100 pg/ml were significantly related to mortality and morbidity, so the patients were stratified into two groups based on cut-off levels of BNP (<100 pg/ml and ≧100 pg/ml).

The primary endpoint was a composite of cardiovascular events (hospitalization and death). Components of the endpoints included the following: heart failure, coronary heart disease events (acute myocardial infarction, unstable angina), stroke (ischemic, hemorrhagic), arrhythmia, dissecting aneurysm, peripheral arterial disease, infective endocarditis, acute myocarditis, renal infarction, pulmonary infarction, embolism of the superior mesenteric artery, and sudden cardiac death. The first of these events was noted as the primary event. Any component of a composite primary endpoint, for which a patient could be counted once in each category, was treated as a second endpoint. Death from any cause was also designated a secondary endpoint. Furthermore, patients with paroxysmal AF were observed for the development of chronic AF. The study protocol was approved by the Ethics Committee of Tsuchida Clinic of Internal Medicine and Cardiology.

2.3 Statistical analysis

Values are shown as mean±standard deviation (SD). Time-to-event curves for the endpoints were estimated by the Kaplan-Meier method for the entire follow-up period. The log-rank test was used to examine the association of BNP levels. Hazard ratio (HR) and 95% confidence interval (CI) were calculated and adjusted for age, sex, the presence or absence of hypertension, diabetes mellitus, and hyperlipidemia with the Cox's proportional hazards model. All analyses were performed with the use of StatView (version 5.0). Significance levels were $p < 0.05$ in these analyses.

3. Results

3.1 Patient characteristics

Clinical characteristics are summarized in Table 1. This study included 371 patients: valvular disease was found in 57 (15%); congestive heart failure (CHF) in 58 (16%); coronary artery disease (CAD) in 47 (13%), old myocardial infarction (OMI) in 16 (4%), angina pectoris (ANG) in 31 (8%); prior stroke in 35 (9%); hypertrophic cardiomyopathy (HCM) in 19 (5%); dilated cardiomyopathy (DCM) in 10 (3%); prior pacemaker operation in 12 (3%); hypertension in 228 (62%); diabetes mellitus in 63 (17%); dyslipidemia in 104 (28%); including some patients with more than one disease. In comparing chronic AF with paroxysmal AF, there were more valvular disease, CHF, and prior stroke in patients with

	All (n=371)	PAF (n=231)	CAF (n=140)	p Value
Age (years)	69.5±10.8	68.4±10.9	71.3±10.2	0.0119
Male gender	205 (55%)	121 (52%)	84 (60%)	0.1534
BNP (pg/ml)	96	57	160	<0.0001
Cardiovascular disease				
Valvular disease	57 (15%)	22 (10%)	35 (25%)	<0.0001
CHF	58 (16%)	12 (5%)	46 (33%)	<0.0001
CAD	47 (13%)	16 (7%)	13 (9%)	0.1925
OMI	16 (4%)	11 (5%)	5 (4%)	0.5855
ANG	31 (8%)	5 (3%)	8 (6%)	0.1531
Prior stroke	35 (9%)	15 (7%)	20 (14%)	0.0127
HCM	19 (5%)	10 (4%)	9 (6%)	0.3752
DCM	10 (3%)	2 (1%)	8 (6%)	0.0127
Prior pacemaker operation	12 (3%)	4 (2%)	8 (6%)	0.0356
Hypertension	228 (62%)	147 (64%)	81 (58%)	0.2688
Diabetes mellitus	63 (17%)	33 (14%)	30 (21%)	0.0760
Dyslipidemia	104 (28%)	70 (30%)	34 (24%)	0.2121
$CHADS_2$ score	1.43	1.23	1.76	<0.0001
0	82 (22%)	60 (26%)	22 (16%)	
1	138 (37%)	95 (41%)	43 (31%)	
2	86 (23%)	46 (20%)	40 (29%)	
3	38 (10%)	21 (9%)	17 (12%)	
4-6	27 (7%)	9 (4%)	18 (13%)	
Medication				
Warfarin	90 (24%)	38 (17%)	52 (37%)	<0.0001
Antiplatelet drugs	177 (48%)	99 (43%)	78 (56%)	0.0162
Beta-blocker	24 (7%)	20 (9%)	4 (3%)	0.0277
ACEI/ARB	55 (15%)	40 (17%)	15 (11%)	0.1033
Ca blocker	196 (53%)	128 (55%)	68 (49%)	0.2018
Digitalis	270 (73%)	173 (75%)	97 (69%)	0.2408
Antiarrhythmic drugs	77 (21%)	65 (28%)	12 (9%)	<0.0001
Thiazide	72 (19%)	25 (11%)	47 (34%)	<0.0001
Antialdosterone agents	60 (16%)	20 (9%)	40 (29%)	<0.0001
Nitrates	27 (7%)	17 (7%)	10 (7%)	0.9382
Statins	95 (26%)	60 (26%)	35 (25%)	0.8355

* PAF: paroxymal atrial fibrillation, CAF: chronic atrial fibrillation
* ACE: angiotension converting enzyme inhibitor, ARB: angiotensin receptor blocker

Table 1. Characteristics of the Study Population

chronic AF than in those with paroxysmal AF. And BNP levels in patients with chronic AF (160 pg/ml) were about 3 folds compared to with paroxysmal AF (57 pg/ml, during sinus rhythm).

Patients with chronic AF had a mean $CHADS_2$ score of 1.76 compared with 1.23 in those with paroxysmal AF ($p<0.0001$). The reason for the higher mean $CHADS_2$ score in patients

with chronic AF was probably because of older age, the presence of more structural heart disease (valvular disease, DCM, prior pacemaker operation and CHF) and prior stroke.
The prior use of warfarin, wntiplatelet drugs, beta-blocker, thiazide and antialdosterone drugs was significantly higher in chronic AF. And the prior use of antiarrhythmic drugs was significantly higher in paroxysmal AF.

3.2 Kaplan-Meier curves for the endpoints and Incidence of death or cardiovascular events

Patients were stratified into two groups based on cut-off level of BNP (100 pg/ml), and a cumulative cardiovascular event-free curve was constructed according to Kaplan-Meier analysis. Cumulative cardiovascular event-free rate, as evaluated by Kaplan-Meier analysis, was significantly lower with a BNP level≧100 pg/ml ($p<0.0001$) (Figure 1). Similarly, in secondary analyses (cardiovascular mortality, all-cause mortality, heart failure, ischemic stroke, development of paroxysmal AF into chronic AF), cumulative survival rate (event-free rate) was significantly lower with a BNP level≧100 pg/ml (Figure 2, Figure 3, Figure4, Figure 5, Figure 6). But only with regard to coronary heart disease events, the cumulative event-free rate was not significantly associated with the BNP level.

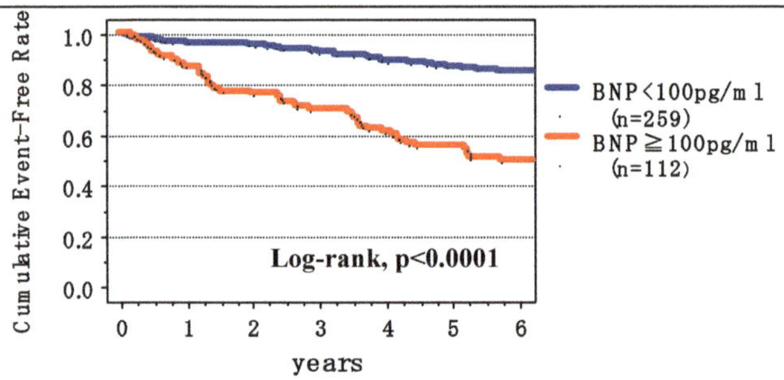

No. at Risk							
BNP<100 pg/ml	259	233	221	207	187	166	148
BNP≧100 pg/ml	112	90	75	64	54	47	40

Fig. 1. Kaplan-Meier Curve for Cardiovascular Events

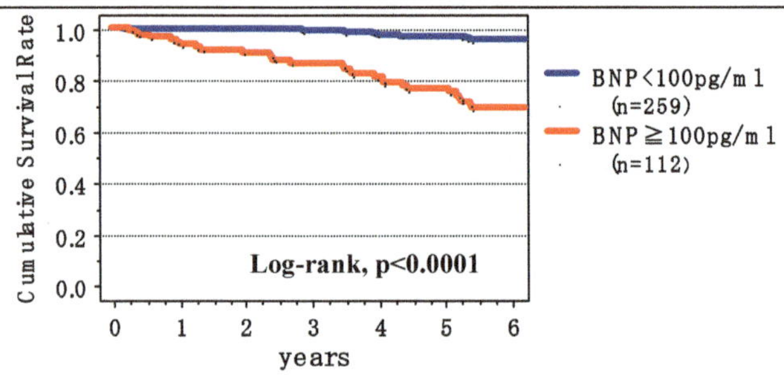

No. at Risk							
BNP<100 pg/ml	259	240	229	220	203	179	160
BNP≧100 pg/ml	112	98	90	77	70	63	54

Fig. 2. Kaplan-Meier Curve for Cardiovascular Mortality

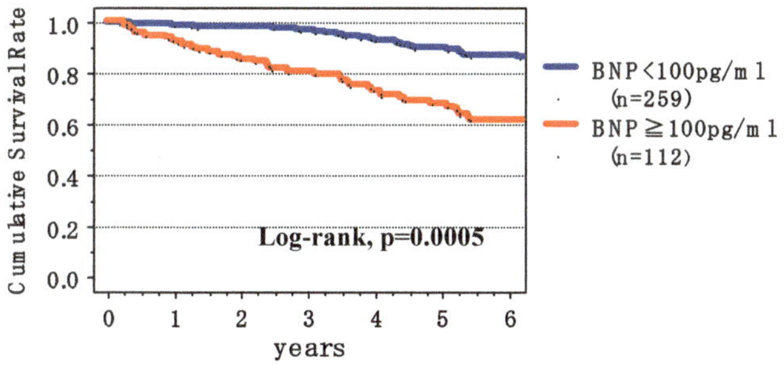

No. at Risk

BNP<100 pg/ml	259	240	229	220	203	179	160
BNP≧100 pg/ml	112	98	90	77	70	63	54

Fig. 3. Kaplan-Meier Curve for All-Cause Mortality

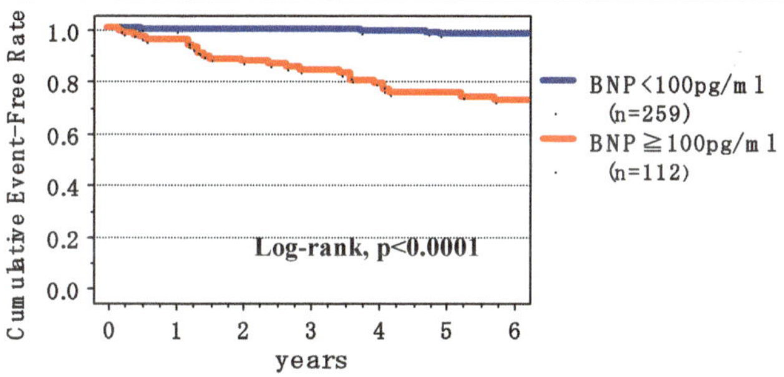

No. at Risk

BNP<100 pg/ml	259	239	228	219	201	178	159
BNP≧100 pg/ml	112	95	82	70	62	55	48

Fig. 4. Kaplan-Meier Curve for Heart Failure

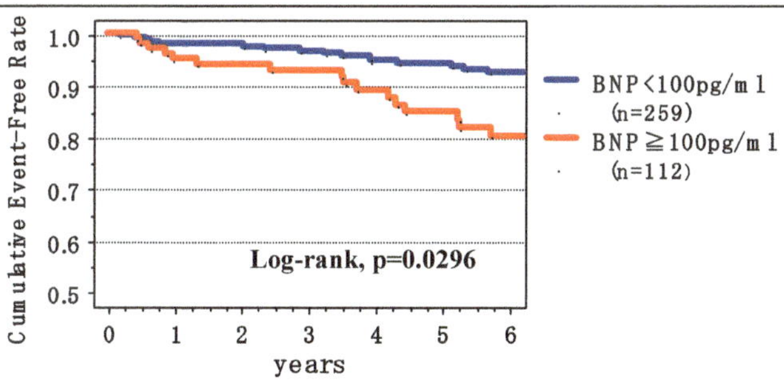

No. at Risk

BNP<100 pg/ml	259	236	225	214	197	172	154
BNP≧100 pg/ml	112	94	86	74	65	58	48

Fig. 5. Kaplan-Meier Curve for Ischemic Stroke

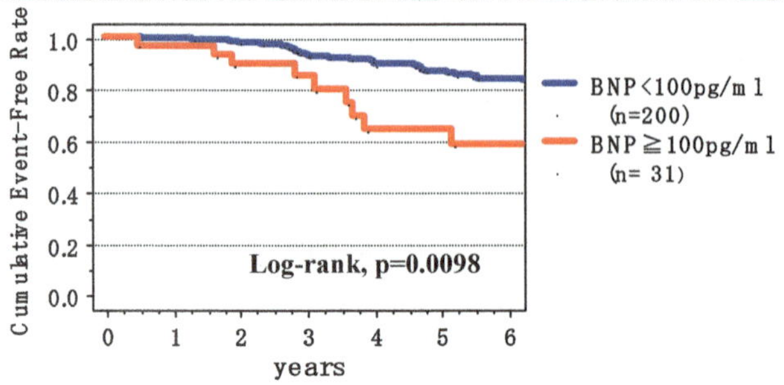

No. at Risk							
BNP<100 pg/ml	200	186	174	161	144	124	107
BNP≧100 pg/ml	31	27	25	17	12	12	8

Fig. 6. Kaplan-Meier Curve for Development of Paroxysmal AF into Chronic AF

	Number of events		HR (95%CI)	p Value
	BNP≧100 (n=112)	BNP<100 (n=259)		
Primary endpoint				
Cardiovascular events	58 (52%)	38 (15%)	3.9 (2.6-6.0)	<0.0001
Secondary endpoints				
Cadiovascular mortality	35 (31%)	11 (4%)	5.2 (2.6-10.5)	<0.0001
All-cause mortality	47 (42%)	33 (13%)	2.3 (1.4-3.7)	0.0005
Heart failure	30 (27%)	8 (3%)	11.0 (4.9-24.5)	<0.0001
Coronary h.d. events	2 (2%)	4 (2%)	0.9 (0.1-5.3)	0.8840
Ischemic stroke	19 (17%)	18 (7%)	2.1 (1.1-4.1)	0.0296
Development of PAF into CAF (PAF, n=231)	10/31 (32%)	29/200 (15%)	2.8 (1.3-6.1)	0.0098

Table 2. Incidence of Cardiovascular Events in Patients with AF

During a mean follow-up of 5.4 years, the number of cardiovascular events was 96/371 (26%): heart failure 38, coronary heart disease events 6 (acute myocardial infarction 6), stroke 38 (ischemic 37, hemorhagic 1), arrhythmia 7 (sick sinus syndrome 4, atrioventricular block 1, ventricular tachycardia 1), embolism of superior mesenteric artery 1, renal infarction 1, others 5. The number of deaths from cardiovascular disease was 46/371 (12%): heart failure 17, coronary heart disease events 2 (acute myocardial infarction 2), stroke 17 (ischemic 16, hemorhagic 1), arrythmia 2 (ventricular fibrillation 2), embolism of superior mesenteric artery 2, dissecting aneurysm 1, others 5. The number of deaths from all causes was 80/371 (22%): cardiovascular disease 46 (as was stated above), malignant tumor 20 (lung 4, stomach 3, colon 5, pancreas 3, esophagus 2, others 3), pneumonia and chronic obstructive pulmonary disease 3, renal failure 2, liver cirrhosis 2, others 7.

A BNP level≧100 pg/ml was associated with a HR (95% CI) of 3.94 (2.57-6.04) for cardiovascular events compared with a BNP<100 pg/ml (p<0.0001), 5.18 (2.55-10.52) for cardiovascular mortality (p<0.0001), 2.32 (1.44-3.72) for all-cause mortality (p=0.0005), 11.01 (4.94-24.54) for heart failure (p<0.0001), 2.11 (1.08-4.14) for ischemic stroke (p=0.0247) , 2.80 (1.28-6.10) for development of paroxysmal AF into chronic AF (p=0.0098); however, it was 0.87 (0.14-5.34) for coronary heart disease events (p=0.8840). In addition, paroxysmal AF developed into chronic AF in 39 of 231 patients (16.9%, 3.1% of patients per year).

3.3 Incidence of stroke in patients with paroxysmal AF and chronic AF

Furthermore, the incidence of ischemic stroke was significantly with BNP≧100 pg/ml than with BNP<100 pg/ml (HR: 5.31, 95%CI: 1.49-18.89, p=0.0812) by univariate analysis (Figure 8), whereas in patients with chronic AF, it was not significantly associated with the BNP levels (HR: 1.02, 95% CI: 0.48-2.18, p=0.3623) (Figure 9).

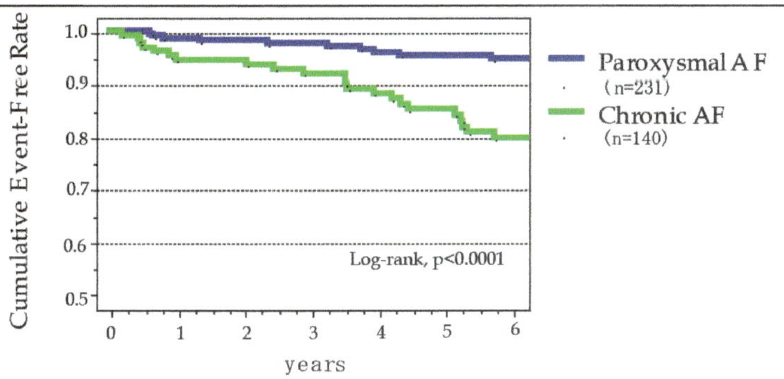

No. at Risk

Paroxysmal AF	231	212	202	188	171	153	133
Chronic AF	140	118	109	100	91	78	69

Fig. 7. Kaplan-Meier Curve for Ischemic Stroke in Patients with paroxysmal AF and chronic AF

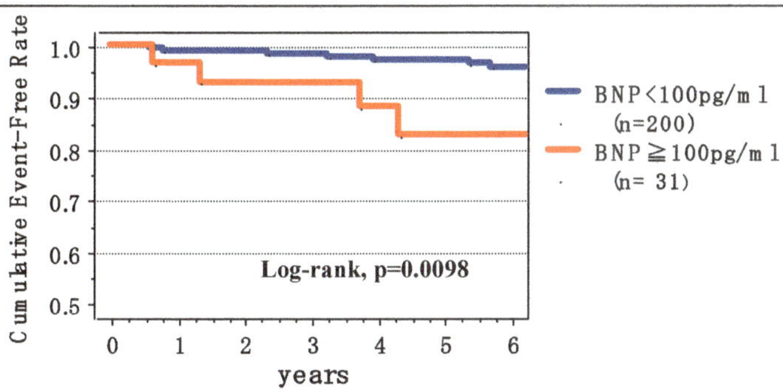

No. at Risk

BNP<100 pg/ml	200	185	176	168	154	138	122
BNP≧100 pg/ml	31	27	26	20	17	15	11

Fig. 8. Kaplan-Meier Curve for Ischemic Stroke in Patients with Paroxysmal AF

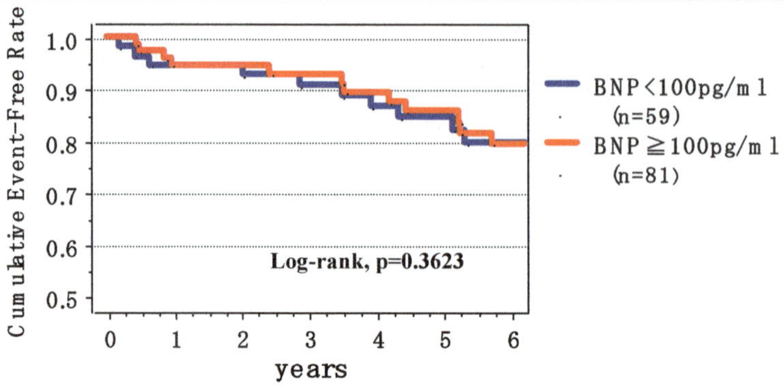

No. at Risk

BNP<100 pg/ml	59	51	49	46	43	34	32
BNP≧100 pg/ml	81	67	60	54	48	43	37

Fig. 9. Kaplan-Meier Curve for Ischemic Stroke in Patients with Chronic AF

3.4 $CHADS_2$ Score and Incidence of Ischemic stroke

Based on Kaplan-Meier analysis of five groups stratified by $CHADS_2$ score (0, 1, 2, 3, 4-6) in Figure 10, it was found that as $CHADS_2$ score was higher, the cumulative event-free rate for ischemic stroke decreased significantly ($p<0.0001$). As detailed in Table 3, there was the number of prior use of warfarin and the incidence of ischemic stroke, stratified by $CHADS_2$ score.

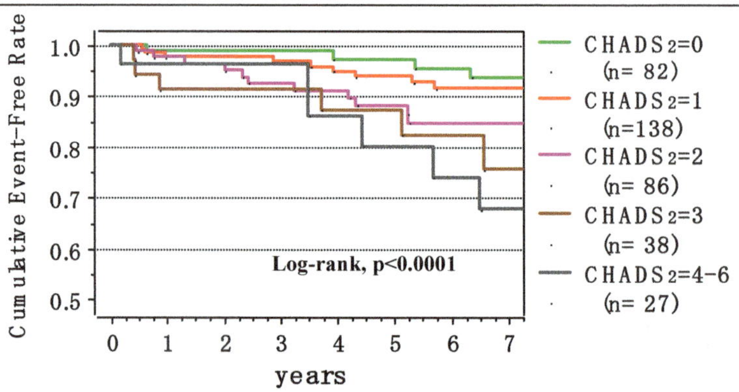

No. at Risk

$CHADS_2$=0	82	77	71	69	65	58	54	44
$CHADS_2$=1	138	123	118	105	96	88	77	66
$CHADS_2$=2	86	80	74	68	65	53	47	38
$CHADS_2$=3	38	31	26	26	21	19	12	10
$CHADS_2$=4-6	27	23	22	20	15	13	12	9

Fig. 10. Kaplan-Meier Curve for Ischemic Stroke, Stratified by $CHADS_2$ Score

$CHADS_2$ score	No. of patients (n=371)	Prior use of warfarin (n=90)	No. of stroke (n=37)
0	82	16 (20%)	3 (4%)
1	138	25 (18%)	9 (7%)
2	86	25 (29%)	13 (15%)
3	38	10 (26%)	6 (16%)
4-6	27	14 (52%)	6 (22%)

Table 3. Incidence of Stroke and Prior Use of Warfarin, Stratified by $CHADS_2$ Score

In patients with $CHADS_2$ score of 0 or 1, a BNP level≧100 pg/ml was associated with a HR (95% CI) of 3.84 (1.18-12.47) for ischemic stroke compared with a BNP < 100 pg/ml (p=0.0254) (Figure 11).

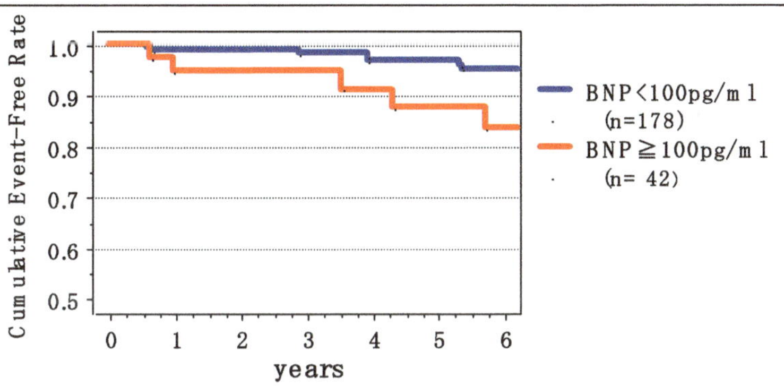

No. at Risk

BNP<100 pg/ml	178	160	154	147	136	123	113
BNP≧100 pg/ml	42	36	35	27	25	23	20

Fig. 11. Kaplan-Meier Curve for Ischemic Stroke in Patients with $CHADS_2$ Score of 0 or 1

4. Discussion

4.1 BNP and the risk of cardiovascular events and death in patients with AF

BNP is a hormone that is secreted by the heart, especially from the ventricle (Sudoh et al., 1988; Yasue et al., 1994), and BNP levels are useful in diagnosis and screening for left ventricular dysfunction and heart failure. Furthermore, during AF, BNP was known to be secreted mainly from the atrium in response to atrial wall stretch (Inoue et al., 2000). Our previous study in outpatients with paroxysmal AF showed that BNP levels during AF attack were increased 2.4 times compared with BNP levels during sinus rhythm (SR) (Tsuchida & Tanabe, 2004). Another study on electric defibrillation in patients with chronic AF showed an increase of about three times during AF than during SR after electric defibrillation (Ohta et al., 2001). These studies revealed that BNP levels during AF (both paroxysmal AF attack and chronic AF) are 2-3 times higher compared to during SR, and therefore BNP level during AF is the sum of the BNP level from the ventricle (reflecting left ventricular function) and the atrium (due to atrial wall stress).

Some studies have shown that BNP levels have a prognostic value of mortality and morbidity in patients with chronic heart failure (Maeda et al., 2000; Anand et al., 2003), in general populations (Wang et al., 2004) and in clinical practice (Tsuchida & Tanabe, 2008). This study shows that BNP level in patients with AF is an important prognostic marker of cardiovascular events, cardiovascular mortality, all-cause mortality, heart failure, ischemic stroke and development of paroxysmal AF into chronic AF, by stratification into two groups based on routinely used cut-off levels of BNP (100pg/ml).

The 14 year follow-up study of paroxysmal AF (Kato T et al., 2004) revealed that paroxysmal AF eventually developed into chronic AF in 132 of 171 patients (77.2%, 5.5% of patients per year), despite changing the drugs as necessary, and the development ratio was significantly increased by aging, an enlarged left atrium, myocardial infarction and valvular disease. In this study (5.4 year follow-up), paroxysmal AF developed into chronic AF in 39 of 231 patients (16.9%, 3.1% of patients per year), and the development ratio was significantly higher in patients with a BNP≧100 pg/ml than a BNP<100 pg/ml. It is conceivable that the reason for lower development ratio in this study than in the former study, is because of less myocardial infarction (5% in this study versus 11% in the former study) and valvular disease (10% versus 20%).

In patients with coronary heart disease, BNP levels were definitely associated with acute phase and outcome of myocardial infarction (Morita et al., 1993; Bibbins-Domingo et al, 2003; Morrow et al., 2003; Suzuki et al., 2004). However, in this study, we did not find an association between BNP levels and the risk of coronary heart disease events in patients with AF, reflecting a similar finding in the report of the Framingham study in a community-based population (Wang et al., 2004).

4.2 Incidence of stroke in patients with paroxysmal AF and chronic AF

Hohnloser et al. (2001) suggested that Warfarin therapy was needed in patients with paroxysmal AF, similarly as in those with sustained AF (Hohnloser et al., 2007). Meanwhile, another study showed that, if SR was maintained with antiarrhythmic therapy, the prognosis of the patients with paroxysmal AF for ischemic stroke was better than those with permanent AF (Komatsu et al., 2004). In this study, the incidence of ischemic stroke was significantly higher in patients with chronic AF than in those with paroxysmal AF. The reason for it was because of older age, the presence of more structural disease (valvular disease, DCM, prior pacemaker operation and CHF), more prior stroke and higher mean $CHADS_2$ score in patients with chronic AF.

This study showed that the incidence of ischemic stroke was significantly higher with a BNP≧100 pg/ml than with a BNP<100 pg/ml. In addition, in patients with paroxysmal AF, the incidence of ischemic stroke was significantly higher with a BNP≧100 pg/ml than with a BNP<100 pg/ml, whereas in patients with chronic AF, it was not significantly associated with the BNP levels.

In our previous study (Tsuchida & Tanabe, 2004), BNP levels during AF attack in patients with paroxysmal AF are 2.4 times higher (due to atrial wall stretch) compared to during SR, and even an asymptomatic AF attack also showed substantial and significant BNP elevation (median BNP levels: 31 pg/ml during SR, 71 pg/ml during AF attack). These findings suggest that BNP elevation of unknown origin could be attributed to the occurrence of asymptomatic AF attack, and the incidence of AF attack may be higher in paroxysmal AF patients with a BNP≧100 pg/ml, besides the degree of left ventricular dysfunction.

Furthermore, in this study, the incidence of development of paroxysmal AF into chronic AF was significantly higher with a BNP≧100 pg/ml, and so paroxysmal AF with a BNP≧100 pg/ml may be going to develop close to chronic AF.
As to the mechanism of association between elevation of BNP levels and development of ischemic stroke in AF patients, there are a few reports. The recent studies demonstrated that BNP levels correlated negatively with left atrial appendage flow velocity in chronic AF patient, and suggested that pathological changes (such as hypertrophy, fibrosis and inflammation) in the atrial myocardium may also be underlying factors in elevated BNP secretion in patients with poor left atrial appendage function, and so BNP as a reflection of left atrial appendage function may be a useful marker to predict vulnerability to thromboembolism in AF patients (Frustaci et al., 1997; Shimizu et al., 2002). Further study needs to be performed as to the mechanism of association between elevation of BNP levels and development of ischemic stroke in AF patients.

4.3 Warfarin therapy in patients with $CHADS_2$ score of 0 or 1

$CHADS_2$ score is known to be very useful to decide the indication of warfarin therapy in patients with AF (Gage et al., 2001). The patients with $CHADS_2$ score of 2 or more are recommended to take warfarin therapy, those with $CHADS_2$ score of 1 to take warfarin or antiplatelet drugs, and those with $CHADS_2$ score of 0 need not take any warfarin.
Based on Kaplan-Meier analysis of five groups stratified by $CHADS_2$ score (0, 1, 2, 3, 4-6), it was found that as $CHADS_2$ score was higher, the cumulative event-free rate for ischemic stroke decreased significantly. Furthermore, in the patients with $CHADS_2$ score of 0 or 1, the incidence of ischemic stroke was significantly higher with a BNP≧100 pg/ml than with a BNP < 100 pg/ml. So in the patients with $CHADS_2$ score of 0 or 1, BNP may be useful as an aid in $CHADS_2$ score to decide the indication of warfarin therapy for prevention to ischemic stroke.

4.4 Study limitations

The study population consisted of 371 outpatients of one local clinic in Japan. Although they were treated according to the accepted guidelines, it was unavoidable that this study showed a certain amount of bias in relation to patient background, diagnosis and treatment.

5. Conclusion

In patients with AF, BNP levels predicted the risk of cardiovascular events and death, except for coronary heart disease. Patients with chronic AF had a higher risk of ischemic stroke than patients with paroxysmal AF. BNP may be useful as an aid in $CHADS_2$ score to decide the indication of warfarin therapy in patients with paroxysmal AF and in patients with $CHADS_2$ score of 0 or 1.

6. Acknowledgment

We thank our patients; and Nobuo Shirahashi (Clinical Epidemiology, Osaka City Graduate School), for statistical support; Joukichi Suzuki (Suzuki Clinic) and Takashi Tomidokoro

(Nagaoka Chuo General Hospital), for helpful discussions; Akiko Tsuchida, for her assistance with this manuscript; Steve Hampton, for his advice concerning English usage; Shigeko Sasaki (Wakaba Pharmacy), for her pharmaceutical support; and staff in Tsuchida Clinic, for their contributions (Yukiko Kawano, Akemi Fujita, Nobue Ohya, Natsuki Komura, Tomoko Koga, Kayoko Ishidaira, Yumiko Tanaka and Aiko Tsuchida).

7. References

Anand IS, Fisher LD, Chiang YT, Latini R, Masson S, Maggioni AP, Glazer RD, Tognoni G & Cohn JN; Val-HeFT Investigators. (2003). *Changes in brain natriuretic peptide and norepinephrine over time and mortality and morbidity in the valsartan heart failure trial.* Circulation 2003; 107: 1278-83.

Bibbins-Domingo K, Ansari M, Schiller NB, Massie B & Whooley MA. (2003). *B-type natriuretic peptide and ischemia in patients with stable coronary disease.* Circulation 2003; 108:2987-92.

Frustaci A, Chimenti C, Bellocci F, Morgante E, Russo MA, Maseri A. (1997). *Histological substrate of atrial biopsies in patients with lone atrial fibrillation.* Circulation. 1997; 96:1180–1184.

Gage BF, Waterman AD, Shannon W, Boechler M, Rich MW & Radford MJ. (2001). *Validation of clinical classification schemes for predicting stroke: results from the National Registry of Atrial Fibrillation.* JAMA 2001 Jun 13; 285(22):2864-70

Hohnloser SH, Pajitnev D, Pogue J, Healey JS, Pfeffer MA, Yusuf S & Connolly SJ; ACTIVE W Investigators. (2007). *Incidence of stroke in paroxysmal versus sustained atrial fibrillation in patients taking oral anticoagulation or combined antiplatelet therapy: an ACTIVE W Substudy.* J Am Coll Cardiol. 2007 Nov 27; 50(22):2156-61.

Inoue S, Murakami Y, Sano K, Katoh H & Shimada T. (2000). *Atrium as a source of brain natriuretic polypeptide in patients with atrial fibrillation.* J Card Fail. 2000 Jun; 6(2):92-6.

Kato T, Yamashita T, Sagara K, Iinuma H & Fu LT. *Progressive nature of paroxysmal atrial fibrillation. Observations from a 14-year follow-up study.* Circ J. 2004 Jun; 68(6):568-72.

Komatsu T, Nakamura S, Suzuki O, Horiuchi D, Yomogida K & Okumura K. (2004). *Long-term prognosis of patients with paroxysmal atrial fibrillation depends on their response to antiarrhythmic therapy.* Circ J. 2004 Aug; 68(8):729-33.

Latini R, Masson S, Anand I, Salio M, Hester A, Judd D, Barlera S, Maggioni AP, Tognoni G & Cohn JN; Val-HeFT Investigators. (2004). *The comparative prognostic value of plasma neurohormones at baseline in patients with heart failure enrolled in Val-heft.* Eur Heart J 2004; 25:292-9.

Maeda K, Tsutamoto T, Wada A, Hisanaga T & Kinoshita M. (1998). *Plasma brain natriuretic peptide as a biochemical marker of high left ventricular end-diastolic pressure in patients with symptomatic left ventricular dysfunction.* Am Heart J 1998; 135: 825-32.

Maeda K, Tsutamoto T, Wada A, Mabuchi N, Hayashi M, Tsutsui T, Ohnishi M, Sawaki M, Fujii M, Matsumoto T & Kinoshita M. (2000). *High levels of plasma brain natriuretic peptide and interleukin-6 after optimized treatment for heart failure are independent risk factors for morbidity and mortality in patients with congestive heart failure.* J Am Coll Cardiol 2000; 36:1587-93.

Morita E, Yasue H, Yoshimura M, Ogawa H, Jougasaki M, Matsumura T, Mukoyama M & Nakao K. (1993). *Increased plasma levels of brain natriuretic peptide in patients with acute myocardial infarction.* Circulation 1993; 88: 82-91.

Morrow DA, de Lemos JA, Sabatine MS, Murphy SA, Demopoulos LA, DiBattiste PM, McCabe CH, Gibson CM, Cannon CP & Braunwald E. (2003). *Evaluation of B-type natriuretic peptide for risk assessment in unstable angina/non- ST-elevation myocardial infarction.* J Am Coll Cardiol 2003; 41:1264-72.

Ohta Y, Shimada T, Yoshitomi H, Inoue S, Murakami Y, Shimizu H, Nakamura K, Ohta T, Katoh H & Ishibashi Y. (2001). *Drop in plasma brain natriuretic peptide levels after successful direct current cardioversion in chronic atrial fibrillation.* Can J Cardiol. 2001 Apr; 17(4):415-20.

Price JF, Thomas AK, Grenier M, Eidem BW, O'Brian Smith E, Denfield SW, Towbin JA & Dreyer WJ. (2006). *B-type natriuretic peptide predicts adverse cardiovascular events in pediatric outpatients with chronic left ventricular systolic dysfunction.* Circulation 2006; 114:1063-9.

Shimizu H, Murakami Y, Inoue S, Ohta Y, Nakamura K, Katoh H, Sakne T, Takahashi N, Ohata S, Sugamori T, Ishibashi Y and Shimada T. (2002). *High plasma brain natriuretic polypeptide level as a marker of risk for thromboembolism in patients with nonvalvular atrial fibrillation.* Stroke 2002 Apr; 33(4): 1005-10.

Sudoh T, Kangawa K, Minamino N & Matsuo H. (1988). *A new natriuretic peptide in porcine brain.* Nature 1988; 332: 78-81.

Suzuki S, Yoshimura M, Nakayama M, Mizuno Y, Harada E, Ito T, Nakamura S, Abe K, Yamamuro M, Sakamoto T, Saito Y, Nakao K, Yasue H & Ogawa H. (2004). *Plasma level of B-type natriuretic peptide as a prognostic marker after acute myocardial infarction.* Circulation 2004; 110:1387-91.

Tsutamoto T, Wada A, Maeda K, Hisanaga T, Maeda Y, Fukai D, Ohnishi M, Sugimoto Y & Kinoshita M. (1997). *Attenuation of compensation of endogenous cardiac natriuretic peptide system in chronic heart failure.* Circulation 1997; 96: 509-16.

Tsuchida K & Tanabe K. (2004). *Influence of paroxysmal atrial fibrillation attack on brain natriuretic peptide secretion.* J Cardiol. 2004 Jul; 44(1):1-11.

Tsuchida K & Tanabe K. (2008). *Plasma brain natriuretic peptide concentrations and the risk of cardiovascular events and death in general practice.* J Cardiol. 2008 Dec; 52(3):212-23.

Wang TJ, Larson MG, Levy D, Benjamin EJ, Leip EP, Omland T, Wolf PA & Vasan RS. (2004). *Plasma natriuretic peptide levels and the risk of cardiovascular events and death.* N Engl J Med 2004; 350:655-63.

Yasue H, Yoshimura M, Sumida H, Kikuta K, Kugiyama K, Jougasaki M, Ogawa H, Okumura K, Mukoyama M & Nakao K. (1994). *Localization and mechanism of secretion of B-type natriuretic peptide in comparison with those of A-type natriuretic peptide in normal subjects and patients with heart failure.* Circulation 1994; 90: 195-203.

Yoshimura M, Yasue H, Okumura K, Ogawa H, Jougasaki M, Mukoyama M, Nakao K & Imura H. (1993). *Different secretion patterns of atrial natriuretic peptide and brain natriuretic peptide in patients with congestive heart failure.* Circulation 1993; 87: 464-9.

11

Prognostic Value of P Wave for Developing Atrial Fibrillation

Hideki Hayashi and Minoru Horie
Department of Cardiovascular and Respiratory Medicine, Shiga University of Medical Science, Otsu, Shiga, Japan

1. Introduction

The prevalence of atrial fibrillation (AF) increases as age advances, especially over 65 years old.[1,2] Given AF occurs, the risk of mortality increases because AF is able to cause thromboembolism and heart failure.[3-5] In industrialized countries, a number of patients with AF need medical care, which has brought a social problem in terms of medical expenses. Therefore, it is so important to prevent the occurrence of AF and predict who more likely develop AF. Epidemiological studies[6-8] revealed that the risk factors for AF development are aging, gender, valvular heart disease, hypertension, chronic lung disease, and left atrial size, and so forth. In addition, smoking[9] and obesity[10] are closely associated with the development of AF. Needless to say, 12-lead ECG is used ubiquitously in clinical practice to evaluate patients and provides information on the presence of structural heart disease and heart rhythm abnormality. Moreover, P-wave morphological characteristics deserve noting that the pattern of atrial depolarization is normal or ill. In this chapter, we focus on the relation between P-wave characteristics and AF occurrence.

2. P Mitrale and AF

The P wave reflects electrical depolarization of both the right atrium (RA) and the left atrium (LA). When the P wave is biphasic in lead V_1 (Figure 1), the positive initial portion and the negative terminal portion of the P wave represent depolarization of the RA and the LA, respectively.[11, 12] Since the early description of an asynchrony of atrial depolarization by Reynolds,[13] several studies reported P-wave abnormality suggesting LA enlargement.[14-16] In 1964, Morris et al.[17] advanced this concept as representing LA overload (LAO). They proposed that P terminal force >0.04 second in duration and >0.1 mV in depth at lead V_1 was associated with hemodynamically strained LA in various valvular heart diseases. The magnitude of the negative terminal potion of the P wave, calculated as the algebraic product of the duration and amplitude (P terminal force) in precordial lead V_1, was significantly larger in patients with various valvular heart diseases than in normal subjects. In their study, the P terminal force was associated with mitral valve area and increased LA pressure. The magnitude of the P terminal force has been shown to be associated with LA enlargement as revealed by transthoracic echocardiography.[18, 19] These findings suggest that the negative terminal potion of the P wave in lead V_1 is a sign of pressure and volume overload in the LA, which may lead to structural and functional remodeling in the LA. Because AF often occurs and/or recurs in the remodeled LA,[20] the increased P terminal force may underlie the generation of AF.

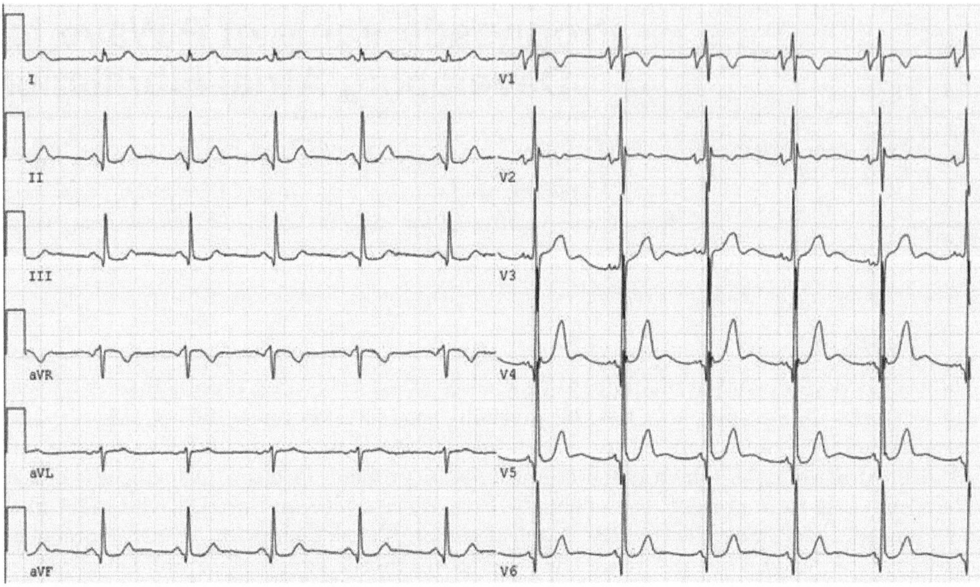

Fig. 1. Twelve-lead ECG showing P mitrale in lead V_1.

The increased P terminal force is observed not only in valvular heart diseases but also in other heart diseases, including hypertension, myocardial infarction, and cardiomyopathy.[21, 22] As patients with such disorders likely suffer from AF, the increased P terminal force in lead V_1 has been considered a probable precursor to development of AF. The terminal portion of the P wave in lead V_1 has been associated with electrical depolarization of the LA alone in humans[23] and in dogs.[24] Using angiocardiography, Miller and Spertus[25] showed a correlation of marked negative component in leads V_1 and V_2 with LA enlargement. Subsequently, Morris et al[17] showed a significant correlation of the magnitude of P terminal force with severity of hemodynamic abnormality. The P terminal portion in lead V_1 is composed of several factors: (1) anatomic shift of the LA to the posterior side by hemodynamic strain, (2) enlarged LA size, (3) LA hypertrophy, and (4) reduced conduction velocity in the LA.[22, 26, 27] These factors are also attributed to prolonged P-wave duration. Ishida et al.[28] studied relation of LAO with development of AF. They found that the rate of AF development was significantly higher in patients with LAO (P terminal force ≥0.06 second×0.2 mV in lead V_1) than in control subjects. In addition, the area of initial portion of P wave in lead V_1 was larger in patients who developed AF than in those who did not. These findings showed that an increased magnitude of P-wave initial force in lead V_1 was associated with a higher rate of AF development. This finding suggests that when a substrate develops in the RA in addition to the LA, susceptibility to the development of AF may increase.

The P-wave features of LAO reflect basic mechanisms underlying AF occurrence in terms of electrophysiologic and structural remodeling of the atrium that predisposes to the development of AF. Increased P-wave duration results from either slow conduction or an enlarged atrium. The former shortens wavelength, and the latter provides a sufficient area for reentry to occur. These pathophysiologic changes are linked to the maintenance of AF.[20] Increased intracardiac pressure of the left ventricle may cause LA remodeling, which is likely to occur in patients with structural heart disease. Disturbed transmitral blood flow due to elevated diastolic pressure in the left ventricle may induce heterogeneous distribution of the atrial refractory period. Structural remodeling, as occurs with interstitial fibrosis and connexin redistribution, causes anisotropic conduction or discontinuous propagation. In hypertrophied atrial myocytes, triggered activity, such as early and delayed afterdepolarizations, is prone to occur, thus AF ensuring in the remodeled atrium.[29, 30]

3. P Pulmonale and AF

It was reported that chronic obstructive pulmonary disease (COPD) complicated AF.[31-33] A recent study[34] acknowledged that multivariate analysis revealed that heart failure, advanced age, prior cerebrovascular events, COPD, and hypertension were independently associated with progression of paroxysmal to persistent AF in pharmacologically treated patients. When chronic obstructive pulmonary disease (COPD) develops, intimal thickening of arterioles, intravascular thrombosis, loss of capillaries occur in addition to perivascular inflammation and fibrosis,[35] causing pulmonary hypertension.[36, 37] Under these pathophysiological conditions, the right atrial pressure increases, which results in right atrial enlargement, being responsible for P pulmonale. In an autopsy study, Berliner and Master reported that subjects with isolated left atrial hypertrophy had normal P-wave amplitude; while those with biatrial hypertrophy had an increase in P-wave amplitude, although in four cases of isolated right atrial hypertrophy, no P-wave abnormalities were noted. Caird and Wilcken[38] found a right atrial abnormality at autopsy in patients with COPD. Tall P waves with the amplitude ≧0.25 mV in inferior leads have been regarded as an ECG sign representing RA overload (RAO).[39] Typically, patients with COPD exhibit vertical P-wave axis with peaked P wave in leads II, III, and aVF (P pulmonale) (Figure 2).[40, 41]

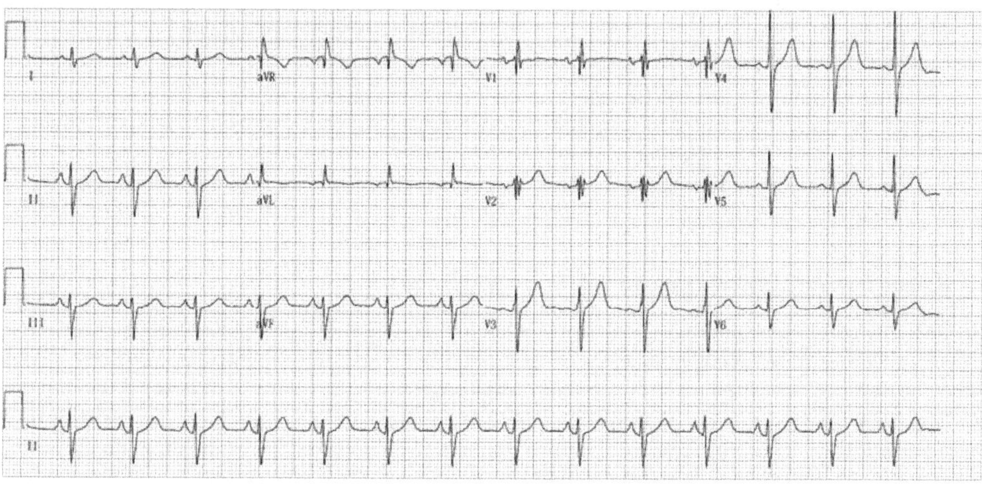

Fig. 2. Twelve-lead ECG showing P pulmonale in inferior leads.

It was reported that P pulmonale was associated with impaired pulmonary function worsens.[42] Asad et al.[43] reported that P-wave amplitude in inferior leads decreased in most patients with COPD after the acute exacerbations subsided. Saha et al.[44] reported that right atrial enlargement or increased right atrial pressure or both are important factors for the change of the P waves in cor pulmonale. However, little correlation between P pulmonale and abnormality of ventilator function in patients with chronic bronchitis was reported[38]. Maeda et al.[45] measured intracardiac pressure using Swan-Ganz catheter in patients with P pulmonale. In these, no significant increase of intracardiac pressure in right-sided chambers was found. However, there was a significant inverse relation between the presence of P pulmonale and the cardiothoracic ratio. These findings indicated that a vertical anatomical position of the heart was attributed to generation of P pulmonale in COPD rather than hemodynamic stress in the right-sided chambers.

As mentioned above, traditional ECG criteria for P pulmonale are increased amplitudes of P waves ≧2.5 mm in leads II, III, and aVF. Such characteristics, however, have been criticized as nonspecific for COPD. Chou and Helm[46] used the term "pseudo P pulmonale" to explain cases where left atrial forces contributed to increased P-wave amplitude in lead II, indicating that P pulmonale is not so specific as has been generally believed. Alternative criteria were proposed for identifying RAO. Macruz et al.[47] investigated that the ratio of P-wave duration to PR interval (P/PR) in normal subjects and patients with RAO and LAO. In RAO, the P/PR increases because of increased transit time from the sinus node to the atrioventricular node. In LAO, the terminal portion of the P wave is delayed because of the prolonged transit time of the depolarization impulse through the enlarged left atrial wall. Hence, the P-wave duration is prolonged, but P-R interval remains unchanged, resulting in the P/PR above the normal limit. Several investigators studied the feasibility of the RAO criteria by determining the size of the RA on imaging. Reeves et al.[48] determined RA size with two-dimensional echocardiography using the apical four-chamber view. They found that RA enlargement was present only in 18% of patients with P pulmonale. However, a qR pattern in lead V_1 was a significant marker for detecting RA enlargement and a positive linear correlation of RA size with the ratio of total QRS amplitude in lead V_2 compared with lead V_1. Kaplan et al.[49] determined the size of the right atrium using quantitative two-dimensional echocardiography in patients with right atrial enlargement. They found that traditional ECG criteria for RAO were insensitive. Instead, a P wave height >0.15 mV in lead V_2 and, a QRS axis >90 degree and an R/S ratio >1 in lead V_1 in the absence of complete right bundle branch block best predicted right atrial enlargement. Recently, Tsao et al.[50] compared anatomic atrial enlargement as determined by volumetric cardiovascular magnetic resonance with ECG findings concurrent to criteria of RAO. They found that the presence of at least one ECG criteria for P pulmonale is sensitive but not specific for anatomic enlargement.

4. Atrial conduction delay and AF

Delayed inter- or intra-atrial conduction time predisposes subjects to the development of AF.[51-53] Histology marked by interstitial fibrosis,[54-56] uncoupling of muscle bundle,[57] altered distribution of gap junction,[58, 59] and inflammation[60] underlies slow conduction, giving rise to P wave prolongation. Several studies[61-68] determined P-wave duration. The maximum P-wave duration varied approximately from 90 ms to 120 ms. Prolonged P-wave duration is a useful predictor of AF development.[63, 69] Prolonged P-wave duration phenotypically represent conduction delay in the atria (Figure 3). A positive correlation between advancing age and P-wave duration was noted.[70, 71] Slowed interatrial conduction velocity has been demonstrated in a cohort with a history of AF, underscoring the importance of atrial conduction delay.[72] Many studies reported intimate association of P-wave duration and occurrence of AF.[63, 73, 74] In addition to P-wave duration, P-wave dispersion, as is reflected as the interval between the longest and the shortest duration of P wave in any of 12-lead ECG leads, is an invariable maker in relation to AF occurrence and recurrence.[73] Both indices are associated with conventional risk factors of AF. Patients with uncontrolled hypertension had significantly prolonged P-wave duration and increased P-wave dispersion as compared to controls or controlled hypertension.[75, 76] Likewise, patients with diabetes had significantly prolonged P-wave duration and increased P-wave dispersion as compared to normal controls.[77] Several studies showed that individuals with obesity had significantly prolonged P-wave duration and increased P-wave dispersion as compared with control groups.[78, 79] Because those risk factors are independently related to AF occurrence, P-wave duration can be used as a noninvasive marker predicting AF occurrence.

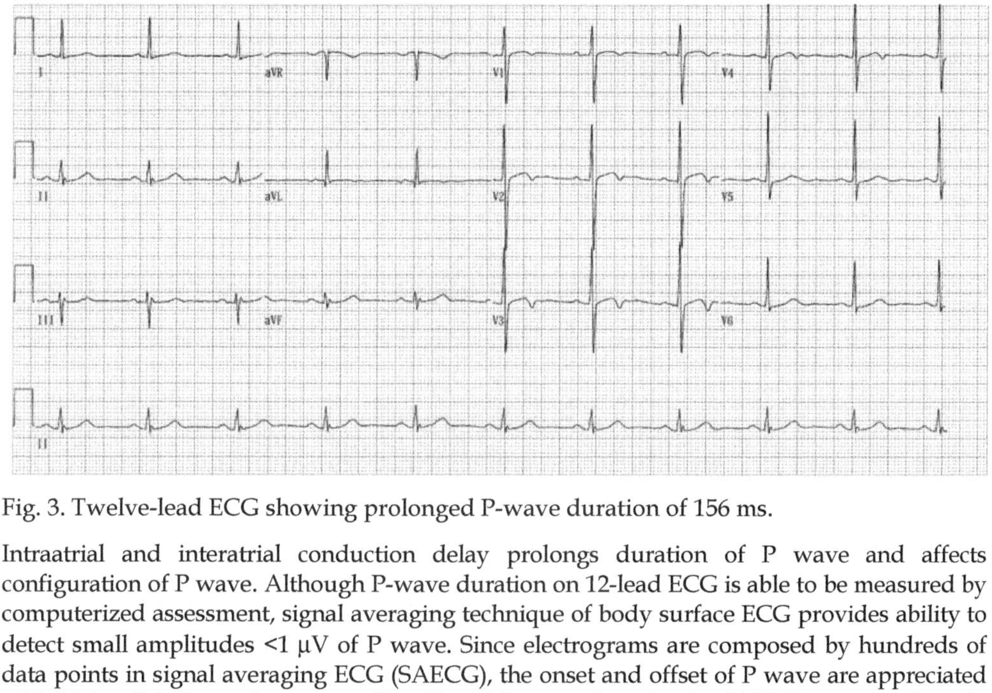

Fig. 3. Twelve-lead ECG showing prolonged P-wave duration of 156 ms.

Intraatrial and interatrial conduction delay prolongs duration of P wave and affects configuration of P wave. Although P-wave duration on 12-lead ECG is able to be measured by computerized assessment, signal averaging technique of body surface ECG provides ability to detect small amplitudes <1 μV of P wave. Since electrograms are composed by hundreds of data points in signal averaging ECG (SAECG), the onset and offset of P wave are appreciated with high reliability and accuracy. The filtered P-wave duration by SAECG was significantly longer in patients with paroxysmal AF than in controls, and the amplitude of atrial late potential for the last 10-20 ms of P wave significantly lower in patients with paroxysmal AF than in controls.[80] Thus, patients at risk for paroxysmal AF can be evaluated by SAECG while in sinus rhythm.[81] The role of P-wave SAECG was further investigated. Prolonged P wave on SAECGs was associated with recurrence of AF after cardioversion[82] and occurrence of AF after cardiothoracic surgery.[83] In addition, P-wave duration on SAECG was longer in hypertensive patients with paroxysmal AF than in those without.[84] Prolonged P-wave duration on SAECG exerted to predict future transition from paroxysmal to persistent AF.[85]

5. Conclusion

P-wave measures can be noninvasively obtained from patients having any disease, if they have sinus rhythm. In clinical practice, it is possible to utilize data of ECG recordings for various study designs such as cross-sectional, case-control, and intervention studies. Therefore, the P-wave analysis needs to be used not only for a diagnostic tool but also to evaluate the prognostic value for AF development in the future study.

6. References

[1] Wolf PA, Benjamin EJ, Belanger AJ, Kannel WB, Levy D, D'Agostino RB. Secular trends in the prevalence of atrial fibrillation: The Framingham Study. Am Heart J 1996;131:790-5.

[2] Go AS, Hylek EM, Phillips KA, et al. Prevalence of diagnosed atrial fibrillation in adults: national implications for rhythm management and stroke prevention: the AnTicoagulation and Risk Factors in Atrial Fibrillation (ATRIA) Study. JAMA 2001;285:2370-5.

[3] Benjamin EJ, Wolf PA, D'Agostino RB, Silbershatz H, Kannel WB, Levy D. Impact of atrial fibrillation on the risk of death: the Framingham Heart Study. Circulation 1998;98:946-52.

[4] Kannel WB, Wolf PA, Benjamin EJ, Levy D. Prevalence, incidence, prognosis, and predisposing conditions for atrial fibrillation: population-based estimates. Am J Cardiol 1998;82:2N-9N.

[5] Wolf PA, Abbott RD, Kannel WB. Atrial fibrillation as an independent risk factor for stroke: the Framingham Study. Stroke 1991;22:983-8.

[6] Benjamin EJ, Levy D, Vaziri SM, D'Agostino RB, Belanger AJ, Wolf PA. Independent risk factors for atrial fibrillation in a population-based cohort. The Framingham Heart Study. JAMA 1994;271:840-4.

[7] Okin PM, Wachtell K, Devereux RB, et al. Regression of electrocardiographic left ventricular hypertrophy and decreased incidence of new-onset atrial fibrillation in patients with hypertension. JAMA 2006;296:1242-8.

[8] Psaty BM, Manolio TA, Kuller LH, et al. Incidence of and risk factors for atrial fibrillation in older adults. Circulation 1997;96:2455-61.

[9] Heeringa J, Kors JA, Hofman A, van Rooij FJ, Witteman JC. Cigarette smoking and risk of atrial fibrillation: the Rotterdam Study. Am Heart J 2008;156:1163-9.

[10] Huxley RR, Lopez FL, Folsom AR, et al. Absolute and attributable risks of atrial fibrillation in relation to optimal and borderline risk factors: the Atherosclerosis Risk in Communities (ARIC) study. Circulation 2011;123:1501-8.

[11] Abildskov JA, Cronvich JA, Burch GE. An analysis of activation in human atria. Circulation 1955;11:97-105.

[12] Haywood LJ, Selvester RH. Analysis of right and left atrial vectorcardiograms. Timed records of 100 normal persons. Circulation 1966;33:577-87.

[13] Reynolds G. The atrial electrogram in mitral stenosis. Br Heart J 1953;15:250-8.

[14] Martins De Oliveira J, Zimmerman HA. Auricular overloadings; electrocardiographic analysis of 193 cases. Am J Cardiol 1959;3:453-71.

[15] Soloff LA, Zatuchni J. Relationship of the P wave to left atrial volume in rheumatic heart disease with mitral stenosis. Am J Med Sci 1958;235:290-6 passim.

[16] Arevalo AC, Spagnuolo M, Feinstein AR. A simple electrocardiographic indication of left atrial enlargement. A study of young patients with rheumatic heart disease. JAMA 1963;185:358-62.
[17] Morris JJ, Jr., Estes EH, Jr., Whalen RE, Thompson HK, Jr., McIntosh HD. P-Wave Analysis in Valvular Heart Disease. Circulation 1964;29:242-52.
[18] Munuswamy K, Alpert MA, Martin RH, Whiting RB, Mechlin NJ. Sensitivity and specificity of commonly used electrocardiographic criteria for left atrial enlargement determined by M-mode echocardiography. Am J Cardiol 1984;53:829-32.
[19] Hazen MS, Marwick TH, Underwood DA. Diagnostic accuracy of the resting electrocardiogram in detection and estimation of left atrial enlargement: an echocardiographic correlation in 551 patients. Am Heart J 1991;122:823-8.
[20] Allessie M, Ausma J, Schotten U. Electrical, contractile and structural remodeling during atrial fibrillation. Cardiovasc Res 2002;54:230-46.
[21] Shettigar UR, Barry WH, Hultgren HN. P wave analysis in ischaemic heart disease. An echocardiographic, haemodynamic, and angiographic assessment. Br Heart J 1977;39:894-9.
[22] Josephson ME, Kastor JA, Morganroth J. Electrocardiographic left atrial enlargement. Electrophysiologic, echocardiographic and hemodynamic correlates. Am J Cardiol 1977;39:967-71.
[23] Wenger R, Hofmann-Credner D. Observations on the atria of the human heart by direct and semidirect electrocardiography. Circulation 1952;5:870-7.
[24] Puech P, Esclavissat M, Sodi-Pallares D, Cisneros F. Normal auricular activation in the dog's heart. Am Heart J 1954;47:174-91.
[25] Miller HI, Spertus I. P Wave Changes Reflecting Atrial Morphology. Dis Chest 1964;46:578-91.
[26] Sutnick AI, Soloff LA. Posterior rotation of the atrial vector. An electrocardiographic sign of left ventricular failure. Circulation 1962;26:913-6.
[27] Gooch AS, Calatayud JB, Gorman PA, Saunders JL, Caceres CA. Leftward shift of the terminal P forces in the ECG associated with left atrial enlargement. Am Heart J 1966;71:727-33.
[28] Ishida K, Hayashi H, Miyamoto A, et al. P wave and the development of atrial fibrillation. Heart Rhythm 2010;7:289-94.
[29] Benjamin EJ, Chen PS, Bild DE, et al. Prevention of atrial fibrillation: report from a national heart, lung, and blood institute workshop. Circulation 2009;119:606-18.
[30] Nattel S. New ideas about atrial fibrillation 50 years on. Nature 2002;415:219-26.
[31] Corazza LJ, Pastor BH. Cardiac arrhythmias in chronic cor pulmonale. N Engl J Med 1958;259:863-5.
[32] Kleiger RE, Senior RM. Longterm electrocardiographic monitoring of ambulatory patients with chronic airway obstruction. Chest 1974;65:483-7.
[33] Senior RM, Lefrak SS, Kleiger RE. The heart in chronic obstructive pulmonary disease: Arrhythmias. Chest 1979;75:1-2.
[34] de Vos CB, Pisters R, Nieuwlaat R, et al. Progression from paroxysmal to persistent atrial fibrillation clinical correlates and prognosis. J Am Coll Cardiol 2010;55:725-31.

[35] Wright JL, Petty T, Thurlbeck WM. Analysis of the structure of the muscular pulmonary arteries in patients with pulmonary hypertension and COPD: National Institutes of Health nocturnal oxygen therapy trial. Lung 1992;170:109-24.
[36] Magee F, Wright JL, Wiggs BR, Pare PD, Hogg JC. Pulmonary vascular structure and function in chronic obstructive pulmonary disease. Thorax 1988;43:183-9.
[37] Han MK, McLaughlin VV, Criner GJ, Martinez FJ. Pulmonary diseases and the heart. Circulation 2007;116:2992-3005.
[38] Caird FI, Wilcken DE. The electrocardiogram in chronic bronchitis with generalized obstructive lung disease. Its relation to ventilatory function. Am J Cardiol 1962;10:5-13.
[39] Surawicz B, Uhley H, Borun R, et al. The quest for optimal electrocardiography. Tast Force I: standardization of terminology and interpretation. Am J Cardiol 1978;41:130-45.
[40] Kilcoyne MM, Davis AL, Ferrer MI. A dynamic electrocardiographic concept useful in the diagnosis of cor pulmonale. Result of a survey of 200 patients with chronic obstructive pulmonary disease. Circulation 1970;42:903-24.
[41] Spodick DH. Electrocardiographic studies in pulmonary disease. I. Electrocardiographic abnormalities in diffuse lung disease. Circulation 1959;20:1067-72.
[42] Calatayud JB, Abad JM, Khoi NB, Stanbro WW, Silver HM. P-wave changes in chronic obstructive pulmonary disease. Am Heart J 1970;79:444-53.
[43] Asad N, Johnson VM, Spodick DH. Acute right atrial strain: regression in normal as well as abnormal P-wave amplitudes with treatment of obstructive pulmonary disease. Chest 2003;124:560-4.
[44] Saha NC. Study of the P wave in normal and obstructive lung disease in Delhi. Am Heart J 1970;80:154-61.
[45] Maeda S, Katsura H, Chida K, et al. Lack of correlation between P pulmonale and right atrial overload in chronic obstructive airways disease. Br Heart J 1991;65:132-6.
[46] Chou TC, Helm RA. The Pseudo P Pulmonale. Circulation 1965;32:96-105.
[47] Macruz R, Perloff JK, Case RB. A method for the electrocardiographic recognition of atrial enlargement. Circulation 1958;17:882-9.
[48] Reeves WC, Hallahan W, Schwiter EJ, Ciotola TJ, Buonocore E, Davidson W. Two-dimensional echocardiographic assessment of electrocardiographic criteria for right atrial enlargement. Circulation 1981;64:387-91.
[49] Kaplan JD, Evans GT, Jr., Foster E, Lim D, Schiller NB. Evaluation of electrocardiographic criteria for right atrial enlargement by quantitative two-dimensional echocardiography. J Am Coll Cardiol 1994;23:747-52.
[50] Tsao CW, Josephson ME, Hauser TH, et al. Accuracy of electrocardiographic criteria for atrial enlargement: validation with cardiovascular magnetic resonance. J Cardiovasc Magn Reson 2008;10:7.
[51] Magnani JW, Williamson MA, Ellinor PT, Monahan KM, Benjamin EJ. P wave indices: current status and future directions in epidemiology, clinical, and research applications. Circ Arrhythm Electrophysiol 2009;2:72-9.
[52] Magnani JW, Johnson VM, Sullivan LM, et al. P wave duration and risk of longitudinal atrial fibrillation in persons >/= 60 years old (from the Framingham Heart Study). Am J Cardiol 2011;107:917-21 e1.

[53] Agarwal YK, Aronow WS, Levy JA, Spodick DH. Association of interatrial block with development of atrial fibrillation. Am J Cardiol 2003;91:882.
[54] Spach MS. Mounting evidence that fibrosis generates a major mechanism for atrial fibrillation. Circ Res 2007;101:743-5.
[55] Kamkin A, Kiseleva I, Wagner KD, et al. Mechanically induced potentials in fibroblasts from human right atrium. Exp Physiol 1999;84:347-56.
[56] Everett THt, Olgin JE. Atrial fibrosis and the mechanisms of atrial fibrillation. Heart Rhythm 2007;4:S24-7.
[57] Davies MJ, Pomerance A. Pathology of atrial fibrillation in man. Br Heart J 1972;34:520-5.
[58] Spach MS, Josephson ME. Initiating reentry: the role of nonuniform anisotropy in small circuits. J Cardiovasc Electrophysiol 1994;5:182-209.
[59] Polontchouk L, Haefliger JA, Ebelt B, et al. Effects of chronic atrial fibrillation on gap junction distribution in human and rat atria. J Am Coll Cardiol 2001;38:883-91.
[60] Chung MK, Martin DO, Sprecher D, et al. C-reactive protein elevation in patients with atrial arrhythmias: inflammatory mechanisms and persistence of atrial fibrillation. Circulation 2001;104:2886-91.
[61] Aytemir K, Ozer N, Atalar E, et al. P wave dispersion on 12-lead electrocardiography in patients with paroxysmal atrial fibrillation. Pacing Clin Electrophysiol 2000;23:1109-12.
[62] Andrikopoulos GK, Dilaveris PE, Richter DJ, Gialafos EJ, Synetos AG, Gialafos JE. Increased variance of P wave duration on the electrocardiogram distinguishes patients with idiopathic paroxysmal atrial fibrillation. Pacing Clin Electrophysiol 2000;23:1127-32.
[63] De Bacquer D, Willekens J, De Backer G. Long-term prognostic value of p-wave characteristics for the development of atrial fibrillation in subjects aged 55 to 74 years at baseline. Am J Cardiol 2007;100:850-4.
[64] De Sisti A, Leclercq JF, Stiubei M, Fiorello P, Halimi F, Attuel P. P wave duration and morphology predict atrial fibrillation recurrence in patients with sinus node dysfunction and atrial-based pacemaker. Pacing Clin Electrophysiol 2002;25:1546-54.
[65] Dogan A, Avsar A, Ozturk M. P-wave dispersion for predicting maintenance of sinus rhythm after cardioversion of atrial fibrillation. Am J Cardiol 2004;93:368-71.
[66] Padeletti L, Santini M, Boriani G, et al. Duration of P-wave is associated with atrial fibrillation hospitalizations in patients with atrial fibrillation and paced for bradycardia. Pacing Clin Electrophysiol 2007;30:961-9.
[67] Ariyarajah V, Frisella ME, Spodick DH. Reevaluation of the criterion for interatrial block. Am J Cardiol 2006;98:936-7.
[68] Gialafos E, Psaltopoulou T, Papaioannou TG, et al. Prevalence of interatrial block in young healthy men<35 years of age. Am J Cardiol 2007;100:995-7.
[69] Ciaroni S, Cuenoud L, Bloch A. Clinical study to investigate the predictive parameters for the onset of atrial fibrillation in patients with essential hypertension. Am Heart J 2000;139:814-9.
[70] Kistler PM, Sanders P, Fynn SP, et al. Electrophysiologic and electroanatomic changes in the human atrium associated with age. J Am Coll Cardiol 2004;44:109-16.

[71] Asad N, Spodick DH. Prevalence of interatrial block in a general hospital population. Am J Cardiol 2003;91:609-10.
[72] Xia Y, Hertervig E, Kongstad O, et al. Deterioration of interatrial conduction in patients with paroxysmal atrial fibrillation: electroanatomic mapping of the right atrium and coronary sinus. Heart Rhythm 2004;1:548-53.
[73] Montereggi A, Marconi P, Olivotto I, et al. Signal-averaged P-wave duration and risk of paroxysmal atrial fibrillation in hyperthyroidism. Am J Cardiol 1996;77:266-9.
[74] Magnani JW, Gorodeski EZ, Johnson VM, et al. P wave duration is associated with cardiovascular and all-cause mortality outcomes: the National Health and Nutrition Examination Survey. Heart Rhythm 2011;8:93-100.
[75] Dagli N, Karaca I, Yavuzkir M, Balin M, Arslan N. Are maximum P wave duration and P wave dispersion a marker of target organ damage in the hypertensive population? Clin Res Cardiol 2008;97:98-104.
[76] Guntekin U, Gunes Y, Tuncer M, Simsek H, Gunes A. Comparison of the effects of quinapril and irbesartan on P-wave dispersion in hypertensive patients. Adv Ther 2008;25:775-86.
[77] Yazici M, Ozdemir K, Altunkeser BB, et al. The effect of diabetes mellitus on the P-wave dispersion. Circ J 2007;71:880-3.
[78] Kosar F, Aksoy Y, Ari F, Keskin L, Sahin I. P-wave duration and dispersion in obese subjects. Ann Noninvasive Electrocardiol 2008;13:3-7.
[79] Seyfeli E, Duru M, Kuvandik G, Kaya H, Yalcin F. Effect of obesity on P-wave dispersion and QT dispersion in women. Int J Obes (Lond) 2006;30:957-61.
[80] Fukunami M, Yamada T, Ohmori M, et al. Detection of patients at risk for paroxysmal atrial fibrillation during sinus rhythm by P wave-triggered signal-averaged electrocardiogram. Circulation 1991;83:162-9.
[81] Guidera SA, Steinberg JS. The signal-averaged P wave duration: a rapid and noninvasive marker of risk of atrial fibrillation. J Am Coll Cardiol 1993;21:1645-51.
[82] Budeus M, Hennersdorf M, Perings C, Wieneke H, Erbel R, Sack S. Prediction of the recurrence of atrial fibrillation after successful cardioversion with P wave signal-averaged ECG. Ann Noninvasive Electrocardiol 2005;10:414-9.
[83] Steinberg JS, Zelenkofske S, Wong SC, Gelernt M, Sciacca R, Menchavez E. Value of the P-wave signal-averaged ECG for predicting atrial fibrillation after cardiac surgery. Circulation 1993;88:2618-22.
[84] Aytemir K, Amasyali B, Abali G, et al. The signal-averaged P-wave duration is longer in hypertensive patients with history of paroxysmal atrial fibrillation as compared to those without. Int J Cardiol 2005;103:37-40.
[85] Budeus M, Felix O, Hennersdorf M, Wieneke H, Erbel R, Sack S. Prediction of conversion from paroxysmal to permanent atrial fibrillation. Pacing Clin Electrophysiol 2007;30:243-52.

Part 4

Management

12

Stepwise Ablation of Permanent Atrial Fibrillation

Michala Pedersen, Daniel Scherr and Méléze Hocini
Hôpital Cardiologique du Haut-Lévêque & University Bordeaux 2 Victor Segalen, France

1. Introduction

The stepwise technique for ablation permanent atrial fibrillation (AF) is a combination and cumulative effect of several strategies (Calkins et al., 2009); pulmonary vein isolation (PVI), ablation of complex fractionated potentials, and linear lesions. This approach leads to termination of AF in 85% of cases without the need for pharmacological or electrical cardioversion and also produces unprecedented clinical outcomes in terms of maintaining sinus rhythm (SR) in the medium term, although more than 50% of patients require repeat procedures (Haissaguerre et al., 2005; O'Niell et al., 2006; Takahashi et al., 2007, Hocini et al., 2010). The cumulative effect of each step can be visualized as in figure 1. Termination of AF may occur at any point throughout the stepwise approach. The endpoint of ablation is termination of AF directly to SR (15%) or through intermediate atrial tachycardias (AT) with a mean of 2.6 atrial ATs per patient (Haissaguerre et al., 2005). With sinus rhythm successfully restored, the PVI and integrity of any linear ablation should be confirmed and if incomplete finished by further ablation as necessary, now in sinus rhythm.

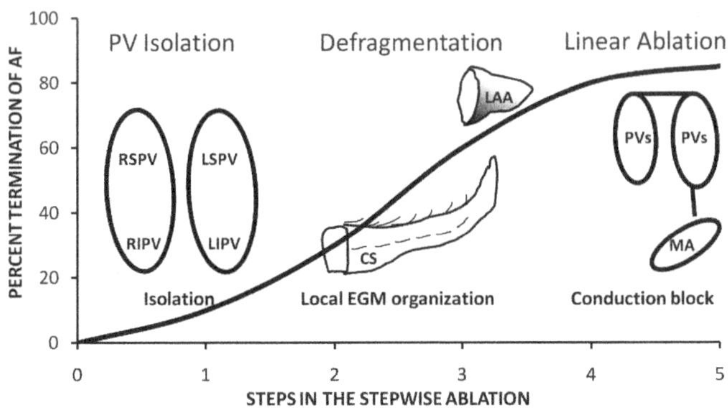

Fig. 1. Shows the cumulative effect of the stepwise ablation: with each next step, more termination of AF. The incremental benefit of each next step has a progressively smaller effect, until a ceiling of about 85% after which more ablation will not result in a higher success rate for AF termination (Hocini et al., 2010). PV Pulmonary Veins, RSPV and RIPV right superior and right inferior pulmonary veins respectively. LSPV and LIPV left superior and left inferior pulmonary veins respectively. MA mitral annulus. CS coronary sinus.

This chapter will go through in detail each step of this ablation approach. In addition, patient selection and preparation as well as post procedural care and complications will be described. Atrial tachycardia mapping and ablation will be described although it is not in the scope of this chapter to give a full description of this large topic. Finally, procedural outcomes and predictors of success will be discussed.
It should be emphasized that this chapter will describe the way the authors carry out their ablation procedures, there are many variations between centers, but generally the similarities in approach far outweigh any differences.

2. Patient selection and pre-procedural preparation

Persistent AF is defined as AF which that is sustained beyond seven days, or lasting less than seven days but necessitating pharmacologic or electrical cardioversion to restore sinus rhythm. Included in the category of persistent AF is "longstanding persistent AF" which is defined as continuous AF of greater than one year duration. Patients with symptomatic persistent AF who are refractory to antiarrhythmic drug therapy are candidates for the procedure if they accept the benefits and risks, as well as a >50% chance of requiring a second procedure. Catheter ablation of AF is a demanding procedure that may result in severe complications, a fact that should be explained to the patient prior to signing any consent form. Patients are not excluded on the basis of LA size or the presence of concomitant structural heart disease. On the contrary, selected patients with heart failure and/or reduced ejection fraction especially seem to benefit from restoration of SR.

2.1 Patient preparation

All patients undergo cardiac evaluation with imaging pre-procedure. A standard two-dimensional echocardiogram is most commonly used. Besides standard parameters such as atrial dimensions and ventricular function, other abnormalities such as an interatrial septal aneurysm or a persistent foramen ovale are actively sought for by the echocardiographer.
A transesophageal echocardiogram (TEE) is performed in all patients prior to the procedure to exclude LA thrombus, which is present in approximately 1% of cases despite appropriate anticoagulation and irrespective of the patients' $CHADS_2$ score (Scherr et al., 2009). The TEE is usually performed the day before to the procedure.
All antiarrhythmic drugs are stopped for at least 5 half lives prior to ablation except in the case of amiodarone, which is continued.

2.2 Pre-procedural advanced cardiac imaging

Computed tomography (CT) and magnetic resonance imaging (MRI) are increasingly used pre-procedure in order to gain more detailed atrial anatomical knowledge as well as for possible merging with 3-D electroanatomical mapping systems (see below). In addition, MRI can assess for areas of delayed enhancement (suggesting fibrosis/scar areas) but for now this additional information is usually part of research. However, neither current evidence nor personal experience has convinced us to routinely use pre-procedural 3D imaging and/or 3D electroanatomic mapping for every AF ablation procedure.

2.3 Anticoagulation

Patients are treated with oral anticoagulants to maintain an international normalized ratio (INR) between 2 and 3 for at least four weeks leading up to the ablation, with cessation 48 hours prior to the procedure. Patients with a contraindication to warfarin or who refuse oral anticoagulation are treated at the physician's discretion. Patients do not routinely receive bridging therapy with low molecular weight heparin between the cessation of warfarin and the procedure. However, in selected patients with major risk factors, e.g. prior embolic event or an enlarged LA with spontaneous contrast, low molecular weight heparin is administered as a bridging therapy.

3. Patient preparation and ablation set-up

The vast majority of our patients undergo the AF ablation procedure under conscious sedation and not under general anaesthesia, aiming to prevent and monitor for any complications such as cerebrovascular embolic events. Sedation is with midazolam and morphine, if any deeper sedation needed, this should be anaesthetist-guided. Arterial lines, urinary catheters or esophageal temperature probes are not routinely used.

One 6 French sheath and two 8 French sheaths (one of which is later replaced with the transseptal sheath) are placed in the right common femoral vein and a decapolar steerable catheter is placed in the CS such that its tip is at the 3 o'clock position in the 30° LAO view.

3.1 Rotational atriography and pulmonary vein angiography

Prior to the transseptal puncture 3D rotational atriography of the LA and pulmonary veins is usually performed (using a Philips Xper FD 10 system (Philips Medical Systems, Best, The Netherlands)). This is done by placing a 6 Fr pigtail catheter in the upper end of the inferior caval vein, with the C-arm carefully isocentered over the LA, and then injecting contrast. After a standard delay, usually 14 seconds (pulmonary transit time), the fluoroscopy is initiated and the C-arm rotates over a 240° arc with an X-ray acquisition speed of 30 frames/sec. The 3D data are automatically transferred and merged onto the workstation to enable on-line 3D reconstruction and as such catheter visualisation in 3D on-line. Details of rotational atriography are described elsewhere (Knecht et al., 2010). This gives very useful acute and precise anatomical definition of the ostia and hence help guide the ablation and minimises complications such as pulmonary vein stenosis, which can occur if ablating too distal into the vein.

A (less ideal) alternative to 3D atriography is selective angiography of the pulmonary veins. This is done by selectively engaging each of the four PV ostia with a multipurpose angiography catheter and injecting contrast media into each vein under fluoroscopy.

3.2 Transseptal puncture

Several different techniques are used to obtain a safe transseptal puncture. Centers should probably continue what they are experienced with and feel competent with. Here we suggest one way of proceeding: an antero-posterior X-ray position is used for the pull-down (usually started with a 4- to 5 o'clock needle position) and, once the jump onto the foramen ovale is seen, for the transseptal puncture. Before puncturing and crossing the needle into the left atrium, the monoplane fluoroscopy system is briefly positioned in a left-lateral position to check for needle position in the sagittal plane (ideally between 12 and 1 o'clock).

Single transseptal puncture is performed with pressure monitoring and using contrast injection through the needle tip to confirm LA access prior to advancing the dilator and sheath assembly. A guidewire is advanced through the dilator and sheath assembly into a left PV and the dilator and sheath are pulled back into the RA to allow passage of the ablation catheter through the same puncture site into the LA (hence a single puncture technique). The dilator and sheath are then advanced over the guidewire into the LA alongside the ablation catheter, the sheath is aspirated and initially flushed with a bolus and subsequently continuously with heparinized saline at 200 ml/hr. Immediately after LA access, a bolus of heparin (50U/kg) is given intravenously. The ACT is checked every 30 to 60 minutes during the procedure and repeat boluses of heparin is administered to achieve a constant activated clotting time (ACT) between 250-300 seconds.

3.3 Sheaths and catheters

A 10-pole, 20 mm circular decapolar catheter is advanced via a transseptal sheath (SL-0, St. Jude Medical, St. Paul, Minnesota) and positioned just distal to the PV ostia to map the PV perimeter during PVI. An externally irrigated tip ablation catheter (eg Thermocool 3.5 mm-tip catheter, Biosense Webster Inc, Diamond Bar, CA) is used, usually with an F-curve, however, the size of the curve used should depend on the size of the atrium.

3.4 Radiofrequency delivery

Radiofrequency energy is delivered using a Stockert generator (Biosense Webster) with the power settings shown in Table 1. These power settings have been determined empirically to provide effective lesions while also minimizing the risks of PV stenosis, steam pops, cardiac tamponade and collateral damage to the phrenic nerve, esophagus and circumflex coronary artery. Target temperatures of 40-42°C are achieved (maximum temperature 45°C) by manual titration of irrigation rates from 5-60 ml/minute (0.9% saline via CoolFlow pump, Biosense Webster).

Ablation site	Power (Watts)	Usual total duration of radiofrequency delivery (mins)
Coronary Sinus	15 -25	4-8
Posterior wall LA	25 - 30	3-6
Anterior wall LA	30 - 35	3-6
Inferior LA	30 – 40	5-10
Roof LA	25 – 30	10-15
PVs	30	25-40
Septum LA	30	3-6
Right atrium	20 – 35	0-20
Mitral Isthmus	30 – 35	10-20

Table 1. The power settings and usual RF delivery time at each anatomic region.

3.5 Signal processing

During AF ablation procedures, 12 lead surface electrocardiograms and bipolar endocardial electrocardiograms are continuously monitored and stored using a digital amplifier and computer recording system (LabSystem Pro, Bard Electrophysiology, Lowell, MA, USA). All signals are sampled at 1Khz with filter settings from 30 to 250Hz for intracardiac signals and 0.1 to 50Hz for surface electrocardiograms. Intracardiac signals are displayed at an amplification of 0.1mV/cm and with a gain of x16 for the mapping/ablation catheter, and 0.2mV/cm with a gain of x8 for the Lasso catheter and coronary sinus catheter.

3.6 Three dimensional mapping

While not routinely required, various 3-D electroanatomic mapping technologies may be used for assessment of anatomy, electrogram analysis, and quantification of the impact of ablation on LA and RA voltages. Occasionally, these technologies are useful for mapping ATs that may arise after AF termination or during subsequent procedures. Any electroanatomic mapping system may be used (EnSite NavX Navigation & Visualization Technology, St. Jude Medical, St. Paul, MN; CARTO3 System, Biosense Webster, Diamond Bar, CA), which allow real-time display of any cardiac catheter during ablation. The ability to display a lasso catheter allows for very rapid creation of a left atrial map and direction of the ablation catheter toward the desired poles on the lasso catheter.

3.7 Atrial Fibrillation cycle length

Assessment of the atrial fibrillation cycle length (AFCL) is an important tool in guiding the ablation procedure. Electrograms (EGMs) in persistent AF are complex and the cycle length cannot be reliably measured, except in the right and left appendages (Figure 2). Throughout the stepwise ablation the AFCL will gradually prolong and once a critical prolongation has been achieved, usually in the region of 180 to 200 ms, the atrium can no longer sustain the fibrillatory process and AF terminates to either SR or, as in the majority of cases, to an atrial tachycardia (AT) that can then be mapped and ablated conventionally.

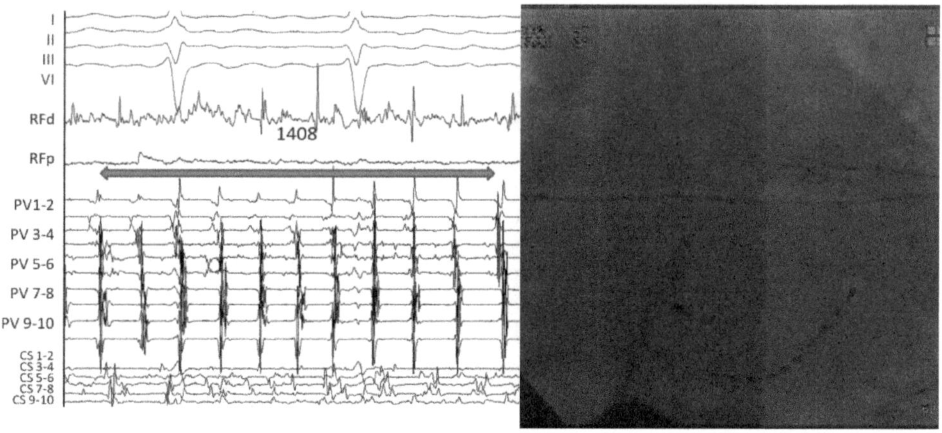

Fig. 2. Surface leads I, II, III and V1. Then the EGMs of the radiofrequency (RF) catheter, RFp (proximal) and RFd (distal), placed in the inferior LA. PV1-PV10 are the EGMs from a LASSO catheter placed in the left atrial appendage (LAA). CS 1-10 are the EGMs from a decapolar catheter in the coronary sinus. The AFCL cannot be measured on the surface ECG nor in the coronary sinus. However the LASSO catheter in the LAA enables measurement a more exact AFCL, here 10 cycle lengths are counted, giving an AFCL of 141ms.

4. Pulmonary vein isolation

Ablation strategies which target the isolation of the PVs are the cornerstone for most AF ablation procedures. The PVs can be isolated individually or as ipsilateral pairs, generally dependent on venous anatomy, catheter stability and operator preference. When the PVs are targeted, complete electrical isolation and elimination of all electrical near-field signals around the PVs is the goal. An example of isolation of the left superior pulmonary vein (LSPV) can be seen in Figure 3.

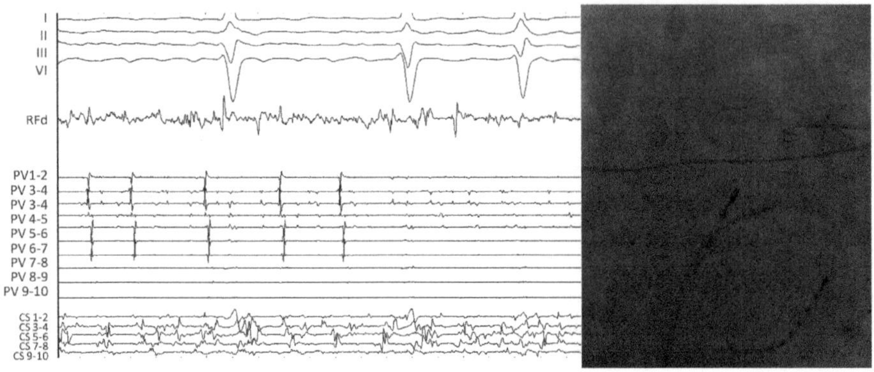

Fig. 3. Left panel shows surface ECG I, II, III and V1. Then, the RF ablation EGMs, followed by the poles 1-10 of the Lasso catheter and the lowest 5 EGMs are the bipoles of the decapolar catheter in the CS. The right panel shows fluoroscopy of the decapolar catheter in the coronary sinus, the Lasso catheter in the LSPV, and the RF catheter ablating just proximal to the ostium of the vein. There is 2:1 entry block into the vein prior to isolation.

Ablation is performed 1 to 2 cm proximal to the PV ostia. The ablation is typically started on the posterior wall towards the LSPV. Ablation can be done in a continuous manner, delivering energy at any given site for 30 - 60 seconds, until the local electrical signals have diminished, before moving on to the next site in a continuous fashion, slowly creating a posterior ablation line (vertical line from high to low) on the left side, followed by ablation within the first millimeters of the venous ostia to target the fascicles lying anteriorly until electrical PV isolation. Circumferential ablation is then repeated around the right PVs with a continuous circular lesion. It is unusual to achieve PV isolation after circumferential coalescent lesions without further ablation targeting the earliest PV activity or sites of reverse PV polarity as recorded on the circumferential mapping catheter indicating the residual anatomical connection. During ongoing AF, the sequence of PV activation is incessantly changing because (i) multiple breakthroughs are present in the most veins, (ii) changing incident wavefronts of activation at the PV ostia and (iii) rate-dependent conduction properties of the LA-PV connections. A consistent activation sequence usually means discrete sites of breakthrough, either spontaneous or following prior ablation. Delivery of RF narrows the width or number of LA-PV connections resulting in progressive consistency of the PV activation sequence. The endpoint of this step is complete electrical isolation of all pulmonary veins evident in the form of entrance block.

During AF, it can be difficult to distinguish far field potentials from local pulmonary vein potentials, both seen on the circular catheter at the PV ostium. Some guides to the differentiation are as follows:

- PV potentials represent local myocardial activation and therefore exhibit sharper electrograms with more rapid deflection than the far-field potentials.
- Activation sequence of PV potentials is constantly changing during ablation, while that of far-fields is relatively stable.
- Consistent prolongation of PV CL may be observed due to reduction of LA to PV connections with radiofrequency applications.
- If doubt remains, far-field potentials can be unmasked by putting a recording catheter in the suspected structure, in particular the LAA. Synchronous activity between LAA and PV potentials confirms an external origin of potentials recorded on the circumferential catheter.

As previously explained, long-standing persistent AF will terminate after PVI alone only in a small minority of patients although the global AFCL usually increase by 8ms (Haissaguerre et al., 2005a). Once sinus rhythm is restored, after the stepwise ablation approach, it is important to confirm complete PVI, this is best done by re-inserting the circumferential lasso catheter into each vein.

Figure 4 shows the AFCL prolongation achieved following pulmonary vein isolation. This tracing is from the same patient as who had an AFCL of 141ms in figure 2 and PVI in figure 3.

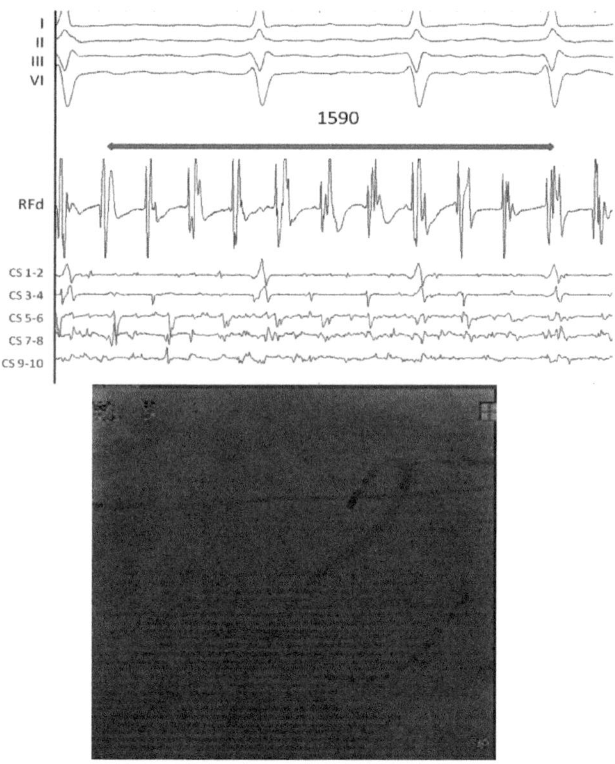

Fig. 4. Upper panel shows the surface leads I, II, III and V1. The EGMs from the RF catheter (placed at the base of the LAA) and lowest the EGMs from the 5 bipoles of the decapolar catheter in the CS. The AFCL is now 159ms. Lower panel shows the catheter placement on fluoroscopy.

5. Electrogram- based ablation during disorganized left atrial activity

The next step in the approach is electrogram based ablation, also colloquially called defragmentation. Following pulmonary vein isolation left atrial activity is usually chaotic with disorganized sites everywhere and the overall activity is too complex to map in terms of activation, morphology or local cycle length. The aim is to ablate favorable areas that would result in slowing and organization of global LA activity.

5.1 Targets for EGM-based ablation

Favorable areas in the left atrium for ablation are continuous electrograms with complex fractionated potentials that are noted at first sight, especially when the AFCL is around 140-150ms. When the AFCL prolongs significantly, we search for sites with a gradient of activation (significant electrogram offset between the distal and proximal recording bipoles on the map electrode), or regions with a cycle length that are shorter that the mean LAA cycle length (Haissaguerre et al., 2005). A recent study found that ablation of areas with continuous activity had the greater impact on AFCL prolongation and AF termination than ablation of areas with high fractionation index, EGM voltage and local cycle length (Takahashi et al., 2008).

The various zones of complex atrial electrograms may be explained by several different underlying etiologies. They may represent areas of colliding wave fronts, pivot points of moving wavelets or collision with barriers such as scars or existing structures for instance valves or appendages. Complex electrograms are seen in the periphery of sites of rapid activity, often with a frequency gradient to surrounding tissue. These sites are usually located at the base of the LAA, the PV ostial region and in the inferior LA along the CS. Figure 5 shows examples of complex electrograms.

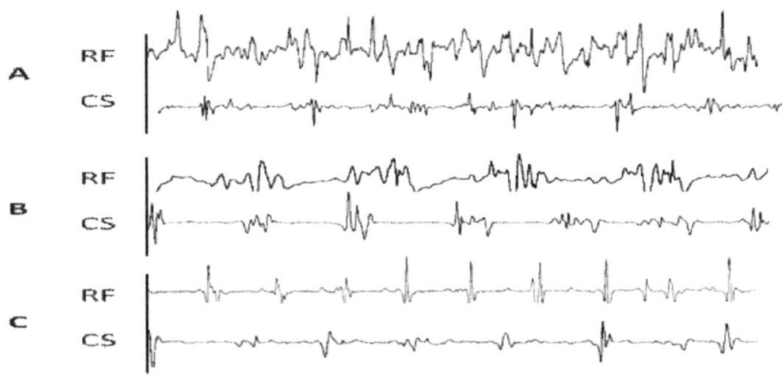

Fig. 5. Shows simultaneous recordings from the RF (in the LA) and CS catheters ; panel A is a recording of continuous activity on the RF catheter without a return to baseline, panel B shows a fractionated potentials on the RF catheter with an interposed isoelectric interval and panel C is an example of rapid activity recorded on the RF catheter with a frequency gradient to the CS.

5.2 Facilitating tools in localizing targets for ablation

Localizing and mapping areas for electrogram based ablation can be difficult. To facilitate this, various methods have been tried, including anatomical guided ablation, the use of multipolar catheters and the use of 3 dimensional mapping systems.

5.2.1 Anatomical guidance to defragmentation

Studies have been done to try determine anatomical areas within the left atrium where ablation has the greatest impact (rise in the LAA-AFCL by at least 5ms) on the AF process; in addition to the pulmonary vein isolation, the base of the left atrial appendage and the interface between inferior LA and the coronary sinus has the greatest impact (Haissaguerre et al., 2005). Figure 6 illustrates this concept. Figure 7 is an example of ablation of chaotic EGMs in the inferior left atrium.

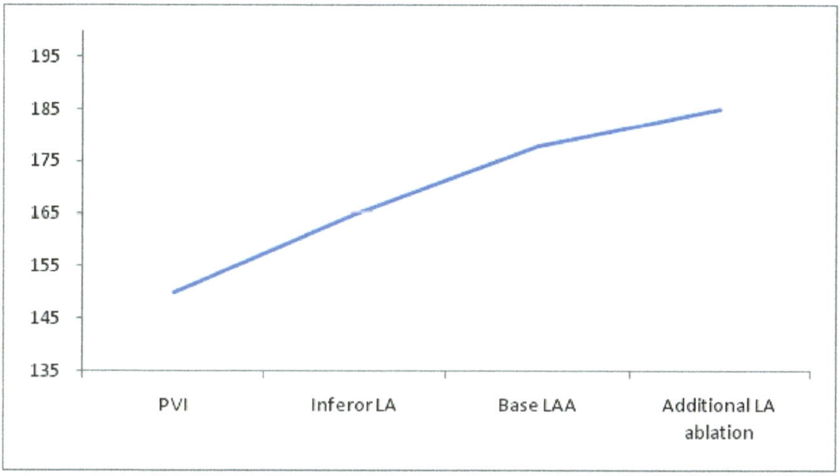

Fig. 6. With ablation of each anatomical area the AFCL gradually prolongs – a cumulative effect.

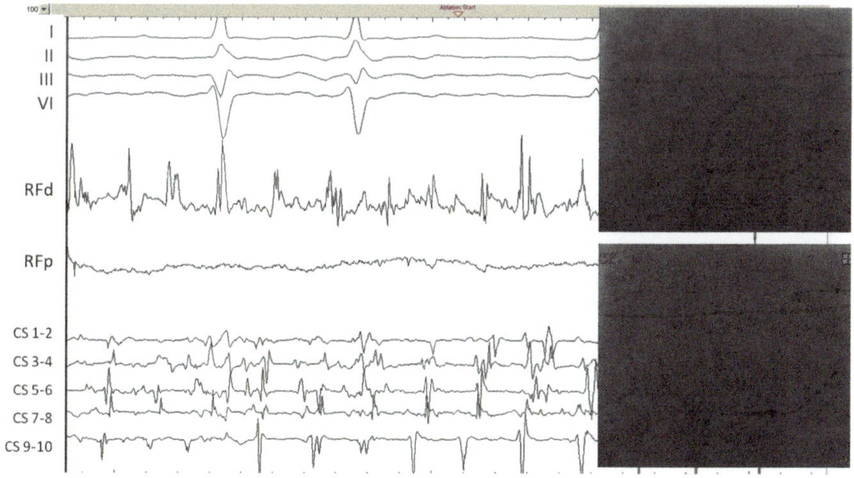

Fig. 7. Surface leads I,II III and VI. The EGMs on the RF catheter are of a complex nature. The decapolar catheter in the CS confirms AF. Ablating in the inferior LA can be done by dragging the catheter along the floor of the atrium, either from left to right (upper insert) or from right to left (lower insert).

5.2.2 Multipolar catheters

Another aid in determining left atrial areas/zones for ablation is the use of multipolar catheters, such as the LASSO catheter or the PENTA-RAY catheter (Biosense Webster, Inc, Diamond Bar, CA, USA), with 10 and 20 poles respectively (figure 8). The advantage, apart from the high density of electrograms, is the temporal and directional information such closely organized catheter poles can provide. These catheters are particularly useful in organized atrial fibrillation, as well as in mapping focal and localized re-entrant tachycardias (an example described below).

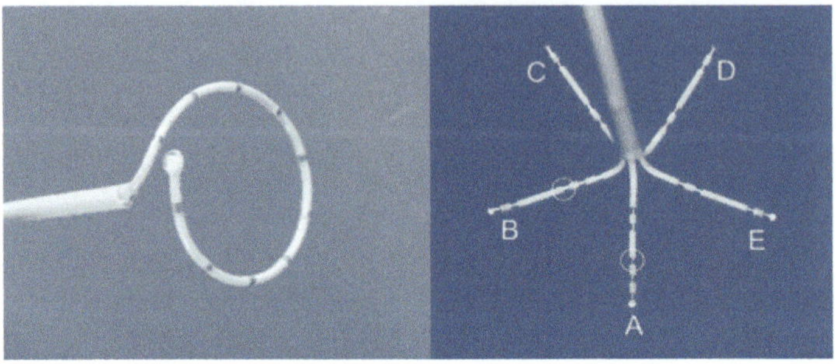

Fig. 8. Examples of multipolar catheters that can be used for mapping, to the left a spiral catheter, to the right a penta-ray catheter.

5.2.3 Three dimensional mapping systems

Finally, an aid can be 3 dimensional mapping systems that have algorithms to compute (on-line) areas of very short cycle lengths and fragmentation. Figure 9 shows an example of a NAVx (St Jude Medical, Inc., MN, USA) eletroanatomic fractionation map of the left atrium during atrial fibrillation. The most fractionated (fastest cycle length) areas are represented by red, the least represented by blue, and grey represents scar or inactive areas.

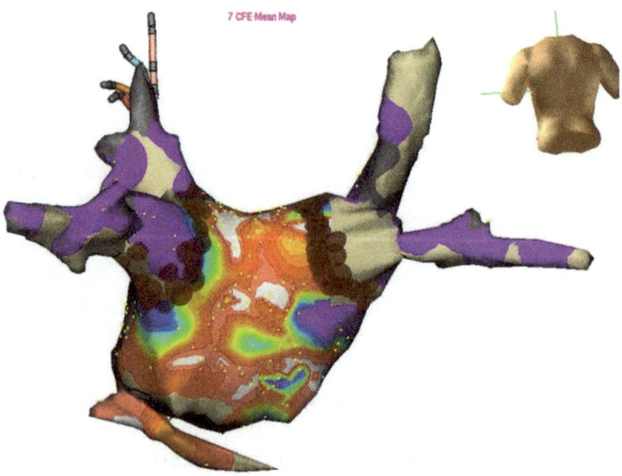

Fig. 9. Shows a NAVx electroanatomic fractionation map of the left atrium (postero-anterior view). Circumferential PVI can be seen represented by brown ablation points.

5.3 Cycle length prolongation

Throughout the defragmentation the AFCL is prolonging and it useful to assess the AFCL after each step of ablation. Figure 10 illustrates the prolongation during defragmentation in the same patient as earlier. He had an initial AFCL of 141ms (figure 2) which prolonged to 159ms after PVI (figure 4). During defragmentation in the inferior LA, base of LAA and septum the AFCL prolonged to 183ms and during roof ablation converted to an AT (figure 10).

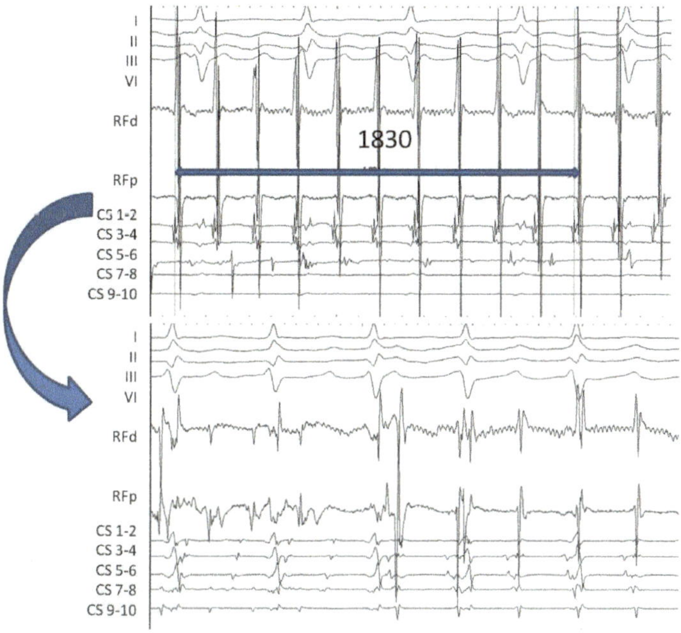

Fig. 10. Both panels show surface leads I, II, III, VI and a decapolar catheter in the CS. In the upper panel the RF catheter is in the LAA and the AFCL is measured over 10 cycles to be 183ms. With further ablation the AF converts to an AT (lower panel).

6. Linear ablation

If the patient is still in AF after the previous steps, the next stride in the stepwise ablation procedure is linear ablation. Linear ablation is an important tool in the step wise ablation procedure (Knecht et al., 2008). The efficacy of linear lesions may be related to interruption of wavelets and macro re-entries, ablation of autonomic innervations and atrial debulking. The left atrial roof and the lateral mitral isthmus are the most common sites for linear ablation. Linear ablation is often done during AF but proving bidirectional block can only be done in SR, usually towards the end of the procedure when SR has been reestablished. It is possible that that the previous steps have rendered the patient in an atrial tachycardia, in which case the lines are ablated (if appropriate) during the AT.

In general, linear ablation is the last step in the stepwise approach. This is because they can be very difficult, they may require not only a long time but also a large amount of radiofrequency to successfully achieve bidirectional block. This alone increases the risk for complications such as perforation and tamponade. In addition incomplete lines are associated with arrhythmia recurrence and pro-arrhythmic effects (Gerstenfeld etal., 2004; Chugh et al., 2005). The 2 left atrial lines will be discussed separately.

6.1 Linear ablation at the left atrial roof

The left atrial roof line is relatively short, forming a continuous line between the already isolated left and right superior pulmonary veins. In the vast majority of patients this step is done during AF and the end point (during AF) is 85-90% diminution or complete abolition of local electrograms along the line. The line is performed as cranially as possible to avoid ablating the posterior LA, hence aiming to avoid complications such as damage to the esophagus.

The electrophysiological endpoint of roof ablation is the creation of a complete line of conduction block between the superior PVs. If the ablation is done during AF, supplementary ablation during sinus rhythm is usually required. Electrical block is confirmed in all patients following restoration of SR using a well described technique (Hocini et al., 2005).

6.1.1 The creation of the roof line

The ablation catheter is curved and dragged along the line with the tip of the irrigated catheter positioned parallel to the roof, either from right to left or left to right. A large loop in the LA is often helpful (figure 11). If the orientation of the catheter tip is perpendicular to the roof power settings should be reduced (to 25W) to lessen the possibility of steam pops and perforation.

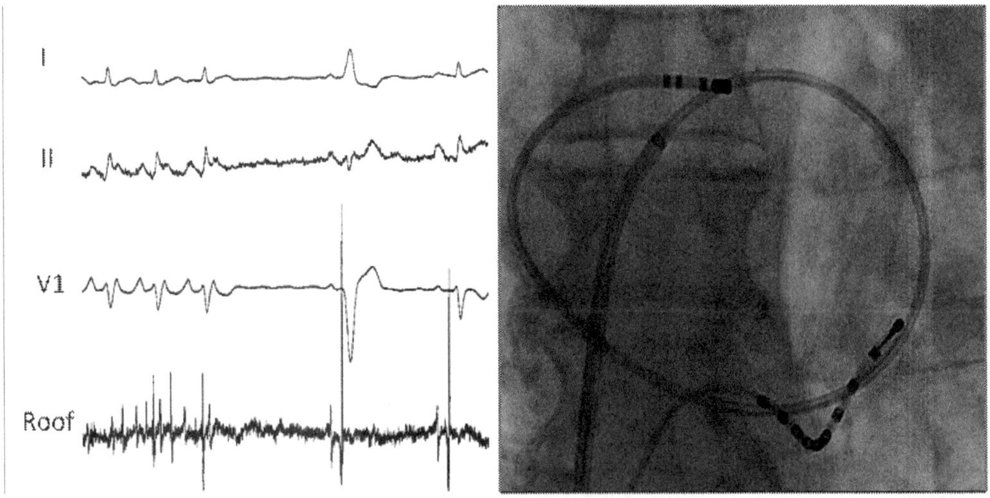

Fig. 11. Surface lead I, II and VI together with the EGMs from the RF. This roof line is carried out during roof dependent atrial tachycardia; fractionated EGMs can be seen on the RF catheter prior to completion of the line when the SR is restored.

6.2 Linear ablation at the mitral isthmus

Ablation of the mitral isthmus, achieving bidirectional conduction block further increases the success rate of catheter ablation in persistent AF (Jais et al., 2004). In general this ablation step in only carried out if deemed necessary; if the previous steps have not terminated the atrial fibrillation or if the patient is in an mitral isthmus dependent atrial tachycardia. If the line is carried out during AF, the endpoint is the same as that for the roof line; abolition of all local electrograms along the line, usually with the creation of double potentials all along the line. If carried out during atrial tachycardia (mitral isthmus dependent flutter) the goal is arrhythmia termination. Once in SR, the electrical block must be confirmed using bidirectional pacing and sensing from the CS catheter and the mapping catheter (see below). Again, it is likely that more ablation is needed once in sinus rhythm to achieve bidirectional block. It must be noted that even in the best pair of hands, block of the mitral isthmus cannot be achieved in about 10% of patients.

6.2.1 The creation of the mitral isthmus line

The mitral isthmus is short, 2-4cm, from the mitral annulus to the left inferior pulmonary vein ostium (or the left atrial appendage). It is often needed to extend the line from the ostium of the inferior pulmonary vein to the base of the LAA in order to achieve block as well as it is needed in up to 80 % to ablate within in coronary sinus to achieve block (Jais et al., 2004). The mitral isthmus line is begun at the ventricular aspect of the mitral annulus, see figure 12. With clockwise rotation on the sheath and catheter the lesion is extended to the left inferior PV and further to the base of the LAA if needed. If mitral isthmus block is not achieved by this, the ablation is extended to the epicardial aspect of the mitral isthmus, via the coronary sinus (Jais et al., 2004). The overall goal remain the same for all linear lesions, elimination of local EGMs along a line connecting 2 electrically inactive sites, e.g. the mitral valve annulus and the encircling lesion of the LIPV.

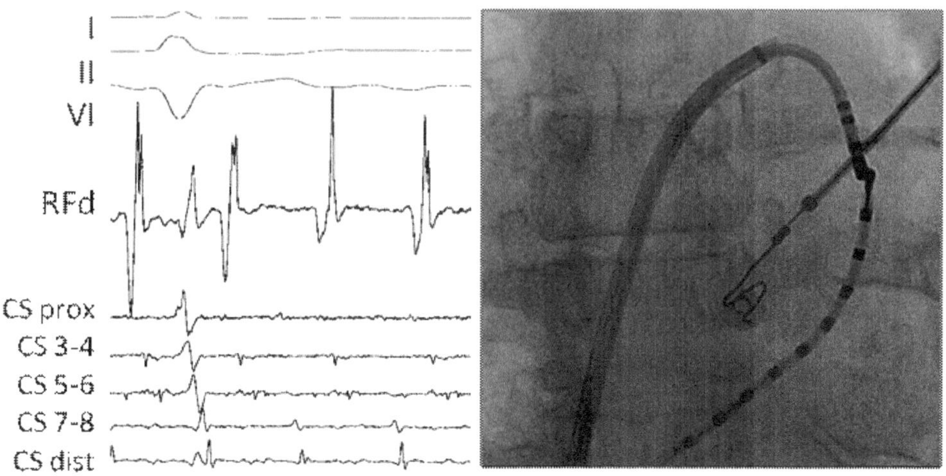

Fig. 12. Surface leads I, II and VI, the RF catheter and the bipolar EGMs of the decapolar catheter in the CS. The RF catheter is at the start of the linear ablation of the mitral isthmus. Often there are high amplitude EGMs at the mitral isthmus pre ablation.

7. Right atrial ablation

In 15% of patient with persistent AF, SR cannot be restored by ablation in the LA and the presence of perpetuators in the RA should be considered (Hocini et al., 2010). This state of affairs should be suspected when the AFCL in the RAA prolongs less than the AFCL in the LAA during ablation; a shorter AFCL in the RAA compared to LAA can be due to the drivers of AF originating in the RA (figure 13). Similarly, pauses in activity in the LA electrograms without corresponding pauses in the RA electrograms would suggest the RA as the driving chamber. The approach to mapping and the electrogram ablation within the RA is the same as for the LA. Preferential anatomical areas at which there is a higher incidence of AF termination during ablation of complex fractionated atrial electrograms are the right atrial appendage, the intercaval region, the SVC and the CS ostium.

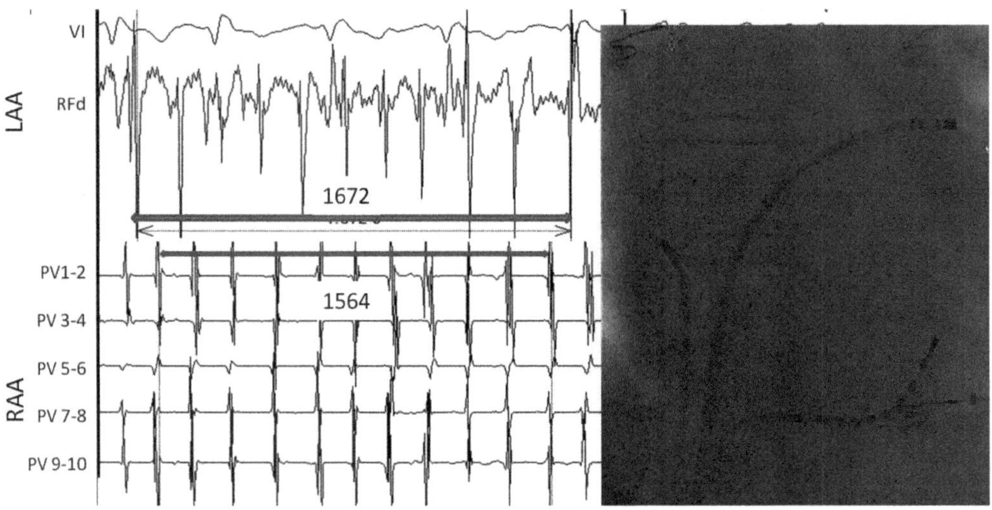

Fig. 13. Shows surface lead VI, EGM from the RF catheter placed in the LAA and the 5 bipolar EGMs from the LASSO catheter placed in the RAA as the lower 5 rows. The LAA AFCL is 167 and the RAA AFCL 156 suggestive of a driving source in the right atrium. The right hand panel is a fluoroscopy of the catheter placement.

8. Atrial tachycardia in the context of atrial fibrillation ablation

Atrial tachycardia may occur at any point throughout the stepwise ablation for atrial fibrillation; when the AFCL is so prolonged that the LA can no longer sustain the fibrillatory process. As described in the introduction, the endpoint of the stepwise ablation is restoration of sinus rhythm, and this re-establishment of sinus rhythm usually occurs via 1 or more ATs (Haissaguerre et al., 2005). In addition, AT is the dominant mode of arrhythmia recurrence in patients in whom AF was terminated during the index procedure (O'Neill et al., 2009).

Atrial tachycardia is characterized by a monomorphic P-wave and a consistent intracardiac activation sequence. In the context of AF ablation, we classify AT into three categories:

Macro re-entry is defined as a circuit involving 3 or more atrial segments, and where more than 75% of the circuit can be mapped.
Focal tachycardia is defined as centrifugal activation originating from a discrete site, and where <75% of the cycle length can be mapped. This tachycardia can be due to any of increased automaticity, triggered activity or re-entrant mechanisms.
Localized re-entry constitutes a circuit involving 1 or 2 adjacent segments, usually smaller than 2 cm in diameter and spanning more than 75% of the cycle length within the involved segments.
A recent series of 238 ATs occurring after ablation of persistent atrial fibrillation found that 46% were macroreentrant and 54% focal or microrentrant ATs. Of the macroreentrant tachycardias the commonest were perimitral circuits (56%), followed by roof dependent circuits (28%), and with a smaller proportion of tricuspid isthmus dependent circuits (16%) (Jais et al., 2009). More complex macro-reentrent circuits are less common e.g. double loop re-entry and circuits passing through gaps between the pulmonary veins and/or the LAA.

8.1 Mapping atrial tachycardias

An approach to mapping atrial tachycardias is shown in figure 14. The first step is to assess atrial tachycardia cycle length variation, if > 15% variable the AT is likely to be of focal or local re-entry aetiology, if < 15% the tachycardia can be of any of the 3 categories (Jais et al., 2009). Fig 15 is an example of a tachycardia with very little cycle length variation. If the cycle length variation is less than 15% the first aim is to deduct whether it is a macroreentrant tachycardia or of a focal source. This requires activation mapping and entrainment mapping. If the cycle length variation is more than 15% and the atrial tachycardia mechanism therefore most likely a focal or localized re-entry source, the aim then is to map the source.

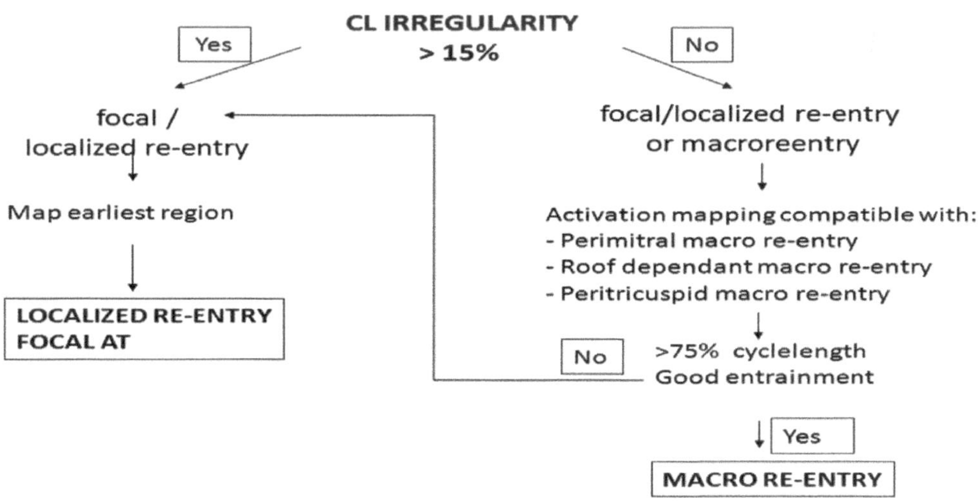

Fig. 14. Shows an algorithm for the diagnosis of atrial tachycardias.

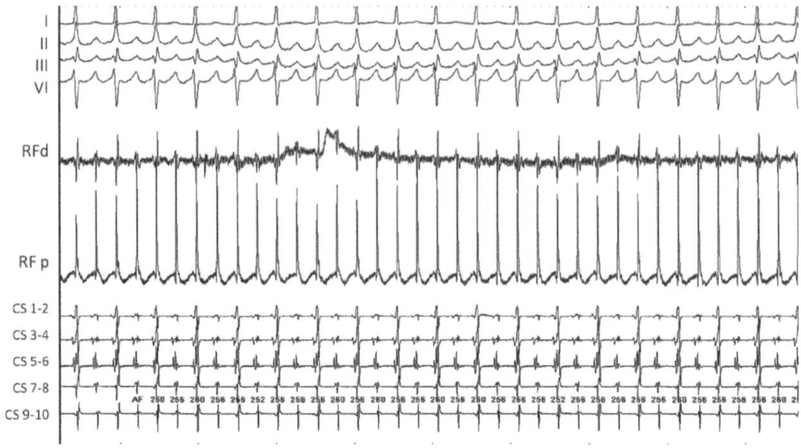

Fig. 15. Shows a tracing of an atrial tachycardia with very little cycle length variation, in this case 3%. The AT can therefore be either any of the 3 categories of AT: focal, localized re-rentry and macroreentrant. In such case, the first step is to rule in, or rule out, a macroreentrant tachycardia using activation mapping and entrainment. This tracing is from the same patient as in figures 2, 3, 4 and 10.

8.1.1 Mapping macro reentrant tachycardias

If the AT CL variation is more than 15%, the first aim is to rule in or rule out a macro re-entrant tachycardia. Given that the majority of macroreentrant AT are one of the following three: 1) Mitral isthmus dependent flutter (Perimitral AT), 2) Roof dependent flutter and 3) Cavotricuspid isthmus dependent flutter (Peritricuspid AT); activation mapping around the mitral annulus, anterior and posterior LA, the roof and the tricuspid annulus are mapped to look for the presence of activity all through the period of one tachycardia cycle length. Each of the 2 left atrial circuits has their own distinct activation sequence of the LA (figure 16):

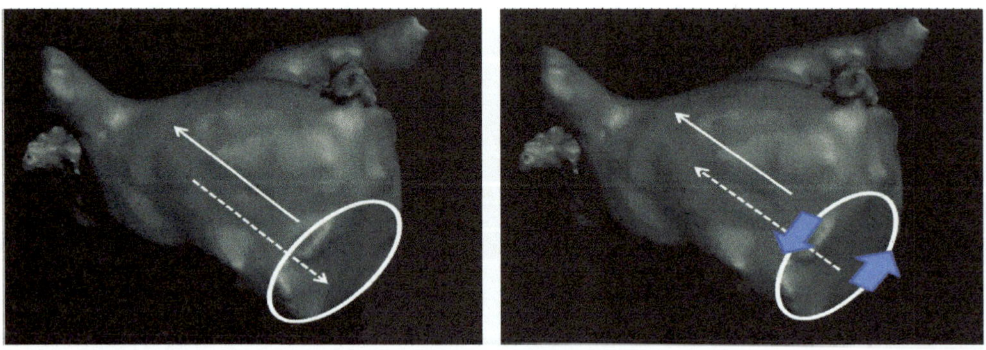

Fig. 16. Depicts the left atrial activation pattern of the macro reentry circuits: counterclockwise peri-mitral (A) and roof dependant (B)

Once the activation pattern of the macro-reentrant tachycardia has been established, entrainment from at least 2 opposite segments should be done to confirm (or rule out) the diagnosis. If macro re-entrant circuits are ruled out the algorithm leads back to the top of the arm for focal and localised re-entrant tachycardias.

8.1.2 Ablating macroreentrant tachycardias

The perimitral atrial tachycardia passes through the mitral isthmus between the mitral valve annulus and the left inferior pulmonary vein, and hence ablation with complete isthmus block abolishes this arrhythmia. The roof dependent flutter is dependent on the relatively narrow part between the 2 upper pulmonary veins and a complete ablation line would terminate roof dependent flutter. The ablation of these two lines is described above. It is not in the scope of the chapter to describe the ablation of the right atrial peritricuspid flutter.

8.1.3 Confirming bidirectional block following line ablation – roof line

This very important step is undertaken after the SR has been restored, either from the stepwise ablation, or form direct current cardioversion. Following a complete roof line, pacing of the LAA will result in the activation of the posterior LA from inferior to superior direction as the activation front cannot travel posteriorly over the blocked roof. Figure 17 illustrates this concept.

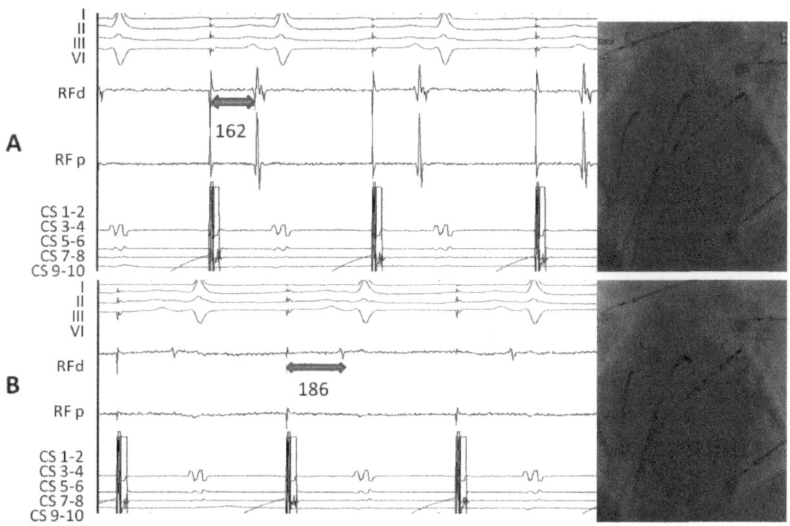

Fig. 17. The left panels show the surface leads I, II, III and VI. Then the EGMs of the RF catheter and lowest the 5 bipoles of the decapolar catheter - now placed though the transseptal puncture to the LAA. Pacing is done from the distal CS (LAA). In Panel A the RF catheter is placed low on the posterior wall and in panel B high on the posterior wall. During pacing from the LAA the time to low posterior wall is 162ms and to high posterior wall 184ms - thereby proving roof block.

8.1.4 Confirming bidirectional block following line ablation – mitral line

Following a mitral isthmus line, block is confirmed using differential CS pacing and pacing from the RF catheter at the lateral LA just anterior to the mitral line or in the LAA. In the presence of block the activation front moves along the anterior wall to the septum and then along the posterior wall, septal to laterally, during LAA pacing. This gives a proximal to distal activation sequence of the CS. Figure 18A illustrates this. In the other direction, block is assessed by pacing the first the distal poles of the CS catheter, which is near the mitral line and measuring the delay to LAA. The pacing is then changed to a more proximal pole wherefrom the delay to the LAA should be shorter in the presence of blocked linear lesion. Figure 18B illustrates this.

18 A

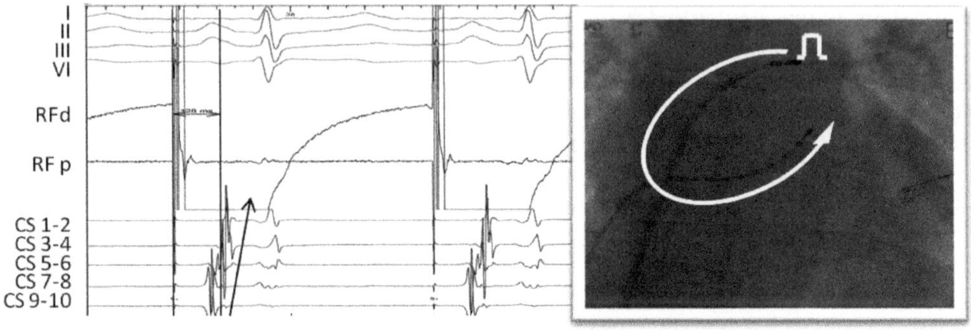

18 B

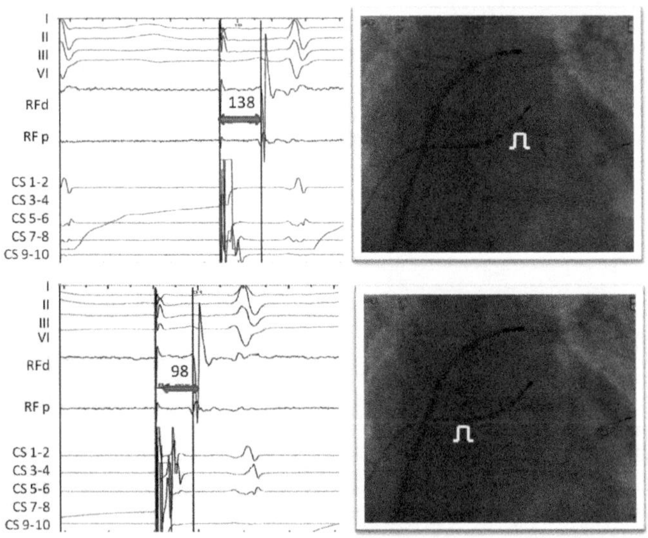

Fig. 18. A and B. The left panels show surface leads I, II, III and VI, then the RF catheter placed just anterior to the mitral line. Lowest is the EGMs of the bipoles of the decapolar catheter in the CS. In figure 18A pacing from the RF catheter confirms clockwise block over the mitral line by activating the CS catheter in a proximal to distal manner. Figure 18B confirms counterclockwise block by differential pacing, the pacing to RF is longer (138ms) when pacing the distal CS than when pacing the more proximal CS (98ms).

8.2 Focal and localized reentrant tachycardias

After macroreentrant tachycardias have been ruled out the next step is tracking the earliest potentials for a focal or localized re-entry AT. Once the suspected region of origin has been found, careful mapping will suggest whether it is a focal or localized reentrant tachycardia. Local activity spanning most of the AT CL suggest local re-entry whereas if only a limited part of the CL can be mapped, the likely etiology is a focal tachycardia. Overall, these 2 tachycardias are mapped and ablated in a similar manner.

8.2.1 Mapping focal and localized reentrant tachycardias

The aim is to gradually 'pinpoint' on the earliest spot. Often multipolar catheters can be helpful in localizing the earliest spot, simply by their ability to cover a larger area. Figure 15 was an example of an AT with a cycle length variation of 3% (same patient as in figure 2, 3, 4 and 10), where activation mapping and entrainment ruled out a macro reentrant circuit. The earliest region was found to be on the posterior wall and to aid localize the very earliest site of activation a LASSO catheter was used to map the posterior wall in detail. Figure 19 illustrates this:

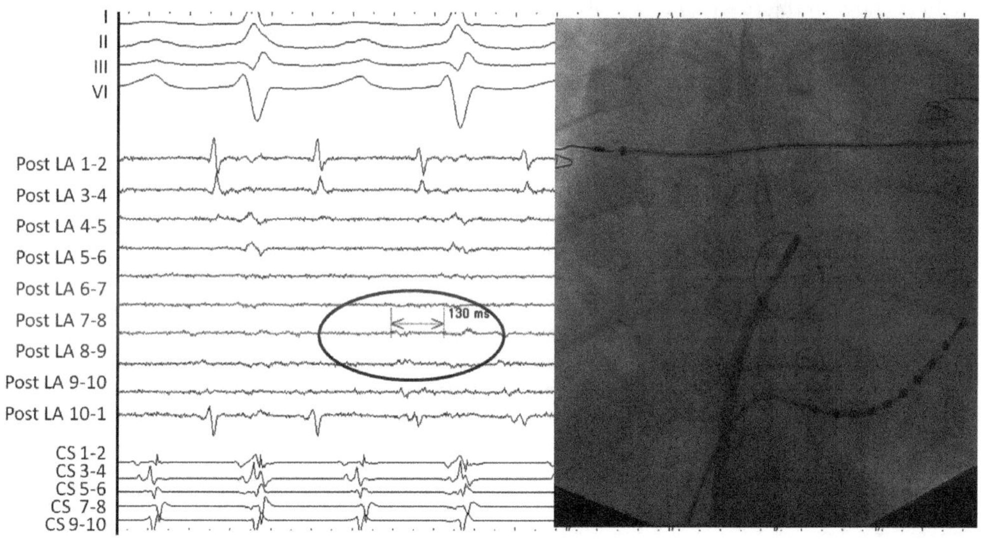

Fig. 19. Right panel shows the LASSO catheter on the posterior wall of the LA. The left panel shows surface leads I, II, III and VI at the top and the EGMs from a decapolar catheter in the CS at the bottom. The EGMS from the posterior wall shows the earliest potentials on the posterior wall to be near LASSO pole 7-8.

8.2.2 Ablating focal and micro reentrant tachycardias

Once the earliest potentials are located, be it a focal or localized reentrant tachycardia, ablation at the earliest point or at the site covering more than 90% of the tachycardia cycle length should eliminate the arrhythmia. Figure 20 shows the successful ablation of the tachycardia mapped in figure 19 with the lasso catheter to the posterior wall.

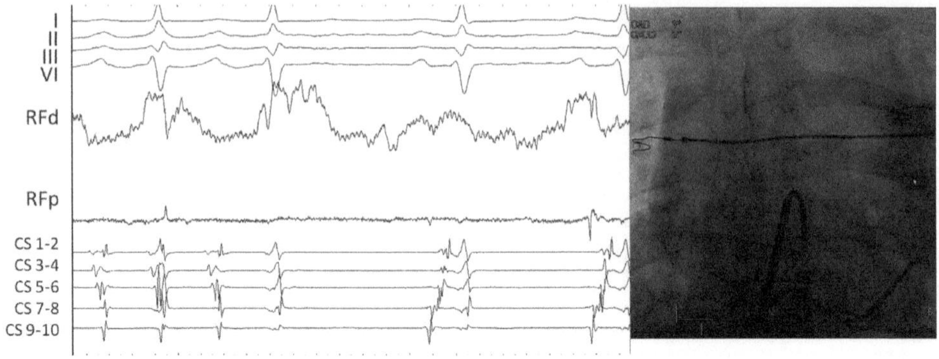

Fig. 20. Shows the successful ablation of the tachycardia mapped in figure 19. The LASSO catheter is replaced by an RF catheter and RF energy is applied to where the poles 7-8 were and the tachycardia converts to SR. This example is the same patient as in figures 2, 3, 4, 10 and 11, and he has now completed the stepwise ablation. However, before leaving the catheter laboratory it is paramount to ensure complete PVI and complete electrical block of any lines, now in the re-established SR.

9. Post procedural care

Following ablation, the guiding sheaths are pulled out of the left atrium and heparin is stopped. Patients will typically lie flat for 6 hours after sheaths are pulled due to the large sheaths used. All patients are treated with warfarin after ablation. Patients receive subcutaneous heparin injections beginning on the evening of the ablation and continuing until the INR is therapeutic. Patients are usually subjected to echocardiography and observed 48-72 hours post-procedure prior to discharge.

Patients are followed up closely for the year following an ablation procedure. At 3, 6 and 12 months, patients are admitted to hospital for 24 hours and undergo clinical evaluation including exercise stress testing, ambulatory Holter monitoring and transthoracic echocardiography. After the procedure, warfarin is continued for at least six months, and guided thereafter by the presence or absence of conventional risk factors for thromboembolism and maintenance of sinus rhythm. Patients with a CHADS2 score ≥2 are kept on warfarin regardless of their rhythm outcome. All antiarrhythmic drugs are discontinued by 3-6 months except in case of recurrence. In such case, patients are offered a repeat procedure.

10. Complications

Serious complications can occur during an ablation for permanent atrial fibriallation, and it is important that these (and their rate of occurrence) are carefully discussed with the patients prior to him or her signing the consent form. The major complications are described in detail in the task force on atrial fibrillation (Calkins et al., 2007) and anybody carrying out these ablations should probably familiarize themselves with this document. Overall, tamponade, pulmonary vein stenosis, atrio-esophageal fistula and/or death (so far not existent at our centre), air emboli and cerebrovascular or peripheral-vascular complications compile to a cumulative 2-3% complication rate.

11. Procedural outcomes

The stepwise ablation of permanent atrial fibrillation leads to termination in 87% of patients (Haissaguerre et al., 2005a). In this series 23 of 53 patients had a repeat procedure for arrhythmia recurrence (mainly for 1 or more atrial tachycardias). After repeat ablation 95% of all patients were in sinus rhythm at 11+- 6 months.

O'Neill (O'Neill et al, 2009) report similar results from a larger cohort (156 patients) achieving atrial fibrillation termination in 85% using the stepwise ablation approach in patients with persistent AF (ie termination by ablation alone, not requiring pharmacological and/or DC cardioversion). After 34 months follow up 95% of these patients were still in stable sinus rhythm, albeit 49% needed a repeat procedure. If AF termination was not achieved from ablation during the index procedure stable sinus rhythm was only found in 52% at 34 months, again albeit a redo procedure in 70%. In the AF termination group 89% have stopped anti-arrhythmic medication, whereas in the non-termination group only 25% stopped their AADs. Subsequent studies both from our group (Takahashi et al., 2007; Hocini et al, 2010) as well as studies published form other groups (Rostock et al., 2011) have reported the same findings; that the stepwise approach to ablation of persistent AF leads to unprecedented good clinical outcome.

11.1 Predictors of success

The duration of uninterrupted AF and AFCL has been shown to be independent factors predicting AF termination (O'Niell et al., 2009, Matsuo et al., 2009). If the duration of AF is less than 12 months there is a 90% chance of AF termination. This success rate gradually decreases to 54% if the duration of AF is more than 48 months. Similarly, the AFCL is a predictor of success, with a likelihood of AF termination of 95% if the AFCL is more than 161ms, gradually decreasing to 50% likelihood of success with AFCL of less than 120ms. Left atrial size is also predictor for termination of AF (Matsuo et al., 2009). Left ventricular ejection fraction, amiodarone use, troponin, procedure time and RF time did not reach statistical significance.

Termination of AF by ablation is also a strong predictor of success with up to 95% of patients remaining in SR after almost 3 years after 1.5 procedures (Takahashi et al., 2007; Rostock et al., 2011).

Fine atrial fibrillation, as measured by the fibrillatory (F-) wave on the surface ECG, has been shown to be a marker of longer lasting atrial fibrillation and larger left atrial size compared to patients with a more coarse AF. Coarse atrial fibrillation with F-waves ≥0.1mV in leads V1 and II of the surface ECG are correlated to younger age, a shorter AF history and a smaller left atrium. An F-wave amplitude of ≥ 0.7 mV predicts AF termination by ablation with a sensitivity and specificity of about 80%. Lastly, the smaller amplitude F-wave (<0.05mV) is associated with a higher AF recurrence rate as compared with higher F-waves (≥0.5mV) (Nault et al., 2009).

12. Conclusion

The stepwise ablation of permanent atrial fibrillation is a logical, patient tailored approach that is guided by electrophysiological endpoints. The method can lead to termination of AF in up to 85% of patients and render them arrhythmia free at least in the medium term, albeit more than 50% of patients need more than 1 procedure to achieve sustained sinus rhythm. Termination of AF by ablation, mapping and ablation of all intermediate ATs, and linear blocks confirmed is associated with a better long-term clinical outcome than when AF is not terminated by ablation.

Predictors of success in restoration of acute and sustained sinus rhythm include the duration of the continuous AF, mean baseline AFCL, age and the amplitude of the surface ECG fibrillatory waves. Understanding further baseline characteristics, both clinically and electrophysiologically, may help improving outcome and lead towards better patient selection criteria.

It is not known how to forecast which patients will experience arrhythmia recurrence, but predictors are incomplete lines, either from recovery of conduction or deficient line-block at the time of creation. Both recovery of pulmonary vein conduction (Ouyang et al., 2005) and incomplete left atrial linear lesions (Knecht et al., 2008) are important factors for arrhythmia recurrence. However, this is by no means the cause of all recurrences, for example, about 20% of recurrence of atrial tachycardia following the index procedure occurred from sites not previously ablated (O'Neill et al., 2009).

Despite unprecedented success of the stepwise approach to catheter ablation of permanent AF, ignorance remains particularly interpreting signals during chaotic activation in the atrium and this needs much more work. We still have only rudimentary tools to help identify the individual elements involved in AF and there is still a long way to go until we fully understand and master this arrhythmia.

13. References

Calkins, H., Brugada, J., Packer, D.L., Cappato, R., Chen, S.A., Crijns, H.J., Damiano, R.J, Davies, D.W., Haines, D.E., Haissaguerre, M., Iesaka, Y., Jackman, W., Jais, P., Kottkamp, H., Kuck, K.H., Lindsay, B.D., Marchlinski, F.E., McCarthy, P.M., Mont, J.L., Morady, F., Nademanee, K., Natale, A., Pappone, C., Prystowsky, E., Raviele, A., Ruskin, J.N. & Shemin, R.J. (2007). European Heart Rhythm Association (EHRA); European Cardiac Arrhythmia Scoiety (ECAS); American College of Cardiology (ACC); American Heart Association (AHA); Society of Thoracic Surgeons (STS), HRS/EHRA/ECAS expert Consensus Statement on catheter and surgical ablation of atrial fibrillation: recommendations for personnel, policy, procedures and follow-up. A report of the Heart Rhythm Society (HRS) Task Force on catheter and surgical ablation of atrial fibrillation. *Heart Rhythm.* Vol 4(6), pp. 816-61. Erratum in: *Heart Rhythm*. 2009. Vol 6(1), pp. 148.

Chugh, A., Oral, H., Lemola, K., Hall, B., Cheung, P., Good, E., et al. (2005). Prevalence, mechanisms, and clinical significance of macroreentrant atrial tachycardia during and following left atrial ablation for atrial fibrillation. *Heart Rhythm.* Vol 2(5), pp. 464-471.

Gerstenfeld, E. P., Callans, D. J., Dixit, S., Russo, A., Nayak, H., Lin, D., et al. (2004). Mechanisms of organized left atrial
tachycardias occurring after pulmonary vein isolation. *Circulation*. Vol 110(11), pp. 1351-1357.

Haissaguerre, M., Sanders, P., Hocini, M., Takahashi, Y., Rotter, M., Sacher, F., Rostock, T., Hsu, L., Bordachar, P., Reuter, S., Roudaut, R., Clementy, J. & Jais, P. (2005).

Catheter Ablation of Long-Lasting Persistent Atrial Fibrillation: Critical Structures for Termination. *Journal of Cardiovascular Electrophysiology*, Vol 6(11), pp. 1125-37. (a)

Haissaguerre, M., Hocini, M., Sanders, P., Sacher, F., Rotter, M., Takahashi, Y., Rostock, T., Hsu, L.-F., Bordachar, P., Reuter, S., Roudaut, R., Clementy, J. & Jais, P. (2005). Catheter Ablation of Long-Lasting Persistent Atrial Fibrillation: Clinical Outcome and Mechanisms of Subsequent Arrhythmias. *Journal of Cardiovascular* Electrophysiology. Vol 16(11), pp. 1138-47. (b)

Hocini, M., Jais, P., Sanders, P., Takahashi, Y., Rotter, M., Rostock, T., et al. (2005). Techniques, evaluation, and consequences of linear block at the left atrial roof in paroxysmal atrial fibrillation: A prospective randomized study. *Circulation*. Vol 112(24), pp. 3688–3696.

Hocini, M., Nault, I., Wright, M., Veenhuyzen, G., Narayan, S. M., Jais, P,. Lim, K.-Y., Knecht, S., Matsuo, S., Forclaz, A., Miyazaki, S., Jadidi, A., O'Neill, M.D., Sacher, F., Clementy, J. & Haissaguerre M. (2010). Disparate Evolution of Right and Left Atrial Rate During Ablation of Long-Lasting Persistent Atrial Fibrillation *Journal of American College of Cardiology*. Vol 55, pp. 1007-1016

Jais, P., Shah, D., Haïssaguerre, M., Hocini, M., Peng, J.-T., Takahashi, A., Garrigue, S., Le Métayer, P. & Clémenty, J. (2000). Mapping and Ablation of Left Atrial Flutters. *Circulation*. Vol 101, pp. 2928-2934

Jais, P., Hocini, M., Hsu, L.F., Sanders, P., Scavee, C., Weerasooriya, R., et al. (2004). Technique and results of linear ablation at the mitral isthmus. *Circulation*. Vol 110(19), pp. 2996–3002.

Jais, P., Seiichiro, M., Knecht, S., Weerasooriya, R., Hocini, M., Sacher, F., Wright, M., Nault, I., Lellouche, N., Klein, G., Clementy, J. & Haissaguerre, M. (2009). A Deductive Mapping Strategy for Atrial Tachycardia Following Atrial Fibrillation Ablation: Importance of Localized Reentry. *Journal of Cardiovascular Electrophysiology*. Vol. 20, No. 5, May pp 480-491.

Knecht, S., Wright, M., Spyridon Akrivakis, S., Nault, I., Matsuo, S., Chaudhry, M., Haffajee, C., Sacher, F., Lellouche,N., Miyazaki, S., Forclaz, A., Jadidi, A., Hocini, M., Ritter, P., Clementy, J., Haïssaguerre, M., Orlov, M. & Jaïs, P. (2010) Prospective randomized comparison between the conventional electroanatomical system and three-dimensional rotational angiography during catheter ablation for atrial fibrillation. *Heart Rhythm*. Vol 7, pp 459-465.

Knecht, S., Hocini, M., Wright, M., Lellouche, N., O'Neill, M.D., Matsuo, S., Nault, I., Chauhan, V.S., Makati, K.J., Bevilacqua, M., Lim, K.T., Sacher, F., Deplagne, A., Derval, N., Bordachar, P., Jais, P., Clementy, J. & Haissaguerre, M. (2008). Left atrial linear lesions are required for successful treatment of persistent atrial fibrillation. *European Heart Journal*. Vol 19, pp. 2359–2366.

Matsuo, S., Lellouche, N., Wright, M., Bevilacqua, M., Knecht, S., Nault, I.,Lim, K.-T., Arantes, L., O'Neill, M. D., Platonov, P. G., Carlson, J., Sacher, F., Hocini, M., Jais, P. & Haïssaguerre, M. (2009). Clinical Predictors of Termination and Clinical Outcome of Catheter Ablation for Persistent Atrial Fibrillation. *Journal of American College of Cardiology*. Vol 54(9),pp. 788–95

Nault, I., Lellouche, N., Matsuo, S., Knecht, S., Wright, M., Lim, K., Sacher, F., Platonov, P., Deplagne, A., Bordachar, P., Derval, N., O'Neill, M., Klein, G., Hocini, M., Jaïs, P., Clémenty, J. & Haïssaguerre, M.(2009). *J Interv Card Electrophysiol* Vol 26; pp 11–19.

O'Neill, M.D., Jais, P., Takahashi, Y., Jonsson, A., Sacher, F., Hocini, M., Sanders, P., Rostock, T., Rotter, M., Pernat, A., Clementy, J. & Haissaguerre, M. (2006). The stepwise ablation approach for chronic atrial fibrillation–evidence for a cumulative effect. *Journal of Interventional Cardiac Electrophysiology*. Vol 16, pp. 153–167.

O'Neill, M.D., Wright, M., Knecht, S., Jais, P., Hocini, M., Takahashi, Y., Jonsson, A., Sacher, F., Matsuo, S., Lim, K., Arantes, L., Derval, N., Lellouche, N., Nault, I., Bordacher, P., Clementy, J. & Haissaguerre M. (2009). Long term follow up of persistent atrial fibrillation ablation using termination as procedural endpoint. *European Heart Journal*. Vol 30, pp. 1105-1112.

Ouyang, F., Antz, M., Ernst, S., Hachiya, H., Mavrakis, H., Deger, F.-T., Schaumann, A., Chun, J., Falk, P., Hennig, D., Liu, X., Bansch, D., Kuck, K.H. (2005). Recovered pulmonary vein conduction as a dominant factor for recurrent atrial tachyarrhythmias after complete circular isolation of the pulmonary veins: lessons from double Lasso technique. *Circulation*. Vol 111, pp.127–135.

Takahashi, Y., O'Neill, M.D., Hocini, M., Reant, P., Jonsson, A., Jais, P., Sanders, P., Rostock, T., Rotter, M., Sacher, F., Laffite, S., Roudaut, R., Clementy, J. & Haissaguerre, M. (2007). Effects of stepwise ablation of chronic atrial fibrillation on atrial electrical and mechanical properties. *Journal of American College of Cardiology*. Vol 49, pp.1306–1314.

Takahashi, Y., O'Neill, M.D., Hocini, M., Dubois, R., Matsuo, S., Knecht, S., Mahapatra, S., Lim, K.T., Jais, P., Jonsson, A., Sacher, F., Sanders, P., Rostock, T., Bordachar, P., Clementy, J., Klein, G.J. & Haissaguerre, M. (2008). Characterization of electrograms associated with termination of chronic atrial fibrillation by catheter ablation. *Journal of American College of Cardiology*. Vol 5, pp 1003–1010.

Rostock, T., Salukhe, T. V., Steven, D., Drewitz, I., Hoffmann, B. A., Bock, K., Servatius, H., Müllerleile, K., Sultan, A., Gosau, N., Meinertz, T., Wegscheider, K. & Willems, S. (2011). Long-term single- and multiple-procedure outcome and predictors of success after catheter ablation for persistent atrial fibrillation. *Heart Rhythm* (in press)

Scherr, D., Sharma, K., Dalal, D., Spragg, D., Chilukuri, K., Henrikson, C., Nazarian, S., Berger, R., Calkins, H. & Marine, J. (2009). Incidenceand predictors of periprocedural cerebrovascular accident in patients undergoing catheter ablation for atrial fibrillation. *Journal of Cardiovascular Electrophysiology*. Vol 20, pp 1357-1363.

13

Surgical Management of Atrial Fibrillation

Bobby Yanagawa, Khaled D. Algarni and Gideon Cohen
Division of Cardiac and Vascular Surgery, Schulich Heart Centre, Sunnybrook Health Sciences Centre, University of Toronto, Toronto, Ontario, Canada

1. Introduction

Atrial fibrillation (AF) is the most common arrhythmia in adults and a major burden of morbidity and mortality in cardiovascular patients (1). The major sequelae are cardiovascular and include heart failure and thromboembolic events, primarily stroke. The prevalence of AF is 0.4-1% in the overall population which rises with age to approximately 15% in those patients 70 years and older (2). The incidence of AF is rising due in part to the increase in the aging population, increase in those living with structural cardiovascular pathology and more frequent diagnosis from the use of ambulatory monitoring devices. Overall, AF affects more than 2.5 million adult in the US and 200,000 to 250,000 in Canada (Heart and Stroke Foundation of Canada statistics; http://www.heartandstroke.com). Overall, this represents a considerable burden of illness in vulnerable populations such as the elderly and those with congestive heart failure.

The Framingham Study found that development of chronic AF was associated with a two-fold increase in mortality from cardiovascular disease (2). Furthermore, AF was an independent risk factor for mortality in this population (3). The risk of stroke with persistent AF is 8% per year and 2% per year with warfarin. This is balanced with a bleeding risk of 2% per year while on warfarin at an INR of 2-3 (4). Of 5070 patients in the Framingham Study followed for 34 years, a two-fold increase in stroke events were found with AF with higher rates in those with heart failure (5). The attributable risk of stroke increases with age from 1.5% for the youngest cohort (50-59 years) to 23.5% for the oldest cohort (80-89 years).

AF is defined based on the clinical presentation, relevant patient characteristics and any associated cardiac pathology. There is considerable variation in the descriptors for types of atrial fibrillation. These include acute, chronic, long-standing, sustained, recurrent, and so forth. The Society of Thoracic Surgeons (STS) has published reporting guidelines to facilitate consistency in reporting which include classification of AF as paroxysmal, persistent and permanent; duration of arrhythmia and patient burden (percentage of overall time in AF) as well as previous interventions and relevant patient characteristics such as association with cardiac pathology (6). The European Society of Cardiology differs in that for AF lasting greater than 1 year, patients undergoing a rhythm control strategy have longstanding persistent AF whereas patients who have accepted the arrhythmia and are not therefore treated with rhythm control therapy have permanent AF. Table 1 provides the descriptors and definitions of AF utilized in this chapter.

AF Subtypes	Definition
Paroxysmal*	>2 episodes, duration < 7 days, spontaneous termination
Persistent*	> 7 days or requires cardioversion
Longstanding Persistent	>1 year with rhythm control treatment; failed or no cardioversion
Permanent	> 1 year without rhythm control treatment
Primary / Lone	Not associated with cardiac pathology, usually MR
Secondary / Concomitant	Associated with cardiac pathology
Post-Operative	Post-cardiac surgery, usually transient

MR, mitral regurgitation
* Characterized by the most frequent presentation

Table 1. Definition of AF Subtypes

Electrophysiologically, AF is characterized by irregular and uncoordinated atrial activation caused by macro re-entry circuits in left and right atria. In paroxysmal AF, 90% of micro re-entry circuits or triggers exist in close proximity to the pulmonary veins (in the context of mildly dilated atria) which trigger large macro-reentrant circuits (7). This is the basis for pulmonary vein isolation (PVI). There is however evidence for extrapulmonary vein sites for initiation of AF which include superior vena cava (8), ligament of Marshall (9), left atrial (LA) posterior wall (10,11), coronary sinus, crista terminalis, interatrial septum, and LA appendage (LAA) (12). An important caveat is that most mapping studies have been performed in lone AF cases and may not be reflective of concomitant AF, particularly in atria with significant structural alterations. Atrial fibrillation may be conceptualized as a spectrum of severity. Paroxysmal AF resulting from macro reentry circuits in the absence of major tissue remodeling. If untreated, this may progress to persistent and then permanent AF with substrate alterations associated with atrial structural remodeling (Figure 1). These later stages of AF may not be sufficiently addressed with PVI and may require a more extensive procedure, to be discussed in later sections.

Patients with concomitant AF may have associated mitral pathology and possibly other valvulopathy as well as coronary disease. This is relevant as the atrial tissue is rendered susceptible to AF secondary to atrial stretch or damage, resulting in loss of myocardium and replacement fibrosis (13). The ultimate end result is electrical remodeling and shortened refractory periods (14). In fact, left atrial size may be utilized as a surrogate marker for atrial remodeling. There also exists some evidence for a role of proinflammatory signaling as seen with active valvular or coronary disease and/or dysfunction of sinoatrial and atrioventricular nodes in AF development (15).

Medical management of AF is based on rate or rhythm control as well as anticoagulation for stroke prevention. The Atrial Fibrillation Follow-up Investigation of Rhythm Management (AFFIRM) trial, a 4060 patient multicentered randomized controlled trial demonstrated no survival difference between rate and rhythm control at 3.5 years, although rate control was associated with fewer adverse events (16). Anticoagulation has been traditionally accomplished with warfarin (INR 2-3) for stroke prophylaxis but is associated with bleeding events. More recently, anticoagulation with the direct thrombin inhibitor dabigatran has shown similar stroke prevention rates with lower bleeding events and without the need for INR monitoring (17).

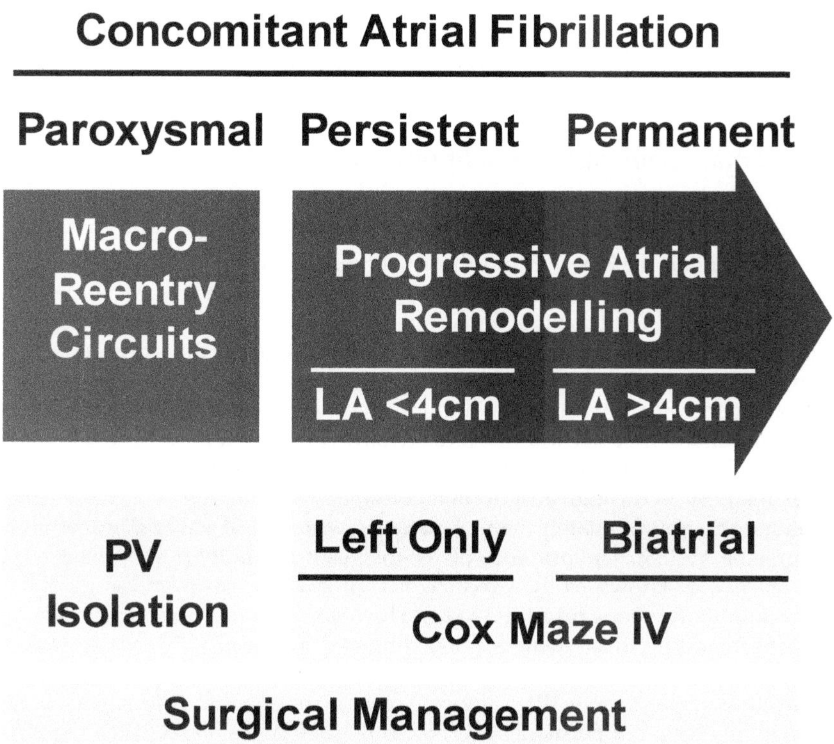

Fig. 1. Pathophysiology and surgical management of concomitant AF. Atrial fibrillation may be described clinically as paroxysmal, persistent or permanent, which is associated with macro reentry circuits plus progressive left atrial remodeling. Surgical management of paroxysmal AF may be limited to pulmonary vein isolation, but more chronic AF types require left-only or complete Maze IV lesion sets.

Another rhythm control strategy is interventional. Generally patients with lone AF who are refractory to medical management are initially considered for catheter ablation. This is best suited for patients with paroxysmal AF where pulmonary vein isolation (PVI) alone may address the ectopic foci. In patients with longstanding persistent or permanent AF, due to atrial substrate alterations, linear and ECG-guided extra pulmonary vein ablation may be necessary but even with these adjuncts, the success of less likely. The major limitation of this technology is inconsistent outcomes due to procedural failure and AF recurrence. For patients with paroxysmal AF, success is approximately 66% after a single procedure (18). Percutaneous LAA closure is also possible as an adjunct to ablation.

Several devices have been developed and tested for percutaneous LAA closure for thromboembolic prevention. In the prospective, randomized controlled trial PROTECT-AF, the WATCHMAN LAA closure device (Atritech, Plymouth, MN) was found to be non-inferior to warfarin alone for the composite endpoint of stroke, cardiovascular death, and systemic embolism (3.0 vs. 4.9/100 patient years) but hemorrhagic stroke was lower in the intervention group (19). There were, however, risk of procedural complications including pericardial effusions and stroke, likely due to air embolism, and less commonly device embolization. Other devices used for percutaneous LAA closure include the PLAATO (Percutaneous LAA Transcatheter Occlusion) membrane-covered self-expandable nitinol cage system and the Amplatzer Septal Occluder (20,21).

2. Surgical management of atrial fibrillation

The underlying basis for surgical management of atrial fibrillation is *targeted synthesis of scar tissue which does not conduct electrical impulses.* We will consider surgical management of patients with primary or lone AF and those with concomitant valvular or coronary disease who are undergoing surgery and are being considered for adjunctive AF surgery.

Of patients with lone AF, those that failed one or more attempts at catheter ablation or those who prefer surgery based on superior published outcomes, are considered for surgical management. Lee et al (22) reviewed AF surgery and correctly identified that patients with lone AF are generally unwilling to undergo sternotomy to address AF alone. In such patients, a minimally-invasive approach to AF surgery offers a reasonable alternative. These approaches include PVI, minimally-invasive Cox-Maze IV procedure or beating heart epicardial ablation, all through a right thoracotomy.

More commonly, approximately half of patients with mitral valve disease have reported some degree of AF (23). The presence of AF increases mortality post-MV surgery. The cut-and-sew maze, also known as the Cox-maze III procedure, has been the gold standard AF surgical technique for sinus restoration (24). However, due to the morbidity of cut-and-sew atrial lesions including those related to bleeding and increased CPB and cross-clamp times, most centers opt for the use of alternative energy sources. For paroxysmal AF without significant atrial enlargement, PVI alone may be a reasonable adjunctive procedure. For patients with persistent or permanent AF, the full Maze IV lesion set offers highest chance of success at sinus restoration. Although other modified lesions sets such as the Cox Mini-Maze and left only-Maze procedure and others have been introduced, we will limit our discussion to the full Maze lesion set (25-27).

2.1 Surgical techniques

Ultimately the success of sinus restoration is dependent on the type and duration of AF, patient-specific and anatomical factors, and the successful creation of a transmural lesion set. Furthermore, for adjunctive procedures, the added surgical morbidity and mortality related to increased time on CPB and increased complications must be taken into consideration. All patients considered for AF surgery should have a careful assessment of their symptoms as well as transthoracic echocardiography for comprehensive assessment of left and right atrial anatomy.

2.1.1 Maze procedure

In 1987, Dr. Cox introduced the maze procedure and subsequently reported outcomes on the first seven patients who were free of AF (28). However, the original maze procedure was complicated by an inability to generate tachycardic response during exercise, left atrial dysfunction as well as surgical complexity and resulting long bypass and cross clamp times (29). Since that time, the maze has undergone several iterations. As mentioned, the Cox Maze III is the gold standard for AF surgery. The Cox-maze III procedure is associated with a higher incidence of sinus restoration, improved sinus node function, fewer pacemaker requirements and improved atrial function compared with its predecessors. Importantly the Cox-Maze III has proven robust effectiveness in the setting of paroxysmal, persistent or permanent AF (30). Although this procedure has not been widely adopted, it is important to appreciate the lesion set which forms the basis of the Cox Maze IV procedure.

The Cox Maze III procedure is generally performed as an adjunct to a mitral procedure. The left-sided lesion set is performed at the time of MV repair/replacement via the left atriotomy, then the right-sided lesion set is performed on the beating heart at the time of patient rewarming. Briefly, the complete lesion set for the Maze III may be performed as follows: The LA is entered via the inter-atrial groove. 1) PVI is performed to prevent the macro-reentry circuits originating from the PVs. To accomplish this, the left atriotomy is extended in a circumferential fashion, until all pulmonary veins are encircled and the left atrium completely detached from its base. 2) Then the LAA is isolated to block re-entry circuits at its base. The LAA is excised and the remaining defect incorporated into the atriotomy closure. 3) The mitral line and coronary sinus (CS) lesion are created to block conduction originating from mitral orifice and the CS, respectively. The PV encircling incision is joined to the mitral annulus at its postero-medial aspect and the CS is spot cryoablated. 4) On the right side, the intercaval lesion circuits originate from the SVC and IVC. To block these circuits, the longitudinal atriotomy is fashioned along the free wall of the right atrium extending from the tricuspid annulus (atrioventricular groove) to the left atriotomy incision. 5) The right atrial counter lesion blocks signals originating from the RAA. A second incision is fashioned along the free wall of the RAA, once again originating at the level of the tricuspid annulus, however extending only partially along the wall of the atrium. The resulting island provides a conduction 'corridor' through which normal stimuli can travel. 6) The T-lesion blocks RA flutter waves and reentry circuits (31). The right atrial isthmus incision is created, once again, using cryoablation.

In cases of concomitant and continuous AF with normal RA size and no evidence of flutter waves, as the source is likely the LA, some groups have suggested that a left-only Maze may be sufficient. This would avoid a more complex operation with incision into the RA. However, the RA isthmus has been identified as a source of atrial flutter. As such, atrial flutter post-left Maze may necessitate additional right atrial catheter ablation (32). If the RA dimension is abnormal, the RA may support two of more macro reentrant circuits and a full Maze lesion set is recommended. Furthermore, a full Maze lesion set is recommended in cases where atrial flutter is present or when the RA is already opened.

In 2004, the Cox-maze IV was introduced which replaced most surgical incisions with alternative energy sources (33). This has significantly shortened cross-clamp times compared with the Cox-maze III (41min vs 93 min) with comparable short term freedom from AF (34). The lesion set of the Cox Maze IV is shown in Figure 2. On the left, the PVs are isolated and two linear ablation lines are used to create a box lesion. Voeller et al (35) found that a box lesion around all four PVs which completely isolates the posterior LA wall led to greater mid-term freedom from AF as opposed to isolation in pairs. The LAA is surgically removed but if performed through a right thoracotomy, the LAA is oversewn from the inside. The mitral line is created and the CS is cryoablated. On the right the intercaval lesion is created. Through the right atriotomy the counter lesion and T-lesion are created.

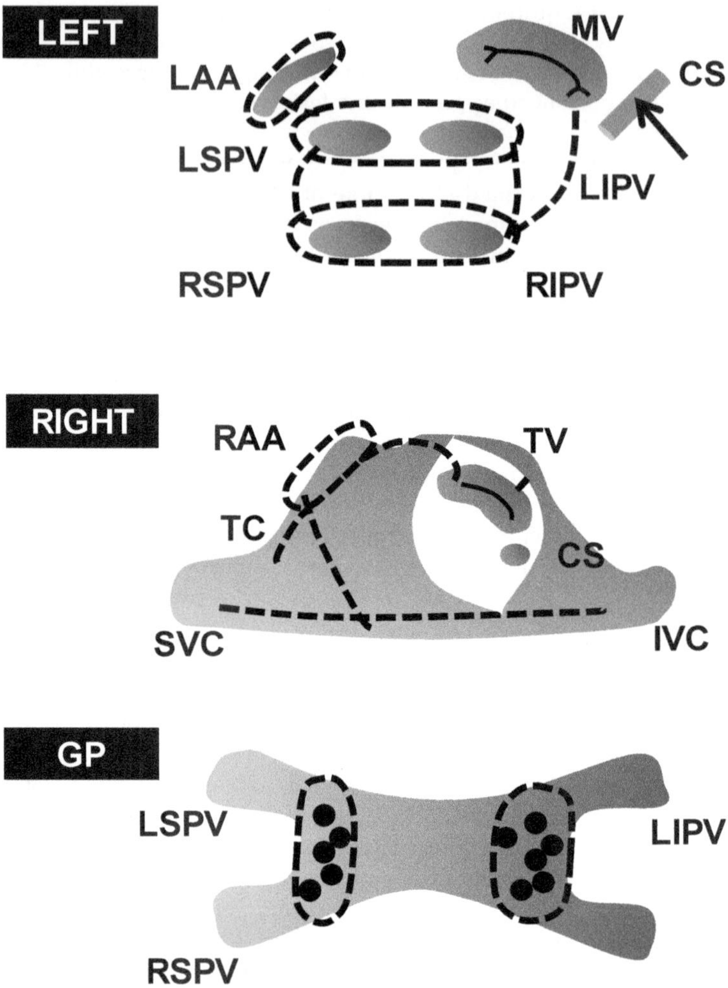

Fig. 2. Illustration of lesion sets for Cox-Maze IV and GP ablation. We illustrate left and right Maze IV lesions (dotted lines) as well as foci for GP (black circles) ablation.

There are several alternative energy sources for the Cox Maze IV at different stages of development and clinical evaluation (Table 2). The major problem with such devices is the challenge of reliably creating a transmural lesion due to loss of energy to circulating blood creating a 'heat sink'. The most commonly utilized ablation devices today are based on bipolar radiofrequency (RF) which addresses this challenge by focusing energy only in tissues between the jaws of the device, thereby eliminating surrounding blood. Radiofrequency can be delivered dry or saline-irrigated, the later may be more likely to deliver a transmural lesion by cooling the surface thereby creating a lesion of greater depth, however esophageal injury is a risk (36). With the use of any alternative energy source, it is important to use some confirmatory technique to ensure establishment of exit block.

Energy Source	Advantage	Disadvantage
High Intensity Frequency Ultrasound	Focused lesion Minimal 'heat sink'	Fixed penetration depth
Unipolar RF	May be irrigated/non-irrigated	Significant 'heat sink'
Bipolar RF	Energy focused between clamps - Minimal 'heat sink'	Costly
Microwave*		Significant 'heat sink' Inconsistent lesion
Cryoablation	Less damage to adjacent critical tissue Reusable probe	Slower Questionable transmurality
Laser*		Significant 'heat sink' Inconsistent lesion

*No longer in clinical use

Table 2. Alternative Energy Devices for Maze IV

2.1.2 Pulmonary vein isolation

The identification of AF triggers adjacent to the PVs is the rationale for PVI (7). This can be performed successfully by a sternotomy, a thoracotomy or completely thoracoscopically. A minimally-invasive procedure via bilateral minithoracotomies for paroxysmal AF is associated with 80.8% freedom from AF at 1 year (37). Thoracoscopic bilateral PVI and LAA exclusion has also been described for treatment of lone AF refractory to cathether ablation (38,39). For patients with concomitant, paroxysmal AF, PVI may be performed using a bipolar RF device to create two lesions separately encircling left and right pulmonary veins for patients undergoing MV repair or replacement, AVR or CABG.

2.1.3 Ganglion ablation

Electrophysiological studies have found that ectopic impulses originating from the autonomic ganglionic plexus (GP) in epicardial fat adjacent to the atria-PV interface to be a source of arrhythmias (7, 40). To address this, GP ablation may be performed as an adjunct to Maze procedure (Figure 2). A prospective randomized trial of 67 patients demonstrated improved freedom from AF with the addition of GP ablation to catheter-based PVI (85.3% vs 60.6% freedom from AF) at 4.3 months follow up (41). Similarly, comparison of patients of GP ablation with Maze vs. a case-matched control Maze cohort found significantly higher freedom from AF at 1 year (90% versus 50%)(42).

2.1.4 Atrial plasty

A subset of patients with AF is those with giant LA (GLA), defined as LA diameter > 65mm. This may occur as a primary defect in the LA wall or secondary to mitral valve pathology, Rheumatic or otherwise. Major complications of GLA include compression of bronchopulmonary and left ventricle, post-operative low output syndrome and respiratory complications. Furthermore, LA enlargement exacerbates macro re-entrant circuits and is a risk factor for thromboembolic disease. Left atrial size was found to be a significant predictor for stroke and death in the Framingham Heart Study (43). Furthermore, GLA (70 vs 58mm, LA diameter) was associated with failure to restore sinus rhythm following Maze procedure at the time of MV surgery (44). Several studies have demonstrated that addition of left atrial plication to mitral valve surgery improved restoration of sinus rhythm compared to mitral valve surgery alone (45, 46). However, others have shown greater than 50% recurrent arrhythmias in patients post-Cox Maze IV with LA size greater than 8cm even with a LA plasty (47).

The surgical approaches for LA plasty include excision of either inferior or inferior and superior walls as well as the autotransplant approach. An added advantage of these techniques is excellent exposure of the mitral valve to facilitate replacement or repair. The classical wall plication targets the inferior LA wall and has since been modified to a para-annular and superior approach (48). The biatrial reduction plasty when utilized with Maze IV during valvular surgery has demonstrated effective sinus restoration (49). In the combined superior-transseptal approach, the interatrial septum is opened at the fossa ovarium and extended to the inferior limbus and towards the LA appendage (50). The inferior wall can then be plicated from the LAA to the posteromedial aspect of the mitral valve using several interrupted sutures and reinforced with an over-and-over stitch. More recently, spiral resection has been proposed which extends a superior-transseptal left atriotomy in the direction of the left atrial appendage, to the inferior wall and then to the right atrial free wall (51). This approach is associated with an extensive suture line with increased bleeding risk but has the advantage of placation of the LA, RA and interatrial septum. Reef imbricate technique used as an adjunct to maze and MV surgery was associated with significant LA size reduction and sinus restoration in patients with LA enlargement and GLA, respectively (52). A 'half-moon' continuous reef imbricate sutureline suture is placed between the left and right PVs and circumferentially around the left atriotomy.

LA size reduction for GLA is associated with lower mitral valve surgical mortality, likely due to reduction in compression effects, low output syndrome, thromboembolic complications and restoration of sinus rhythm (48, 53). Whether reduction in LA size for patients with GLA undergoing mitral valve surgery in the absence of AF reduces the incidence of new onset AF is unknown. We generally do not perform reduction plasty in the absence of AF as LA size may undergo positive remodeling with relief of LA volume load.

2.2 Adverse effects

There has been no significant additive operative mortality with concomitant Maze procedures for patients undergoing coronary or valvular surgery (54). The reported risks of the Maze procedure include bleeding and blood transfusion, need for permanent pacemaker (PPM), impaired left atrial transport and rarely atrioesophageal fistula (54). Sinus node dysfunction immediately post-Maze is often reversible but if there is no recovery within 7-10 days, PPM implantation should be considered. The overall incidence of sinus node dysfunction requiring PPM is approximately 3-4%. It is unlikely that Maze lesion sets cause direct harm to the sinoatrial node and more likely that successful ablation of AF uncovers a sick sinus requiring pacing (55). Importantly, atrial transport may become impaired as scar tissue does not contribute to atrial contractility and as portions of atrial tissue may still fibrillate, depending on the location of the lesion sets.

2.3 Post-operative management

All patients should be monitored by telemetry post-operatively for the duration of hospital admission. Also, all patients, regardless of freedom from AF immediate post-operatively, should continue on oral anticoagulation until comprehensive cardiology assessment at 3 and 6 months time. It is not uncommon for patients to be in AF acutely post-operatively as atrial scar formation takes time to develop and thus success or failure of AF surgery should be assessed at follow-up clinic 3-6 mo post-operatively. If patients are in sinus rhythm at this time, as assessed by the absence of symptoms, ECG or 24 hour Holter monitor, then oral anticoagulation is discontinued. All patients require routine cardiology follow-up to monitor for AF recurrence.

3. Clinical evidence for surgical management of atrial fibrillation

3.1 Sinus restoration

Most evidence for the efficacy of Maze procedures are for concomitant AF during repair or replacement of mitral valve. Several observational studies strongly suggests that surgical intervention is beneficial for return to sinus rhythm (54,56,57). The original Maze III cohort reported by Dr. Cox's group showed 95.9% and 97.5% freedom from AF at 5.4 years performed in lone and concomitant AF, respectfully (54). In another report and perhaps more importantly, the stroke rate in this cohort was 0.1% per year over 11.5 years of follow-up (56). As the authors mention, this is likely the result of 1) sinus restoration, 2) preservation of atrial transport function and 3) removal or obliteration of the LAA. A single center trial comparing patients undergoing mitral valve replacement or repair demonstrated improved conversion to sinus rhythm with concurrent modified radiofrequency maze ablation versus medical treatment (75% vs 39%) at 1 year follow-up (57). Damiano et al (47) recently report 89% freedom success with the Maze IV at 1 year. This outcome is notable in that the results are comparable to those of the Maze III and they utilized a strict definition of success as freedom from AF, A flutter or atrial tachycardia as determined by ECG or 24h Holter monitor and disuse of arrhythmia medications. The predictors of late AF recurrence following with Maze IV were enlarged LA, failure to isolated the posterior LA and presence of early tachyarrhythmias (47). Other groups have recapitulated these results demonstrating similar conversions to sinus rhythm and lowered stroke rates.

Six randomized controlled trials (RCTs) have been performed using various Maze procedures which have all demonstrated higher sinus restoration compared with no maze. The first RCT in 2001 randomized 30 patients with concomitant AF to demonstrate sinus restoration with saline-irrigated-cooled-tip-radiofrequency ablation (SICTRA) or MV surgery alone (58). In 2003, 35 patients who underwent either MV repair with Maze III or MV repair alone (2.5:1 ratio) at one year follow-up demonstrated 92% vs 20% freedom from AF (59). In another study, sixty-seven patients randomized to either adjuvant port-access irrigated radiofrequency Maze procedure demonstrated favorable freedom from AF at 1 year (93.6% vs 9.4%)(60) compared with mitral rahe surgry alone. Another RCT demonstrated that PVI and Maze both demonstrated similar improvements in sinus restoration in patients with mitral valve disease compared with MV surgery alone (61). Yet another RCT in 70 patients with Rheumatic heart disease demonstrated an improvement in sinus restoration (79.4% vs 26.9%) with SICTRA procedure (62). The largest trial included 160 patients in India undergoing surgery for rheumatic valve disease with maze III, left maze, PV isolation or no AF surgery who experienced 62.5%, 57.5%, 67.5% and 20% return to sinus rhythm, respectively (63). Although these clinical trials are relatively small single center experiences with short-term follow up times, they demonstrate a consistent improvement in sinus rhythm restoration regardless of the underlying MV pathology and procedure used including maze III, Left Maze, Maze with alternative energy sources and PVI. Importantly, no clinical trial has yet demonstrated survival benefit with a Maze procedure. Clearly, a large multicenter RCT with long term follow up is necessary to conclusively demonstrate freedom from AF and survival benefit. Regarding survival benefit, considering that medical therapy leading to sinus restoration has not demonstrated improved survival, it may not be surprising if surgery for AF does not show this (22).

Two meta-analyses have been performed to date. The first is a meta-analysis of 69 studies, mostly retrospective, included 5885 patients with persistent, concomitant AF report that Maze III was associated with greater freedom from AF at 1-3 years and that biatrial Maze III was more effective than Left Maze III (92.0-87.1% vs 86.1-73.4% range over 1-3 years) (64). However, no significant differences were found in survival between surgical approaches compared to control groups. Forty-two percent of studies were small (<50 patients), only 19% included control populations and most data was extrapolated from Kaplan-Meier plots. The authors made no attempt to screen studies but rather to perform a comprehensive examination of the current literature. Another meta-analysis of four RCT and six retrospective studies demonstrate weak evidence in support of a reduction in stroke but an increase in need for PPM following the Maze procedure (65).

As mentioned, GLA is seen in a significant proportion of patients with AF. Several studies have demonstrated that addition of left atrial plication to mitral valve surgery improved restoration of sinus rhythm compared to mitral valve surgery alone (45, 46). Left atrial size reduction (69 to 55mm) was associated with a significant improvement in sinus restoration at 3 years compared with those that had mitral valve surgery and RF ablation alone (45). Furthermore, LA size reduction at the time of maze procedure improves outcomes. On the other hand, Choo et al (66) demonstrated similar sinus conversion rates comparing patients with GLA vs non-GLA (67.4 vs 61.1mm, LA diameter) undergoing mitral surgery and maze. Interestingly, another report from the same group found that patients under 50 had significantly better 5-year freedom from AF than those older than 50 (87.1% vs 77.3%, respectively) (67). These differences may be attributed, at least in part, to the somewhat arbitrary cut-off of GLA on the spectrum of LA enlargement.

Compared with surgical outcomes, cathether-based ablation has inferior short term outcomes and longterm results are pending. Catheter-based RF ablation may be used for paroxysmal and persistent AF with overall mid-term rates of sinus restoration of approximately 50-80% (68-70). More recently, Weerasooriya et al (71) present single center results demonstrating 5-year freedom from arrhythmia recurrence of 29% with one procedure and 63% with repeat ablation. Consistent with these clinical outcomes, Niv et al (72) demonstrated that 95% of pulmonary veins tested post-catheter ablation at the time of subsequent Maze III/IV were not electrically-isolated. We recommend that catheter ablation be best suited for younger patients with new onset (<6 months) paroxysmal lone AF. This may be combined with percutaneous device closure of LAA which has proven non-inferior to anticoagulation for stroke prevention but as mentioned, initially associated with complications including pericardial effusion, bleeding and device embolization (73-75).

There are several important considerations with respect to outcomes. When evaluating outcomes, it is important to clearly define the patient selection, choice of lesion set, energy source utilized and the use of a confirmatory technique for successful creation of a transmural lesion. Success or failure of AF surgery should be assessed following a blanking period of 3-6 months needed for scar tissue to develop. An important issue is the definition and measurement of procedural success. Early studies utilized mailed questionnaire or telephone interviews to determine if patients had symptoms or clinical events. A more accurate determination is ECG or 24-hour Holter monitor. More recently, the HRS/EHRA/ECAS consensus statement proposed a more stringent definition of success as the following: 1) freedom from AF, atrial fibrillation and atrial tachycardia lasting >30seconds and 2) off Vaughan-Williams class I and III anti-arrhythmic medications (76). Finally, much evidence has come from high-volume expert centers. It is clear that patient selection is key as is the surgical skill and knowledge of anatomy for comprehensive completion of a complete ablation set. It is unclear whether the outcomes in real-world practice at lower volume centers can mimic these results.

3.2 Areas of uncertainty

It is unclear whether patients with lone AF, should undergo percutaneous ablation or minimally invasive surgical ablation. As mentioned, the midterm outcome with catheter ablation is approximately 50-60% with repeat procedures. On the other hand, Weimar et al (77) demonstrated 90% freedom from AF and 84% freedom from AF off antiarrhythmic medication at 24 months. Even with video-assisted, thoracoscopic PVI and LAA exclusion procedure alone, Wang et al (2011) found improved freedom from AF compared to percutaneous ablation at 1-3.9 year follow up (74.7% vs. 59.0%). Yet another option which requires evaluation is off-pump, epicardial ablation for lone AF (78). Ultimately, the patient will have to balance the need for repeat intervention with catheter ablation vs. the upfront risk associated with surgery.

It remains a challenge to identify those patient subsets for which AF surgery is unlikely to be beneficial. These include patients with paper thin LA, calcified walls, cardiothoracic ratio > 70% and a LA diameter > 80 mm (79). With regards to AF characteristics, low amplitude fibrillatory waves and longstanding AF (> 6 months) are associated with poor rates of sinus restoration. In addition, although the risk associated with the Maze procedure may be low, appropriate judgment must be exercised in selecting the most appropriate patients for this procedure. In very elderly or high risk patients, the potential benefits of a successful Maze procedure are unlikely to outweigh the risks of atriotomy and a longer bypass time.

The importance of parasympathetic ganglion ablation to AF pathogenesis and whether such should be addressed is yet unclear. Ganglia plexi are located in epicardial fat pads in close proximity to the left and right PV antrum. The rationale for GP ablation is based on early basic studies which identified efferent parasympathetic and sympathetic processes in the GPs and implicated their involvement in triggering and sustaining AF (80,81). Ablation targets can be identified by vagal response to high-frequency stimulation. However, the additional benefit of adjunctive GP ablation to Maze procedure and the patient subset that is likely to benefit are not known.

The optimal energy source for maze IV is yet unclear. Cryoablation has the advantage that it enables safe creation of the isthmus lesion as use of RF poses a risk of injury to vascular structures such as circumflex coronary artery. All unipolar devices including laser, microwave, unipolar RF and HIFU are limited as blood is not excluded from the interface thereby dissipating heat, thus negatively impacting transmurality, termed the 'heat sink effect' (82). Due to inconsistency in creation of transmural lesion sets, early energy sources such as microwave and laser have largely been discontinued.

4. Guidelines

In 2010, three major guideline revisions were released by the European Society of Cardiology (ESC)(83), by a joint committee of the American College of Cardiology Foundation (ACCF)/American Heart Association (AHA)/Heart Rhythm Society (HRS) and the Canadian Cardiovascular Society (CCS). Then in 2011, focused revisions were released by the American College of Cardiology Foundation (ACCF)/American Heart Association (AHA)/Heart Rhythm Society (HRS) in their respective journals (84). The CCS published their guidelines in 2011 and here we will focus on those that pertain to surgical management (85).

By in large, the recommendations of surgical management of atrial fibrillation are comparable. Bearing in mind that the data does not demonstrate a survival benefit for adjuvant ablation, the rationale for surgery include symptom relief, prevention of thromboembolism, preservation of atrial contraction and support of ventricular function in the setting of CHF. For symptomatic AF, the guidelines suggest a class IIa indication for adjuvant surgical ablation with two exceptions: the ACCF/AHA/HRS suggest a class I indication for paroxysmal AF and the CCS suggest a class I indication for AF with mitral valve disease. The ESC gives a class IIb and CCS suggest a conditional recommendation for surgical management of lone AF.

The guidelines suggest that for patients with recurrent, paroxysmal AF who fail medical management, PV isolation or LA substrate modification may be considered. For patients with persistent AF with symptoms who fail or do not tolerate medical management, LA ablation, the maze and AV nodal ablation and pacing may be considered. AF surgery is indicated for lone AF in patients who 1) prefer surgical management, 2) failed or have a contraindication to catheter ablation or 3) failed (developed thrombus) or have a contraindication to anticoagulation.

5. Summary in points

1. The gold standard surgical treatment for AF is the complete biatrial Cox-Maze lesion set
2. The indications for atrial fibrillation surgery are the following:
   a. Recommendation for patients who i) prefer surgical management, ii) failed or have a contraindication to catheter ablation or iii) failed or have a contraindication to anticoagulation
   b. Recommendation for concomitant AF during a mitral valve procedure
   c. Conditional recommendation for lone AF
3. Randomized controlled trials have consistently demonstrated that surgery for concomitant AF offer improved sinus restoration with very low additive risk.
4. Atrial fibrillation surgery does not offer survival benefit.
5. For lone AF, catheter ablation is currently the preferred technique but minimally-invasive Maze or PVI offers improved freedom from AF with a cosmetically-acceptable incision.
6. Adjunctive procedures to a Maze are ganglia plexus ablation and left atrial plasty. The additive benefit of such still requires careful evaluation.

6. References

[1] Go AS (2001). Prevalence of diagnosed atrial fibrillation in adults: national implications for rhythm management and stroke prevention: the AnTicoagulation and Risk Factors in Atrial Fibrillation (ATRIA) Study. *JAMA*, 285,18,2370-5

[2] Kannel WB (1982). Epidemiologic features of chronic atrial fibrillation: the Framingham study. *N Engl J Med*, 306,17,1018-22.

[3] Benjamin EJ (1998). Impact of atrial fibrillation on the risk of death: the Framingham Heart Study. *Circulation*, 98,10,946-52.

[4] No authors (1996). Adjusted-dose warfarin versus low-intensity, fixed-dose warfarin plus aspirin for high-risk patients with atrial fibrillation: Stroke Prevention in Atrial Fibrillation III randomised clinical trial. *Lancet*,348,9028,633-8.

[5] Wolf PA (1991). Atrial fibrillation as an independent risk factor for stroke: the Framingham Study. *Stroke*,22,8,983-8

[6] Shemin RJ (2007). Guidelines for reporting data and outcomes for the surgical treatment of atrial fibrillation. *Ann Thorac Surg*,2007,83,3,1225-30.

[7] Haissaguerre M (1998). Spontaneous initiation of atrial fibrillation by ectopic beats originating in the pulmonary veins. *N Engl J Med*,339,10,659-66.

[8] Tsai CF (2000). Initiation of atrial fibrillation by ectopic beats originating from the superior vena cava: electrophysiological characteristics and results of radiofrequency ablation. *Circulation*,102,1,67-74.

[9] Hwang C (2000). Vein of marshall cannulation for the analysis of electrical activity in patients with focal atrial fibrillation. *Circulation*, 101,13,1503-5.

[10] Lin WS (2003). Catheter ablation of paroxysmal atrial fibrillation initiated by non-pulmonary vein ectopy. *Circulation*, 107,25,3176-83.

[11] Nademanee K (2004). A new approach for catheter ablation of atrial fibrillation: mapping of the electrophysiologic substrate. *J Am Coll Cardiol*,43,11,2044-53.

[12] Di Biase L (2010). Left atrial appendage: an underrecognized trigger site of atrial fibrillation. *Circulation*,122,2,109-18.

[13] Allissie M (2002). Electrical, contractile and structural remodeling during atrial fibrillation. *Cardiovasc Res*,54,2,230-46.

[14] Allessie MA (1999). Atrial fibrillation-induced electrical remodeling in humans: what is the next step? *Cardiovasc Res*,44,1,10-2.

[15] Tselentakis EV (2006). Inflammation effects on the electrical properties of atrial tissue and inducibility of postoperative atrial fibrillation. J Surg Res,135,1,68-75.

[16] Wyse DG (2002). A comparison of rate control and rhythm control in patients with atrial fibrillation. *N Engl J Med*,347,23,1825-33.

[17] Connolly SJ (2009). Dabigatran versus warfarin in patients with atrial fibrillation. *N Engl J Med*, 361,12,1139-51.

[18] Wilber DJ (2010). Comparison of antiarrhythmic drug therapy and radiofrequency catheter ablation in patients with paroxysmal atrial fibrillation: a randomized controlled trial. *JAMA*,303,4,333-40.

[19] Holmes DR (2009). Percutaneous closure of the left atrial appendage versus warfarin therapy for prevention of stroke in patients with atrial fibrillation: A randomised non-inferiority trial. *Lancet*,374,534-542.

[20] Block PC (2009). Percutaneous left atrial appendage occlusion for patients in atrial fibrillation suboptimal for warfarin therapy: 5-year results of the PLAATO (Percutaneous Left Atrial Appendage Transcatheter Occlusion) Study. *JACC Cardiovasc Interv*,2,594–600.

[21] Meier B (2003). Transcatheter left atrial appendage occlusion with Amplatzer devices to obviate anticoagulation in patients with atrial fibrillation. *Catheter Cardiovasc Interv*,60,417–422.

[22] Lee R (2009). Surgery for atrial fibrillation. *Nat Rev Cardiol*,6,8,505-13.

[23] Ad N (2002). The significance of atrial fibrillation ablation in patients undergoing mitral valve surgery. *Semin Thorac Cardiovasc Surg*,14,3,193-7.

[24] Cox JL (2000). Current status of the Maze procedure for the treatment of atrial fibrillation. *Semin Thorac Cardiovasc Surg*,12,1,15-9.

[25] Cox JL (2003). Atrial fibrillation II: rationale for surgical treatment. *J Thorac Cardiovasc Surg*,126,6,1693-9.

[26] Cui YQ (2008). Intraoperative modified Cox mini-maze procedure for long-standing persistent atrial fibrillation. *Ann Thorac Surg*,85,4,1283-9.

[27] Tuinenburg AE (2000). Mini-maze suffices as adjunct to mitral valve surgery in patients with preoperative atrial fibrillation. *J Cardiovasc Electrophysiol*,11,9,960-7.

[28] Cox JL (1991). The surgical treatment of atrial fibrillation. III. Development of a definitive surgical procedure. *J Thorac Cardiovasc Surg*,101,4,569-83.
[29] Cox JL (1995). Modification of the maze procedure for atrial flutter and atrial fibrillation. I. Rationale and surgical results. *J Thorac* Cardiovasc Surg,110,2,473-84.
[30] Gillinov MA (2005). The Maze procedure in mitral valve disease: predictors of recurrent atrial fibrillation. J Thorac Cardiovasc Surg,130,6,1653-60.
[31] Cox JL (1995). Modification of the maze procedure for atrial flutter and atrial fibrillation. II. Surgical technique of the maze III procedure. *J Thorac Cardiovasc Surg*,110,2,485-95.
[32] Usui A (2002). Repetitive atrial flutter as a complication of the left-sided simple maze procedure. *Ann Thorac Surg*,73,5,1457-9.
[33] Gaynor SL (2004). A prospective, single-center clinical trial of a modified Maze procedure with bipolar radiofrequency ablation. *J Thorac Cardiovasc Surg*,128,4,535-42.
[34] Shen J (2009).The surgical treatment of atrial fibrillation. Heart Rhythm,6,8,S45-50.
[35] Voeller RK (2008). Isolating the entire posterior left atrium improves surgical outcomes after the Maze procedure. J Thorac Cardiovasc Surg,135,4,870-7.
[36] Gillinov AM (2001). Esophageal injury during radiofrequency ablation for atrial fibrillation. *J Thorac Cardiovasc Surg*,122,6,1239-40.
[37] Edgerton JR (2010). Pulmonary vein isolation and autonomic denervation for the management of paroxysmal atrial fibrillation by a minimally invasive surgical approach. *J Thorac Cardiovasc Surg*,140,4,823-8.
[38] Yilmaz A (2010). Completely thoracoscopic pulmonary vein isolation with ganglionic plexus ablation and left atrial appendage amputation for treatment of atrial fibrillation. *Eur J Cardiothorac Surg*,38,3,356-60.
[39] Yilmaz A (2008). Completely thoracoscopic bilateral pulmonary vein isolation and left atrial appendage exclusion for atrial fibrillation. *J Thorac Cardiovasc Surg*,136,2,521-2.
[40] Schauerte P (2001). Focal atrial fibrillation: experimental evidence for a pathophysiologic role of the autonomic nervous system. *J Cardiovasc Electrophysiol*,12,5,592-9.
[41] Katritsis DG (2011). Rapid Pulmonary Vein Isolation Combined with Autonomic Ganglia Modification: A Randomized Study. *Heart Rhythm*,8,5,672-8.
[42] Ware AL (2011). Left atrial ganglion ablation as an adjunct to atrial fibrillation surgery in valvular heart disease. *Ann Thorac Surg*,91,1,97-102.
[43] Benjamin EJ (1995). Left atrial size and the risk of stroke and death. The Framingham Heart Study. *Circulation*,92,4,835-41.
[44] Kosakai Y (1994). Maze procedure for chronic atrial fibrillation associated with mitral valve disease. *J Thorac Cardiovasc Surg*,108,6,1049-54.
[45] Scherer M (2007). Impact of left atrial size reduction and endocardial radiofrequency ablation on continuous atrial fibrillation in patients undergoing concomitant cardiac surgery: three-year results. *J Heart Valve Dis*,16,2,126-31.
[46] Scherer M (2003). Impact of left atrial size reduction on chronic atrial fibrillation in mitral valve surgery. *J Heart Valve Dis*,12,4,469-74.
[47] Damiano RJ Jr (2011). The Maze IV procedure: predictors of late recurrence. J Thorac Cardiovasc Surg,141,1,113-21.
[48] Kawazoe K (1983). Surgical treatment of giant left atrium combined with mitral valvular disease. Plication procedure for reduction of compression to the left ventricle, bronchus, and pulmonary parenchyma. *J Thorac Cardiovasc Surg*,85,6,885-92.

[49] Romano MA (2004). Atrial reduction plasty Maze procedure: extended indications for atrial fibrillation surgery. *Ann Thorac Surg*,77,4,1282-7.

[50] Yuasa S (2003). Surgical treatment of giant left atrium using a combined superior-transseptal approach. *Ann Thorac Surg*,75,6,1985-6.

[51] Sugiki H (2006). Novel technique for volume reduction of giant left atrium: simple and effective "spiral resection" method. *Ann Thorac Surg*,81,1,378-80.

[52] Wang W (2011). Left atrial wall tension directly affects the restoration of sinus rhythm after Maze procedure. Eur J Cardiothorac Surg,40,1,77-82.

[53] Piccoli GP (1984). Giant left atrium and mitral valve disease: early and late results of surgical treatment in 40 cases. *J Cardiovasc Surg (Torino)*,25,4,328-36.

[54] Prasad SM (2003). The Maze III procedure for atrial fibrillation: long-term efficacy in patients undergoing lone versus concomitant procedures. *J Thorac Cardiovasc Surg*,126,6,1822-8.

[55] Barnett SD (2006). Surgical ablation as treatment for the elimination of atrial fibrillation: a meta-analysis. *J Thorac Cardiovasc Surg*,131,5,1029-35.

[56] Cox JL (1999). Impact of the maze procedure on the stroke rate in patients with atrial fibrillation. *J Thorac Cardiovasc Surg*,118,5,833-40

[57] von Oppell UO (2009). Mitral valve surgery plus concomitant atrial fibrillation ablation is superior to mitral valve surgery alone with an intensive rhythm control strategy. *Eur J Cardiothorac Surg*,35,4,641-50.

[58] Khargi K (2001). Saline-irrigated, cooled-tip radiofrequency ablation is an effective technique to perform the maze procedure. *Ann Thorac Surg*,72,3,S1090-5.

[59] Cappato R (2005). Worldwide survey on the methods, efficacy, and safety of catheter ablation for human atrial fibrillation. *Circulation*,111,9,1100-5.

[60] Akpinar B (2003). Combined radiofrequency modified maze and mitral valve procedure through a port access approach: early and mid-term results. *Eur J Cardiothorac Surg*,24,2,223-30.

[61] de Lima GG (2004). Randomized study of surgery for patients with permanent atrial fibrillation as a result of mitral valve disease. *Ann Thorac Surg*,77,6,2089-94.

[62] Abreu Filho CA (2005). Effectiveness of the maze procedure using cooled-tip radiofrequency ablation in patients with permanent atrial fibrillation and rheumatic mitral valve disease. *Circulation*,112,9,I20-5.

[63] Srivastava V (2008). Efficacy of three different ablative procedures to treat atrial fibrillation in patients with valvular heart disease: a randomised trial. *Heart Lung Circ*,17,3,232-40.

[64] Barnett SD (2006). Surgical ablation as treatment for the elimination of atrial fibrillation: a meta-analysis. *J Thorac Cardiovasc Surg*,131,5,1029-35.

[65] Reston JT (2005). Meta-analysis of clinical outcomes of maze-related surgical procedures for medically refractory atrial fibrillation. *Eur J Cardiothorac Surg*,28,5,724-30.

[66] Choo SJ (2004). Excellent results for atrial fibrillation surgery in the presence of giant left atrium and mitral valve disease. *Eur J Cardiothorac Surg*,26,2,336-41.

[67] Lee SH (2011). The influence of age on atrial fibrillation recurrence after the maze procedure in patients with giant left atrium. *J Thorac Cardiovasc Surg*,141,4,1015-9.

[68] Pappone C, Rosanio S, Oreto G, Tocchi M, Gugliotta F, Vicedomini G, et al. Circumferential radiofrequency ablation of pulmonary vein ostia: A new anatomic approach for curing atrial fibrillation. Circulation 2000 Nov 21;102(21):2619-28.

[69] Jais P, Cauchemez B, Macle L, Daoud E, Khairy P, Subbiah R, et al. Catheter ablation versus antiarrhythmic drugs for atrial fibrillation: the A4 study. Circulation 2008 Dec 9;118(24):2498-505.

[70] Ouyang F (2010). Long-term results of catheter ablation in paroxysmal atrial fibrillation: lessons from a 5-year follow-up. *Circulation*,122,23,2368-77.
[71] Weerasooriya R (2011). Catheter ablation for atrial fibrillation: are results maintained at 5 years of follow-up? J Am Coll Cardiol,57,2,160-6.
[72] Ad N (2011). The outcome of the Maze procedure in patients with previous percutaneous catheter ablation to treat atrial fibrillation. Ann Thorac Surg,91,5,1371-7.
[73] Sick PB (2007). Initial worldwide experience with the WATCHMAN left atrial appendage system for stroke prevention in atrial fibrillation. *J Am Coll Cardiol*,49,13,1490-5.
[74] Reddy VY (2011). Safety of Percutaneous Left Atrial Appendage Closure: Results From the Watchman Left Atrial Appendage System for Embolic Protection in Patients With AF (PROTECT AF) Clinical Trial and the Continued Access Registry. *Circulation*,123,4,417-24.
[75] Holmes DR (2009). Percutaneous closure of the left atrial appendage versus warfarin therapy for prevention of stroke in patients with atrial fibrillation: a randomised non-inferiority trial. *Lancet*,374,9689,534-42.
[76] European Heart Rhythm Association (EHRA) (2007). HRS/EHRA/ECAS expert Consensus Statement on catheter and surgical ablation of atrial fibrillation: recommendations for personnel, policy, procedures and follow-up. A report of the Heart Rhythm Society (HRS) Task Force on catheter and surgical ablation of atrial fibrillation. *Heart Rhythm*,4,6,816-61.
[77] Weimar T (2011). The Maze IV procedure for lone atrial fibrillation: a single center experience in 100 consecutive patients. J Interv Card Electrophysiol,31,1,47-54.
[78] Mitnovetski S (2009). Epicardial high-intensity focused ultrasound cardiac ablation for surgical treatment of atrial fibrillation. Heart Lung Circ,18,1,28-31.
[79] Isobe F (1998). The outcome and indications of the Maze III procedure for chronic atrial fibrillation with mitral valve disease. *J Thorac Cardiovasc Surg*,116,2,220-7.
[80] Scherlag BJ (2005). Electrical stimulation to identify neural elements on the heart: their role in atrial fibrillation. J Interv Card Electrophysiol,13,Suppl 1,37-42.
[81] Schauerte P (2001). Focal atrial fibrillation: Experimental evidence for a pathophysiological role of the autonomic nervous system. *J Cardiovasc Electrophysiol*,12,592–599.
[82] Gaynor SL (2006). Microwave ablation for atrial fibrillation: dose-response curves in the cardioplegia-arrested and beating heart. Ann Thorac Surg,81,1,72-6.
[83] European Heart Rhythm Association (2010). Guidelines for the management of atrial fibrillation: the Task Force for the Management of Atrial Fibrillation of the European Society of Cardiology (ESC). *Eur Heart J*,31,19,2369-429.
[84] Fuster V (2011). 2011 ACCF/AHA/HRS focused updates incorporated into the ACC/AHA/ESC 2006 Guidelines for the management of patients with atrial fibrillation: a report of the American College of Cardiology Foundation/American Heart Association Task Force on Practice Guidelines developed in partnership with the European Society of Cardiology and in collaboration with the European Heart Rhythm Association and the Heart Rhythm Society. *J Am Coll Cardiol*,57,11,e101-98.
[85] Pagé P (2011). Canadian Cardiovascular Society atrial fibrillation guidelines 2010: surgical therapy. *Can J Cardiol*,27,1,67-73.

14

Ganglionated Plexi Ablation for Atrial Fibrillation

Yong Zhang, Mei Gao, Jiangrong Wang and Yinglong Hou
Department of Cardiology, Qianfoshan Hospital of Shandong University, Jinan City, China

1. Introduction

With an estimated prevalence of 0.4%~1% in the general population, atrial fibrillation (AF) is the most common cardiac arrhythmia encountered in clinical practice [1]. As an emerging technology, catheter ablation is becoming more and more important in the treatment of AF at present. In a sense, catheter ablation is more superior to the antiarrhythmic drug and surgery treatment, but this technology remains a challenge, because long-term success rate is low, most patients require repeat procedure and there is no established ablation method.

The importance of the autonomic nervous system (ANS) in the initiation of AF has been proved in the early 1990s [2-4], and the ganglionated plexi (GP), found in epicardial fat pads, was subsequently shown to play a role in initiation and maintenance of AF [5, 6]. Studies have shown that chemical or electric stimulation of GP can initiate rapid firing from the pulmonary vein (PV) or PV-atrial junction, which is similar to the focal firing observed in patients with AF [7-9]. Moreover, several studies indicate that ablation of the major atrial GP can suppress the inducibility and maintenance of AF [9].

Therefore the GP ablation has received more and more attentions nowadays, and it promises to be a more superior ablation technology of AF. However, the long-term success rate of GP ablation is quite variable (40%~90%, approximately), and the reasons remain under investigate.

2. Cardiac ANS and its effects on the initiation and maintenance of AF

The cardiac ANS can be divided into the extrinsic and intrinsic components. The extrinsic cardiac ANS consists of the soma in brain nuclei and chains of ganglia along the spinal cord and the axons that course en route to the heart. The intrinsic cardiac ANS is composed of a neural network formed by axons and autonomic ganglia concentrated at the GP embedded within epicardial fat pads on the heart itself and the ligament of Marshall (LOM) [10]. There are four main GPs on the atrium of mammalian hearts [11]: the anterior right GP (ARGP) at the right superior PV (RSPV)-atrial junction; the inferior right GP (IRGP) at the junction of inferior vein cava and both atria; the superior left GP (SLGP) near the left superior PV (LSPV)-atrial junction and left pulmonary artery, and inferior left GP (ILGP) at the left inferior PV (LIPV)-atrial junction (see Figure 1 and 2).

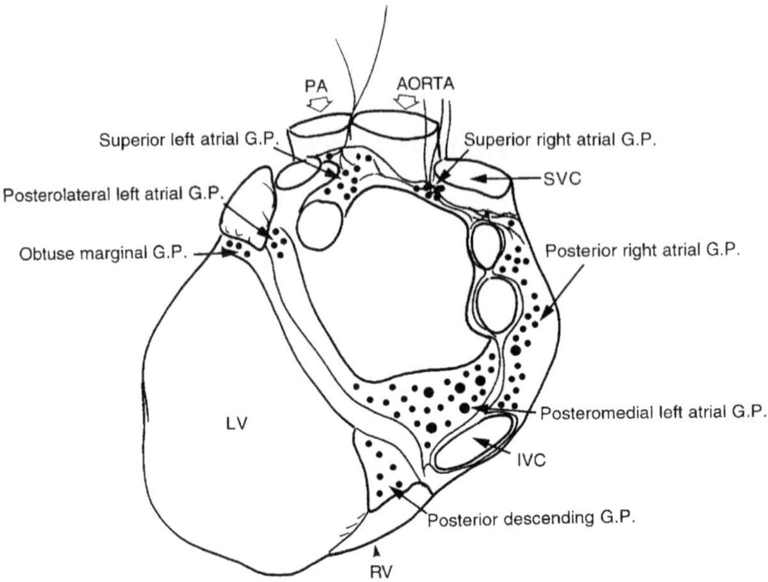

Fig. 1. Drawing of a posterior view of the human heart and major vessels illustrating the locations of posterior atrial and ventricular GP. Note the mediastinal nerves coursing adjacent to the aortic root and joining the two superior atrial GP. SVC = superior vena cava, IVC = inferior vena cava, RV = right ventricle, LV = left ventricle. (Armour JA, et al. Anat Rec 1997; 247(2): 289-98)

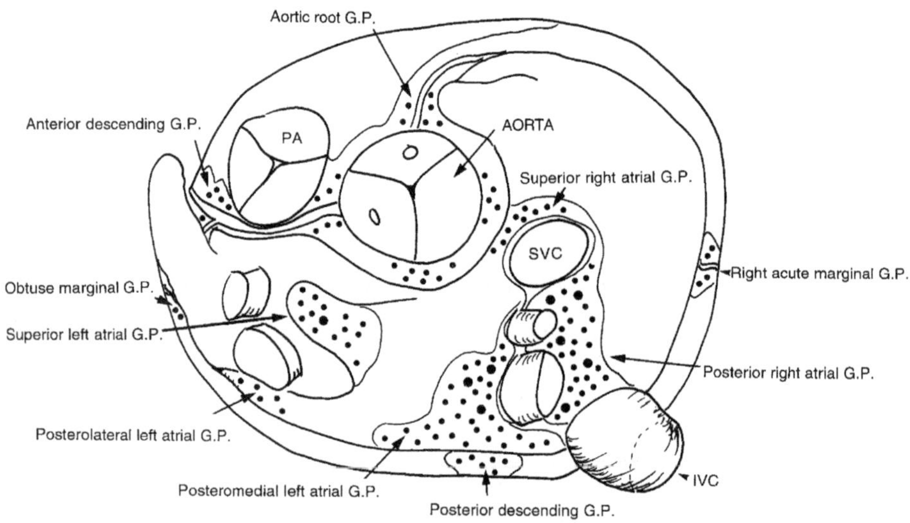

Fig. 2. Drawing of a superior view of the human heart illustrating the distribution of ganglionated plexuses on the surface of the atria and ventricles. For abbreviations, see Figure 1. (Armour JA, et al. Anat Rec 1997; 247(2): 289-98)

In 1947, Scherf [12] found that AF could be induced by application of aconitine to the atrium in the experimental condition. He proposed that a focal firing source could initiate AF. Moe et al. [13] in 1964, using a computer model, hypothesized that AF could exist as a stable mechanism independent of the triggering event. They assumed that this self-sustaining mechanism could be described as multiple wavelets in randomly rotating circuits within the atrial confines. In 1985, Allessie et al. [14] on the basis of an elegant mapping technique, found that at any given time at least three to six self-perpetuating wavelets could be found wandering over the surface of the atrium during AF. The focal mechanism resurfaced, based on Haissaguerre's discovery [15] that rapidly firing foci within the PV could induced AF in 1998, and since then, research on the genetic, trigger, electrophysiology, structure and adjustment of the initiation and maintenance of AF has witnessed considerable breakthrough.
In recent years, with the continuous development of our knowledge, more and more profound researches on the relationship between ANS and AF have been conducted. Moreover, some researchers even studied the difference between the effects of vagus and sympathetic nerves on the initiation of AF. In 2000, Schauerte et al. [16] found that radiofrequency ablation of parasympathetic nerve fibers along right pulmonary artery, inferior or superior vena cava blunted the atrial effective refractory period (AERP) shortening caused by vagal stimulation (VS), and abolished the increase covariance of AERP caused by VS, and led to an increase of the baseline AERP. Before the ablation, VS could induce and maintain AF; while after the ablation, it could not induce AF any more. Further study [5] carried out by this team in 2001 found that high-frequency stimulation (HFS) on pulmonary and superior vena cava could lead to the initiation of atrial premature depolarization, atrial tachycardia (AT) and AF. More importantly, in this study, blockers of autonomic nerves receptor were used to intervene, which were found to blunt or abolish the response of atrial to HFS. Later, more attention was turned to myocardial sleeves of PV. A study [17] in 2005 found that HFS on PV myocardial sleeves could shorten the action potential duration (APD) of myocardial sleeve cells and trigger AF, and this phenomenon could be blocked by atropine and atenolol, which indicated that the rapid discharge of myocardial sleeves of PV was the result of combined action of sympathetic and parasympathetic neurotransmitters. In 2007, the effects of the VS or isoproterenol on the PV tachycardias, which were created by burst pacing from a PV or the application of aconitine onto the PV, were evaluated [18]. The result indicated that VS effects affecting the PVT and atrium facilitate the onset and maintenance of PV-triggered AF, but not isoproterenol. In another study [19], complete atrioventricular block (AVB) was produced by radiofrequency current in 17 dogs. After 8 weeks, the atrial dimensions and the percentage of fibrosis in the atrium were observed significantly greater. However, atrial and PV effective refractory periods were shorter, and atrial conduction velocity increased during sympathetic stimulation, but not during VS, which indicated that contrary to the normal atrium, sympathetic stimulation was crucial for the genesis of AF in the remodeled atrium.
As previously mentioned, the intrinsic cardiac ANS is composed of a neural network formed by axons and autonomic ganglia concentrated at GP. Therefore, GP is certainly quite important during the research of ANS, and there are several studies involving the relationship between GP and AF. According to the study performed by Scherlag et al [7], the HFS at the base of RSPV provide a substrate for the conversion of PV firing into AF, and the more intense the HFS, the easier the conversion became. Study [8] in 2006 pointed out that the injection of acetylcholine and carbachol, two parasympathomimetic agents, into the GP of RSPV could result in autonomic or easily-triggered AF and rapid discharge could be

detected in the PV and atrium near the injected position. Thus, it suggested that the high excitation of GP might be the important link in the transformation from the trigger of PV into AF. In 2009, Lu et al. [9] exerted HFS on atrium and PV in the refractory period of the cardiac muscles of dogs to trigger AF, and GP ablation was conducted to observe its effect. The results showed that HFS could initiate rapid discharge by activating cardiac autonomic nerve network. The GP on both sides could facilitate the initiation of rapid discharge or the trigger of AF by HFS on the same side or the opposite side. What's more, it could increase the trigger threshold of AF through GP ablation, or even prevent AF. A large number of studies have confirmed that GP played an important role in the initiation and maintenance of AF. The advancement of these studies promotes GP ablation to become a therapy, thus providing the theoretical basis for the clinical application of GP ablation.

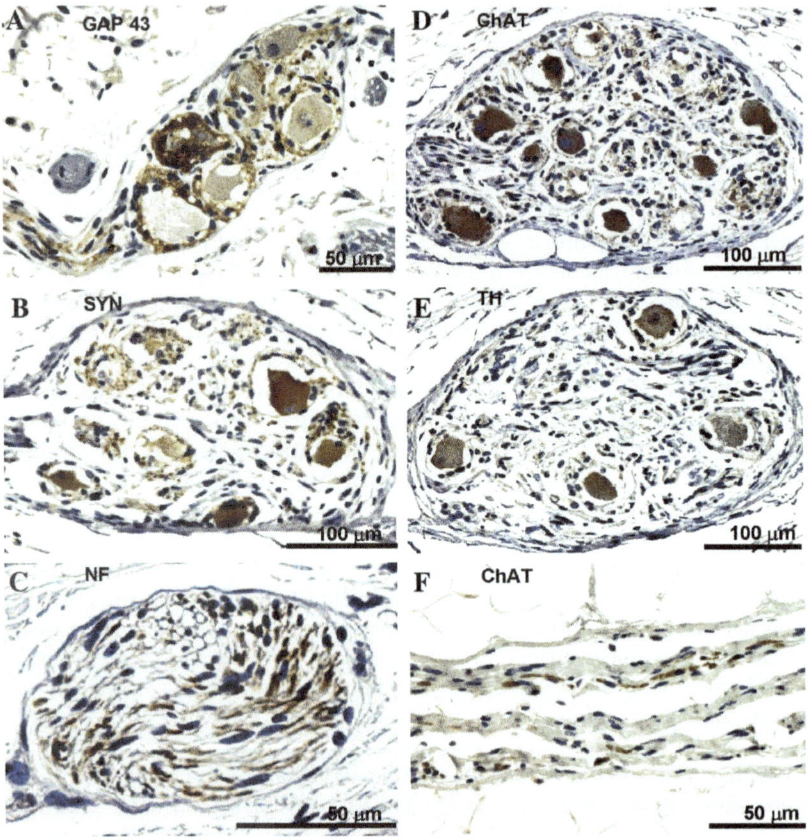

Fig. 3. Examples of immunohistochemical staining results in cardiac ganglia and nerves. (A) Growth-associated protein 43 (GAP 43) demonstrating axonal growth within the ganglion; (B) synaptophysin (SYN) staining demonstrating synaptic endings; (C) neurofilament (NF) staining confirming the presence of nerve fibers; (D) choline acetyltransferase (ChAT) staining showing cholinergic nature of most ganglion cells; (E) tyrosine hydroxylase (TH) staining showing co-localization of adrenergic cells within the same ganglion; and (F) ChAT positivity of nerve adjacent to ganglion. (Tan AY, et al. J Am Coll Cardiol. 2006; 48(1): 132-43)

With the deepening of the functional research, further anatomic studies of ANS have been performed, which have revealed the anatomic basis of the important role of cardiac ANS in the initiation and maintenance of AF. In 2005, Chevalier et al. [20] conducted 43 autopsies and found that there was a high intensity of innervation at the junction of PV and left atrium, and they found the nerve density was significantly higher at the ostia of the PVs than in their distal part, and there were gradients of innervation from right to left and from the front to the rear of the atrium. This study attempted to provide some clinical implications for radiofrequency ablation of AF. In 2006, Tan et al. [21] conducted further research on the heart obtained from the autopsy, which revealed that at the junction of PV and the left atrium, there were a great deal of discontinuous muscles and abrupt fiber orientation changes. And starting from this junction, within a range of 5mm in the left atrium, the density of autonomic nerves reaches its highest, with the coexistence of adrenergic and cholinergic nerves (see Figure 3). The anterior superior walls of two superior PV had a relatively higher density of nerves; the inferior walls of two inferior PV had a higher density of nerves (see Figure 4); the density of nerves of epicardium was higher than that of endocardium.

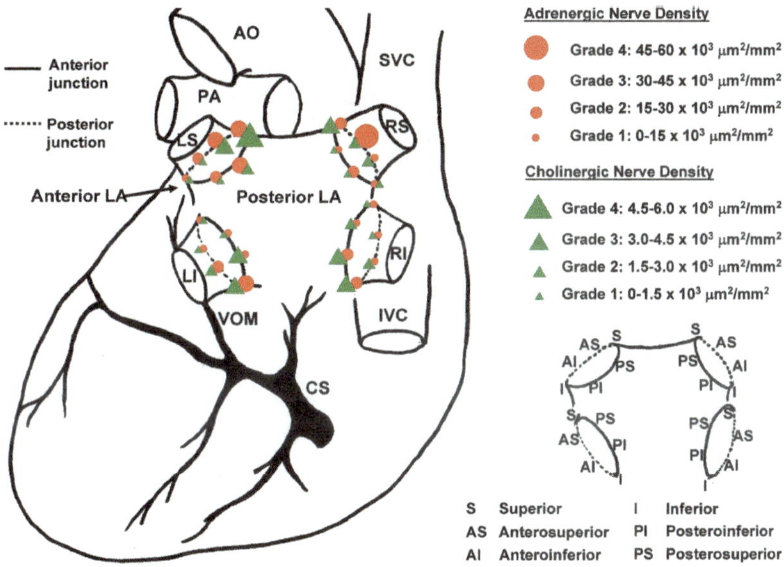

Fig. 4. Circumferential distribution of autonomic nerves at the PV-left atrium junction. AO = aorta; CS = coronary sinus; LA = left atrium; LI = left inferior PV; LS = left superior PV; PA = pulmonary artery; RI = right inferior PV; RS = right superior PV; VOM = vein of marshall, other abbreviations, see Figure 1. (Tan AY, et al. J Am Coll Cardiol. 2006; 48(1): 132-43)

3. GP ablation for AF

Either the adrenergic or vagal arm of the ANS may be involved in atrial electrical instability. Vagal activation shortens AERP and increases their dispersion, and adrenergic stimulation enhances atrial myocardial automaticity. Coumel [3] who studied patients with paroxysmal AF and the relationship between this arrhythmia and ANS, was the first to identify two different clinical patterns: vagal and adrenergic AF. In 2008, a research [22] was conducted in Europe including 1517 patients with paroxysmal AF. In this study, AF was divided into sympathetic, vagal and mixed type in terms of the trigger mode. Observations revealed that the three types of AF constituted 15%, 6% and 12% of the total respectively, suggesting that the cause of AF in at least one third of the patients might have associated with ANS (see Figure 5).

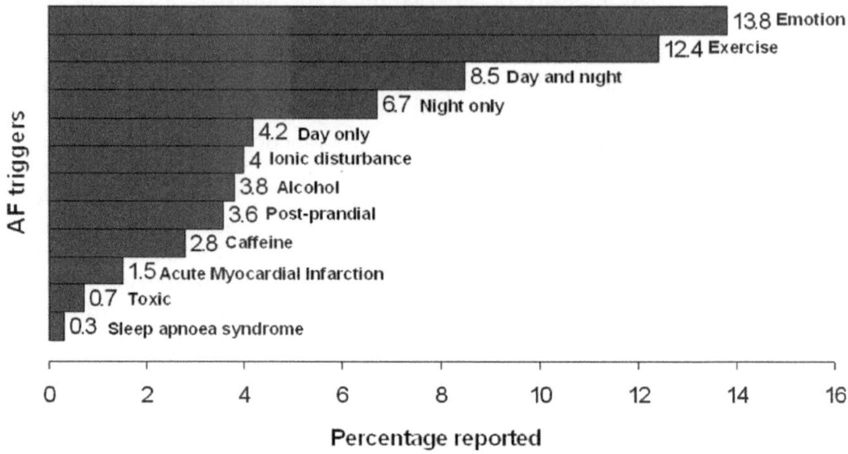

Fig. 5. Percentages of triggers reported in patients with paroxysmal atrial fibrillation in the Euro Heart Survey. (de Vos CB, et al. Eur Heart J. 2008; 29(5): 632-9)

As described above, profound researches have been conducted on the role of cardiac ANS in the initiation and maintenance of AF. In recent years, clinical studies based on these theories have been carried out. Besides traditional radiofrequency ablation therapy of AF (such as circumferential PV ablation and PV isolation), an additional, even independent GP ablation therapy has been attempted with certain curative effect. In this chapter, a brief introduction would be presented on the clinical studies concerning GP ablation recently.

According to the method of localization of GP, there are two different ablation manners: selective ablation of GP identified by HFS and extensive regional ablation targeting the anatomic areas of GP. Each GP contains both parasympathetic and sympathetic neural elements; stimulation of the former typically elicits an immediate response (within 2~4 seconds), while stimulation of the latter induces a delayed response (8~10 seconds). It is the rationale of localization of GP by HFS [23]. Therefore, HFS is usually delivered at each site for only 2~5 seconds, and the sites of positive parasympathetic responses are considered the GP sites. The predominant efferent parasympathetic responses include bradycardia, hypotension and high grade AVB (or obvious increase in mean R-R interval during AF).

In 2004, Pappone et al. [24] conducted radiofrequency ablation for patients with AF. Thirty four percent of 297 patients reported an apparent vagal response such as bradycardia at the high energy radiofrequency current at some sites in the left atrium when receiving circumferential PV ablation. Continuous ablation on these sites could make vagal response disappear. At a mean follow-up of 12 months 99% of the patients who had reported a vagal response suffered from no reoccurrence of AF; while the percentage for those who had not reported vagal response was only 74%. These sites might be the corresponding area of endocardium to GP of epicardium, and in fact, radiofrequency ablation was conducted on GP of epicardium via endocardium, suggesting that GP ablation based on circumferential PV ablation might help to increase the success rate.

In 2004, Platt et al. [25] reported a research involving 26 AF patients receiving only GP ablation without PV isolation. The clinical results were that immediate success rate of the operation was 88% (23/26). For patients who had positive vagal response, GP ablation was performed, and the immediate success rate was 96% (22/23); in the 22 cases of immediate success, 14 needed to take antiarrhythmic drugs which had no effect before the operation and 8 didn't need any drug to maintain sinus rhythm. Follow-up averaging 6 months showed that 85% (22/26) of the patients still maintained sinus rhythm, which indicated GP ablation alone could also obtain a satisfactory effect.

In 2005, Scherlag et al. [26] reported the results of ablation for 60 AF patients. Twenty seven received standard PV isolation and 33 received standard PV isolation + GP ablation. For the standard group, follow-up averaging 12 months showed the non-reoccurrence rate was 71% (19/27); while follow-up averaging 5 months of the group with additional GP ablation indicated a rate of 91% (30/33). Therefore, it was suggested that GP ablation could help to increase the success rate of PV isolation for AF.

In 2006, Lemery et al. [27] localized GP by endocardial HFS. GP ablation was conducted on 14 patients with paroxysmal and persistent AF. The result showed the success rate was only 50%.

In 2006, Scanavacca et al. [28] conducted GP mapping and ablation applying endocardial and epicardial HFS. The results revealed that 7 out of 10 cases showed vagal response; 3 cases failed to show the vagal response but accepted circumferential PV ablation. During the mean follow-up of 8.3 months, 2 out of 7 cases after GP ablation were free from symptoms without taking antiarrhythmic agents; 4 cases underwent circumferential PV ablation for frequent recurrence of AF; and 1 case suffered from slight AF without using antiarrhythmic agents.

In 2008, Pokushalov et al. [29] reported the results of the conduction of GP ablation alone in 58 patients with AF. This concurrently eliminated AF in 94% of cases in the process of the ablation and vagal response was shown in 93% of cases. There were not any arrhythmia episodes in 86% of patients over the mean follow-up of 7.2 months, with no need to take any antiarrhythmic agents.

In 2008, Danik et al. [30] reported the results of GP ablation in 18 cases suspected of vagal AF. After elimination of all vagal response sites from endocardium, 17 cases still suffered from HFS-induced AF. The researchers believed in that GP ablation could not prevent the immediate induction of AF.

In 2008, Katritsis et al. [31] also conducted GP ablation in 19 cases of paroxysmal AF by means of anatomically based GP ablation, and compared the results with 19 cases of age, gender-matched patients with conventional circumferential PV ablation. The results showed that in the process of ablation, vagal response occurred only in 4 cases, and during the mean follow-up of 1 year, the recurrent rate of arrhythmia was 74% and 37% in GP ablation group and circumferential PV ablation group, respectively. Among them, 2 patients suffered from atrial flutter besides the recurrence of AF, suggesting that anatomically-based GP ablation might be inferior to circumferential PV ablation.

In 2009, Pokushalov et al. [32] compared the results of the selective GP ablation identified by applying HFS with those of the anatomically based regional GP ablation in 80 cases (40 cases in each group) of paroxysmal AF. Ablation targets of selective GP were the vagal response sites evoked by HFS. The end point of the procedure was marked by the failure to evoke vagal responses by HFS. Regional GP ablation was defined as the more extensive ablation conducted at the anatomic sites of GP for anatomical damage. During the mean follow-up of 13.1 months, no symptomatic paroxysmal AF occurred in 42.5% and 77.5% of the cases in the two groups, respectively, indicating that the anatomic ablation might improve the success rate of AF ablation.

In 2009, Han et al. [33] reported the results of applying thoroscopic pulmanory vein isolation + GP ablation + Marshal liganents ablation + left auriculectomy therapy in 45 cases (33 cases of paroxysmal AF and 12 cases of persistent AF). The results showed that, during the mean follow-up of 1 year, 65% of the patients did not suffer from atrial tachyarrhythmias that lasted for more than 30 seconds; in most of the cases where atrial tachyarrhythmias reoccurred, another ablation procedure or application of antiarrhythmic agents were effective.

In 2009, Po et al. [23] also reported the therapeutic results of 83 cases of AF after GP ablation and PV isolation. Patients who did not suffer from AF or AT after the single procedure of ablation accounted for 80% during the mean follow-up of 1 year and 86% during the mean follow-up of 22 months. The researchers held that the benefits of GP ablation based on PV isolation increased with time, especially 12 months after ablation, and suggested that this later benefits might be due to the irreversible damage of the autonomic neuron in GP.

In 2010, Pokushalov research group [34] also reported the results of anatomic GP ablation therapy in 89 cases of chronic AF, of which 29 needed additional circumferential PV isolation and 5 cases needed circumferential PV isolation once more. The follow-up averaged 2 years. The maintenance rate of sinus rhythm without medications following the single procedure of anatomic GP ablation was 38.2%.

And in the same year, Pokushalov research group [35] reported the results of the ablation of left atrial GPs in 56 patients with paroxysmal AF. Seventy one percent of the patients (40/56) did not suffer from the recurrence of arrhythmia over the mean follow-up of 12 months, suggesting that local ablation applying to the left atrial GPs might become an alternative therapy for paroxysmal AF.

In 2010, Mikhaylov et al. [36] reported the long-term follow-up results of a group undergoing GP ablation. The case control study included 70 cases of paroxysmal AF, of which 35 cases underwent GP ablation and 35 circumferential PV ablation. The incidence of arrhythmia over the mean follow-up of 36.3 months was 34.3% in GP ablation group and 65.7% in circumferential PV ablation group, respectively, suggesting that the long-term therapeutic effect of GP ablation was not as good as that of circumferential PV ablation.

In 2011, Krul et al. [37] reported the curative effect of thoracoscopic PV isolation + GP ablation in 21 cases of AF. Eighty six percent (19/21) of the patients were free of the reoccurrence of AF, atrial flutter, and AT over the mean follow-up of 1 year, without the use of antiarrhythmic agents.

In 2011, Katritsis et al. [38] reported a randomized controlled trial between a group with PV isolation alone and the group with PV isolation + GP ablation. It was found during the mean follow-up of 1 month that 60.6% (20/33) of the patients in the PV isolation group and 85.3% (29/34) of patients in the PV isolation +GP ablation group were free of arrhthymia, respectively, suggesting that adding GP ablation to PV isolation might help improve the efficacy of ablation.

Thus, studies on GP ablation in the treatment of AF are increasing year by year. In addition, the types of researches are shifting from retrospective ones to randomized controlled trials, initiating an in-depth exploration of the safety of GP ablation, such as the canine model by Cui et al [39], which observed whether GP ablation produced acute effect on the functions of sinoatrial node and atrioventricular node.

It has been found that, in the process of AF ablation, GP ablation, whether single or additional, direct or indirect, is effective to certain extent. It has also been found that there exist significant curative differences among GP ablation therapies, the reason of which will be discussed in the next section. GP ablation in the treatment of AF is now in its initial stage, lacking large-scale clinical researches and the number of randomized controlled trials is very small. However, related works are now being carried out. Several issues are yet to be addressed, such as whether GP ablation is beneficial at all, which type of patients with AF is more suitable for GP ablation, which method is more acceptable in terms of GP localization, etc. We believe that, in near future, GP ablation will be better understood through large number of randomized controlled trials as well as meta-analysis.

4. Possible reasons for the variable long-term success rate of GP ablation

As stated above, the efficacies of GP ablation differs significantly, for which there are many possible reasons, including the clinical features of the cases selected, methods to apply ablation, localization for GP sites, the extent of denervation, criteria to judge success, time and index for follow-up, and the performer's experiences, etc. Among them, localization of GP sites has attracted more attention. Most of the existing studies target GP by HFS-induced vagal responses, however, either GP mapping through endocardium or epicardium cannot result in ideal success rate. It is assumed that the sites where vagal responses occur are not necessarily the anatomic GP sites.

Chen et al. [40] believed that HFS mapping primarily revealed the sites of ANS afferent nerves, because only stimulation of the afferent nerves could explain the vagal responses such as reflex bradycardia and vasodilatation. Therefore, the sites presented by vagal responses were not necessarily consistent with those of GP and efferent nerves (see Figure 6). Moreover, according to the "octopus theory" hypothesized by Po et al. [41] explaining from another point of view, there existed within the atrium a highly integrated neural network and neurotransmitters would be secreted after GP activation, further causing AF. And the activation of axons would excite GP reversely and also cause neurotransmitter release, inducing AF. Similar in shape to octopus, activation of GP (octopus's head) might trigger neurotransmitter release, inducing AF, while axons (octopus's cirrus), when stimulated, might activate GP (octopus's head) reversely and cause neurotransmitter release, thus also triggering AF (see Figure 7).

Therefore, many studies have come up with reasonable explanations regarding the differences between positive vagal response sites and actual anatomic GP sites. Just as mentioned above, some studies [32, 34] have applied radiofrequency ablation on anatomic GP sites and obtained satisfactory effect. However, even with the same anatomically based GP mapping, the above mentioned research results by Katritsis et al. [31] are disappointing.

For this, we also did a series of research. In our first study [42], with vagosympathetic trunk stimulation, sinus rate, and ventricular rate during AF were compared before and after sequential ablation of SLGP, ARGP, and IRGP in dogs, and in our second study [43], sinus rate, AH interval during atrial pacing, and ventricular rate during AF were compared before and after GP stimulation and after their ablation. We found that GP is the "integration center" not only between extrinsic and intrinsic cardiac ANS (see Figure 8), but also within the intrinsic cardiac ANS (see Figure 9), and the integration is substantially more complicated than previously thought, which may lead the variable long-term success rate of GP ablation. Moreover, in the second study, we also optimized the GP ablation strategy. As described above, one or more of the GP may serve as the "integration center" in the complex neural network, so a carefully designed ablation strategy targeting the "integration center" would have substantial impact on the outcome of AF ablation. If the "integration center" was ablated before HFS is applied to other GP, stimulation may fail to induce ventricular rate slowing during AF and subsequently decreases the ability to localize the GP. Therefore the "integration center" needs to be ablated after other clinically relevant GP have been localized in order to achieve sufficient attenuation of the intrinsic cardiac ANS. For instance, the IRGP should not be ablated until the SLGP has been localized. Based on this postulation, Po et al. [23] stimulated and ablated the GP in 83 cases of AF in the following order: (1) SLGP, (2) ILGP, (3) ARGP, and (4) IRGP, and obtained satisfactory success rate.

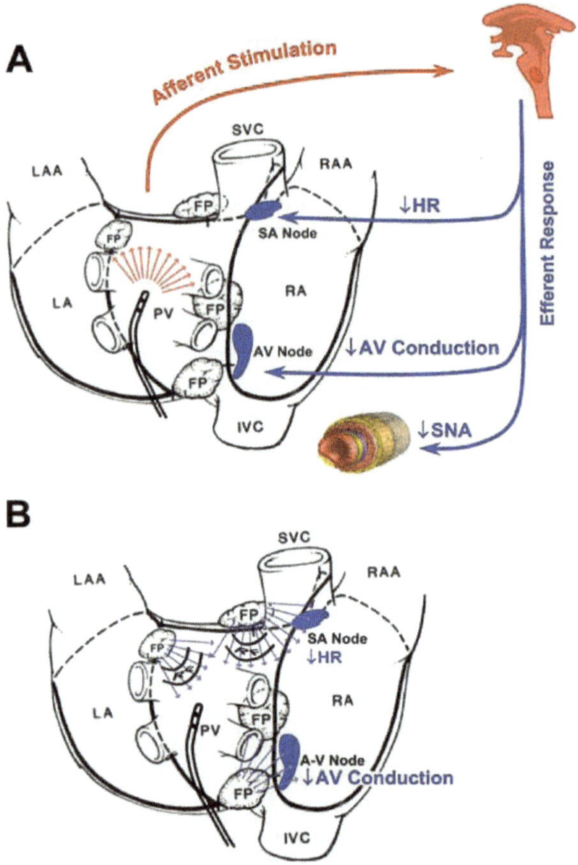

Fig. 6. Illustration of the possible mechanisms of denervation associated with RF ablation. Posterior view of the heart. (A) RF ablation applied at the pulmonary vein ostia stimulating vagal afferent nerve fibers, inducing reflex bradycardia, atrioventricular block, and decreased efferent sympathetic nerve activity leading to hypotension. Repeated RF ablation at these sites could result in damage to the afferent limb of the reflex. (B) RF ablation applied at the pulmonary vein ostia stimulating postganglionic efferent parasympathetic fibers. Repeated RF ablation at these sites could potentially damage efferent postganglionic parasympathetic fibers. RA = right atrium; LAA = left atrial appendage; RAA = right atrial appendage; FP = fat pad, other abbreviations, see Figure 1 and 4. (Chen J, et al. PACE. 2006; 29(4): 413-21)

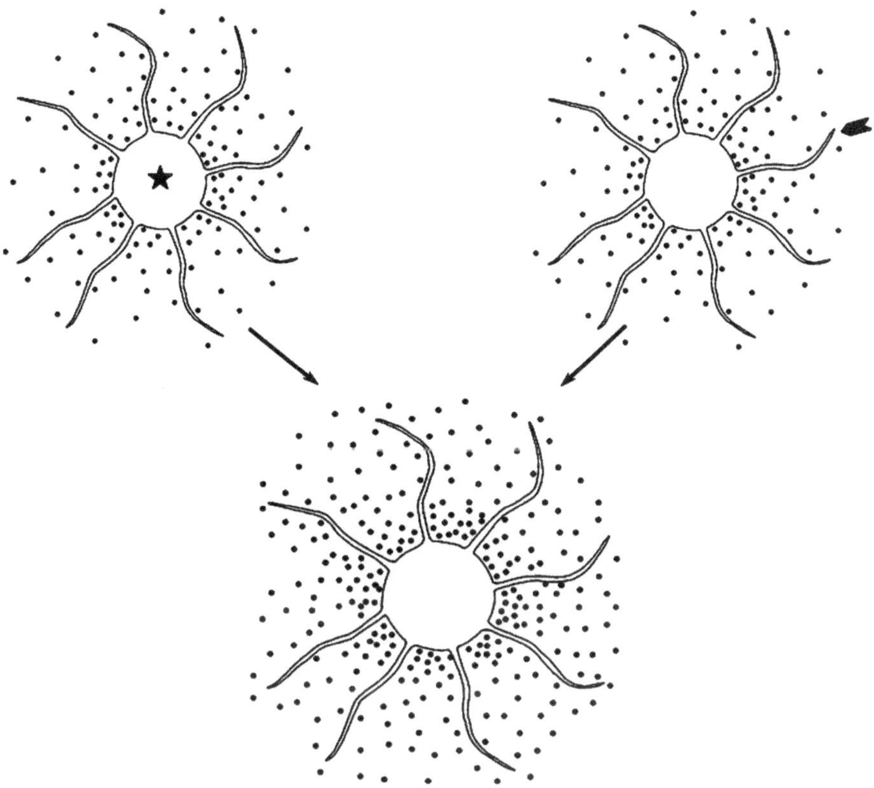

Fig. 7. The "Octopus" hypothesis. A hyperactive state of the GP (head of octopus, left upper panel) may trigger local release of a gradient of excessive amounts of neurotransmitters and subsequently initiate AF (lower panel). When the axons (tentacles) are excited (right upper panel), the GP can be retrogradely activated and elicit a similar response. Star: a hyperactive of the GP. Arrowhead: axons are excited. Black dots: local release of neurotransmitters. (Zhou J, et al. J Cardiovasc Electrophysiol. 2007; 18(1): 83-90)

Recently, Po's research group [44] has continued their study, trying to make a breakthrough in traditional GP mapping methods. They blocked GP by means of superparamagnetic nanoparticles (MNPs) carrying neurotoxicity drug N-isopropylacrylamide monomer (NIPA-M), and achieved satisfactory results. The agent was found to be potentially targeting to IRGP. It does open a new train of thought, though research in this field has just begun.

Apart from the localization of GP, many researches with respect to mechanism in the curative differences in GP ablation therapy have been conducted. Studies by Zhao et al. [45] revealed that local increases occurred to the concentration levels of TNF-α and iterleukin-6 after GP ablation might be considered as a factor that increases the vulnerability to AF. This also provides us with a new train of thought. There are many issued, such as whether there is any other high expression of inflammatory factors besides TNF-α and iterleukin-6 in local GP ablation and whether these inflammatory factors can be blocked by certain means and therefore improving the effectiveness of GP ablation, remain to be addressed.

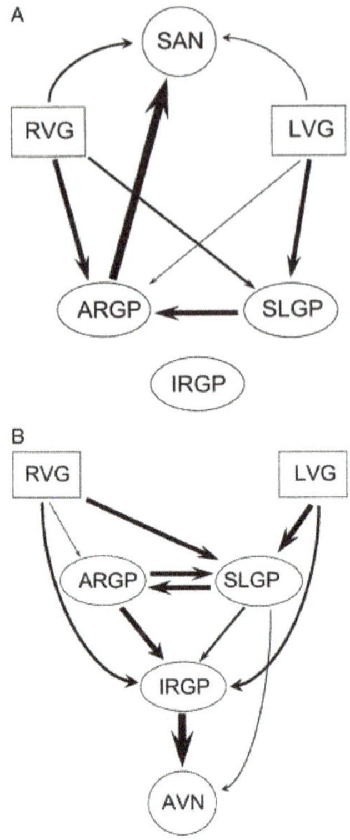

Fig. 8. Interactions among vagosympathetic trunks, ARGP, IRGP, and SLGP on SAN and AVN function (A) Modulation of sinus rate by vagosympathetic stimulation. (B) Modulation of ventricular rate during atrial fibrillation by vagosympathetic stimulation. Thick lines and thin lines indicate strong and weak regulatory effects, respectively. ARGP = anterior right GP, IRGP = inferior right GP, SLGP = superior left GP, AVN = atrioventricular node; LVG = left vagosympathetic trunk; RVG = right vagosympathetic trunk; SAN = sinoatrial node. (Yinglong Hou, et al. J Am Coll Cardiol, 2007; 50(1): 61–8).

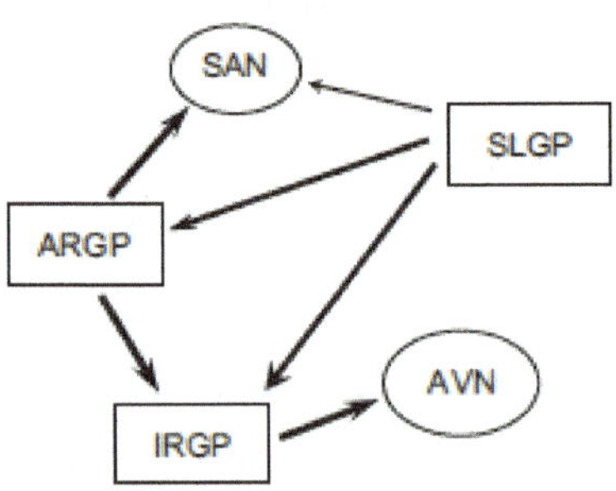

Fig. 9. Summary of the interactions among ARGP, IRGP, and SLGP on SAN and AVN function. Thick lines and thin lines indicate strong and weak regulatory effects, respectively. The abbreviations, see Figure 8 (Yinglong Hou, et al. Heart Rhythm, 2007; 4(1): 56–63).

5. Regeneration of nerve tissues after GP ablation

Regeneration of nerve tissues after ablation may be associated with long-term curative effect of GP ablation. However, scientists' opinions diverge on the existence of regeneration.

In 2006, studies by Oh et al. [46] revealed that responsiveness to VS by both sinoatrial and atrioventricular nodes as well as the inductivity of AF had declined significantly immediately after radiofrequency ablation of dog fat pads, yet inductivity returned to pre-ablation levels 4 weeks after ablation, suggesting that fat pad ablation did not have the long-term preventive effect on AF.

In 2007, Verma et al. [47] studied 20 cases of patients who accepted PV isolation once more for recurrent AF. The mean interval between two ablations was 4 months. No vagal response was observed after this ablation, suggesting that there was no more regeneration of GP tissues.

In 2009, Po et al. [23] reported 83 cases of patients who received GP ablation and single PV ablation. The incidence of post-procedure non-AF or non-AT were 80% during 1-year follow-up and 86% during 22-month follow-up, suggesting that the benefits of GP ablation based on PV ablation increased with time, especially 12 months after ablation, with no regeneration of ablated GP.

In 2010, Sakamoto et al. [48] divided 18 dogs into three groups, to perform GP ablation, GP ablation + PV isolation, and GP ablation + left atrial posterior wall isolation, respectively. The results showed that GP ablation could significantly reduce vagal innervation, while vagal response restored 4 weeks after the procedure, suggesting that there might be early regeneration of atrial nerve tissues.

In 2010, Zhao et al. [49] put forward the concept of post-GP ablation autonomic nerve reconstruction. They randomized, in their studies, 13 dogs into GP ablation group and sham-operated group, performing ARGP ablation and IRGP ablation, respectively. The results showed that it was extremely easy to induce AF 8 weeks after GP ablation and that growth-associated protein 43-positive, tyrosine hydroxylase-positive, and choline acetyltransferase-positive nerve densities in the right atrium in GP ablation group were significantly lower than those of the sham-operated group. The researchers held that the reconstruction of the atrial autonomic nerves might be the mechanism of the AF reoccurrence after GP ablation. The study also revealed that unilateral GP ablation might lead to imbalanced nerve reconstruction and therefore the reoccurrence of AF.

The information above revealed that it is still an unsolved issue whether nerves regenerate after GP ablation. There have been no sufficient evidence so far to demonstrate that ANS regeneration is directly associated with the recurrence of AF. However, if the nerves regeneration really exists, are there some certain substances, such as the inflammatory factors mentioned above, contributing to nerve regeneration after GP ablation? And can these substances be suppressed in some ways to further improve the efficacy of GP ablation? These issues leave much space for research.

6. References

[1] Go A, Hylek E, Phillips K, et al. Prevalence of diagnosed atrial fibrillation in adults: national implications for rhythm management and stroke prevention: the AnTicoagulation and Risk Factors in Atrial Fibrillation (ATRIA) Study. JAMA. 2001; 285(18): 2370-5.

[2] Coumel P. Cardiac arrhythmias and the autonomic nervous system. J Cardiovasc Electrophysiol. 1993; 4(3): 338-55.
[3] Coumel P. Paroxsysmal atrial fibrilation: a disorder of autonomic tone? Eur Heart J. 1994; 15 Suppl A: 9-16.
[4] Coumel P. Autonomic influence in atrial tachyarrhythmias. J Cardiovasc Electrophysiol. 1996; 7(10): 999-1007.
[5] Schauerte P, Scherlag BJ, Patterson E, Scherlag MA, Matsudaria K, Nakagawa H, et al. Focal atrial fibrillation: experimental evidence for a pathophysiological role of the autonomic nervous system. J Cardiovasc Electrophysiol. 2001; 12(5): 592-9.
[6] Scherlag BJ, Po S. The intrinsic cardiac nervous system and atrial fibrillation. Curr Opin Cardiol. 2006; 21(1): 51-4.
[7] Scherlag BJ, Yamanashi WS, Patel U, et al. Autonomically induced conversion of pulmonary vein focal firing into atrial fibrillation. J Am Coll Cardiol. 2005; 45(11): 1878–86.
[8] Po SS, Li Y, Scherlag BJ, et al. Experimental model for paroxysmal atrial fibrillation arising at the pulmonary vein-atrial junctions. Heart Rhythm. 2006; 3(2): 201-8.
[9] Lu Z, Scherlag BJ, Lin J, et al. Autonomic mechanism for initiation of rapid firing from atria and pulmonary veins: evidence by ablation of ganglionated plexi. Cardiovasc Res. 2009; 84(2): 245-52.
[10] Ardell JL: Structure and function of mammalian intrinsic cardiac neurons. In: Armour JA and Ardell JL, eds. Neurocardiology. Oxford Univ. Press: New York, 1994, pp. 95-114.
[11] Armour JA, Murphy DA, Yuan B-X, et al. Gross andmicroscopic anatomy of the human intrinsic cardiac nervous system. Anat Rec 1997; 247(2): 289-98.
[12] Scherf D. Studies on auricular tachycardia caused by aconitine administration. Proc Soc Exp Biol Med. 1947; 64(2): 233-9.
[13] Moe GK, Rheinboldt WC, Abieldskov JA. A computer model of atrial fibrillation. Am Heart J. 1964; 67: 200-20.
[14] Allessie M, Lammers WJEP, Bonke FIM, et al. Experimental evaluation of Moe's multiple wavelet hypothesis of atrial fibrillation. In: Zipes DP, Jalife J, editors. Cardiac Electrophysiology and Arrhythmias. New York, NY: Grune and Stratton, 1985; 265-75.
[15] Haissaguerre M, Jais P, Shah DC, et al. Spontaneous initiation of atrial fibrillation by ectopic beats originating in the pulmonary veins. N Engl J Med. 1998; 339(10): 659-66.
[16] Schauerte P, Scherlag BJ, Pitha J, et al. Catheter ablation of cardiac autonomic nerves for prevention of vagal atrial fibrillation. Circulation. 2000; 102(22): 2774-80.
[17] Patterson E, Po S, Scherlag BJ, et al. Triggered firing in pulmonary veins initiated by in vitro autonomic nerve stimulation. Heart Rhythm. 2005; 2(6): 624-31.
[18] Horikawa-Tanami T, Hirao K, Furukawa T, et al. Mechanism of the conversion of a pulmonary vein tachycardia to atrial fibrillation in normal canine hearts: role of autonomic nerve stimulation.J Cardiovasc Electrophysiol. 2007; 18(5): 534-41.
[19] Furukawa T, Hirao K, Horikawa-Tanami T, et al. Influence of autonomic stimulation on the genesis of atrial fibrillation in remodeled canine atria not the same as in normal atria. Circ J. 2009; 73(3): 468-75.
[20] Chevalier P, Tabib A, Meyronnet D, et al. Quantitative study of nerves of the human left atrium. Heart Rhythm. 2005; 2(5): 518-22.

[21] Tan AY, Li H, Wachsmann-Hogiu S, et al. Autonomic innervation and segmental muscular disconnections at the human pulmonary vein-atrial junction: implications for catheter ablation of atrial-pulmonary vein junction. J Am Coll Cardiol. 2006; 48(1): 132-43.
[22] de Vos CB, Nieuwlaat R, Crijns HJ, et al. Autonomic trigger patterns and anti-arrhythmic treatment of paroxysmal atrial fibrillation: data from the Euro Heart Survey. Eur Heart J. 2008; 29(5): 632-9.
[23] Po SS, Nakagawa H, Jackman WM. Localization of left atrial ganglionated plexi in patients with atrial fibrillation. J Cardiovasc Electrophysiol. 2009;20(10):1186-9.
[24] Pappone C, SantinelliV, Manguso F, et al. Pulmonary vein denervation enhances long-term benefit after circumferential ablation for paroxysmal atrial fibrillation. Circulation. 2004, 109(3): 327-34.
[25] Platt M, Mandapati R, Scherlag BJ, et al. Limiting the number and extent of radiofrequency applications to terminate atrial fibrillation and subsequently prevent its inducibility [abstract]. Heart Rhythm 2004; 1: IS–II.
[26] Scherlag BJ, Nakagawa H, Jackman WM, et al. Electrical stimulation to identify neural elements on the heart: their role in atrial fibrillation. J Interv Card Electrophysiol. 2005; 13 Suppl 1:37-42.
[27] Lemery R, Birnie D, Tang A, et al. Feasibility study of endocardial mapping of ganglionated plexuses during catheter ablation of atrial fibrillation. Heart Rhythm 2006; 3(4): 387-96.
[28] Scanavacca M, Pisani CF, Hachul D,et al. Selective atrial vagal denervation guided by evoked vagal reflex to treat patients with paroxysmal atrial fibrillation.Circulation. 2006; 114(9): 876-85.
[29] Pokushalov E, Turov A, Shugayev P, et al. Catheter ablation of left atrial ganglionated plexi for atrial fibrillation. Asian Cardiovasc Thorac Ann. 2008; 16(3): 194-201.
[30] Danik S, Neuzil P, d'Avila A, et al. Evaluation of catheter ablation of periatrial ganglionic plexi in patients with atrial fibrillation. Am J Cardiol. 2008; 102(5): 578-83.
[31] Katritsis D, Giazitzoglou E, Sougiannis D, et al. Anatomic approach for ganglionic plexi ablation in patients with paroxysmal atrial fibrillation. Am J Cardiol. 2008; 102(3): 330-4.
[32] Pokushalov E, Romanov A, Shugayev P, et al. Selective ganglionated plexi ablation for paroxysmal atrial fibrillation. Heart Rhythm. 2009; 6(9): 1257-64.
[33] Han FT, Kasirajan V, Kowalski M, et al. Results of a minimally invasive surgical pulmonary vein isolation and ganglionic plexi ablation for atrial fibrillation: single-center experience with 12-month follow-up. Circ Arrhythm Electrophysiol. 2009; 2(4): 370-7.
[34] Pokushalov E, Romanov A, Artyomenko S, et al. Ganglionated plexi ablation for longstanding persistent atrial fibrillation. Europace. 2010; 12(3): 342-6.
[35] Pokushalov E, Romanov A, Artyomenko S, et al. Left atrial ablation at the anatomic areas of ganglionated plexi for paroxysmal atrial fibrillation. Pacing Clin Electrophysiol. 2010; 33(10): 1231-8.
[36] Mikhaylov E, Kanidieva A, Sviridova N, et al. Outcome of anatomic ganglionated plexi ablation to treat paroxysmal atrial fibrillation a 3-year follow-up study. Europace. 2011; 13(3): 362-70.

[37] Krul SP, Driessen AH, van Boven WJ, et al. Thoracoscopic video-assisted pulmonary vein antrum isolation, ganglionated plexus ablation, and periprocedural confirmation of ablation lesions. Circ Arrhythm Electrophysiol. 2011; 4(3): 262-70.
[38] Katritsis DG, Giazitzoglou E, Zografos T, et al. Rapid pulmonary vein isolation combined with autonomic ganglia modification a randomized study. Heart Rhythm. 2011; 8(5): 672-8.
[39] Cui B, Lu Z, He B, et al. Acute effects of ganglionated plexi ablation on sinoatrial nodal and atrioventricular nodal functions. Auton Neurosci. 2011; 161(1-2): 87-94.
[40] Chen J, Wasmund S, Hamdan M, et al. Back to the future: the role of the autonomic nervous system in atrial fibrillation. PACE. 2006; 29(4): 413-21.
[41] Zhou J, Scherlag B, Ewards J, et al. Gradients of atrial refractoriness and inducibility of atrial fibrillation due to stimulation of ganglionated plexi. J Cardiovasc Electrophysiol. 2007; 18(1): 83-90.
[42] Yinglong Hou, Benjamin J Scherlag, Jiaxiong Lin, et al. Ganglionated Plexi Modulatextrinsic Cardiac Autonomic Nerve Input. J Am Coll Cardiol, 2007; 50(1): 61–8.
[43] Yinglong Hou, Benjamin J Scherlag, Jiaxiong Lin, et al. Interactive atrial neural network: Determining the connections between ganglionated plexi. Heart Rhythm, 2007; 4(1): 56–63.
[44] Yu L, Scherlag BJ, Dormer K, et al. Autonomic denervation with magnetic nanoparticles. Circulation. 2010; 122(25): 2653-9.
[45] Zhao Q, Zhang S, Huang H, et al. Inflammation abnormalities and inducibility of atrial fibrillation after epicardial ganglionated plexi ablation. Arch Cardiovasc Dis. 2011; 104(4): 227-33.
[46] Oh S, Zhang Y, Bibevski S, et al. Vagal denervation and atrial fibrillation inducibility: epicardial fat pad ablation does not have long-term effects. Heart Rhythm 2006; 3(6):701–708.
[47] Verma A, Saliba WI, Lakkireddy D, et al. Vagal responses induced by endocardial left atrial autonomic ganglion stimulation before and after pulmonary vein antrum isolation for atrial fibrillation. Heart Rhythm. 2007; 4(9): 1177-82.
[48] Sakamoto S, Schuessler RB, Lee AM, et al. Vagal denervation and reinnervation after ablation of ganglionated plexi. J Thorac Cardiovasc Surg. 2010; 139(2): 444-52.
[49] Zhao QY, Huang H, Zhang SD, et al. Atrial autonomic innervation remodelling and atrial fibrillation inducibility after epicardial ganglionic plexi ablation. Europace. 2010; 12(6): 805-10.

15

Non- Isolation Treatment of Atrial Fibrillation: Does Autonomic Nerve Modulation Really Act?

Hong-Tao Wang et al.,*
Tangdu Hospital, Fourth Military Medical University, Xi' an, China

1. Introduction

Atrial fibrillation (AF) is an abnormal heart rhythm that originates in the top chambers of the heart (atria). Pulmonary vein (PV) ablation is an effective treatment for AF, which has been used widely in clinic; however, significant side effects are difficult to avoid including potential recurrence, pulmonary vein stenosis, systemic thromboembolism, pericardial effusion, cardiac tamponade, esophageal perforation, and phrenic nerve paralysis.

These limitations suggest that PV isolation is not a majority determinant of clinical success and promote research toward the development of less aggressive, but equally effective, procedures. First, researchers focus on some non-anti-arrhythmic drug therapy. There is accumulating evidence in support of the anti-arrhythmic effects of non-anti-arrhythmic drugs. Treatments with angiotensin-converting enzyme inhibitors, angiotensin-receptor blockers, statins, and omega-3 fatty acids all seem promising, over and above any effect related to the treatment of underlying heart disease. Despite exciting results from animal experiments and promising outcomes from retrospective analyses, there is no robust evidence of specific effects of these drugs to transform current clinical practice (Ardell et al., 2001). Therefore, autonomic nerve modulation has recently become a new strategy for AF management.

This chapter aims to study the relationship between ANS and AF; and to investigate the effect of autonomic nerve modulation on AF.

2. The relationship between ANS and the atrial fibrillation

2.1 Innervation of ANS to the heart

The cardiac ANS contains two main components: the extrinsic and intrinsic ANS. The extrinsic ANS is defined as the nerves coming from the brain and thoracic paravertebral ganglia, consisting mainly of ganglia and their axons located outside the heart.

The extrinsic ANS is composed of the sympathetic system and the parasympathetic system. The cardiac sympathetic ganglia include a superior cervical ganglion, which communicates with C1-3, and the cervicothoracic (stellate) ganglion, which communicates with C7-8–T1-2. In addition, the thoracic ganglia (as low as the seventh thoracic ganglion) contribute to sympathetic innervation of the heart. The superior, middle, and inferior cardiac nerves from

---

* Qiang-Sun Zheng, Xiong-Tao Liu, Jun Li, Fu-Jun Shang, Fei-Fei Su, Bo-yuan Fan and Dong-Bo Ou
The first 3 authors contributed equally to this work.

these ganglia innervate the heart by following a simple course along the brachiocephalic trunk, common carotid and subclavian arteries. On the other hand, the thoracic cardiac nerves in the posterior mediastinum must follow a complex course to reach the heart in the middle mediastinum. Parasympathetic innervation comes from the vagus and is divided into superior, middle, and inferior branches. Although both sides of the autonomic branches run through the ventral and dorsal aspects of the aortic arch, the right autonomic cardiac nerves tend to follow a ventral course. The main vagal trunk then continues along the esophagus to reach the gut.

The intrinsic ANS is composed mainly of ganglionated plexi (GP) and their axons situated on the heart itself or along the great vessels in the thorax (Scherlag et al., 2006). These GPs usually are embedded in the fat pads located on the epicardium. Prior studies showed multiple GPs located on the atria of mammalian hearts, including the anterior right GP located at the caudal end of the sinoatrial (SA) node, the inferior right GP situated at the junction of inferior vein cava and both atria, and the superior left GP located adjacent to the base of the left superior pulmonary vein between the left atrial appendage and the left pulmonary artery (another appellation is right pulmonary artery ganglionated plexi; RPA GP, because this GP is also adjacent to the right pulmonary artery). The anterior right GP is also referred to as the right superior pulmonary vein fat pad or SA fat pad because of its close proximity to the right superior pulmonary vein and SA node; the inferior right GP is sometimes called the AV node fat pad because of its role in modulating the AV conduction; and the superior left GP is often referred to as the left superior pulmonary vein fat pad because of its close proximity to the left superior pulmonary vein (Hou, et al., 2007). However, the specific intrinsic autonomic efferent pathway to the atrium and PVs remains unknown when reaches to the region of superior vena cava (SVC). This area is adjacent to the aortic root, contains the SLGP, the surrounding fat tissues and some dispersed GPs.

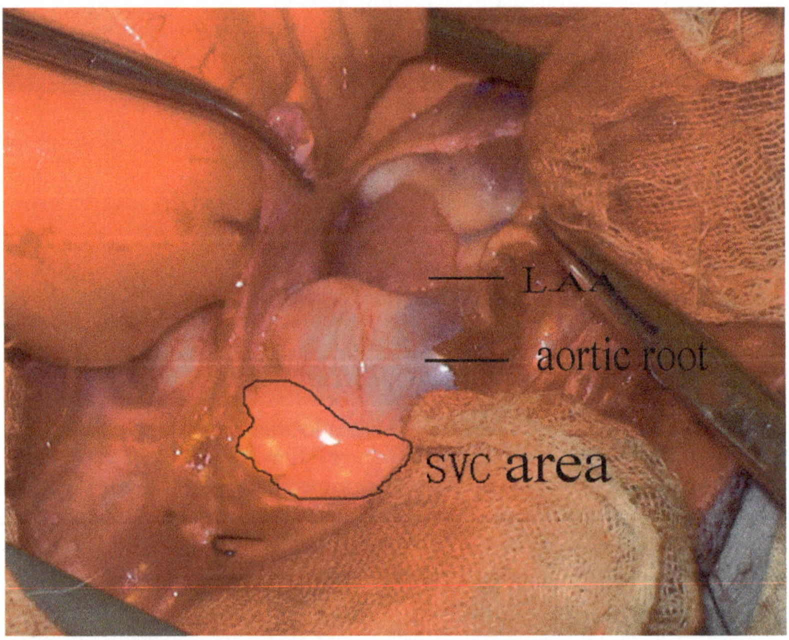

Fig. 1. Location of the SVC area.

Illustration: The SVC area is adjacent to the aortic root, contains superior vena cava and aortic root ganglionated plexi, surrounding fat tissues and some dispersed GPs.

3. The function of the SVC area

3.1 Identifying the neuron cell type of the SVC area

Hearts were excised from the mongrel dogs, and a cannula was infused into the aorta ascendent. This procedure was followed by perfusion with 250 ml physiologic saline to clean the hearts. The SVC area was isolated from the aortic root, perfused and fixed with 1 L 4% formalin, and stored in 30% sucrose overnight after an additional post-fixation for 4 h in 4% formalin. The tissues were cut into three parts and embedded in OCT. Tissues were cut into 20-mm sections at -25 °C with a cryostat.

The SVC area was cut into 3 parts, and Nissl's staining was used to determine the location of the GPs. The results reveal that neurons mix with fat cells, are widely distributed in the GPs, and are present in small clusters of 3 to 15 cells with most embedded in the right part of SVC area (Figure 2).

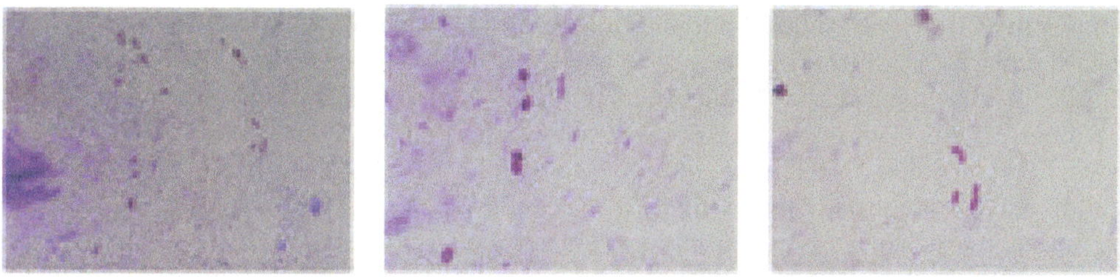

Fig. 2. Location of the ganglionated plexuses in SVC area.

Illustration: Nissl's staining was performed to reveal the distribution of ganglionated plexuses (GPs). Figure 2A (1×20 eye lens) shows that GPs are widely distributed in the SVC area and are surrounded by many fat cells. Figures 2B and 2C (1×40 eye lens) show that GPs are present in small clusters of 7 and 5 cells, respectively.

The study by Chiou et al (Chiou et al., 1997) showed that the SVC FP receives most vagal nerves to both atriums. Chiou et al. claimed that stimulation of this FP shortened ERP of atriums, prolonged spontaneous cycle length, and induced AV block. Catheter ablation of this FP could vagally denervate the atrium. This GP located in the right side of the aortic root, and did not include the surrounding fat tissues. Therefore, the right part was more likely to be the location of SVC-Ao FP. There were also GPs in the middle and left part of the aortic root. These GPs and the surrounding fat tissues were also important components of the SVC area that could not be ignored.

Fluorescent dual-labeling with antityrosine hydroxylase (TH) and anticholine acetyltransferase (ChAT) antibodies was performed to determine the neuron cell types in the GPs and to determine whether both adrenergic and cholinergic nerves co-exist within the GPs. Fluorescein-labeled anti-mouse IgG was used as the secondary antibody. Fluorescein isothiocyanate (FITC) was conjugated to TH, and Rhodamine-Labeled Anti-Goat IgG was conjugated to ChAT. The dual-labeled sections were then visualized with a laser-scanning confocal microscope.

Fluorescent double staining showed complex categories of neurons in the SVC area: adrenergic and cholinergic neurons were both observed, but the majority of neurons in the

GP were of the cholinergic subtype (Figure 3A, 3B). Moreover, a proportion of neurons expressed dual adreno-cholinergic phenotypes (Figure 3C).

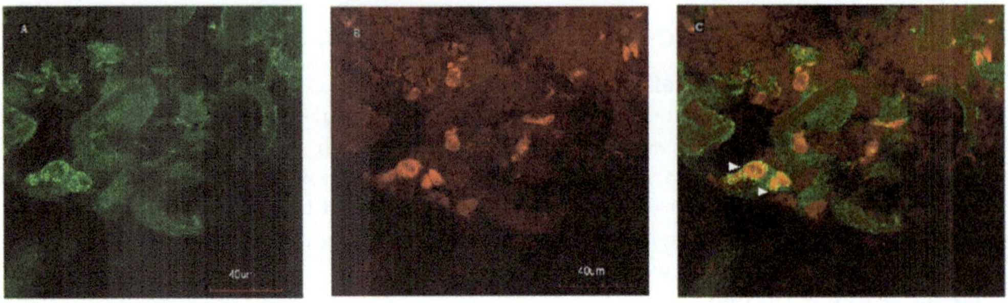

Fig. 3. Neuronal cell types in the ganglionated plexuses of SVC area.

Illustration: Fluorescence photomicrographs show that TH and ChAT are co-expressed in GPs of the SVC area. Figure 3A shows the TH (green)-labeled cholinergic neurons; Figure 3B shows the ChAT (red)-labeled adrenergic neurons; and Figure 3C shows the co-expression of TH and ChAT (white arrow).

These results suggest that ganglion cells can potentially simultaneously express both cholinergic and adrenergic markers, which may occur in the process of a neurochemical switch in response to external stimuli. These cells have also been observed in human pulmonary vein-atrial junction (Tan et al., 2006). This result indicates that stimulation/excision of GPs actually influenced the whole ANS, neither the vagal nor the sympathetic system alone, and the vagal effect was predominant because cholinergic neurons were the majority.

3.2 Efferent autonomic pathway to the atrium and PVs

Five microliters of 10% (w/v) biotinylated dextran amine (BDA) anterograde tracer (MW 10,000; lysine fixable; Molecular Probes, Invitrogen) dissolved in 0.05 M PBS was injected into the SVC area with micropipettes. A total of 5 injection sites —being adjacent to the root of the right part of the SVC area— were selected, and the micropipettes were used at each injection site for 5 min. The dogs were sacrificed 3 days after BDA injection.

Both the atria and the four pulmonary veins were cut into 10-µm-thick sections on a cryostat. The series of sections were then processed for BDA, TH, and ChAT triple immunofluorescence histochemistry. Avidin-conjugated CY5 was used to label BDA, and both TH and ChAT were labeled as described above. Finally, the labeled slides were examined under a laser-scanning confocal microscope.

Injection of an anterograde tracer into the SVC area showed that BDA-containing varicose fibers (Figure 4, A) projected directly into the LA and LPV, while TH-labeled (Figure 4, B) and ChAT labeled (Figure 4, C) axons and varicosities were observed within the same traced varicose fibers. A total of 101 BDA-positive varicose fibers were counted in the LA and LPVs of five animals, and the counts were obtained for 20 sections (four sections in each animal). Of the fibers, 23 (22.7%) were only ChAT-immunoreactive, and 20 (19.8%) displayed both TH and ChAT-like immunoreactivity. Double-immunostaining of TH and ChAT in the absence of BDA was also observed in both the LA and LPV (Figure 4, D).

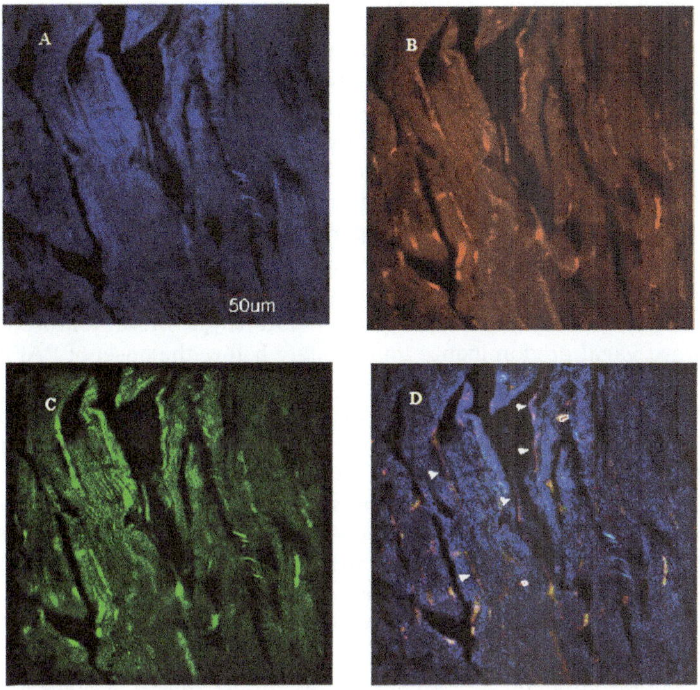

Fig. 4. Co-expression of TH and ChAT in the left atrium and left pulmonary veins.

Fluorescence photomicrographs showed BDA-labeled autonomic fibers projected from the SVC AREA to both the LA and LPV. BDA, ChAT, and TH immunoreactivities were visualized with Avidin-conjugated CY5 (A, blue), Rhodamine (B, red), and FITC (C green,) antibodies, respectively. The merged digital image (D) showed triple staining of ChAT, TH, and BDA (white arrow).

In contrast to our initial predictions, BDA-positive varicose fibers were not found in the RA or RPV. It is possible that the nerve fibers travel to other GPs (i.e., SLGP, ARGP, or IRGP) first and then project into the RA and RPV.

From the above study, we demonstrated parasympathetic and sympathetic neural elements were highly co-localized in the SVC area and mixed with fat cells. We could not separate cholinergic neurons from adrenergic ones or neuron cells from fat cells. This result explains why the whole SVC area, including the fat cells, needs to be all excised to eliminate the intrinsic ANS effect.

4. The effect of ANS modulation on atrial fibrillation

4.1 Review of ANS modulation

Autonomic GPs play an important role in the initiation and maintenance of AF. Several observations suggest that the ANS is crucial in both the initiation and/or the maintenance of AF in humans. Changes in autonomic tone, especially the vagal tone, may be involved in the generation of ectopic PV activity (Schauerte et al., 2001; Sharifov et al., 2004). Vagal nerve stimulation shortens AERP, decreases the wavelength of atrial reentrant circuits and increases dAERP, thus, promoting the stability of AF (Li et al., 2007). However, SLGP acts as the "head station" of vagal inputs to both atria and the sinus and AV nodes in the dog. Most patients with idiopathic PAF appear to be vagally dependent, with heightened susceptibility to vasovagal cardiovascular response. Studies have demonstrated that modification of GPs affected atrial vagal inputs and prevented AF initiation (Lemola et al., 2008). In contrast, in most patients with organic heart diseases, the PAF episodes appear more sympathetically dependent (Huang J.L. et al., 1998). A shift toward an increase in sympathetic tone or a loss of vagal tone has been observed before postoperative PAF, before the onset of atrial flutter, and before PAF occurring during sleep, whereas a shift toward vagal predominance was observed in young patients with lone AF and nocturnal episodes of PAF. More recently, it has been observed that a primary increase in adrenergic drive followed by marked modulation toward vagal predominance immediately before the onset of PAF (Chen P.S. et al., 2007).

Atrial autonomic nerve density is highest in the region of the PVs. One area rich in autonomic innervation is the PV–LA junction which may contribute to the initiation of AF (Chen et al., 2007). Recently, some progresses have been made in ANS modulation. Support for the autonomic basis of paroxysmal and persistent forms of atrial fibrillation have been forthcoming from several clinical series. In 2004, Platt et al. (Platt M et al., 2004) reported that 22 of 23 patients (96%) with persistent atrial fibrillation who had ganglionated plexi ablation alone (no pulmonary vein isolation) were non-inducible immediately after the procedure and at a short follow-up period (median 6 months). Importantly, the number of radiofrequency applications delivered ranged from 5 to 17 (Pappone C et al., 2004) reported that during the application of radiofrequency to induce linear lesions to encircle the pulmonary veins, a 'vagal' response was noted in 100 patients in a series of 297 consecutive cases. This took the form of slowing of the sinus rate during sinus rhythm or a slowing of the ventricular response during atrial fibrillation. While continuing the radiofrequency application, these responses disappeared. A 12-month follow-up showed that the 34.4% who appeared the vagal response had a 99% freedom from atrial fibrillation recurrence whereas the other group had an 85% success rate, that is, freedom from recurrence. Scherlag (Scherlag et al., 2006) stated that ablation of only the ganglionated plexi in the cadiac fat pads may result in higher success rates and may reduce damage incurred to healthy myocardium.Tan (Tan et al., 2008) further demonstrated that cryoablation of extrinsic sympatho-vagal nerves eliminated paroxysmal atrial fibrillation.

These results indicate that rapid ANS modulation does act in the treatment of AF. However, the effect and mechanism of ANS modulation on AF originating in PVs is still unclear. We all know that facal repetitive activities arise from PVs, conduct to the left atria through P-A junction and initiate AF. The following study will investigate Whether ANS modulation can decrease these facal activities in PVs and prevent AF occurrence?

4.2 SLGP stimulation and ablation

To stimulate the SLGP in this FP, a self-made electrode with eight metal electrode heads was used.

The radiofrequency energy was delivered to the SLGP through a 7F deflectable quadripolar catheter with a 4-mm-tip electrode. The catheter tips were placed manually on the surface of the SLGP and the surrounding fat tissues under direct visualization to ensure ideal tissue contact and energy delivery. Continuous unmodulated radiofrequency current (300 to 750 kHz) with a power output setting of 30 to 35 W was delivered from a radiofrequency generator for a duration of 60 seconds.

The results (Wang HT et al., 2010) showed that SLGP stimulation changed atrial electrophysiological properties. Compared with the baseline group, stimulation shortened AERP, LSPVERP, LIPVERP, RSPVERP, and RIPVERP while it increased dAERP .

Catheter ablation reversed the changes in electrophysiological properties caused by SLGP stimulation. Compared with the baseline group, ablation prolonged AERP, LSPVERP, LIPVERP, RSPVERP, RIPVERP, and decreased dAERP (Figure 5).

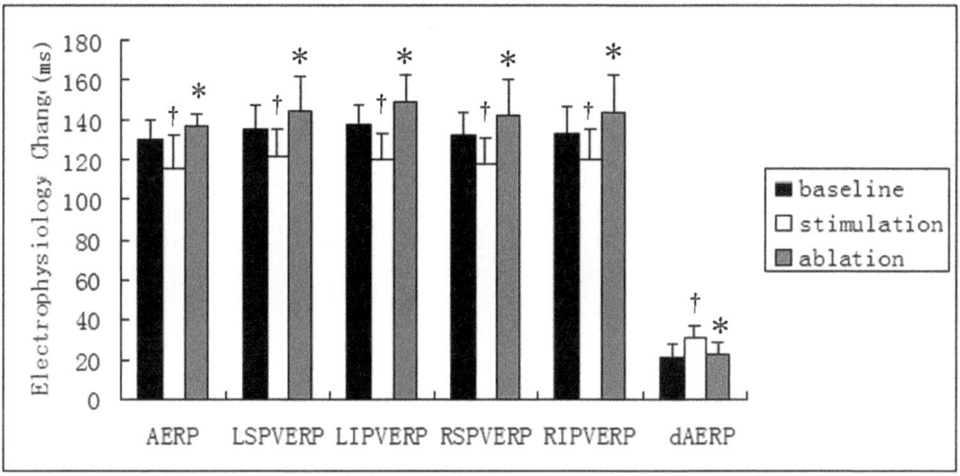

Fig. 5. Electrophysiological changes during RPA FP/GP modification.

Illustration: Changes of AERP, dAERP, PVERP at baseline, during RPA FP/GP stimulation or after ablation. RPA FP/GP stimulation significantly shortened AERP and PVERP and increased dAERP at all atrial sites compared with baseline (P<0.01). After ablation, AERP and PVERP increased and dAERP decreased significantly compared with baseline (P<0.05). *P<0.05 vs., baseline; † P<0.01 vs., baseline.

4.3 Induction of AF

AF was initiated from the distal part of the four PVs. The recording electrode was placed in the proximal PV, and the distance between the stimulating electrode and the recording electrode was about 2cm. AF was first provoked by programmed electrical stimulation (S1S2). If S1S2 failed to induce arrhythmia, burst pacing (S1S1) at a cycle length of 200 ms for 30 seconds was applied to provoke AF in the remaining dogs, and the cycle length was decreased to 160 and 120 ms in turn if 200 ms was ineffectual. The percent of AF induced was measured to evaluate AF inducibility.

The results (Wang HT et al., 2010) showed that AF was induced in 11 of 20 dogs from distal LSPV (Table 1) at baseline without VS stimulation. S1S2 provoked 3 AF episodes, and S1S1 provoked the other 8 (Table 1). vagosympathetic stimulation (VS) significantly increased AF episodes to 18. S1S2 provoked 11 AF episodes, and S1S1 provoked the other 7 (Table 1). After ablation during VS stimulation, AF was no longer inducible by S1S2 in any dogs. S1S1 could still induce AF in 8 of 20 dogs, but the percent induced decreased to 40% (Table 1).

The same protocol was performed at distal LIPV, RSPV, and RIPV at baseline without VS stimulation, and the percent of AF induced was 45%, 50%, and 50%, respectively (Table 1). In contrast, at baseline with VS stimulation, the percent induced increased to 80%, 75%, and 70%, respectively (Table 1). However, after ablation during VS stimulation, AF episodes decreased to 30%, 30%, and 25%, respectively, compared with baseline values (Table 1), and these episodes were all induced by S1S1.

		S1S2	S1S1	Total	(%) n=20
LSPV					
Baseline	VS-	3	8	11	55
	VS+	11	7	18	90*
Ablation		0	8	8	40
LIPV					
Baseline	VS-	2	7	9	45
	VS+	8	8	16	80
Ablation		0	6	6	30
RSPV					
Baseline	VS-	2	8	10	50
	VS+	7	8	15	75
Ablation		0	6	6	30
RIPV					
Baseline	VS-	1	9	10	50
	VS+	7	7	14	70
Ablation		0	5	5	25

Table 1. Comparison of AF incidence before and after RPA FP/GP ablation.

% refers to the percent induced of AF. VS + indicates baseline with vagosympathetic stimulation and VS - indicates baseline without vagosympathetic stimulation. Ablation refers to vagosympathetic stimulation post ablation of GP * P<0.01 vs. baseline.

Programmed stimulation (S1S2) and burst stimulation (S1S1) were performed in turn to provoke AF from distal PVs. In 20 dogs, the percent of AF induced decreased significantly after RPA FP/GP ablation compared with baseline groups.

In conclusion, AF was less likely to be induced from PVs after SLGP ablation. Although the mechanism is unclear, the results may be relevant not only for the independent modulation of the intrinsic autonomic system, but also for the improvement of electrophysiological properties after ablation—less dAERP and longer AERP and PVERP, which decreased the number of atrial reentrant circuits and made re-entry more difficult. Recently, studies showed that ablating only SLGP or SLGP plus IVC-LA GP partially denervates atrial autonomic nerves and increases the incidence of AF (Hirose et al., 2002; Oh et al., 2006). Partial denervation of the atrium was therefore avoided in AF treatment. However, our findings demonstrate that partial denervation of atrial autonomic nerves by ablating SLGP decreased inducibility of AF originating in PVs. This finding suggests that the three major FPs play different roles in AF initiation, and partial denervation is not always harmful to control AF.

5. Prospect-the role of the parasympathetic signal pathway in AF

Except the above mass electrophysiology and histological study, we also studied muscarinic type-2 receptors (M2R) and inward rectifying K+ current (IKACh), which were the key roles of parasympathetic signal pathway.

The M2 muscarinic receptors reside in both the atria and ventricles but have a greater density in the former. The known effects of the parasympathetic nervous system on cardiac function, heart rate, and atrioventricular nodal conduction appear modulated generally via M2 R. The M2R plays an important role in AF. The densities of M2R was spatial heterogeneity combined with the heterogeneous distribution of parasympathetic innervations of the atria, which may contribute to the proarrhythmic ability of vagal nerve stimulation. Cong-Xin Huang (Huang CX et al., 2006) found the density densities of M2R in LAA, RAA and LA were higher than that in RA, PV and SVC. Furthermore, we demonstrated (Hong et al., 2009) that autoantibodies against M2R (M2-AAB) can induce atrial electrophysiology remodeling, atrial fibrosis and upregulation of the M2R and IKACh. These results suggest that the presence of M2-AAB may participate in the induction and perpetuation of AF. And we also demonstrated (Yang et al., 2009) that the distribution of atrial M2R was heterogeneous and had the greatest density in the left atrial free wall (LAFW).The epicardial side had greater M2R density than the endocardial side. We found the distribution of atrial M2R changed with age. Increased density of the M2R in the LAFW accompanied senescence. This variation may enhance the heterogeneity of the M2R distribuion and may contribute to age-related changes in AF vulnerability.

The IKACh is present in the sinoatrial node, atria, atrioventricular node, and Purkinje fibers of the mammalian heart and coupled to muscarinic type-2 receptor and adenosine type-1 receptors through pertussis toxin (PT) or select-activating protein -sensitive G-proteins (GK). The IKACh possesses three distinct open/closed states. IKACh is comprised of two homologous proteins: GIRK1 and GIRK4. In the heart, only the expression of Kir3.1 and Kir3.4 mRNAs is detected. GIRK4 is the functional subunit of IKACh and ablation of GIRK4 typically results in the functional elimination of IKACh. Moreover, GIRK1 cannot form a functional ion channel in the absence of GIRK4.

The cardiac acetylcholine-sensitive K+ channel plays a major role in the parasympathetic regulation of heart rate, and is also crucial in the generation and maintenance of AF. First, IKACh was spatial heterogeneity in the atria which facilitated the generation and maintenance of AF. Cong-Xin Huang (Huang CX et al., 2006) found the densities of IKACh in LAA, RAA and LA were higher than that in RA, PV and SVC in LAA, RAA. Sarmast F (Sarmast F et al., 2003) found a greater abundance of Kir3.x channels and higher IKACh density in LA than RA myocytes result in greater ACh-induced speeding-up of rotors in the LA than in the RA. A canine form of constitutively active IKACh(called IKH) shows regional heterogeneity (larger in PV cardiomyocyte sleeves).Secondly, the IKACh participated the electric remodeling of atrial fibrillation. Kir3.1 mRNA levels are downregulated in human AF. In contrast to reduced functional IKACh and Kir3 subunit mRNA content, an increase in a constitutively active form of this current has been described as a potentially important contributor to the AF substrate.Furthermore, IKACh is a potentially interesting target for atrial-selective anti-AF therapy. The suggested activation of IKACh predisposed to AF and lack of IKACh prevented AF. But it is still unknown the precise mechanism of IKACh inhibition to the antiarrhythmic potency of these drugs and selective inhibitors are not yet available for clinical application. We successfully used (Liu et al.,2009) adenovirus-delivered short hairpin RNA targeting GIRK4 not only decreased the expression of GIRK4 in human atrial myocytes, but also affected IKACh densities. If we attempted to acquire more effective and persistent RNAi effects in human atrial myocytes and use adenovirus-delivered small hairpin RNA against GIRK4 in clinic, there are a great deal challenges to be overcome.

Although the role of the parasympathetic signal pathway is accpepted both in initiation and maintenance of AF. It is less clear in AF patients whether inhibition of parasympathetic activity have an anti-arrhythmic effect. Furthermore, persistent and selective inhibition was still difficult.

In conclusion, ANS modulation plays an important role in the treatment of AF. The mechanism remains unclear. And the change of ion-channel current should be investigated to disclose the mechanism of ANS modulation in the control of AF. Maybe more penetrating studies are needed to associate ANS modulation with ion-channel inhibition to probe a new way to improve the treatment of AF.

6. References

Armour J.A., & Ardell J.L. (1994). Neurocardiology (Second edition.). Structure and function of mammalian intrinsic cardiac neurons. Oxford University Press, New York, pp, 95–114.

Chen P.S., & Tan AY. (2007). Autonomic nerve activity and atrial fibrillation. Heart Rhythm, 4, S61- S64.

Chiou C.W., Eble J.N., & Zipes D.P. (1997). Efferent vagal innervation of the canine atria and sinus and atrioventricular nodes. Circulation, 95, 2573-2584.

Hirose M, Leatmanoratn Z, Laurita K.R., & Carlson M.D. (2002). Partial vagal denervation increases vulnerability to vagally induced atrial fibrillation. J Cardiovasc Electrophysiol,13, 1272-1279.

Hong C.M., Zheng Q.S., Liu X.T., Shang F.J., Wang H.T., & Jiang W.R. (2009). Effects of Autoantibodies against M2 Muscarinic Acetylcholine Receptors on Rabbit Atria in vivo. Cardiology, 112,180–187.

Hou Y, Scherlag B.J., Lin J, Zhou J, Song J, Zhang Y, Patterson E, Lazzara R, Jackman W.M., & Po S.S. (2007). Interactive atrial neural network: Determining the connections between ganglionated plexi. Heart Rhythm, 4, 56-63.

Huang C.X., Zhao Q.Y., Liang J.J., Chen H, Yang B, Jiang H, & Li G.S. (2006). Differential densities of muscarinic acetylcholine receptor and I_{KACh} in canine supraventricular tissues and the effect of amiodarone on cholinergic atrial fibrillation and I_{KACh}. Cardiology, 106, 36–43.

Huang J.L., Wen Z.C., Lee W.L., Chang M.S. & Chen S.A.(1998).Changes of autonomic tone before the onset of paroxysmal atrial fibrillation, Int J Cardiol, 66 , 275–283.

Lemola K, Bsc D.C., Yeh Y.H., Dubuc M, Cartier R, Armour A, Ting M, Sakabe M, Shiroshita-Takeshita A, Comtois P, & Nattel S. Pulmonary Vein Region Ablation in Experimental Vagal Atrial Fibrillation. Role of pulmonary veins versus autonomic ganglia. Circulation. 2008; 117:470-477.

Li Y, Li W, Yang B, Han W, Dong D, Xue J, Li B, Yang S, & Sheng L. (2007). Effects of Cilazapril on atrial electrical, structural and functional remodeling in atrial fibrillation dogs. J Electrocardiol, 40, e1-e6.

Liu X.T, Yang J, Shang F.J, Hong C.M., Guo W.G., Wang B, & Zheng Q.S. (2009). Silencing GIRK4 expression in human atrial myocytes by adenovirus-delivered small hairpin RNA. Mol Biol Rep,36, 1345–1352.

Oh S, Zhang Y, Bibevski S, Marrouche N.F., Natale A, & Mazgalev T.N. (2006).Vagal denervation and atrial fibrillation inducibility: Epicardial fat pad ablation does not have long-term effects. Heart Rhythm, 3,701-708.

Pappone C, Santinelli V, Manguso F, Vicedomini G, Gugliotta F, Augello G, Mazzone P, Tortoriello V, Landoni G, Zangrillo A,Lang C, Tomita T, Mesas C, Mastella E, Alfieri O.(2004). Pulmonary vein denervation enhances long-term benefit after circumferential ablation for paroxysmal atrial fibrillation. Circulation, 109,327-334.

Platt M, Mandapati R, Scherlag B.J. (2004). Limiting the number and extent of radiofrequency applications to terminate atrial fibrillation and subsequently prevent its inducibility [abstract]. Heart Rhythm, 1, S11.

Sarmast F, Kolli A, Zaitsev A, Parisian K, Dhamoon A.S., Guha P.K., Warren M, Anumonwo J.M., Taffet S.M., Berenfeld O, & Jalife J. (2003).Cholinergic atrial fibrillation: I_{KACh} gradients determine unequal left/right atrial frequencies and rotor dynamics. Cardiovasc Res, 59,863-873.

Scherlag B.J., & Po S. (2006). The intrinsic cardiac nervous system and atrial fibrillation. Curr Opin Cardiol, 21, 51-54

Scherlag B.J., Patterson E, & Po S. (2006). The neural basis of atrial fibrillation. J Cardiovasc Electrophysiol, 39, S180-183.

Sharifov O.F., Fedorov V.V., & Beloshapko G.G., Glukhov A.V., Yushmanova A.V., & Rosenshtraukh L.V. (2004). Roles of adrenergic and cholinergic stimulation in spontaneous atrial fibrillation in dogs.J Am Coll Cardiol, 43, 483-490.

Schauerte P, Scherlag B.J., Patterson E, Scherlag M.A., Matsudaria K, Nakagawa H, Lazzara R, & Jackman W.M. (2001). Focal atrial fibrillation: experimental evidence for a pathophysiologic role of the autonomic nervous system. J Cardiovasc Electrophysiol, 12,600-601.

Tan A.Y., Zhou S, Ogawa M, Song J, Chu M , Li H.M., Fishbein M.C., Lin S.F., Chen L.S., & Chen P.S.(2008).Neural mechanisms of paroxysmal atrial fibrillation and paroxysmal atrial tachycardia in ambulatory canines. Circulation, 118,916-925.

Tan A.Y., Li H, Wachsmann-Hogiu S, Chen L.S., Chen P.S., Fishbein M.C. (2006). Autonomic innervation and segmental muscular disconnections at the human pulmonary vein-atrial junction: implications for catheter ablation of atrial-pulmonary vein junction. J Am Coll Cardiol, 48,132-143.

Wang H, Li J, Hong C, Liu X, Shang F, He Y, Wang Z, & Zheng Q. (2010) Epicardial ablation of right pulmonary artery ganglionated plexi for the prevention of atrial fibrillation originating in the pulmonary veins. J Electrocardiol, 43, 367-372

Yang Y.H., Zheng Q.S., Li J, Shang F.J., Liu T, Wang H.T., Liu X.T., & Liu L. (2009). Age-related changes in the atrial muscarinic type 2 receptor and their effects on atrial fibrillation vulnerability in rabbits. Experimental Gerontology 44, 572–578.

16

Clinical Result of Epicardial Pulmonary Vein Isolation (LAVIE) by Cryoablation as Concomitant Cardiac Operation and Clinical Application of New Ablation Device (KIRC-119 Infrared Coagulator) to Treat Atrial Fibrillation

Hiroshi Kubota[1], Kenichi Sudo[1], Shinichi Takamoto[2], Hidehito Endo[1], Hiroshi Tsuchiya[1], Akihiro Yoshimoto, Yu Takahashi, Yusuke Inaba[1] and Akira Furuse[3]

[1]*Dpt of Cardiovascular Surgery, Kyorin University, Tokyo,*
[2]*Mitsui Memorial Hospital, Tokyo,*
[3]*JR Tokyo General Hospital, Tokyo,*
Japan

1. Introduction

Maze surgery is widely used to treat atrial fibrillation but requires cardiopulmonary bypass and longer aortic cross-clamping time. Percutaneous transcatheter pulmonary vein isolation or catheter-based maze procedure are time consuming and relies on fluoroscopy and contrast media, and pulmonary vein obstruction and cardiac tamponade are still major problems. Although thoracoscopic minimally invasive epicardial pulmonary vein isolation using a radiofrequency device is also widely accepted, the device has the weakness to ablate the free wall of the atrium. To overcome these drawbacks, new ablation devices and techniques were developed using two kinds of energy source.

2. Epicardial cryoablation and epicardial infrared ablation

As energy sources, cryothermia and infrared were used. They were applied experimentally and clinically.

2.1 Epicardial cryoablation

First, to enable circumferential epicardial PV ablation, a hook-shaped cryoprobe was developed. Its efficacy was examined in canine model.

Second, a new operative procedure using a conventional cryo-system was also developed and applied clinically.

2.1.1 Epicardial pulmonary vein isolation with a hook-shaped cryoprobe to treat atrial fibrillation

After it was shown that a rapidly firing focus in a pulmonary vein (PV) can cause atrial fibrillation, percutaneous endocardial PV isolation (ablation) using radiofrequency became an established method of treatment. However, the technique is time consuming. It requires fluoroscopy and contrast media to identify the PV, and cardiac tamponade and PV stenosis (obstruction) are major complications. To overcome these drawbacks, we tried using cryoablation. Although the effectiveness of cryoablation has already been demonstrated in the modified maze procedure, its effectiveness by the epicardial approach in the beating heart was unknown. We developed a hook-shaped cryoprobe to circumferentially ablate PV orifices epicardially. The aim of this study was to confirm the efficacy of this method electrophysiologically in an experimental study in dogs.

We used a cryosurgical system PCG12R (CO_2, −60 degrees; Spembly Medical Ltd. Hampshire, UK) to create the cryolesions. A novel hook-shaped cryoprobe, 20-mm long and 3-mm wide, was developed to facilitate the PV ablation (Fig 1-A, B).

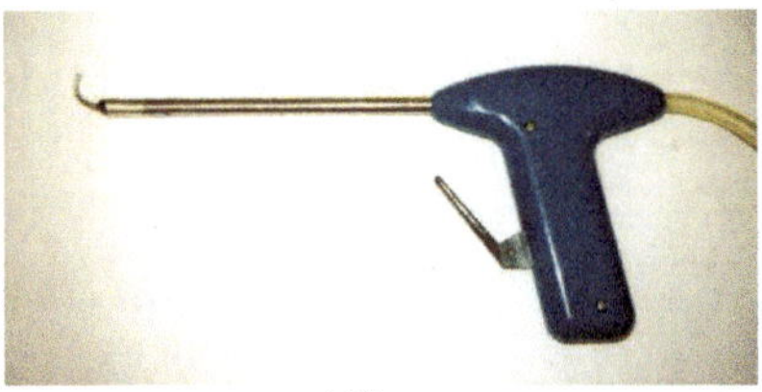

(A)

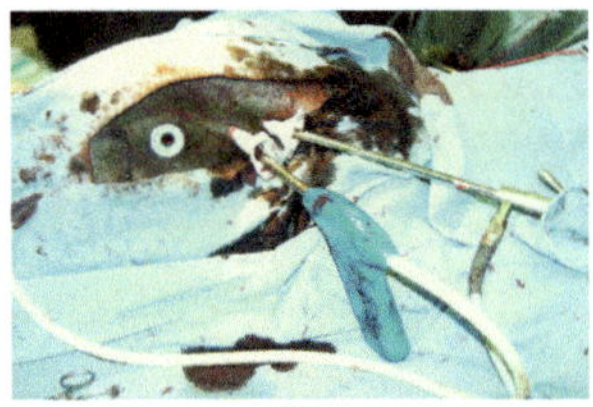

(B)

Fig. 1. The hook-shaped cryoprobe. (A) The hook is 20-mm long and 3-mm wide. (B) Thoracoscopic experiment using a canine model.

Material and methods

Five adult mongrel dogs weighing 14.2 ± 2.5 kg were anesthetized with ketamine hydrochloride (20 mg/kg, IM) and sodium pentobarbital (16 mg/kg, IV), and ventilated. The pericardium was opened through a median sternotomy, and the surrounding tissue was dissected to expose all PVs and their orifices into the left atrium. Since each dog had six or seven PVs, a total of 32 PVs were examined.

Before cryoablation, the pacing threshold of the left atrium was determined by stimulation with a bipolar electrode. Next, each PV was stimulated. The electrode was slid from the ostium to the distal site of the PV little by little, and the area of each PV that had the same pacing threshold as the left atrium was identified. Encircling cryoablation was then performed with the hook-shaped cryoprobe to circumferentially ablate the orifice of each PV epicardially. The circumferential cryolesions were created by passing the probe behind the orifice of the PV. The PV was compressed and flattened by pulling the probe upward when the cryoablation was done. The probe was applied to each orifice for 90 seconds (Fig 2, 3).

Chnges in PV potential

Before and during cryoablation, bipolar electrodes were placed on the PV, left atrium, left atrial appendage, and right atrium, and electrical potentials were recorded (n = 16). Two hours later, the electrical potentials were also recorded.

Changes in cardiac rhythm

Before and during ablation, bipolar electrodes were placed on the PV, left atrium, left atrial appendage, and right atrium, and the heart was paced through the electrode on the PV. The electrical potentials at each site were recorded (n = 16), and they were also recorded during PV pacing two hours later.

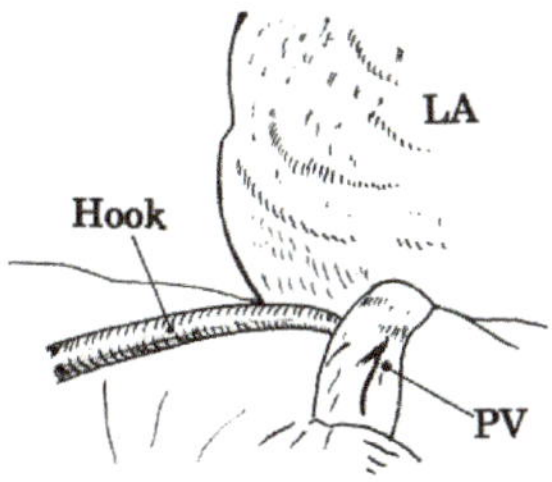

Fig. 2. Diagram of the area where cryoablation is performed with the assistance of the probe. (LA = left atrium; PV = pulmonary vein.)

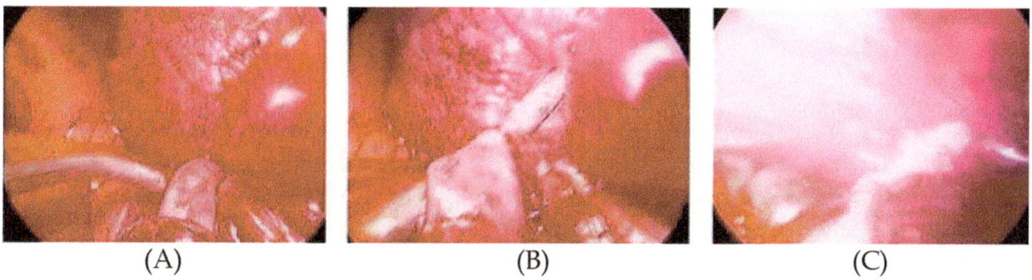

Fig. 3. Procedure for creating a circumferential cryolesion (Thoracoscopic view).(A) The probe is passed behind the PV and pulled upward. (B) The PV is compressed and flattened by the probe. (C) Cryoablation is performed for 90 seconds.

Results

The mean distance between the PV orifice and the pacing boundary was 8.9 ± 1.3 mm (Fig. 4).

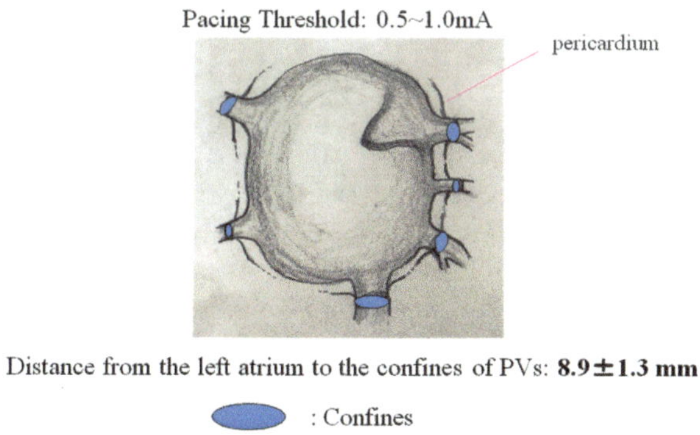

Fig. 4. Electriphysiological characteristics of canine PVs

Canine PVs showed same electrophysiological characteristics as the atrium in some extention.

All PVs had the same pacing threshold as the left atrium at some distance. Twenty-nine of the pacing boundaries were present on the pericardial reflection or in the pleural cavity; the pacing boundaries of only three PVs (left superior) were in the pericardial space. When a pacing site was positioned beyond the boundary, the pacing threshold suddenly became extremely high.

Immediately after commencing the cryoablation, the potential of the PV diminished (Fig. 5), and it had not recovered two hours later. Immediately after commencing the cryoablation, the cardiac rhythm converted from the pacing rhythm to the sinus rhythm (Fig. 6). The effectiveness of the ablation persisted two hours later.

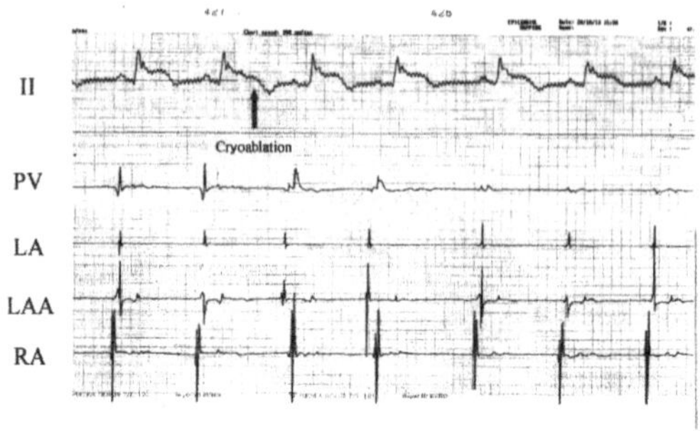

Fig. 5. Atrial and PV potentials during ablation (spontaneously beating heart).
Immediately after the start of cryoablation, the PV potential decreased rapidly and became almost flat. A couple of ectopic beats, which may have arisen from the cryosite, were observed. (LA = left atrium; LAA = left atrial appendage; PV = pulmonary vein; RA = right atrium.)

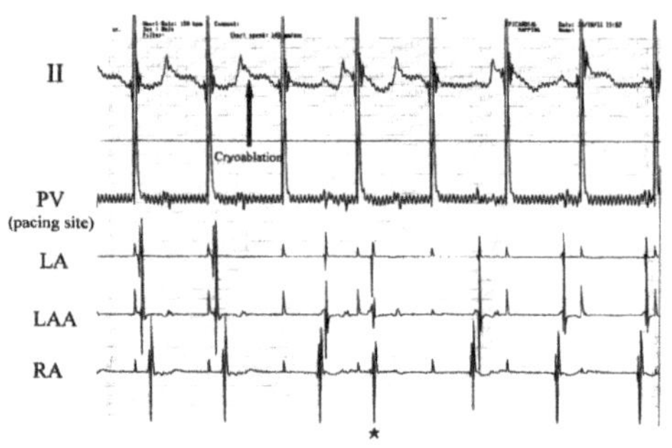

Fig. 6. Atrial and PV potentials during ablation (pacing from the PV).
Before ablation, pacing signals from the PV were conducted to both atria. Immediately after commencing the cryoablation, the cardiac rhythm converted from pacing rhythm to sinus rhythm. An ectopic potential (★), which may have arisen from the cryosite, is seen.

Comment

Radiofrequency endocardial PV ablation became widely adopted after reporting that rapidly firing foci could be identified in and around the PVs, and that ablation of such foci might lead to resolution of paroxysmal AF (Haissaguere et al., 1998; Pappone et al., 2000). However, the procedure depends on fluoroscopy and the use of contrast medium to identify the PVs. The electrophysiologic studies are time consuming, and cardiac tamponade and PV obstruction are still major problems. Our experiment was designed to overcome these problems.

We first investigated whether the PVs of mongrel dogs have the same electrophysiological characteristics as human PVs. Most dogs have 6 to 7 PVs, and a total of 32 PVs were studied. All PVs were found to have the same electrical characteristics as the left atrium at some distance, and almost all PVs had their electrical boundary on the pericardial reflection on the

PVs or after they passed into the thoracic cavity. Although no histopathologic examinations were performed in this study, these findings suggested that the myocardium extends into the PVs of dogs, the same as in humans. Based on these findings, we concluded that mongrel dogs could be used as a model to verify the efficacy of ablation.
The potential of the PVs diminished immediately after the start of ablation, and the PV pacing rhythm immediately converted to sinus rhythm. These phenomena demonstrate that the epicardial cryoablation had created a bidirectional conduction block. Although the irreversibility of the effectiveness of ablation was confirmed two hours later, a chronic study is needed to demonstrate the permanence of the effect of the cryolesion.
The effect of epicardial cryoablation does to not reach the endocardium of the beating heart, because the normothermic blood flow within it weakens the cryoeffect (Kubota, et al., 2002). However, we have shown that the cryoablation in the warm beating heart is effective only at sites that can be compressed by the cryoprobe, thereby eliminating blood flow with it. When the hook probe was pulled upward, the PV was flattened and the blood flow within it was completely eliminated. Flattening a PV can create a "local arrested heart," that may be why cryoablation is able to produce an encircling lesion in a "single" application and create a bidirectional electrical block at PV orifices. Although no histopathologic examinations were performed in our study, the electrophysiologicl findings suggest that the PV wall was ablated transmurally. These results of our preliminary experiment suggest that cryoablation is capable of overcoming some of the drawbacks of the percutaneous endocardial approach. Modification of the device will allow thoracoscopic epicardial ablation of the PVs (Kubota et al. 2004).

2.1.2 Epicardial pulmonary vein isolation by cryoablation as concomitant cardiac operation to treat nonvalvular atrial fibrillation: "LAVIE" procedure

How should patients with nonvalvular atrial fibrillation who require cardiac operation be managed? We developed an epicardial technique to isolate the left atrial posterior wall and pulmonary veins. The first clinical case is presented and postoperative clinical course of 16 patients' series are described.
Case presentation
On March 29, 2001, an 82-year-old woman was transferred to our hospital with a diagnosis of acute aortic dissection, DeBakey II, Stanford A. Preoperative echocardiography revealed normal cardiac function, and aortic regurgitation was trivial. There was no mitral regurgitation and no enlargement of the left atrium. A preoperative electrocardiogram showed AF, and the amplitude of the f-wave in V_1 was 0.1 mV. The patient's AF had initially been diagnosed about 3 years previously. An operation was performed on the day after admission.
The pericardium was opened through a median sternotomy. A mild bloody pericardial effusion was aspirated, and tapes were passed around the SVCand the IVC. A cardiopulmonary bypass was established by cannulations through the left femoral artery and both vena cavae, and the left ventricle was vented through the right superior PV. During cooling, the tissue behind the SVC and IVC was carefully dissected to expose the left atrium. When the tympanic temperature reached 20°C, both vena cavae were snared, and epicardial cryoablation was started with N_2O at −60 °C (Cardiac Cryosurgical System CCS-200; Cooper Surgical, Shelton, CT). A pencil-type probe (20 mm × 9 mm) and a T-shaped probe (20 mm × 5 mm) were used. The right side of the left atrium was cryoablated first. The roof of the left atrium behind the SVC was then ablated by pulling the snared tape anteriorly, and the left atrium behind the IVC was ablated pulling the snared tape anteriorly (Fig 7A). At a tympanic temperature of 18°C, the ascending aorta was incised under circulatory arrest and retrograde cerebral perfusion. Antegrade blood cardioplegia was

infused. A 26-mm woven Dacron graft (Hemashield®, Boston Scientific Medi-Tech, Wayne, NJ) was anastomosed. The graft was clamped, and the antegrade perfusion was started through a side branch of the graft. The retro-aortic portion of the left atrial roof was easily cryoablated because the proximal ascending aorta was left transected. Reinforcement of the proximal aorta and an anastomosis were carried out. The cryoablation of the remaining part of the left atrium was continued while warming. A tape was passed around the pulmonary artery, and as the tape was pulled anteriorly, the cryoprobe was passed into the transverse sinus, thereby enabling ablation of the left side of the roof of the left atrium. Great care was taken not to ablate the left coronary artery system to prevent reactive hypertrophy of the intima, which might cause serious ischemia of the myocardium. The ablation was extended to the left side of the left atrium, the inferior wall of the left atrium parallel to the coronary sinus, and was finally connected to the retro-IVC lesion that had been made before circulatory arrest (Fig 7B, C). The left atrial appendage was ligated, and the orifices of the left superior and inferior pulmonary vein were cryoablated (Fig 7D). All applications of the probe were epicardial, and the cryolesions were always created so that they overlapped by 2~3 mm to produce a continuous lesion. The duration of each application was 1.5 minutes.

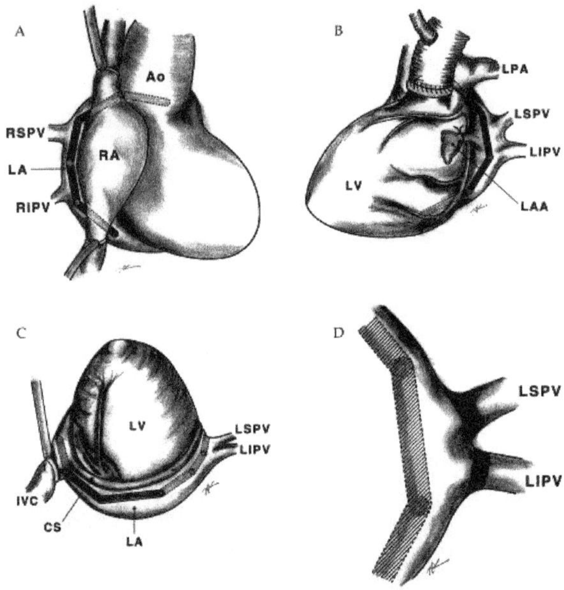

Fig. 7. Epicardial encircling cryoablation of the left atrium.

The cryolesions were made with 2~3 mm overlaps to obtain a continuous linear lesion. The duration of each application was 1.5 min. Two kinds of cryoprobe were used. (A) Tapes were passed around the SVC and the IVC. The right side of the left atrium was cryoablated. The left atrium behind the IVC and the roof of the left atrium behind the SVC were ablated while the snared tape was pulled anteriorly. (B) Before the proximal anastomosis, the retro-aortic portion of the left atrium was ablated. The cryoablation of the remaining part of the left atrium was continued while warming. Great care should be taken not to ablate the left coronary artery. The ablation was extended to the left side of the left atrium. (C) The inferior wall of the left atrium parallel to the coronary sinus was ablated and it was connected to the retro IVC lesion that was made before circulatory arrest. (D) The left atrial appendage was ligated. The orifices of the left superior and inferior pulmonary vein were cryoablated respectively. (LPA; left pulmonary artery, CS; coronary sinus)

The heart beat recovered spontaneously and was in sinus rhythm from the start. Weaning from the cardiopulmonary bypass was easy. Total cardiopulmonary bypass time was 199 minutes. Aortic cross-clamping time was 99 minutes. Circulatory arrest time was 40 minutes. Operation time was 5 hours.

The patient was extubated the next day and returned to a general ward on postoperative day 2. The postoperative electrophysiological examination revealed that overdrive pacing inside of the encircling lesion with a bipolar pacing wire left behind the left atrium did not affect the cardiac rhythm, even when the output was set at maximum (Fig. 8). Atrial electrical potential within the encircling lesion was recorded with the same pacing wire, and no atrial potential was found within the encircling lesion. A Holter electrocardiogram recorded 4 months after the operation showed a regular sinus rhythm without any supraventricular tachycardia. The patient is alive and well, an electrocardiogram ten years after the operation showed that the regular sinus rhythm had been maintained without drugs.

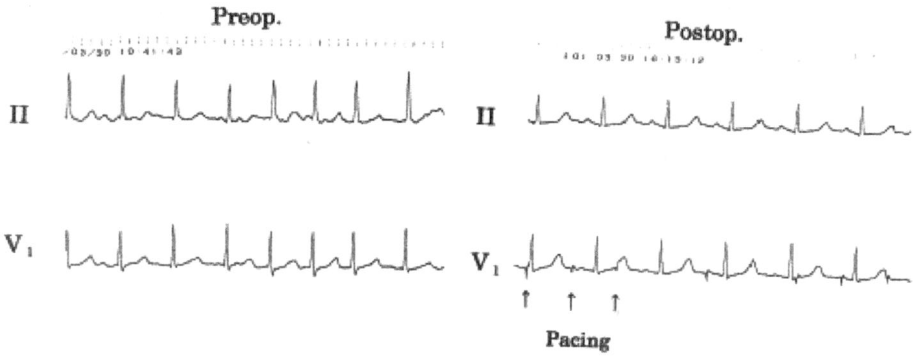

Fig. 8. Postoperative electrophysiological study.
When the posterior wall inside the encircling lesion was paced, pacing failed to affect the cardiac rhythm.

Comment

The maze procedure is usually performed to treat AF secondary to atrial overload mainly caused by valvular disease and is not commonly used to treat paroxysmal or lone AF because full sternotomy, cardiopulmonary bypass, and dual atriotomy are too invasive. On the other hand, we are often faced with elderly patients who are surgical candidates and have AF plus nonmitral disease (eg, coronary artery disease, aortic stenosis, aortic dissection, and aortic aneurysm). Until now we have tended not to perform the maze procedure concomitant with operation for the primary disease in such patients because it prolongs aortic cross-clamp time and requires additional atriotomy. To overcome these problems, we developed the technique previously described and called it the "LAVIE" (left atrium and vein isolation: epicardial) procedure. Although a preoperative electrophysiological study was not performed, in view of the patient's advanced age and echocardiographic findings her AF was thought to be lone AF, very probably of the pulmonary vein origin. The postoperative electrophysiological study showed that the encircling pulmonary vein lesion had produced a bi-directional block. The posterior wall of the left atrium, including the pulmonary veins, had been electrically isolated. We added the cryoablation of the orifice of the left pulmonary veins to isolate the ectopic focus with greater certainty. In nonopen cardiac operation, such as coronary bypass procedures, the entire length of the left atrial roof can be ablated by pulling up a tape passed around the ascending aorta and the pulmonary trunk through the transverse sinus.

The left atrium and vein isolation technique does not require atriotomy and does not prolong the aortic cross-clamp time. Since two cryoprobes can be used simultaneously, total ablation time can be shortened. Both vena cavae were snared to reduce blood flow in the left atrium. Reducing the blood flow, which weakens the cryo effect, is quite important to producing transmural cryolesions. The left ventricular venting is also effective to reduce the blood in the left atrium. This technique should be applied only during cardiac operations with total cardiopulmonary bypass (Kubota et al., 2003).

2.1.3 Clinical result of epicardial pulmonary vein isolation (LAVIE) by cryoablation as concomitant cardiac operation to treat atrial fibrillation

From April 2002 to April 2010, 16 patients underwent LAVIE technique concomitant with non-valvular cardiac operation. The primary diseases were: coronary artery disease, acute aortic dissection, and aortic stenosis. The conversion ratio to sustained sinus rhythm was verified and compared with the result of modified Kosakai maze procedure performed in the same period.

Results: The postoperative EPS revealed that overdrive pacing from inside of the box lesion did not affect the cardiac rhythm, and no atrial potential was found within the lesion (Fig. 9). Sustained sinus rhythm, including atrial-based paced rhythm was present in 75.0 % in LAVIE performed patients.

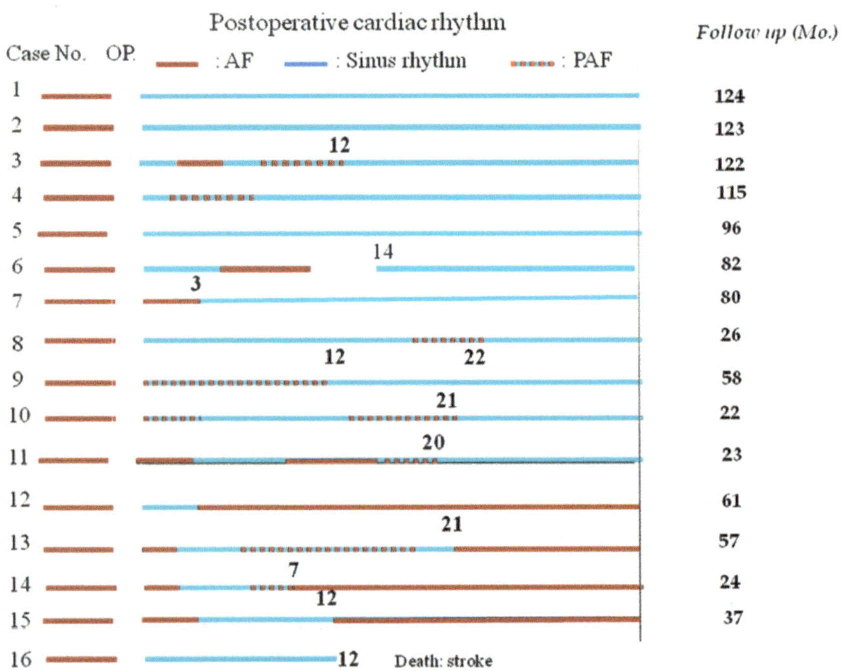

Fig. 9. Postoperative cardiac rhythm after "LAVIE" procedure
Sinus rhythm was restored in 75%. Note that in eight patients, after the "irritable" period, stable sinus rhythm restored.

2.2 Epicardial infrared ablation

Infrared is one of the effective energy sources to ablate the myocardium. To realize transmural atrial ablation, KIRC-119 was developed. Its efficacy was examined in canine model and applied clinically.

2.2.1 Fundamental experiment of atrial ablation using a prototype infrared coagulator

The ideal method for atrial ablation has not yet been reported. In the infrared coagulator, the distal exit plane of the light-conducting rod is connected to a tip. We made three kinds of artificial sapphire tips for this device to obtain linear photocoagulation. When each tip is touched to the epicardium, light energy is absorbed by the myocardium, which becomes photocoagulated. In this study, the characteristics of the three kinds of tip were first compared in a canine heart. The depth and width of the myocardial lesions were measured, and their histopathologic features were observed. Changes in the atrial conducting pathway immediately after and 3 months after ablation then were recorded by epicardial mapping.

Material and methods

The IRK-151 infrared coagulator (Infrarot-Kontaktkoagulator; Messerschmidt-Bolkow-Blohn, Frankfurt, Germany) was originally developed to secure hemostasis in bleeding parenchyma as an alternative to high-frequency electrocoagulation or laser coagulation (Fig 10A). The single-application time is limited to within 3 seconds by a timer. In this device, light from a tungsten-halogen lamp is focused by a reflector into a light-conducting quartz rod with a diameter of 10 mm. It emerges as 35 W/cm2 of near-infrared light energy (wavelength, 400 to 1600 nm; peak wavelength, 850 nm). The distal exit plane of the light-conducting rod is connected to the tip. We made three kinds of original tips using artificial sapphire (tapered, coated, and angled) by polishing the surface of a cylindrical sapphire slantwise (Fig 10B). All the tips have a rectangular (1.5 × 10.0 mm) edge to allow linear atrial myocardial ablation.

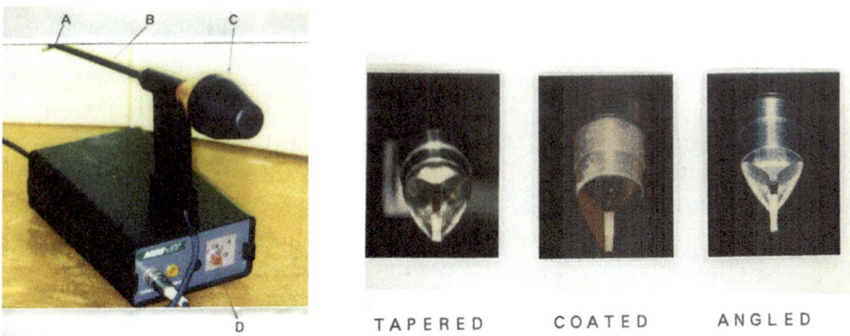

(A) (B)

Fig. 10. (A) The IRK-151 infrared coagulator (a = tip; b = light-conducting quartz rod; c = reflector; d = timer). (B) Three kinds of artificial sapphire tips: (left) tapered, (middle) coated, and (right) angled. The coated tip has the same shape as the tapered tip, but the slanting surfaces are coated with nickel and tin dichloride. The angled tip has a 4-mm straight nose to prevent unnecessary ablation caused by direct contact of the slanting surface. When these sapphire tips are pressed into tissue, light energy is absorbed by the myocardium, which is then photocoagulated.

The coated tip has the same shape as the tapered tip, and the slanting surfaces are coated with nickel and tin dichloride to prevent leakage of unnecessary energy in a lateral direction. The angled tip has a 4-mm straight nose to prevent unnecessary ablation resulting from direct contact with the slanting surface.

Methods

Developing a suitable tip for obtaining linear atrial ablation

Nine adult mongrel dogs weighing 13.5 ± 1.7 kg were anesthetized using ketemine hydrochloride (20 mg/kg) intramuscularly and sodium pentobarbital (16 mg/kg) intravenously and were ventilated. Through a right thoracotomy, the beating right ventricular myocardium was ablated using the IRK-151 from the epicardium. The tip was compressed 2 to 3 mm into the epicardium unless this induced paroxysmal ventricular contraction. Four lesions were created using different durations of application (3, 9, 15 and 21 seconds). The three different sapphire tips were applied to 3 dogs each. Therefore, a total of 36 lesions were created. After ablation, the hearts were rapidly excised and the myocardium was fixed in 10% formalin. After adequate fixation, thin sections were cut and stained (hematoxylin-eosin and azan). The width, depth, and shape of ablation, and the resulting histopathologic changes were observed by light microscopy. To obtain linear coagulation, the ideal tip should create deep and narrow coagulation. Therefore we devised the linear index, to describe this: Linear index=depth of coagulation/width of coagulation. The linear indices using the three kinds of tips at 21 seconds of application were calculated and compared for each tip. Ventricular myocardium was used instead of atrial myocardium to assess the depth of coagulation because the atrial myocardium is too thin for this evaluation.

To evaluate the influence of tip pressure on the epicardium, the depth of the lesion when the tapered tip was compressed 2 to 3 mm into the epicardium and that when the same tip merely touched the epicardium were compared for various durations of application (3, 9, 15 and 21 seconds) using 3 adult dogs.

Atrial ablation with an infrared coagulator

In 3 dogs a linear lesion on the beating right atrial free wall was created from the annulus of the tricuspid valve to the intraatrial sulcus by using the tapered tip. This lesion was created by several overlapping applications (15 seconds for each application) from both the epicardial and endocardial sides (Fig.11). First, the endocardial ablation was performed by insertion of the light-conducting rod into the right atrium through a purse-string suture on the right atrial appendage. After that, epicardial ablation was performed on the same line as endocardial ablation. To ensure complete coverage, 2.0 mm of overlapped lesions were made. Before and after ablation, epicardial plaque–electrode mapping (24-channel bipolar electrodes, 33 × 45 mm) was performed to determine the conduction pathway in the right atrial free wall. The recording conditions were spontaneous beating and overdrive pacing from the low right atrium (R = 140/min). In two other dogs, the same line as that to be ablated was clamped with a Satynsky clamp. The atrial wall was then cut and sutured. After unclamping, epicardial mapping was performed in the same way. The result of postablation epicardial mapping was contrasted with the mapping of the cut and sutured atrial wall. The collected data were recorded and analyzed by the HPM-7100 mapping system (Fukuda Denshi, Tokyo, Japan). After the experiment, the chest wall was closed. Three months later, right atrial epicardial plaque–electrode mapping was performed again through another thoracotomy. After the completion of mapping, the right atrial free wall was excised, fixed, and stained in the same way as the ventricle, and the histopathologic changes were observed by light microscopy.

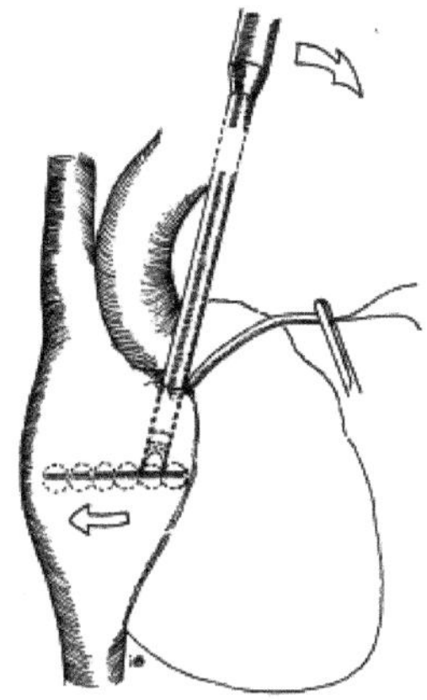

Fig. 11. A linear lesion was created by several overlapping applications from both the epicardial and endocardial sides.

Results

Developing a suitable tip for obtaining linear atrial ablation

Depth of lesion

The depth of the lesion was correlated with increased coagulation time (Fig. 12). The maximum depth was 10.3 ± 0.8 mm at 21 seconds using the tapered tip, which was significantly deeper than with the other kinds of tips. The depth of the lesion using the angled tip was 5.2 ± 0.3 mm, and that with the coated tip was 7.7 ± 0.3 mm at 21 seconds.

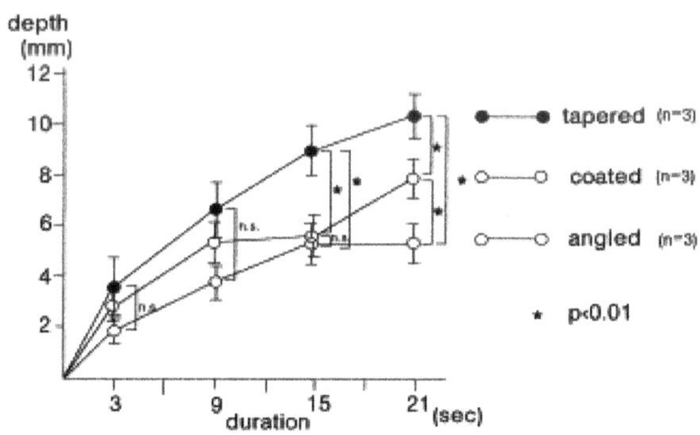

Fig. 12. Average depth of the lesion.
The maximum average depth of the lesion was 10.3 ± 0.8 mm at 21 seconds with use of the tapered tip. (n.s. = not significant.)

Width of lesion

The narrowest lesion width, 13.7 ± 1.5 mm at 21 seconds of ablation (Table 1), was created by the tapered tip. The linear index obtained using the tapered tip (0.76 ± 0.13 mm) was higher than that for the other tips (angled tip, 0.25 ± 0.02 mm; coated tip, 0.43 ± 0.03 mm).

Tip	Depth (mm)	Width (mm)	Linear Index[b]	n
Angled	5.2 ± 0.3	21.0 ± 1.0	0.25 ± 0.02	3
Coated	7.7 ± 0.3	18.0 ± 1.0	0.43 ± 0.03	3
Tapered	10.3 ± 0.8	13.7 ± 1.5	0.76 ± 0.13	3

[a] All comparisons between tips were statistically significant ($p < 0.05$).
[b] Linear index = myocardial depth of lesion/epicardial width of lesion.

Table 1. Lesion Measurements and Linear Indexa

Shape of lesion
Longitudinal sections showed that the longitudinal length of the lesions created by the three kinds of tips was preserved from the surface to the bottom. The cross-section of the lesion created by the tapered tip showed an elliptical shape. The coated tip created a cone-shaped lesion and the angled tip created a convex lesion at the center (Fig. 13).

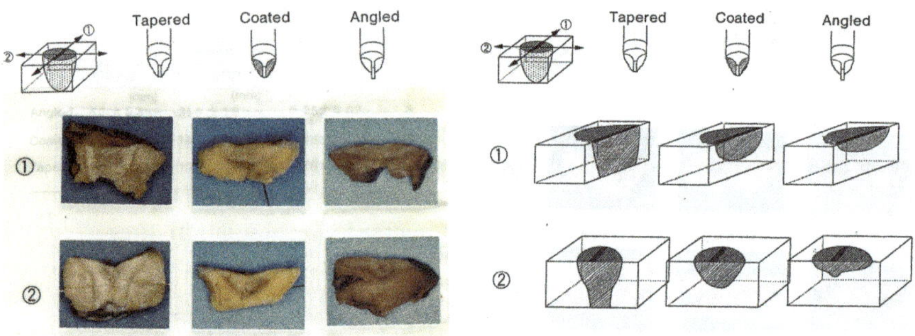

Fig. 13. Three kind of tips and shape of the lesion of the canine right ventricle
The cross-section of the lesion created by the tapered tip showed a transmural lesion.

Influence of tip pressure on the epicardium
When the probe merely touched the epicardium, the maximum depth of the lesion was 5.7 ± 0.3 mm at 21 seconds. By compressing the tip into the epicardium, it was possible to obtain a maximum of 1.8 times this depth at 21 seconds of ablation (Fig. 14).

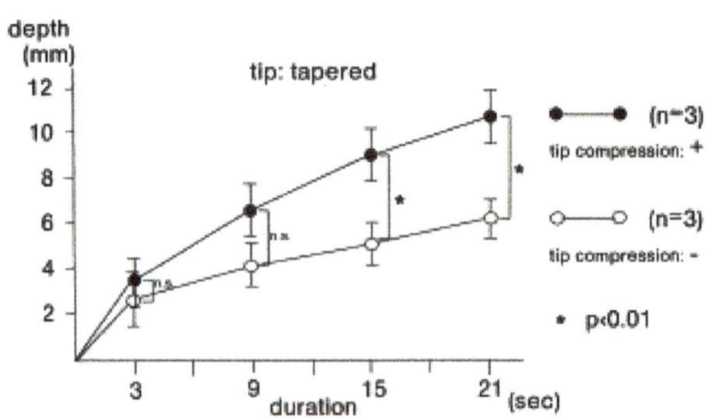

Fig. 14. Influence of tip pressure on the epicardium.
When the tip was pressed into the epicardium, the deeper lesion was created.

Histopathologic findings

The epicardium was preserved, and the ablated myocardium had well-demarcated photocoagulation necrosis without carbonization or vaporization. The nuclei of the myocardial fibers were concentrated. The myocardial fibers were atrophic and degenerated. The fundamental histopathologic structure was the same irrespective of whether ablation time was short or long (Fig. 15). All of the vessels were patent.

epicardium

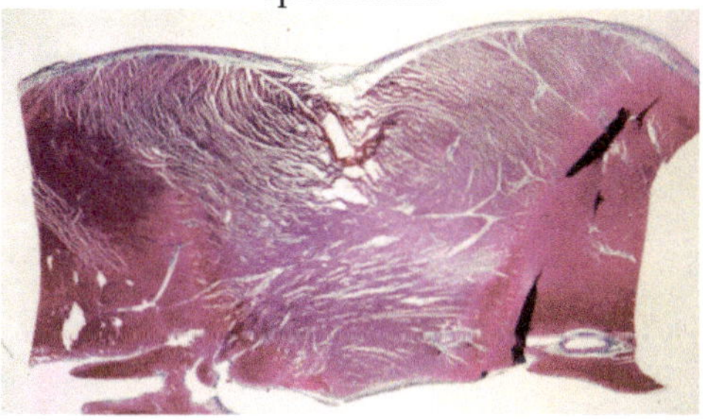

Fig. 15. Histopathologic findings of ventricular myocardium.
The ablated myocardium had well-demarcated photocoagulation. The vessels were patent. The lesion reached the endocardium with use of the tapered tip at 21 seconds.

Epicardial mapping

Before linear ablation on the right atrial wall, electrical potential was conducted regularly from the sinus node. After ablation, it was conducted from the node to the annulus of the tricuspid valve through the lateral side (intraatrial sulcus side) of the ablation area. Under overdrive pacing from the low right atrium, it was conducted from the low right atrium to the right atrial appendage through the lateral side of the ablation area (Fig. 16). Mapping after cutting and suturing the atrial wall showed the same pattern of conduction. Mapping 3 months after ablation also showed the same pattern of conduction.

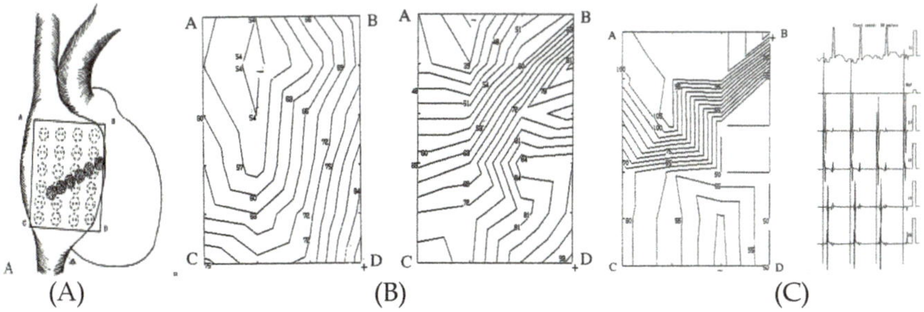

Fig. 16. Right atrial epicardial mapping
(A). Location of the electrodes. (B) The preablation map (left) and the postablation map (right) (sinus rhythm). The electrical conduction of the right atrium was blocked by the linear zone of photocoagulation. (C) Right atrial epicardial mapping (overdrive pacing from the low right atrium) (left) and electrocardiogram (right). Electrical potential conducted from the low right atrium to the right atrial appendage. The electrical conduction was blocked by the same area as in B. Electrodes 17 and 18 were on the lower side, and 19 and 20 were on the higher side near the lesions.

Histopathologic findings
The atrial epicardium was preserved. The ablated myocardium had well-demarcated transmural photocoagulation necrosis without carbonization or vaporization, as in the ventricular myocardium. The deposition of hemosiderin, invasion of macrophages, increased capillary vessels, and increased juvenile elastic fibers were observed in chronic phase. The myocardium did not revive. The endocardium was thickened, and elastic fibers also appeared (Fig. 17).

epicardium

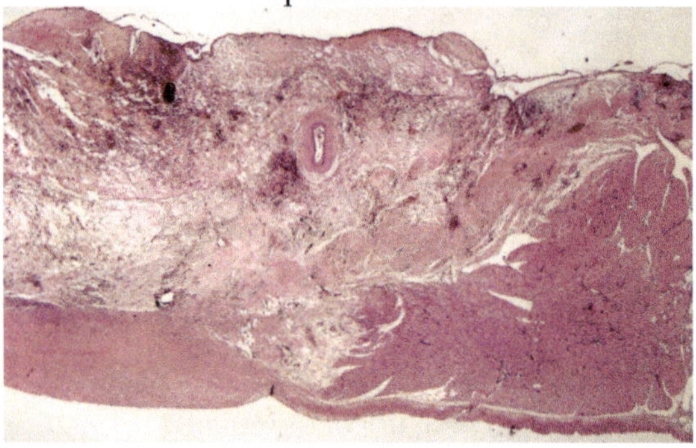

Fig. 17. Right atrial free wall 3 month after ablation
The endocardium was thickened. Density of juvenile elastic fibers was higher. The vessels were patent.

Comment
Since the maze procedure for treating atrial fibrillation was published (Cox et al., 1991), surgical treatment for atrial fibrillation has attracted considerable attention and become widespread.
An IRK-151 infrared coagulator was developed in Germany (Nath et al., 1976). In relation to arrhythmia, The electrocardiographic changes after photocoagulation using the IRK-151 were examined on sinus node, right bundle branch, and His bundle in canine heart (Nakajima, et al., 1982). Because the atrial wall is thinner than the ventricular wall, atrial coagulation should not cause carbonization or vaporization, to prevent perforation. In our experiment, infrared photocoagulation caused well-demarcated and homogeneous necrosis within the lesions, without carbonization or vaporization, and the epicardium remained intact. Comparison of precoagulation and postcoagulation atrial epicardial electrode mapping confirmed that transmural degeneration of the atrial wall caused electrical block concurrently.
Linear ablation is more efficient than continuous overlapped ablation with a round tip. Usually, the volume of the lesion is calculated according to a formula using the epicardial radius (a) and myocardial depth (b): Volume (oblate)=(1/2)(4/3) π a2b, and Volume (prolate)=(1/2)(4/3) π ab2, where for oblate, a > b and for prolate, a < b (Holman et al., 1983, Markovitz et al., 1988). This formula is not suitable for evaluating the efficacy of linear ablation as it is neither oblate nor prolate. A compact index (linear index=myocardial depth of lesion [mm]/epicardial width of lesion [mm]) was therefore devised. As the index increases, the ablation approaches linearity. Unexpectedly the tapered tip showed the highest index (0.76), and the coated tip the lowest index (0.43). This result may have

occurred because the nickel and tin dichloride coating the surface could not reflect the infrared rays perfectly, leading to heating of the tip surface. The degree of tip pressure on the myocardium is also important for determining the depth of the lesion. Our experiment showed that compressing the myocardium created a deeper lesion than merely touching it. The argon laser and neodymium:yttrium-aluminum garnet laser are used clinically for treatment of arrhythmia (Hendry et al., 1993, Svenson et al., 1987). These instruments are expensive and large, and it is difficult to obtain linear ablation. Furthermore, lasers may cause perforation of the thin atrial wall. The IRK-151 infrared coagulator produces well-demarcated lesions that are easily detected with the naked eye and whose depth is controllable by adjusting the duration of application. The depth was found to be adequate for atrial ablation aimed at blocking the conduction pathway. An average depth of 5 mm is created when a cryoprobe is applied to perfused dog epicardium for 90 to 120 seconds (Mikat E. et al., 1977). When the infrared coagulator was used, it took only 6 seconds to obtain the same depth of the lesion. The infrared-maze procedure can be done in a short time compared with the cryo-maze. Although the maximum length of the cryolesion at one application is 15mm, the infrared coagulator is capable to elongate the lesion length at one application by modifying the shape of the sapphire tip, light-conducting rod, and a reflector (Kubota et al., 1998).

2.2.2 Conventional maze procedure using an IRK- 151 infrared coagulator in canine model

The IRK- 151 infrared coagulator was employed to electrophysiologicany confirm the efficacy of this device under arrested heart in canine model.

Methods. The MAZE-Ill procedure was performed in four mongrel dogs. Instead of a pulmonary vein-encircling incision, IRK-151 was applied endocardially to create a continuouously overlapping circular lesion under the arrested heart using a cardiopulmonary bypass. After aortic declamping, the potentials of both atria were recorded using 18 bipolar electrodes implanted in the atrial wall (Fig. 18). The recording conditions were: 1) sinus rhytlm, 2) overdrive pacing from outside the encircling coagulation, and 3) overdrive pacing from inside the encircling coagulation. After the experiment, the bronchus and esophagus behind the coagulation point were excised, fixed and stained (HE, Azan).

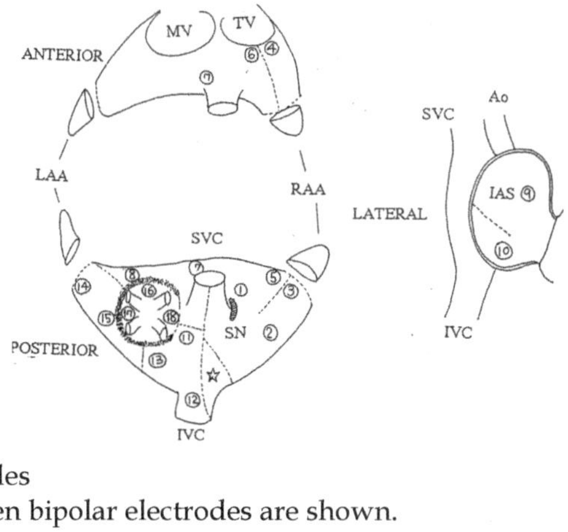

Fig. 18. Sites of electrodes
Inserted sites of eighteen bipolar electrodes are shown.

Results.
The mean aortic cross-clamping time was 26±10 min. The total infrared coagulation time was 4.1±0.6 min.
1) There was no detectable potential with the pulmonary vein-encircling coagulation. 2) There was no conduction of paced atrial potential inside the encircling coagulation. 3) Only the area within the encircling coagulation was activated by the stimulus. Other parts of the atrium showed sinus rhythm simultaneously (Fig. 19 A, B, C).

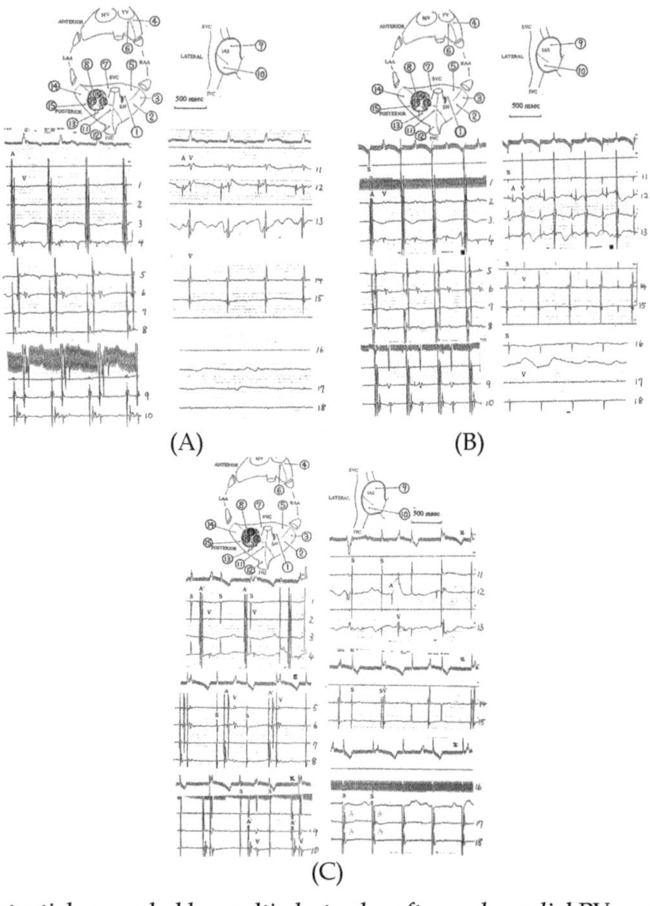

Fig. 19. Atrial potentials recorded by multi-electrodes after endocardial PV-encircling ablation (A) With the heart beating spontaneously, electrode no. 1 was the earliest activating point. The synchronous atrial potentials were detected in electrodes nos. 2-12. With electrodes nos. 13-18, no atrial potentials were detected. (B) With stimulation by electrode no. 1 (S-S interval: 500 msec), synchronous atrial potentials were detectedby electrodes nos. 1-13. No atrial potentials were detected by electrodes nos. 16-18. (C) With stimulation by electrode no. 16 (S-S interval: 500 msec), synchronous atrial potentials were detected by electrodes nos. 17 and 18. Electrodes nos 1-12 showed sinus rhythm. The bronchus and the esophagus near behind the coagulated left atrium showed no histopathological change.

Comment

Based on above results, it can be said that the pulmonary vein encircling area could be electrically isolated by endocardial coagulation under the cardioplegic arrested heart without collateral tissue damage (Kubota et al., 2000).

2.2.3 Epicardial maze procedure on the beating heart with an infrared coagulator KIRC-119

To make the treatment of AF less invasive, we applied this device to epicardial maze procedure on the beating heart in canine model, and in this study we attempted to electrophysiologically and pathologically confirm the efficacy of the method.

Material and Methods

Because the original IRK-151 contains a 3-second timer and the plastic body of the IRK-151 is not strong enough to tolerate the long coagulation time, we modified the coagulator to make it strong enough for atrial ablation by substituting a 40-second timer and changing the body from plastic to metal (Fig. 20).

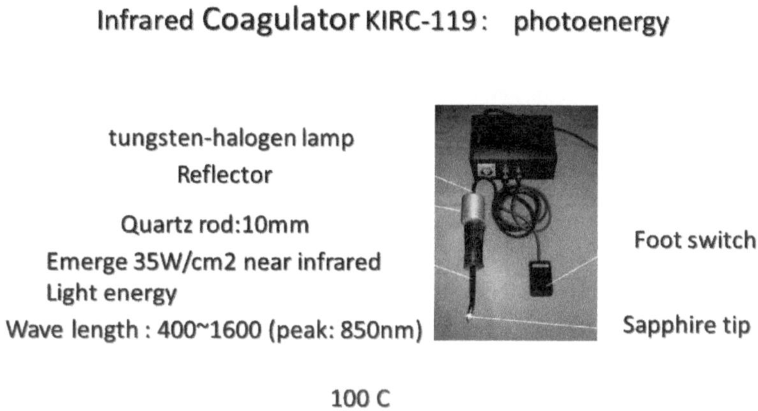

Fig. 20. KIRC-119: the plastic body has been replaced by a metal body to enable it to tolerate the long duration of the coagulation

Five mongrel dogs weighing 14.5 ± 2.3 kg were anesthesized with ketamine hydrochloride (20 mg/kg, intramuscularly) and sodium pentobarbital (16 mg/kg, intravenously), and were ventilated. After median sternotomy, both pleural cavities are openand the vagal nerves are exposed. The pericardium was then opened, and a bipolar electrode was attached to the right atrium. Sustained AF was induced preoperatively by bilateral vagal nerve stimulation (pulse width 0.2 ms, 3 V, 10 Hz) followed by 2 hours of burst stimulation of the atrium. A tape was passed around the SVC, another around the IVC, and a third around the ascending aorta and the main pulmonary artery through the transverse sinus. The tissue behind the SVC and IVC was carefully dissected to expose the left atrium; and after ligating and dividing the azygos vein, the infrared coagulation was performed. Instead of all the incisions of the maze III procedure, except the intraatrial septal incision, the infrared coagulator was applied epicardially to create continuous overlapping linear lesions. The duration of application for each ablation was 9 seconds, and a 10-mm lesion was created. After completion of all of the lesions, 11 bipolar electrodes were attached to the wall of each atrium (Fig 21 A). An electrocardiogram (ECG) and atrial potentials were recorded with an HPM 4500 polygraph (Fukuda Denshi, Tokyo, Japan).

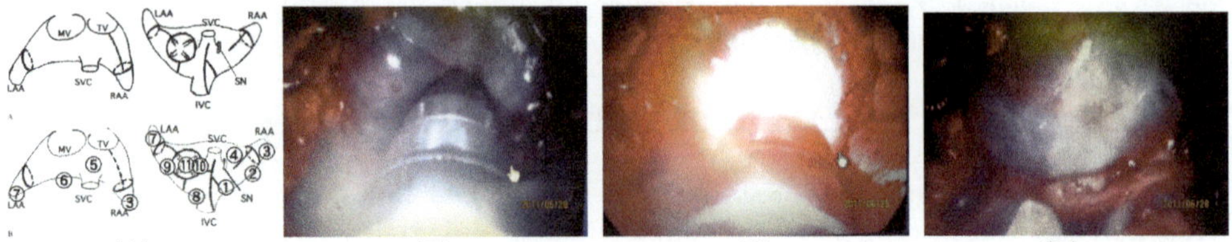

(A) (B) (C) (D)

Fig. 21. Lesion pattern and thoraciscopic view of infrared ablation
(A) Coagulation was performed along the incision line of the Maze III procedure, except intraatrial septal incision. After the procedure, 11 bipolar electrodes were placed in the atrial wall, and the potentials were recorded. (B-D) After the infrared ablation, atral free wall was discolored.

The recording conditions were as follows: (1) spontaneous beating; (2) overdrive pacing from the right atrial appendage (RAA); (3) overdrive pacing from the left atrial appendage (LAA); and (4) overdrive pacing from inside the PV encircling lesion.
After recording the atrial potentials, burst stimulation was applied in an attempt to induce AF. If it failed the first time, we tried two more times. After the experiment, the coagulated left atrial wall was excised, fixed, and stained (hematoxylin-eosin, AZAN), and histologic sections were examined microscopically.
Results
No potentials were detectable within the RAA, LAA, or PV encircling lesion during spontaneous beating, but other areas of the atrium exhibited sinus rhythm (Fig. 22 A). During overdrive pacing from the RAA, the atrial potential subsequent to the pacing was detected only in the RAA. Other areas exhibited sinus rhythm (Fig. 22 B). During overdrive pacing from the LAA, only the area within the LAA lesion was activated by the stimulus. Other areas exhibited sinus rhythm (Fig 22 C). During overdrive pacing from inside the PV encircling lesion, only the area within the PV encircling lesion was activated by the stimulus. Other areas exhibited sinus rhythm (Fig 22 D)

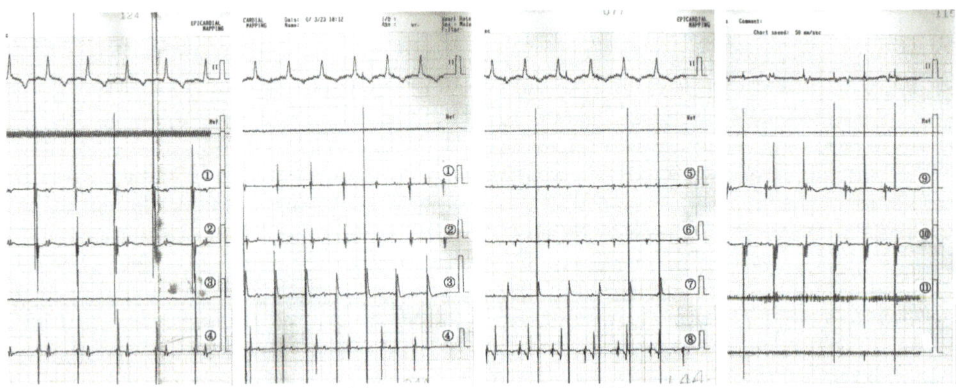

(A) (B) (C) (D)

Fig. 22. Atrial potential recorded by multi-electrodes.

(A) Atrial potential during spontaneous beating. No potential was detected within the right atrial appendage ([RAA] electrode no. 3). Other areas of the atrium exhibited sinus rhythm. No potentials were detected with the electrodes within the left atrial appendage (LAA) or pulmonary vein (PV) encircling lesion (electrodes nos. 7, 10, and 11) either. (B) During overdrive pacing from the RAA (electrode no. 3), only the area within the RAA lesion was activated by the stimulus. Other areas exhibited sinus rhythm.

(C) During overdrive pacing from the LAA (electrode no. 7), only the area within the LAA lesion was activated by the stimulus. Other areas exhibited sinus rhythm. (D) During overdrive pacing from inside the PV encircling lesion, only the area within the PV encircling lesion (electrode no. 10) was activated by the stimulus. Other areas exhibited sinus rhythm. Electrode no. 11 was used to stimulate the atrium.

None of the three areas inside the encircling lesion exhibited any potentials during sinus rhythm, and only these lesions were activated by the overdrive stimulus from inside the lesions. Other areas always exhibited sinus rhythm with or without the pacing from inside the encircling lesions. Although we tried to induce AF three times in each dog after completing the ablation, burst stimulation failed to induce AF in any of the dogs. Histologic examination showed preservation of both the endocardium and epicardium of the coagulated lesion. Well-demarcated transmurally degenerated myocardium was demonstrated (Fig.23).

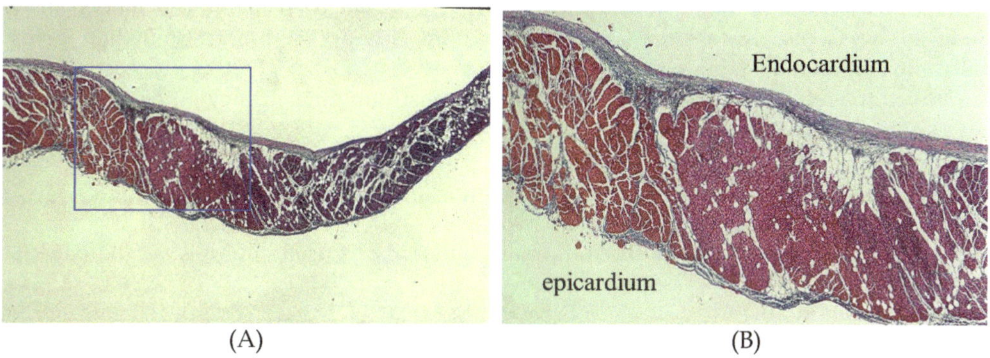

Fig. 23. Histologic changes in the left atrium.
(A) Well-demarcated transmurally degenerated myocardium was demonstrated. Both the endocardium and the epicardium were intact. (B) High-power field.

Burst stimulation did not induce AF in any of the dogs. No ST-T changes or arrhythmias occurred during ablation.

Comment

Is the warm beating heart more suitable for infrared coagulation than the cardioplegic arrested heart? The depth, width, and volume of the myocardium coagulated with a Nd-YAG laser were compared in the warm red beating heart and in the cold white nonbeating heart infused with 0°C saline (cardioplegic model) through the coronary artery (Ohtake et al., 1992). The depth, width, and volume of red myocardium coagulated were significantly greater than in the white myocardium, and the volume of white myocardium coagulated was about 60% of the volume of the red myocardium that was coagulated. They concluded that Nd-YAG laser energy was absorbed by the blood (red color indicates hemoglobin) and that a higher temperature was transmitted to the myocardium. Accordingly, because infrared rays are capable of producing photocoagulation that is equivalent to laser coagulation, the beating heart is preferable for obtaining efficient myocardial coagulation with infrared rays.

To develop a new ablation device, it is important to preserve the endocardium to prevent thromboembolism. Histologic examination revealed photonecrosis in the ablated myocardium without carbonization or vaporization, and the epicardium and the endocardium were intact. The photoenergy passes through them because both of them are translucent and when the energy reaches the myocardium, a higher temperature is transmitted. There are three encircling lesions in our procedure, one each in the RAA, LAA, and PV encircling lesion. All three lesions in our experiment were confirmed to be isolated electrophysiologically in all dogs, suggesting that the coagulator is capable of being used to make continuous transmural lesions in both atria. The intraatrial septum was not ablated in our procedure because cardiopulmonary bypass is necessary to expose the intraatrial septum. Although the contribution of the intraatrial incision to the effectiveness of the maze procedure is not well known, omitting the intraatrial ablation in our experiment did not interfere with prevention of AF induction. Vagus nerve and atrial burst stimulation were used to create a model of AF. Since the earliest mRNA induction that modifies the atrial potassium channel and shortens the atrial refractory period begins only 30 minutes after continuous burst stimulation (Yamashita et al., 2000), we tried creating a model of AF induced by vagus nerve stimulation followed by 2 hours of burst stimulation before ablation. A model of stable sustained AF was achieved in all dogs by this procedure, and it improved the reliability of our experiment in demonstrating the efficacy of the treatment of AF (Kubota et al., 2004).

2.2.4 Epicardial electrical isolation of the right atrial appendage on the beating heart with an infrared coagulator KIRC-119

We present a 1st case in which the infrared coagulator was used clinically on the patient's beating heart.

Case presentation

On August 25, 2005, a 63-year-old man was referred to our hospital because of a complaint of chest oppression. He was diagnosed with unstable angina pectoris. Emergency coronary angiography revealed 75% stenosis of the left main trunk, 60% stenosis of the proximal left anterior descending artery, and 60% stenosis of the middle portion of the left circumflex artery. The left ventricular ejection fraction was 0.40. Echocardiography showed anteroseptal hypokinesis of the left ventricle but no valvular dysfunction. The diameter of the left atrium was 34 mm. The electrocardiogram (ECG) showed ST depression in leads II, III, aVF, and V_2through V_6. No Q waves were detected. The ECG also showed atrial fibrillation (AF), and the maximum voltage of the f wave in V_1 was 0.2 mV. The serum creatine kinase-MB fraction level was 3.4 IU/L, and the serum troponin-I level was 0.96 ng/mL. According to his family physician, the patient had an 18-month history of AF. Because of his hemodynamic instability, an intraaortic balloon pump was inserted. After obtaining his informed consent, including to the use of the infrared coagulator to treat the AF, the patient was transferred to the operating room immediately after the coronary angiography and emergency coronary artery bypass grafting was performed. The pericardium was opened through a median sternotomy, and the cardiopulmonary bypass was established. The left ventricle was vented with a cannula inserted through the right superior pulmonary vein. Two CABGs with saphenous vein were performed, one to the left anterior descending coronary artery and the other to the left circumflex coronary artery. A left internal thoracic artery was not used because enzyme leakage was detected and it was thought that earlier revascularization would be better. Next, tapes was passed around the SVC, IVC, and the transverse sinus to achieve good left atrial exposure. A total CPB was established by snaring the tapes around the SVC and IVC.

Epicardial ablation was performed by applying the KIRC-119 infrared coagulator. The duration of the each application was 10 seconds: two ablations of 4 seconds, 2 seconds apart. Ablation was started in the RA. The root of the RAA was encircled, and the free wall of the RA was ablated from the RAA-encircling lesion to the IVC. Vertical ablation was performed from this coagulated line to the tricuspid annulus. The opposite side of the RA was ablated from the RAA-encircling lesion to the roof of the left atrium (LA), and a box lesion encircling the PV was created. Finally, the LAA was encircled, and a linear connecting lesion between the LAA-encircling lesion and the LA box lesion was created. After all of the lesions were completed, a pair of electrodes was sutured to the RAA and another pair to the free wall of the RA. Soon after returning the patient to the intensive care unit, an ECG and atrial potentials were recorded with an HPM 4500 polygraph (Fukuda Denshi, Tokyo, Japan). Two weeks later, ECGs were recorded in the same manner. The recording conditions were (1) spontaneously beating heart, (2) overdrive pacing from the RA free wall, and (3) overdrive pacing from the RAA.

The AF spontaneously converted to sinus rhythm during the operation. No potentials were detected within the RAA-encircling lesion during spontaneous beating, but the free wall of the RA exhibited potentials synchronous with the sinus rhythm (Fig.24 A). During overdrive pacing from the RA, the cardiac rhythm was synchronous with the pacing. Overdrive pacing from the RAA did not affect the cardiac rhythm, which was a sinus rhythm (Fig 24 B).

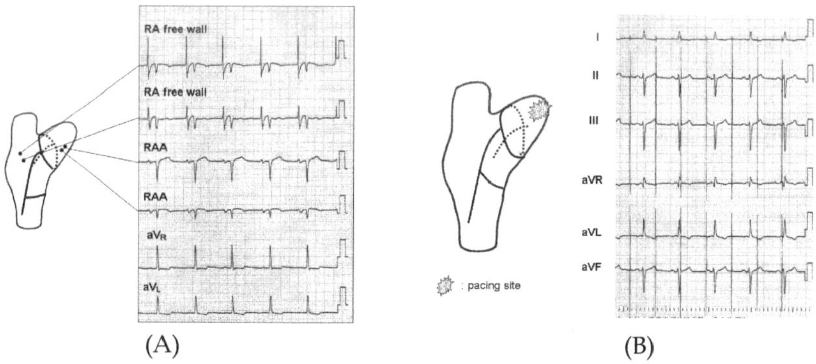

Fig. 24. Atrial potentials recorded by the attached electrodes.
(A) Atrial potentials synchronous with the sinus rhythm were detected at the right atrial free wall. No atrial potentials were detected within the right atrial appendage encircling lesion. Only the small smooth curve caused by RAA movement was seen. (B) Overdrive pacing from the right atrial appendage. The pacing did not affect the cardiac rhythm.

The results of the electrophysiologic study performed 2 weeks after the operation were the same. Persistent bidirectional block was confirmed. Regular sinus rhythm was confirmed by a postoperative 24-hour Holter monitor, and no supraventricular tachyarrhythmia was observed. An antiplatelet drug (aspirin, 81 mg/d) was started and continued. The patient recovered well, with no complications, and as of 3 years after the operation, his sinus rhythm has been maintained without the use of any antiarrhythmia drugs.

Second clinical application was performed under on-pump beating condition after ASD closure + TAP (Fig. 25). The right-side maze ablation was done epicardially. The patient restored sinus rhythm and it is maintained without antiarrhythmia drugs.

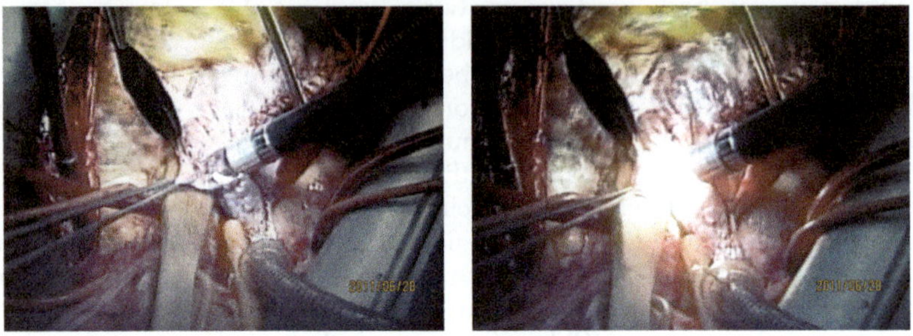

(A)

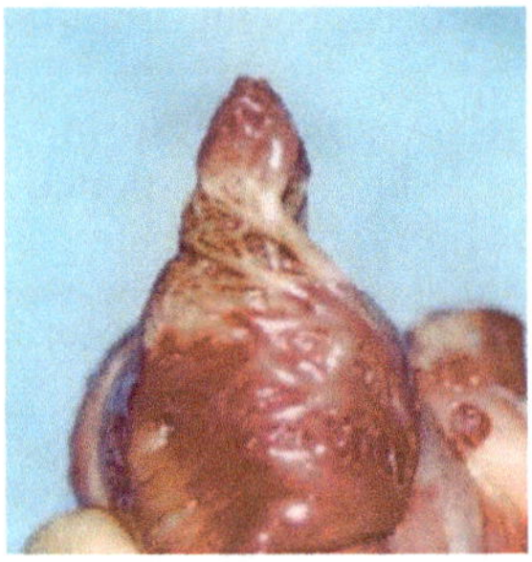

(B)

Fig. 25. Clinical application and internal appearance of the right atrial appendage in canine experiment.
(A) KIRC-119 enabled the creation of a continuous encircling transmural lesion. (B) Well-demarcated degenerated myocardium is seen. Note that all the complicated trabecular structures are discolored.

Comment

In the case reported here, the RAA was electrophysiologically isolated and the heart converted to sinus rhythm during the operation. The electrical block was confirmed immediately after the operation and again 2 weeks after the operation. We can conclude that the KIRC-119 coagulator created a continuous encircling transmural lesion in the RAA (Kubota et al., 2009).

3. Conclusions

In this chapter, the efficacy of two kinds of myocardial ablation energy source were examined and applied clinically. Using a hook-shaped cryoprobe, it was possible to create a bidirectional conduction block in canine PVs. LAVIE technique using a conventional cryo-system was capable to a certain extent to treat non-valvular AF without prolonging aortic cross-clamp time.

Infrared energy also could make a continuous transmural lesion on the atrium in a short time. Its efficacy was confirmed experimentally, clinically and electrophysiologically. It could make a transmural lesion even on the free wall of the beating warm atrium where the cryoablation is difficult to obtain enough depth of the lesion. As next steps, accumulation of clinical cases of beating maze procedure, and development of thoracoscopic maze procedure using KIRC-119 will be considered.

4. Acknowledgement

We thank Dr Isabelle Brazzalotto, Anesthesia Service, for her assistance in preparing the drawings, and Prof Eliane Albuisson, Biostatistics and Medical Informatics Service, University of Clermont-Ferrand, France, for statistical assistance. We are grateful for the assistance of Dr Bruno Miguel, Dr Benoit Legault, Prof Lionel Camilleri and Prof Charles de Riberolles, Cardiovascular Surgery, University of Clermont-Ferrand, in the preparation of the manuscript. We are also greatful to cardiac surgeons, University of Tokyo. These works were supported by a Grant-in-Aid for Scientific Research from the Japanese Ministry of Education and Science in 1994, 1995, 2000, and 2001 to 2003; a Japan Heart Foundation/Pfizer Grant for Cardiovascular Disease Research in 2000; and by the Fujita Memorial Fund for Medical Research in 2001.

5. References

Cox JL, Schessler RB, & Boineau JP. (1991) The surgical treatment of atrial fibrillation. I. Summary of the current concepts of the mechanisms of atrial flutter and atrial fibrillation. *J Thorac Cardiovasc Surg* 101, pp. 402–405. ISSN 00225223

Cox JL, Canavan TE, Schessler RB, Cain ME, Lindsay BD, Smith PK, Corr PB, & Boineau JP. (1991) The surgical treatment of atrial fibrillation. II. Intraoperative electrophysiologic mapping and description of the electrophysiologic basis of atrial flutter and atrial fibrillation. *J Thorac Cardiovasc Surg* 101, pp. 406–425. ISSN 00225223

Cox JL, Schessler RB, Dagostino HJ, Stone CM, Chang BC, Cain ME, Corr PB, & Boineau JP. (1991) The surgical treatment of atrial fibrillation. III. Development of a definitive surgical procedure. *J Thorac Cardiovasc Surg* 101, pp. 569–583. ISSN 00225223

Cox JL, The surgical treatment of atrial fibrillation. IV. Surgical technique. (1991) *J Thorac Cardiovasc Surg* 101, pp. 584–592. ISSN 00225223

Haïssaguerre M, Jaïs P., Shah DC, Takahashi A, Hocini M, Quiniou G, Garrigue S, Le Mouroux A,

Le Métayer P, & Clémenty J. (1998) Spontaneous initiation of atrial fibrillation by ectopic beats originating in the pulmonary veins, New Engl J Med 339, pp. 659–666., ISSN 00284793

Holman WL, Ikeshita M, Douglas JM, Smith PK, & Cox JL. (1983) Cardiac cryosurgery: effects of myocardial temperature on cryolesion size. *Surgery* 93, pp. 268–272. ISSN 00396060

Hendry PJ, Mikat EM, Anstadt MP, Plunkett MD, & and Lowe JE. Argon beam coagulation compared with cryoablation of ventricular subendocardium. *Ann Thorac Surg* 55 (1993), pp. 135–139. ISSN 00034975

Kubota H, Furuse A, Takeshita M, Kotsuka Y, & Takamoto S. (1998) Atrial ablation with an IRK- 151 infrared coagulator, Ann Thorac Surg 66, pp. 95–100. ISSN 00034975

Kubota H, Takamoto S, Takeshita M, Miyaji K, Kotsuka Y, & Furuse A. (2000) Atrial ablation using an IRK-151 infrared coagulator in canine model, *J Cardiovasc Surg* 4, pp. 835–847. ISSN 00219509

KubotaH, Takamoto S, Ohtsuka T, Nonaka K, Sato M, Fujiki K, & Sudo K. Efficacy of cryoablation in the beating heart in the treatment of atrial fibrillation, (2002) *Cardiovasc surg* 10 Suppl 1. P. 17 ISSN 09672109

Kubota H, Takamoto S, Morota T, Ohtsuka T, Motomura N, Kotsuka Y, & Sudo K. (2003) Epicardial pulmonary vein isolation by cryoablation as concomitant cardiac operation to treat nonvalvular atrial fibrillation, Ann Thorac Surg 75 pp. 590-593. ISSN 00034975

Kubota H, Takamoto s, Ohtsuka T, Endo H, Sato M, Fujiki T, & Sudo K. (2004) Epicardial pulmonary vein isolation with a hook-shaped cryoprobe to treat atrial fibrillation, *Ann Thorac Surg* 78, pp. 1056-1059. ISSN 00034975

Kubota H, Takamoto S, Furuse A, Sato M, Endo H, Fujiki T, & Sudo K. (2005) Epicardial maze procedure on the beating heart with an infrared coagulator, *Ann Thorac Surg* 80, pp. 1081–1086. ISSN 00034975

Mikat E, Hackel DB, Harrison L, Gallagher JJ, Wallace AG. (1977) Reactionof the myocardium and coronary arteries to cryosurgery. Lab. Invest 37: pp. 632-641. ISSN 00236837

Markovitz LJ, Frame LH, Josephson ME, & Hargrove WC. (1988) Cardiac cryolesions: factors affecting their size and a means of monitoring their formation. *Ann Thorac Surg* 46, pp. 531–535. ISSN 00034975

Nakajima M, Atsumi K, Furuse A, Shindo G, Kotsuka Y, & Saegusa M (1982), Studies on photocoagulation of accessory conduction pathway. *Kyobu Geka* 35, pp. 109–115. ISSN 00215252

Nath G, Kreitmair A, Kiefhaber P, & Moritz K. (1976) In: Neue infrarot-Koagulationsmethode. 9. Kongress der deutchen Gesellschaft für Endoscopie Perimed Verlag, *Erlangen*, p. 17.

Ohtake H, Watanabe G, Mukai K, Misaki T, Matsunaga Y, Matsumoto I et al. (1992) Basic study of myocardial coagulation by intraoperative laser ablation: In the presence and absence of blood. *Kyobu Geka* 45: 870-872. ISSN 00215252

Pappone C, Rosanio S, Oreto G, Tocchi M, Gugliotta F, Vicedomini G, Salvati A, Dicandia C, Mazzone P, Santinelli V, Gulletta S, & Chierchia S. (2000) Circumferential radiofrequency ablation of pulmonary vein ostia: a new anatomic approach for curing atrial fibrillation, *Circulation* 102 , pp. 2619–2628., ISSN 00097322

Svenson RH, Gallagher JJ, Selle JG, Zimmern SH, Fedor JM & Robicsek F. (1987) Neodymium: YAG laser photocoagulation: a successful new map-guided technique for the intraoperative ablation of ventricular tachycardia. Circulation 76, pp. 1319–1328. ISSN 00284793

Yamashita T, Murakawa Y, Hayami N, et al. (2000) Short-term effects of rapid pacing on mRNA level of voltage-dependent K(+) channels in rat atrium: electrical remodeling in paroxysmal atrial tachycardia. *Circulation* 25; 101: 2007-14. ISSN 00097322

17

Treatment of Atrial Fibrillation in Patients Undergoing Mitral Valve Surgery

Carlo Rostagno[1], Maria Brigitte Berioli[1] and Pier Luigi Stefàno[2]
[1]*Dipartimento Area Critica Università Firenze,*
[2]*Cardiochirurgia AOU Careggi Firenze,*
Italia

1. Introduction

Spontaneous sinus rhythm recovery occurs in not more than 10% of patients with preoperative atrial fibrillation and mitral valve disease who undergo mitral valve surgery (Kernis et al, 2004). In a recent review Lee et al (2009) reported that less than 20% of patients with permanent atrial fibrillation undergoing surgery without treatment of atrial fibrillation were in sinus rhythm at 6-8 months from operation. Persistence of atrial fibrillation (AF) is associated with a decreased exercise tolerance, an increased risk of systemic embolization (Reston & Shuahaiber, 2005) and an higher long-term mortality (Khargi et al 2005). Moreover 15% of patients in sinus rhythm before surgery are discharged in atrial fibrillation after treatment of mitral valve disease. At multivariate analysis an enlarged left atrium is associated with an increase risk of development of AF.

The surgical treatment of AF was proposed by James Cox in the1980s and evolved into the Maze III procedure (Cox et al, 1991). The aim of the intervention was to create numerous atrial surgical incisions that form a maze-like pattern, with the scar tissue providing a conduction block to interrupt propagation of the arrhythmia from sites of electrical instability and favouring the conduction from sinus node to atrio-ventricular node. The procedure involves surgical encircling of pulmonary veins at their entry in left atrium. A lesion between an inferior pulmonary vein and the mitral annulus, and a lesion joining the coronary sinus and the inferior vena cava are usually added to block other trigger zones, in particular in patients with permanent atrial fibrillation The left atrial appendages is excised or closed to prevent thromboembolism in the event of postoperative AF.

The surgical treatment proposed by Cox has been mainly used in patients with other heart disease with indication to surgery, however it was used also in patients with invalidating "lone atrial fibrillation " not responsive to pharmacological treatment.

Despite an high success rate, from 70% to 90% in relation to population treated, surgical Maze procedure has an elevated technical difficulty, prolongs significantly the times of cardiopulmonary by-pass, increases the risk of post-operatory bleeding and has a not negligible risk of mortality. The need for permanent pacing is close to 6%.

Sinus rhythm recovery allows the maintenance of atrial mechanic activity and prevents the development or worsening of tricuspid regurgitation (Je et al, 2008).

Preoperatory duration of atrial fibrillation and left atrial volume were independent factors related to sinus rhythm recovery (Benussi et al, 2002; Beukema et al, 2005; Chan et al, 2005).

In the following years, due to the complexity of the "cut and saw" Maze procedure, the research was directed to create the maze pattern with energy ablation rather than incisions (Benussi et al, 2001). These methods have simplified the procedure and increased its application. Energy sources used for intraoperative ablation include cryotherapy, radiofrequency, microwave, laser, and ultrasound.

Radiofrequency probes may be unipolar or bipolar (Williams et al, 2001; Gaynor et al, 2004). The main limitation of monopolar probes is the high probability to not obtain transmural lesions. Bipolar probes have an higher chance to obtain transmural lesions and a reduced risk of damaging adjacent structures such as the esophagus. (Bugge et al, 2005; Benussi et al, 2005). Moreover have been introduced devices for epicardial treatment which allows treatment for example in patients undergoing off-pump coronary revascularization. Irrigated radiofrequency probes have greater efficiency because the cooling effect on the surface of the tissue drives the focus of energy deeper into the tissue and prevents char accumulation on the surface. Radiofrequency treatment of atrial fibrillation usually prolongs the times of the intervention by no more of 20 minutes.

More recently bipolar radiofrequency probes have been introduced to treat "lone atrial fibrillation " through a mini invasive bilateral thoracotomy , thus avoiding the need for sternotomy and related complications (Wolf et al , 2005). Preliminary results are similar to that obtained with the traditional surgical approach.

Microwave energy creates deeper lesions than does radiofrequency energy in a similar length of time and may have more potential for epicardial application. Laser and ultrasound energy are still relatively new energy sources, but both may produce transmural lesions even through epicardial fat (Saltman et al, 2003).

2. Literature review

In patients undergoing combined mitral valve and Cox maze surgery, Cox et al (2004) reported 98% cure of AF, Prasad et al (2003) observed a greater than 90% freedom from AF in patients having a Cox maze procedure with concomitant surgery. In contrast, others have used a classic cut-and-sew technique and reported less success. Raanani et al (2001) recorded sinus rhythm in only 75% of patients a mean of 26 months after Cox maze and mitral valve surgery, which is similar to the Mayo Clinic experience of 74% freedom from AF at 2 years (Handa et al ,1999; Shaff et al 2000).

The use of RF energy for the creation of the atrial lesions of the Cox maze procedure was associated with significantly less freedom from AF both at hospital discharge and at follow-up (Stulak et al 2007).

The differences of the long-term success rate could be influenced other than by the differences among intraoperative variables, mainly by preoperative variables, such as concomitant valvular surgery and rheumatic valvular heart disease.

The surgical results of the maze procedure for AF associated with rheumatic mitral valve disease have been known to be less effective than for lone or non-rheumatic AF (Raanani et al, 2001). Few clinical studies in the literature compared the results of concomitant AF maze in open heart surgery with those of a concurrent control arm (that is leaving the AF untreated). A control is important to eliminate confounding variables that may influence results of the maze procedure and the determination of clinical outcomes. Absence of a control arm also does not allow discernment of the absolute effect of the maze surgery because we cannot know how many of the patients would convert to sinus rhythm spontaneously.

Wogk and Mak (2006) examited the results of seven matched-controlled and four randomized trials of Maze procedure associated with concomitant mitral valve surgery. In the matched-controlled studies freedom from AF was 77% to 95% in the maze group versus 4% to 53% in the control group at 2 to 8 years of follow-up. In matched-controlled studies 12-lead electrocardiography was used for rhythm evaluation. The four randomized studies reported a 78% to 88% freedom from AF in the maze group versus 20% to 40% in the control group at 1- to 1.5-year follow-up

About 20—30% of the patients who underwent maze procedures have shown recurrence of AF during the follow-up periods, and there are few reports showing mid- to long-term results and reporting predictors of the maze failure.

Je et al, (2008) showed that preoperative size of the LA larger than 60 mm, cardiothoracic ratio over 60%, fine AF wave in preoperative ECG, no early sinus restoration and SSA were found as independent predictors of maze failure in mid-term follow-up period at multivariate analysis. Patients with left atrial dimension 50 mm or greater had almost twice probability of experience late recurrence of AF.

Besides the acute end point (for example, PV isolation, demonstration of bidirectional block of linear lesions, non-inducibility of AF, etc), the more important result of any ablation strategy is the clinical efficacy in restoring SR without the need for further antiarrhythmic medication. However, comparison of clinical success has been hampered by the absence of a clear AF classification, adequate reporting of underlying cardiac conditions (such as coronary artery disease, heart failure, etc), and the use of symptomatic only follow-up. "Rhythm at last follow-up" may underestimate the recurrence of atrial arrhythmias in the follow-up period, and thus overestimate the success of the procedure. In a consent statement (Calkins et al, 2007) a minimum of sequential Holter recordings is advised, with more stringent recommendations for prospective trials (for example, 7 days of Holter recording or even implantable loop recording).

Finally a "prophylactic" maze procedure has been proposed for patients with preoperative sinus rhythm and a dilated left atrium undergoing surgery for mitral valve disease. The altered atrial tissue in these patients represents an arrhythmogenic substrate, with an high risk (approximately 40%) for the development of postoperative AF even after correction of the mitral valve disease. Clearly, the risks and benefits should be weighed before an additional procedure is performed, which carries intraoperative and long-term (Saad et al, 2003) adjuntive risks other the need of PPM implantation (new permanent pacemakers are required in 10% to 15% of patients) (Gillinov et al, 2004). The indication in almost all was bradycardia due to sinus node dysfunction. Technical modifications to the original Cox-maze operation may however reduce injury to the sinoatrial node.

2.1 Personal experience

In our Department the fist Cox maze radiofrequency (RF) ablation was performed in 2002 in one patient undergoing mitral valve repair. Since then at least 350 procedures, initially with monopolar thereafter with bipolar probes, have been performed, usually in association with mitral valve surgery but also with more complex interventions. In present paper we report the results of monopolar radiofrequency ablation in patients with atrial fibrillation undergoing mitral valve surgery.

At present, long terms results of AF radiofrequency ablation associated with mitral valve surgery are poorly defined in literature not allowing the definition of classes of recommendation and levels of evidence concerning the utility and efficacy of the procedure (Padalinam et al., 2005).

In present investigation we evaluated: overall mortality; cause and time of death ; incidence of stroke; maintenance of sinus rhythm; persistence of sinus rhythm during follow-up; eventual relapse of AF or the onset of other types of arrhythmias; the necessity of permanent pacing after the procedure; further hospitalization due to cardiac complications; . We even evaluated the relationship between several clinical and echocardiographic parameters and long term clinical outcome.

2.1.1 Material and methods

Patient population.

From 1/1/2002 to 31/12/2007, 173 patients with AF and mitral valve disease underwent monopolar radiofrequency ablation procedure, associated with mitral valve surgery in the heart surgery Deparment of the Azienda Ospedaliera Universitaria di Careggi (AOUC).

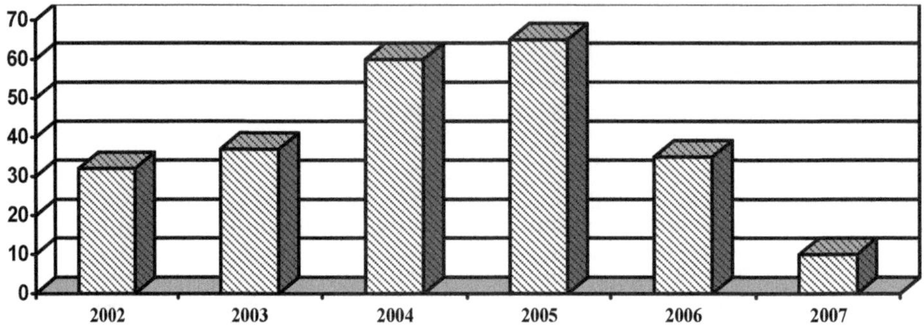

Fig. 1. Monopolar radiofrequency ablation at Florence Heart Surgery Department

In the study were included 101 men and 72 women, with a mean age of 67 +/- 9 years.
81.7% were in permanent AF (mean duration 38 +/- 43 months) while 18.3% suffered from paroxysmal AF.

A careful clinical evaluation was performed before surgery in order to establish time of onset of AF and NHYA functional class. Electrocardiographic examination was performed to confirm the presence of the arrhythmia.

All patients underwent transthoracic echocardiography using a 2.5 and 3.5 MHz probe (Sequoia C256 Acuson Siemens Mount View, California). Parameter measured were : left atrium M-mode AP diameter (mm) and 2D area (cm^2) and right atrium 2D area (cm^2) from four chamber projection, left ventricular ejection fraction (LVEF)- average value of three measurements. End-diastolic and end-systolic images were synchronized on ECG tracings.

Pulmonary systolic pressure (PAP) was calculated adding RV/RA pressure gradient to estimated right atrial pressure.

For statistical analysis were recorded:

- the surgical procedure (valve replacement with mechanical or biologic valve vs. mitral valve repair; associated surgical procedures).
- associated tricuspid valve repair
- need for electrical cardioversion before discharge.
- need for permanent pacing
- ECG rhythm at the time of discharge. After surgery patients were evaluated after the first and sixth months and later once a year. At every visit we performed a clinical, electrocardiographic and echocardiographic examination. In addition to previously reported parameters in patients in sinus rhythm right and left E and A waves amplitude and E/A ratio were measured to evaluate atrial mechanical activity.

The study was terminated on December 31 2010. Overall duration of follow-up has been 1743 +/- 845 days.

Maze Procedure

The Medtronic Cardioblate surgical ablation system consists of a power generator and a pen. The pen is a handheld, unipolar RF ablation device. The electrode tip is irrigated with saline that cools the tissue and provides a low-impedance path, which allows creation of deeper lesions with less damage to the surrounding tissue The patient is grounded by an indifferent electrode applied to the skin. After median sternotomy, cardiopulmonary bypass (CPB) was established with bicaval and aortic cannulation under moderate hypothermia (32°C); myocardial protection was assured by antegrade crystalloid cardioplegia. The aorta was cross-clamped and the heart was arrested with cold cardioplegic solution. Access to the inside of the left atrium was gained through a standard atriotomy in the interatrial groove, as for a mitral valve (MV) procedure. After the LAA was excised and sutured, an ablation line from the LAA to the left superior pulmonary vein was created. In addition to the incision in the interatrial groove, isolation of the right pulmonary veins was completed by a circular ablation line. The left pulmonary veins were encircled. Two linear ablations were performed endocardially. The first connected the two encirclings on the posterosuperior atrial wall. This lesion was kept cranial, opposite the transverse sinus, to prevent any possible damage to the esophagus. The last ablation connected the left appendage to the posterior aspect of the mitral annulus. To protect the circumflex artery from heat trauma, the lesion line reached the mitral posterior annulus far from the antero-lateral commisure (figure 2). The transesophageal echocardiographic probe was removed during the ablation to prevent any

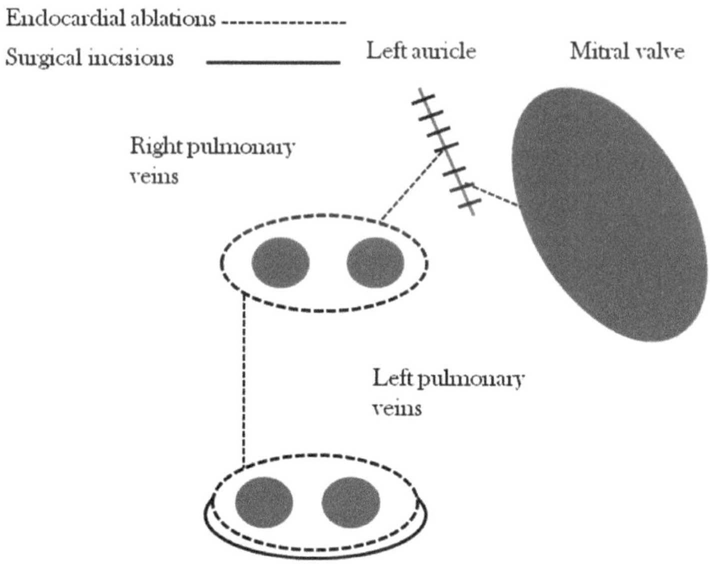

Fig. 2. Modified RF Maze procedure - schematic representation of ablation lines

damage by the transmission of the heat waves to the esophagus. The mitral valve procedure was completed and the left atriotomy was sutured in the standard fashion.

Postoperative Management

Antiarrhythmic prophylaxis was carried out on a routine basis. Amiodarone, intravenous bolus of 300 mg, followed by a continuous infusion of 1,200 mg/24 h f was administered in the first 48 hours; thereafter were prescribed 200 mg every 8 hours until discharge, followed by a maintenance regimen of 200 mg/day for 1 month. Recurrences of the arrhythmia after surgery were treated by optimizing the medical treatment. Patients who had AF despite optimal medical therapy had at least one attempt of external cardioversion by biphasic DC-shock Successful treatment of the arrhythmia was defined as the absence of refractory AF in patients with chronic AF before operation and absence of any episode of sustained arrhythmia in patients with paroxysmal AF preoperatively. Six months after surgery, oral anticoagulants were discontinued in patients with stable SR and with documented atrial contraction after mitral valve repair or replacement with a biological prosthesis.

2.1.2 Statistical analysis

Data are presented as means +/- SDs for continuous variables and as percentages for categorical variables. Continuous variables were compared through the use of Student's 2 tailed unpaired-sample test. Categorical variables were compared using the chi-square test or Fisher's exact test if appropriate.Kaplan-Meier curves were used for the survival analysis. Differences between groups were compared using Log-Rank test.

A probability value < 0.05 was considered significant. Statistical analysis were performed with SPSS 18.0 software (SPSS, Inc., Chicago, IL, USA).

2.1.3 Results

Four patients died in the immediate postoperative period (2,3%). One patient died for cerebral hemorrhage, one for myocardial infarction, the other 2 for septic shock.

Therefore 169 patients, 99 men and 70 women, were included in the study. Clinical and echocardiographic characteristics are reported in table 1.

Sex (M/F)	99/70
Age (years)	67 +/-9
AF duration before surgery (months)	38 +/- 43
Left ventricular EF (%)	52 +/- 10
Left atrium diameter (mm)	53.6 +/- 7
Left atrium area (cm^2)	32.5 +/- 10
Right atrium area (cm^2)	22.3 +/- 6.7
Systolic pulmonary pressure (mmHg)	45 +/- 15
NHYA class	3 +/- 0.55

Table 1. Clinical and echocardiographic characteristics

	N°	%
Mitral valve prolapse	48	28.6
Rheumatic mitral valve disease	57	33.9
Mitro-aortic rheumatic valve disease	25	15
Ischemic mitral regurgitation	20	11.9
Mitral regurgitation associated with DCM	6	3.5
Other	12	7.1

Table 2. Etiology of mitral valve disease. DCM= dilated cardiomyopathy

Rheumatic mitral valve disease, alone or associated with aortic valve disease, was the most frequent indication to surgery (73/169), followed by mitral valve prolapse (table 2)
Mitral valve repair was performed in 46 %. In combined mitro-aortic valve disease, aortic valve replacement was combined with mitral valve replacement in more than 60% of patients and with mitral valve repair in the remaining cases. Twenty (12%) patients underwent associated CABG (figure 2).

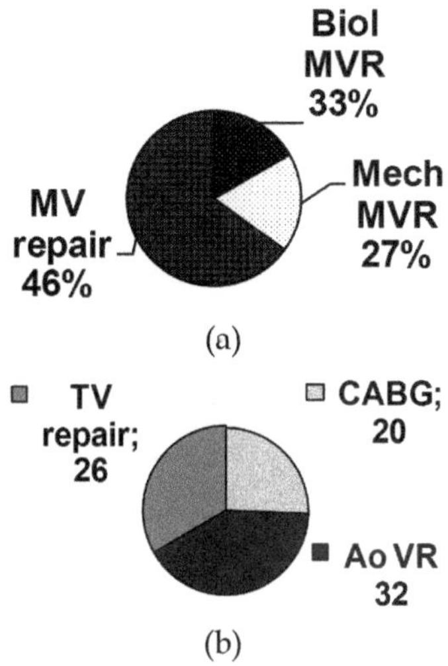

Fig. 3. a) Main surgical procedure (%) b) associated surgery (n°).

26/169 (15%) patients underwent tricuspid valve repair for severe tricuspid regurgitation most (>85%) according to Kay technique. At the time of surgery almost 80% of patients had severe functional impairment (III-IV NHYA class).

NYHA class before surgery		%
I	0	0
II	27	16
III	116	69
IV	24	15

Table 3. Functional NYHA class before surgery

Rhythm analysis.
119/169 subjects (70%) were in sinus rhythm at hospital discharge , while sinus rhythm was present in 100 at the end of follow up period. Atrial fibrillation was never resolved in 39. During the period of follow up 42% of patients has been in stable sinus rhythm, while 34 % had at least one symptomatic AF recurrence. 7,8% developed arrhythmias different from AF.

Stable sinus rhythm N (%)	AF recurrence N (%)	Permanent AFN (%)
72 (42%)	58 (34%)	39 (24%)

Table 4. Number an percentage of patients with stable sinus rhythm (SR), with AF recurrence and persistent atrial fibrillation (AF)

	Stable sinus rhythm	AF recurrences	Permanent AF	P
Age (years)	68.1 +/- 9.6	67.7 +/- 9.8	71.5 +/- 8	0.0494
Left atrium diameter (mm)	51.6 +/- 6.6	54.2 +/- 8.3	55.5 +/- 8.2	<0.0001
Left atrium area (cm^2)	30.4 +/- 7.2	32.8 +/- 8.5	36.9 +/- 14.5	<0.0001
Right atrium area (cm^2)	20.6 +/- 4.5	22.2 +/- 6.3	23.7 +/- 6.2	<0.0159
Systolic PAP (mmHg)	41.2 +/- 12.8	44.7 +/- 15.3	45.3 +/- 15.8	<0.0001
Electrical CV before discharge (%)	9.5	20.5	28.6	0.0092
Hospitalizations (%)	17.4	48.4	30.8	<0.0001

Table 5. Comparison of baseline clinical and echocardiographic parameters in patients with stable sinus rhythm (SR), with AF recurrence and permanent atrial fibrillation (AF)

On average AF recurrence occurred 750 days after surgery.

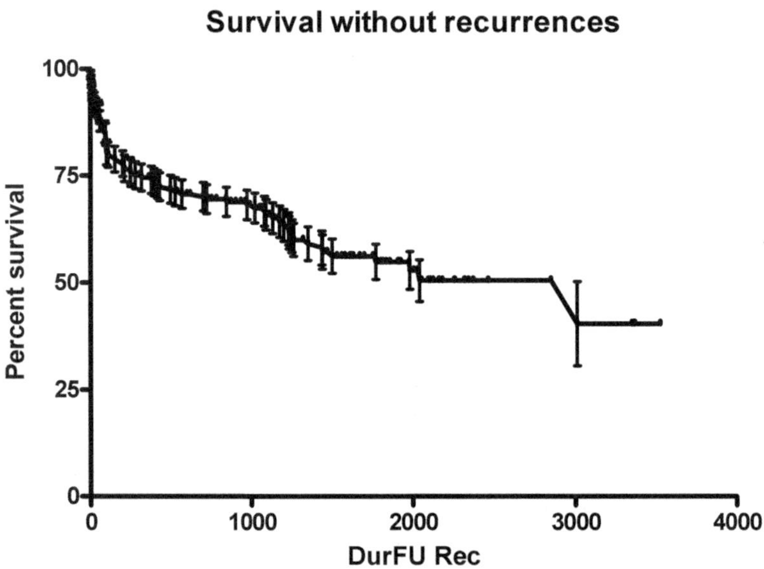

Fig. 4. Survival free from AF recurrences in patients with SR at hospital discharge

In table 5 are reported the clinical and echocardiographic characteristics of the three groups of patients (stable sinus rhythm; AF recurrences; permanent AF) at enrolment.
Patients who were in chronic AF were on average older (3 years) than those who never had AF recurrences or who remained in permanent sinus rhythm (p=0,0494; figure 5).

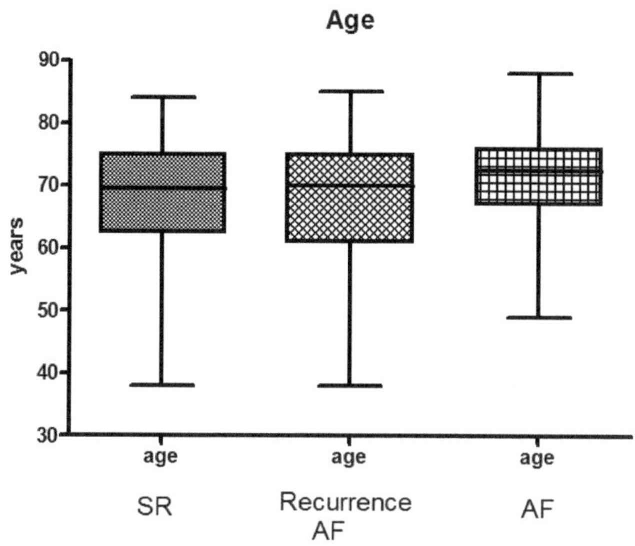

Fig. 5. Baseline mean age in patients in stable sinus rhythm (SR), with AF recurrence and permanent atrial fibrillation (AF)

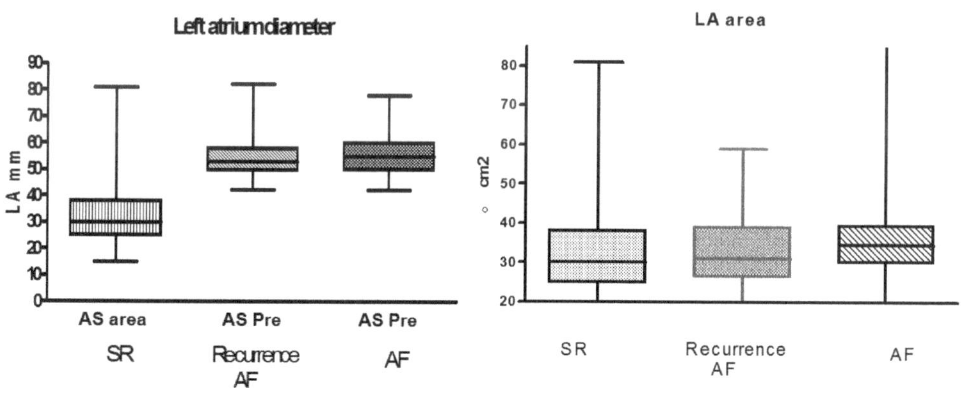

Fig. 6. Baseline left atrium diameter (left) and area (right) in patients in stable sinus rhythm (SR), with AF recurrence and permanent atrial fibrillation (AF)

Left atrium diameter ($p=0,0001$; figure 6,a), left atrium area ($p<0,0001$; figure 6,b) and right atrium area ($p<0,0159$) resulted significantly lower in patients with permanent sinus rhythm in comparison with the other two groups.

Estimated systolic pulmonary artery pressure was higher in patient with AF recurrences or in chronic AF than in those with permanent sinus rhythm ($p<0,0001$; figure 7).

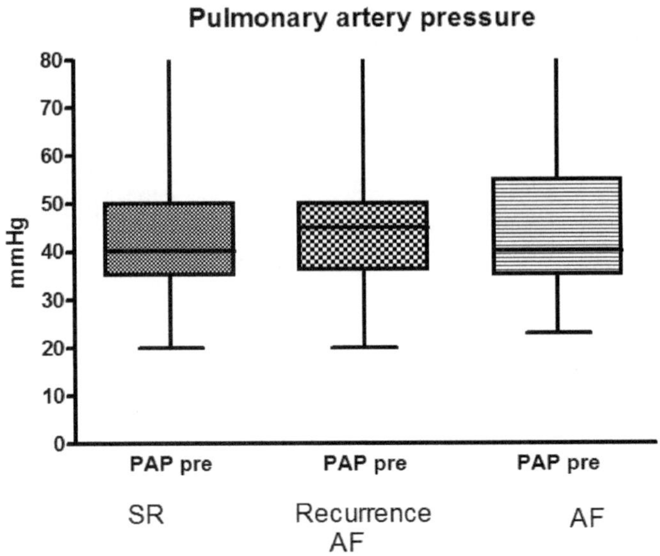

Fig. 7. Baseline systolic pulmonary artery pressure in patients in stable sinus rhythm (SR), with AF recurrence and permanent atrial fibrillation (AF)

The number of patients who needed electrical cardioversion before hospital discharge was significantly lower in the group with stable sinus rhythm than in the other groups (p= 0.005). Twenty-three patients underwent definitive cardiac electrical stimulation. In 6 patients permanent pacing was needed during hospitalization. In 17 a pace maker was implanted during follow-up period. 3,5% had at least one cerebrovascular accident during the postoperative period.

Baseline mean NYHA class was 2.96 in SR and 3.3 in AF patients. At follow-up a significant improvement was found in SR patients (average NYHA class 1.31 vs 2.33, $p<0.003$).

	NYHA class before surgery	NYHA class at follow-up
I	0	47
II	27	68
III	116	31
IV	24	5

Table 6. NYHA functional class before surgery and at follow-up

33,9% underwent hospitalization due to cardiac cause during the follow up period. Hospitalization percentage was almost twofold in patients with chronic AF compared to patients in sinus rhythm ($p<0.0001$).

Mortality

At the end of the average five years follow-up period survival was 86.4%.

Twenty three patients died: in 62% death was due cardiac causes, in the other 38% the cause of death was not cardiac or unknown. Death occurred on overage occurred days after surgery.

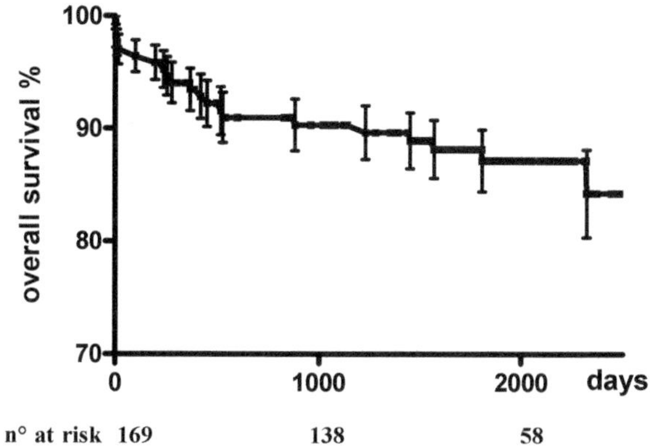

Fig. 8. Actuarial survival curve in patients undergoing RF ablation of AF associated with mitral valve surgery.

Deceased patients were about 5 years older than survivors (mean age of 67 years vs 72 years in the group of deceased patients, p=0.005).
Mortality was higher in men than in women (23% vs 9%).
Time free from AF recurrences, right and left atrial are were related to higher mortality.

	Survived	dead	P
AF duration before surgery (months)	37 +/-48	46 +/-46	0.31
Time free from AF recurrence (day after surgery)	937 +/-738	422 +/-485	0.015
LVEF (%)	52+/- 9	52 +/- 10	0.83
Left atrium diameter (mm)	53,4 +/-9	56 +/- 11	0.17
Left atrium area (cm^2)	31,1 +/- 7	38 +/- 10	0.0116
Right atrium area (cm^2)	21,6 +/- 6	24,5 +/- 9	0.0128
Systolic pulmonary pressure (mmHg)	44 +/- 14	48 +/- 17	0.26

Table 7. Comparison of clinical and echocardiographic parameters between patients survived and went to death

Overall long-term mortality was higher in patients with rheumatic than in those suffering from mitral valve prolapse (table 8).

Etiology	Mortality n (%)
Mitral valve prolapse	4 (8.8%)
Rheumatic mitral valve disease	13 (22%)
Mitro-aortic rheumatic valve disease	2 (8%)
Ischemic mitral regurgitation	3 (15%)
Mitral regurgitation associated with DCM	1 (16%)
Other	0 (0%)

Table 8. Relationship between mortality and etiology of mitral valve disease

Relationship between mortality and type of procedure performed is illustrated in table 9:

Intervention	Mortality n (%)
Mitral valve replacement (mechanical)	5 (20%)
Mitral valve replacement (biological)	5 (17%)
Mitral valve repair	7 (12%)
Mitral valve replacement/repair plus aortic valve replacement	1 (4%)
Mitral valve repair plus CABG	3 (16%)
Mitral valve replacement plus CABG	2 (40%)
Other	0 (0%)

Table 9. Relationship between mortality and type of intervention performed

Tricuspid valve repair was significantly associated with an higher mortality: it was performed in 40% of deceased patients in comparison to 12% of survivors (p= 0.005).
Preoperative NHYA class was not statistically related to survival. The percentage of patients in advanced NHYA class (III-IV) was similar in the two groups (82% of survivors vs 91 % of patients went to death).

NYHA class	Survived (%)	Dead (%)
I	0	0
II	25	2
III	102	15
IV	19	6

Table 10. Relationship between mortality and NYHA class before surgery

Failure to restore sinus rhythm with RF ablation was related to a worse prognosis. Mortality at five years was 30% in patients discharged form hospital in AF in comparison to 10% of those discharged in sinus rhythm.
Moreover survival was higher in patients with stable sinus rhythm during follow up respect to patients with recurrences and finally patients with permanent AF (table 10).
Figure 9 shows the survival curves in patients with persistent sinus rhythm, patients with AF recurrences and patients with permanent AF (Log Rank test-p=0.0022).

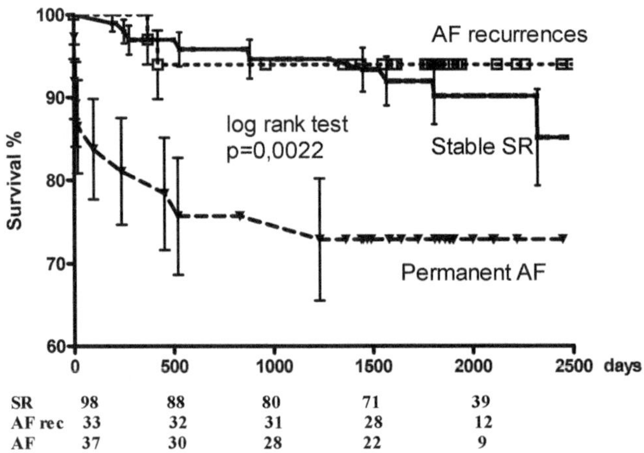

Fig. 9. Kaplan-Meier survival curves in in patients in stable sinus rhythm (SR), with AF recurrence and permanent atrial fibrillation (AF)

3. Conclusion

The ideal goal of AF surgery is a safe, simple, effective, and tailored approach to eradicate the most likely mechanism of AF. New technologies in AF surgery have evolved in creating the lines of block faster, easier, safer, and transmurally.

The merits of various alternative energy sources used to create the lines of block of the maze are subject of debate. But more important AF surgery should be able to demonstrate that mantainance of SR is associated with improved clinical outcomes. Results from our investigation support the hypothesis that in patients remained in sinus rhythm after RF ablation not only the quality of life is improved, as demonstrated by the lower NYHA functional class in patients with stable SR in comparison to patients with permanent AF, but also significantly affects mortality. Properly conducted, larger, randomized studies with adequate follow-up however are needed to determine the true impact of concomitant maze surgery on clinical outcomes.

4. References

Benussi S. (2004). Treatment of atrial fibrillation. *Eur J Cardiothorac Surg.* 26 [suppl 1]:S39-S41.

Benussi S. & Alfieri O. (2006). Off-pump connection of the pulmonary veins with bipolar radiofrequency: toward a complete epicardial ablation. *J Thorac Cardiovasc Surg.* 132:177-178.

Beukema WP, Elvan A, Hauw TS, & al. (2005) Successful radiofrequency ablation in patients with previous atrial fibrillation results in a significant decrease in left atrial size. *Circulation* 112:2089-2095.

Bugge E, Nicholson IA & Thomas SP. (2005) Comparison of bipolar and unipolar radiofrequency ablation in an in vivo experimental model. *Eur J Cardiothorac Surg* 28:76-80.

Calkins H, Brugada J, Packer DL, et al, (2007) Heart Rhythm Society, European Heart Rhythm Association, European Cardiac Arrhythmia Society, American College of Cardiology, American Heart Association, Society of Thoracic Surgeons. HRS/EHRA/ECAS expert consensus statement on catheter and surgical ablation of atrial fibrillation: recommendations for personnel, policy, procedures and follow-up. A report of the Heart Rhythm Society (HRS) Task Force on Catheter and Surgical Ablation of Atrial Fibrillation developed in partnership with the European Heart Rhythm Association (EHRA) and the European Cardiac Arrhythmia Society (ECAS); in collaboration with the American College of Cardiology (ACC), American Heart Association (AHA), and the Society of Thoracic Surgeons (STS). Endorsed and approved by the governing bodies of the American College of Cardiology, the American Heart Association, the European Cardiac Arrhythmia Society, the European Heart Rhythm Association, the Society of Thoracic Surgeons, and the Heart Rhythm Society. *Europace* 9:335–79.

Chen MC, Chang JP, Chang HW & al. (2005) Clinical determinants of sinus conversion by radiofrequency maze procedure for persistent atrial fibrillation in patients undergoing concomitant mitral valvular surgery. *Am J Cardiol.* 96:1553-1557.

Cox JL, Boineau JP, Schuessler RB, & al. (1993) Five year experience with the Maze procedure for atrial fibrillation. *Ann Thorac Surg.* 56:814–824.

Cox JL, Ad N, Palazzo T, Fitzpatrick S, Suyderhoud JP, DeGroot KW & al. (2000). The Maze-III procedure combined with valve surgery. SeminThorac Cardiovasc Surg. 12:53-5.

Cox JL. (2004). Cardiac surgery for arrhythmias. *J Cardiovasc Electrophysiol.* 15:250-262.

Gaynor SL, Diodato MD, Prasad SM, & al. (2004) A prospective, single-center clinical trial of modified Cox maze procedure with bipolar radiofrequency ablation. *J Thorac Cardiovasc Surg.* 128:535-542.

Gillinov AM & McCarthy PM. (2004) Advances in the surgical treatment of atrial fibrillation. *Cardiol Clin.* 22:147-157.

Handa N, Schaff HV, Morris JJ, Anderson BJ, Kopecky SL & Enriquez- Sarano M. (1999) Outcome of valve repair and the Cox maze procedure for mitral regurgitation and associated atrial fibrillation. *J Thorac Cardiovasc Surg.* 118:628-35

Hyung GJ, Jae WL, Sung HJ, Suk JC, Hyun S, Sung CY & Cheol HC. (2009) Risk factors analysis on failure of maze procedure: mid-term results. *Eur J of Cardiothor Surg* 36 272–279

Je HG, Song H, Jung SH, Choo SJ, Song JM, Kang DH, Yun SC, Chung CH, Song JK & Lee JW. (2008) Impact of the Maze operation on the progression of mild functional tricuspid regurgitation.*J Thorac Cardiovasc Surg.* Nov;136(5):1187-92.

Kernis SJ, Nkomo VT, Messika-Zeitoun & al. (2004) Atrial fibrillation after surgical correction of mitral regurgitation in sinus hythm: incidence, outcome, and determinants. *Circulation* 110:2320 –5

Khargi K, Hutten BA, Lemke B &Deneke T.(2005) Surgical treatment of atrial fibrillation: a systemic review. *Eur J Cardiothorac Surg.* 27:258-265.

Lee R, Kruse J & McCarthy PM. (2009) Surgery for atrial fibrillation. *Nat Rev Cardiol.* 6:505-513.

Padalinam BJ, Prystowsky E. (2005) Should ablation be first-line therapy and for whom: The antagonist position. *Circulation.* 112:1223-1229.

Prasad SM, Maniar HS, Camillo CJ, Schuessler RB, Boineau JP, Sundt TM 3rd, & al. (2003) The Cox maze III procedure for atrial fibrillation:long-term efficacy in patients undergoing lone versus concomitant procedures. J Thorac Cardiovasc Surg. 126:1822-8.

Raanani E, Albage A, David TE, Yau TM & Armstrong S. (2001) The efficacy of the Cox/maze procedure combined with mitral valve surgery: a matched control study. *Eur J Cardiothorac Surg.*;19:438-42

Reston JT & Shuhaiber JH (2005) Meta-analysis of clinical outcomes of maze-related surgical procedures for medically refractory atrial fibrillation . *Eur J Cardiothor Surg* 28;724-730

Saad EB, Rossillo A, Saad CP & al (2003) Pulmonary vein stenosis after radiofrequency ablation of atrial fibrillation: functional characterization, evolution, and influence of the ablation strategy. *Circulation.* 108:3102-3107.

Saltman AE &Gillinov AM (2009).Surgical approaches for atrial fibrillation. *Cardiol Clin.* Feb;27(1):179-88

Schaff HV, Dearani JA, Daly RC & al. (2000) Cox maze procedure for atrial fibrillation. The Mayo Clinic experience. *Semin Thorac Cardiovascular Surg* 12:30-37.

Stulak JM, Dearani JA, Sundt TM III, Daly RC, McGregor CGA, Zehr KJ & Schaff HV. (2007) Superiority of cut-and-sew technique for the Cox maze procedure: Comparison with radiofrequency ablation. *J Thorac Cardiovasc Surg* 133:1023-7

Williams MR, Stewart JR, Bolling SF & al. (2001) Surgical treatment of atrial fibrillation using radiofrequency energy. *Ann Thorac Surg.* 71:1939-1944.

Wolf RK & Gillinov AM. (2005) Surgical ablation of atrial fibrillation. *Prog Cardiovasc Dis.* 48(3):169-177.

Wong JJW & Mak KH. (2006) Impact of Maze and Concomitant Mitral Valve Surgery on ClinicalOutcomes *Ann Thorac Surg* 82:1938-1947

18

Acetylcholine-Activated Potassium Channel as a Novel Target for AF Treatment

Norio Hashimoto
Nissan Chemical America Corporation, USA

1. Introduction

Atrial fibrillation (AF) is the most frequently encountered cardiac arrhythmia in the clinical practice with prevalence of over 2,200,000 and 1,300,000 in the United States and Japan, respectively. The prevalence of AF is strongly age dependent; less than 1% of individuals aged <60 years, but approximately 5% of those older than 65 years and about 8% of those older than 80 years are affected by AF (Furberg et al., 1994; Kannel et al., 1998). AF is not lethal arrhythmia but associated with an increased long-term risk of stroke, heart failure, and all-cause mortality (Stewart et al., 2002). One of the most debilitating consequences of AF is the accompanying risk of stroke, which occurs in an estimated 60,000 patients with AF per year in the United States (Go et al., 2001).

Antiarrhythmic drug therapy remains a cornerstone to restore and maintain sinus rhythm for patient both with paroxysmal and persistent AF. However, conventional drugs such as sodium channel blockers (class I antiarrhythmic drugs) and potassium channel blockers (class III antiarrhythmic drugs) have limited efficacy, especially in persistent AF patients. Clinical studies have shown that the potassium channel blockers can terminate AF in only 30% of cases (Ellenbogen et al., 1996; Falk et al., 1997). Sodium channel blockers are more effective than potassium channel blockers, but a potent sodium channel blocker, pilsicainide demonstrated a modest efficacy in converting AF to sinus rhythm, with a conversion rate of 45% within 90 min in patients with recent-onset AF compared with 8.6% on placebo and was ineffective in chronic AF (Okishige at al., 2006). In addition, these conventional drugs have severe problematic risks of ventricular proarrhythmia, such as *torsade de pointes* (TdP) through excessive delay of ventricular replarization (Waldo et al., 1996; Trop-Pederson et al., 1999) and left ventricular contractile dysfunction. Thus, the development of new antiarrhythmic agents which have more effective and safer profile is highly desirable. These days, the pharmaceutical industry has focused on "atrial-specific antiarrhythmic drug" in the search for safer drugs to terminate or prevent AF (Wirth et al., 2003; Vos 2004; Goldstein & Stambler 2005).

The acetylcholine-activated potassium channel (I_{KACh} channel) is one of the most promising targets for atrial-specific antiarrhythmic agent, because the channel is more abundantly expressed in the atrial than ventricle myocytes (Krapivinsky et al., 1995). In this article, the pathophysiolosical roles of I_{KACh} channel in AF are summarized. In addition, the in vitro and in vivo profiles of I_{KACh} blockers and the usefulness for AF treatment are also discussed.

2. Pathophysiological role of I_{KACh} channel in AF

The cardiac I_{KACh} is a ligand-gated inward rectifier potassium current. The cardiac I_{KACh} channel is heterotetramer of two distinct homologous proteins encoded by GIRK1 and GIRK4 (Kubo et al., 1993; Krapivinsky et al., 1995). The current amplitude is small under basal condition, but it is activated by acetylcholine secreted from the vagal nerve or by adenosine through muscarinic M_2 receptor or adenosine A_1 receptor, respectively. Activated M_2 receptor and A_1 receptor stimulate I_{KACh} via $G_{\beta\gamma}$ protein activation (Fig. 1). Vagal nerve activation, acetylcholine or adenosine treatment shortens atrial effective refractory period (ERP), increases atrial ERP dispersion and promotes AF (Kabell et al., 1994; Liu and Nattel 1997), possibly through the I_{KACh} activation. A report with GIRK4 knockout mice showed that the I_{KACh} channel plays a crucial role in the initiation of AF (Kovoor et al., 2001). In addition, it is well known that the enhancement of vagal nerve tone can lead to paroxysmal AF in human (Chen et al., 1998).

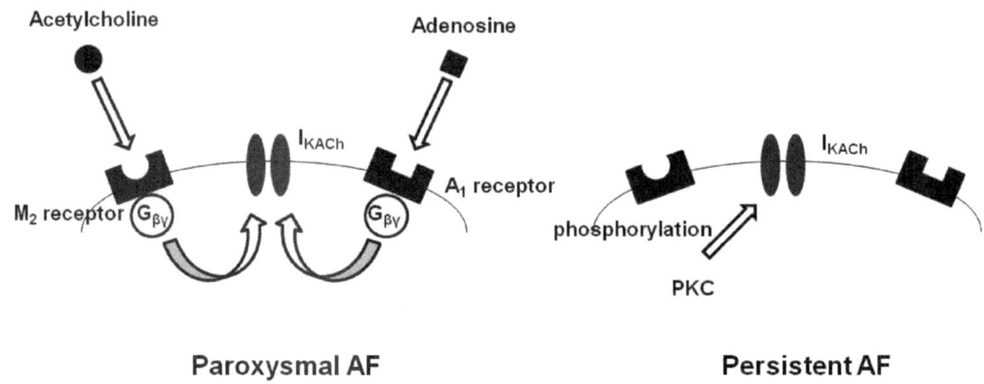

Fig. 1. The different mechanism of I_{KACh} activation mechanism between paroxysmal AF and persistent AF

Although the enhancement of I_{KACh} could be responsible for the initiation of paroxysmal AF in human (Chen et al., 1998), the pathophysiological role of I_{KACh} in patient with persistent AF remains unclear. Dobrev et al. (2001, 2002) showed that the activation of I_{KACh} by muscarinic receptor stimulation is smaller in atria from AF patients compared to those in patients with sinus rhythm. The total acetylcholine-induced inward current in atrial myocytes from AF patients reported to be larger than those from patient with sinus rhythm. However, this increase was due to the increased density of the inward rectifier K^+ current (I_{K1}); the density of I_{KACh} was rather decreased in AF patients than SR patients (Bosch et al., 1999). In addition, reduced muscarinic receptor-related activation of I_{KACh} could be explained by decreased expression of the channel subunits (Dobrev et al., 2001; Brundel et al., 2001a, 2001b). Therefore, it had been thought that the I_{KACh} channel is down-regulated in atrium of persistent AF patients and the effects of the channel blockers might have less effective in persistent AF patients.

However, recent studies suggested that a constitutively active component of I_{KACh} channel exists and it may be upregulated in persistent AF patients. Tertiapin, a selective I_{KACh} blocking peptide, concentration-dependently blocked the whole cell I_{KACh} in persistent AF patients with a higher potency than that in patient with paroxysmal AF or sinus rhythm (Dobrev et al., 2005). The report clearly showed that the basal inward rectifying potassium current was larger in persistent AF patients, although the muscarinic receptor-activated component of I_{KACh} was larger in patients with sinus rhythm or paroxysmal AF. In addition, single channel analysis revealed the presence of constitutively active I_{KACh} channels in persistent AF patients but not in patients with sinus rhythm or paroxysmal AF (Dobrev et al., 2005). Such a tertiapin-sensitive and constitutively active current component contributing to basal outward current was detected in canine left atria and pulmonary vein, and the component was upregulated in preparations from tachycardia-remodeled atria (Ehrlich et al., 2004). In addition, tertiapin prolonged the atrial action potential duration (APD) and prevented AF development in canine tachycardia-remodeled atria (Cha et al., 2006). These results suggest that the receptor-independent I_{KACh} is activated and plays a crucial role in persistent AF patients.

The molecular mechanism underlying constitutive I_{KACh} channel activation in remodeled atria remains unknown. The regulation of I_{KACh} is complex and the channel activity is modulated by levels of intracellular Na^+ concentration (Sui et al., 1996), ATP (Sui et al., 1996; Kim et al., 1997) phosphatidylinositol biphosphate (Huang et al., 1998), and fatty acid (Kim and Pleumsamran, 2000). Recently, Voigt et al. (2007) reported that abnormal PKC function might play important role in the occurrence of constitutive I_{KACh} activation in clinical AF. Although further work will be needed to define the precise signaling mechanisms that enhance the channel activity, modified phosphorylation dependent channel regulation may contribute to the development of constitutive I_{KACh} activity (Fig. 1).

3. In vitro and in vivo profiles of selective I_{KACh} blockers

Several class III antiarrhythmic drugs have been shown to block I_{KACh} in atrial cell (Guillemare et al., 2000; Mori et al., 1995). The blocking effects on I_{KACh} might work additively for their antiarrhythmic efficacy. However, the effects of these drugs on I_{KACh} are not so potent. In addition, the drugs block other cardiac potassium current, including the rapid rectifier potassium current, I_{Kr}. Thus, investigations using more potent and selective blocker are needed to clarify the therapeutic potential, atrial selectivity and safety of I_{KACh} blockers. In this session, the pharmacological profiles of potent I_{KACh} blockers, tertiapin, NIP-141 and NIP-151 are discussed.

3.1 Pharmacological profile of tertiapin, a selective I_{KACh} blocking peptide

Tertiapin is a 21 amino acid residue peptide with two disulfide bonds, isolated from venom of the European honey bee. The peptide was shown to block I_{KACh} potently in cardiac myocyte (Jin and Lu 1998). This peptide inhibits, in a concentration-dependent manner (IC_{50} = ~8 nmol/L), acetylcholine or GTP analogue-induced whole cell current in rabbit atrial myocyte (Kitamura et al., 1994). For the information of selectivity of the peptide, Drici et al. (2000) reported that tertiapin selectively inhibited I_{KACh} at IC_{50} of about 30 nmol/L without significant effects at 1 μmol/L on I_{K1}, I_{Kr}, the transit owtward current (I_{to}), the ultra-rapid delayed rectifier K+ current (I_{Kur}), the slow component of the delayed rectifier K+ current (I_{Ks}), fast sodium current (I_{Na}) and L-type calcium current (I_{Ca}). Tertiapin was the first reported selective I_{KACh} blocker, so we used this peptide to clarify the pathophysiological role of I_{KACh} in AF.

dose (nmol kg^{-1})	*VNS-induced AF*			*aconitine-induced AF*	
	termination of AF	time to AF termination (s)	AF reinduction	termination of AF	time to AF termination (s)
vehicle	0/4	–	–	0/4	–
4	1/5	102	1/1	1/5	137
12	5/5**	88 ± 22	1/5	3/5	49 ± 5
41	n.t.	–	–	4/4*	41 ± 6

n.t. means not tested. Time of AF termination data were expressed as mean ± S.E.M.
**$P<0.01$, *$P<0.05$ vs vehicle-treated group

Table 1. Efficacy of tertiapin in terminating vagal nerve stimulation (VNS)-induced atrial fibrillation (AF) and aconitine- induced AF in dogs (Hashimoto et al., 2006)

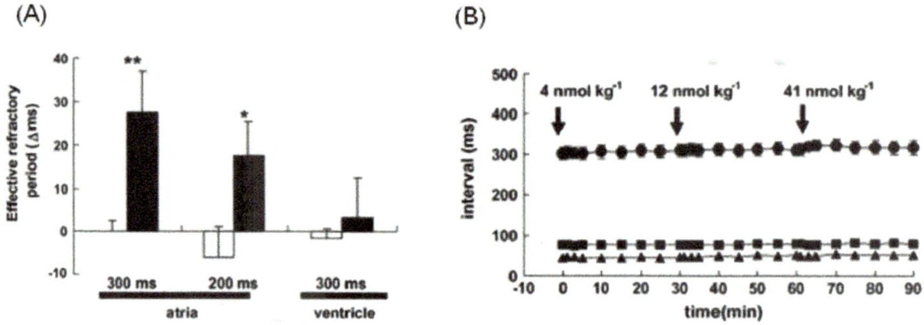

Fig. 2. (A) Effects of tertiapine (12 nmol/kg; solid column) and vehicle (saline; blank column) on atrial and ventricular effective refractory period with vagal nerve stimulation in dogs. Data are expressed as mean ± S.E.M. (n=4) *$P<0.05$, *$P<0.01$ compared with vehicle treated group. (B) Effects of tertiapin (4-41 nmol/kg) on ECG parameters: PQ(■), QRS(▲) intervals and corrected QT value (QTc; ●) in anesthetized beagle dogs. Data are expressed as mean ± S.E.M. (n=4; Hashimoto et al., 2006).

We examined the effects of tertiapin on the two canine AF models: vagal nerve stimulation (VNS)-induced and aconitine-induced AF models, to clarify the antiarrhythmic potential of I_{KACh} blockade. VNS-induced model and aconitine-induced model have been known as different type of paroxysmal AF models; a micro-reentry type AF model and ectopic-focus induced AF model, respectively. Intravenous injection of tertiapin (4-41 nmol/kg) terminated AF in both canine AF models (Hashimoto et al., 2006, Table 1). Tertiapin (12 nmol/kg) significantly prolonged atrial ERP at the basic cycle length of 200 and 300 ms without affecting conduction velocity in atria under VNS condition (Fig. 2A). The result suggests that AF termination by tertiapin is associated with atrial ERP prolongation.

Alternatively, tertiapin at the effective dose ranges (4-42 nmol/kg) had no significant effects on ECG parameters such as PQ, QRS and corrected QT (QTc) intervals and ventricular ERP in anesthetized dogs (Fig. 2B; Hashimoto et al., 2006). These results suggest that I_{KACh} has a crucial role in the maintenance of paroxysmal AF, but has no contribution in ventricular repolarization.

3.2 Pharmacological profile of NIP-142, a multiple channel blocker

The studies using tertiapin clearly suggests that I_{KACh} blocker is effective in some types of AF patients. AF is chronic cardiac disease and the patients have to take medicine for a long term. Thus, the orally active small molecule would be good for the AF treatment. Tertiapin is a peptide and cannot be applied for oral administration. Thus, we conducted the screening of the blocker and found a candidate compound. NIP-142, (3R*, 4S*)-4-cyclopropylamino-3,4- dihydro-2,2-dimethyl-6-(4-methoxyphenylacetylamino)-7-nitro-2H-1-benzopyran-3-ol is synthesized by Nissan Chemical Industries, LTD. (Tanaka & Hashimoto, 2007). The compound has inhibitory effects on multiple potassium channels including I_{KACh} (GIRK1/GIRK4) channel (Table 2). The bioavailability of NIP-142 is about 25-50% in rats and more than 75% in dogs (Tanaka & Hashimoto, 2007), which suggests that the compound would be orally active.

channel	host cell	effect of NIP-142 (IC_{50})	reference
Kv1.5	HEK293	4.8 μM	Matsuda et al. 2001
	Xenopus oocyte	100 μM	-
GIRK1/GIRK4	HEK293	0.64 μM	Matsuda et al. 2006
	Xenopus oocyte	10 μM	Matsuda et al. 2005
hERG	HEK293	44 μM	Matsuda et al. 2004
KCNQ1/KCNE1	HEK293	12 μM	-
Kv4.3, Kv4.2	*Xenopus* oocyte	>100 μM	-

Table 2. Inhibitory effects of NIP-142 on membrane currents

3.2.1 Effect of NIP-142 on the membrane currents

Effects of NIP-142 on various outward membrane currents have been studied by voltage clamp analyses (Table 2). The delayed rectifier current has three components: the rapid component, I_{Kr}, the slow component, I_{Ks} and the ultrarapid component, I_{Kur}. The effects on I_{Kr}, I_{Ks} and I_{Kur} were examined with HEK293 cells expressing the human ether a-go-go (hERG) channel, the human KCNQ1/KCNE1 channel and human K_v 1.5 channel, respectively (Matsuda et al., 2001, 2006). NIP-142 concentration-dependently inhibited these three channel currents. The IC_{50} on I_{Kr}, I_{Ks} and I_{Kur} were 44, 12 and 4.8 μmol/L, respectively (Matsuda et al., 2001; 2006). NIP-142 also inhibited the mouse Kv4.2 and Kv4.3 currents but the potency was very low. This compound had a slight effect on I_{K1}: about 40% inhibition was observed with 10 μmol/L NIP-142.

The effect of NIP-142 on I_{KACh} was examined in HEK293 cells (Matsuda et al., 2006) and Xenopus oocytes (Matsuda et al., 2005) expressing the GIRK1/GIRK4 channel. Concentration- dependent inhibition of the current was observed in both types of cells: the inhibitory effect was 8-10 times potent than those on IKur in both cells (Table 2). The

inhibition of GIRK1/GIRK4 current amplitude in HEK293 cells by 0.1, 1 and 10 μmol/L NIP-142 was 28.9 ± 5.3%, 58.4 ± 6.2% and 76.8 ± 8.4%, respectively (Matsuda et al., 2006). The inhibition was independent from the voltage dependency of the voltage clamp pulse. Among the repolarizing potassium channel currents, NIP-142 inhibited the primarily the GIRK1/GIRK4 channel current which is I_{KACh} (Table 2).
Among other ion currents, NIP-142 at 10 μmol/L inhibited the peak inward current by about 50% and 25% for the L-type and T-type voltage-dependent calcium current in isolated guinea pig ventricular myocytes, respectively. At the same concentration, NIP-142 had no effects on the hyperpolarization- activated inward current (I_f) in isolated rabbit sinoatrial node cells.

3.2.2 Effects of NIP-142 on the refractory period and action potential of isolated myocardium

Effects of NIP-142 on the refractory period were studied in isolated guinea pig atrial and ventricular preparations. At 10 and 100 μmol/L, NIP-142 concentration-dependently prolonged the refractory period in atrium but not in ventricle (Matsuda et al., 2005). The action potential was measured with standard glass microelectrode techniques. NIP-142 concentration-dependently prolonged APD only in the atrium. No significant changes in other action potential parameters, such as resting membrane potential, action potential amplitude and maximum rate of rise (Vmax), were observed (Matsuda et al., 2005).
The effects of NIP-142 on refractory period and action potential were different from those of conventional class III agents. An I_{Kr} blocker E-4031 prolonged APD both in the atrium and the ventricle. In contrast, NIP-142 showed atrial selective prolongation of APD. The prolongation was mimicked by a selective I_{KACh} blocking peptide, tertiapin (Matsuda et al., 2005). These data suggested that the prolongation by NIP-142 was due to the I_{KACh} blockade. Stimulation of the muscarinic receptor in the mammalian atria leads to a shortening of APD through activation of I_{KACh}. NIP-142 (100 μmol/L) completely reversed the carbachol-induced shortening of APD in canine (Nagasawa et al., 2006) and guinea-pig (Matsuda et al., 2006) atrium. Such reversal also observed when NIP-142 was applied after the APD was shortened by adenosine (Matsuda et al., 2006), which also activates I_{KACh} independent of muscarinic receptor.
One of the major problems with existing antiarrhythmic drugs through prolongation of refractory period and APD is "reverse use-dependency", the effect of the drugs are weakened under high stimulation frequency. Such effect is observed both in vitro and in vivo and may explain the ineffectiveness of the drug in high frequency in atrial fibrillation (Nattel, 1999). In guinea-pig atrium, E-4031 at 1 μmol/L prolonged APD when it was applied at pacing frequency less than 1 Hz, but not at frequencies higher than 2 Hz. In contrast, NIP-142-induced prolongation of atrial APD was unaffected by stimulation frequency (Matsuda et al., 2005), suggesting that the APD prolonging effect of the drug may be maintained in atrial fibrillation.

3.2.3 Effects of NIP-142 on AF models

In animal studies, NIP-142 terminated AF in various types of AF models (Table 3). Injection of NIP-142 (3 mg/kg) terminated AF after increase in fibrillation cycle length and prevented reinitiation of AF in VNS-induced model. This compound terminated macroreentry type of atrial flutter induced after placement of an intercaval crush without affecting atrial flutter cycle length (Nagasawa et al., 1999). NIP-142 prolonged atrial ERP by about 10% without affecting intraatrial and interatrial conduction times in these models, which suggested that the antiarrhythmic effects were achieved by the atrial ERP prolongation. We reported NIP-141 (the hydrochloride salt form of NIP-142) at 10 mg/kg terminated AF in aconitine-induced AF model (Hashimoto et al., 2007). Although the mechanism of AF termination in this model remains unclear, the I_{KACh} blocking effect would be mainly involved, because tertiapin was also effective in this model (Hashimoto et al., 2006).

model	effective dose of NIP-142	reference
vagally-induced AF model	3 mg/kg	Nagasawa et al., 1999
intercaval crush-induced AFL model	3 mg/kg	Nagasawa et al., 1999
aconitine-induced AF model	10 mg/kg	Hashimoto et al., 2007
atrial rapid pacing model	2.5 mg/kg/10 min + 2 mg/kg/hr	Hashimoto et al., 2008

Table 3. Effects of NIP-142 in models of atrial fibrillation (AF) and flutter (AFL)

The ERP prolongation by NIP-142 was greater in the presence of VNS than normal condition (Nagasawa et al., 1999). We also reported that this compound at 3 mg/kg prolonged atrial ERP by about 20 ms under VNS, but at doses up to 10 mg/kg it had no significant atrial ERP prolongation effect without VNS (Hashimoto et al., 2007). These findings suggest that the NIP-142-induced atrial ERP prolongation is due mainly to the inhibition of I_{KACh}.

3.2.4 Low proarrhythmic risk with NIP-142

NIP-141 (1-10 mg/kg) produced no significant prolongation of ventricular ERP in the pentobarbital-anesthetized dogs (Hashimoto et al., 2007). NIP-142-induced prolongation of atrial ERP was greater than that of ventricular ERP in AF models (Nagasawa et al., 1999). Because ventricular ERP or QT prolongation is not suitable for drug-induced TdP (Thomsen et al., 2003, 2004), we also evaluated the proarrhythmic risk of NIP-142 using the methoxamine-sensitized rabbit model, known as Carlsson model (Carlsson et al., 1990). By intravenous infusion, NIP-142 (30 mg/kg over 30 min) induced no ventricular arrhythmia in eight rabbits. In contrast, an I_{Kr} blocker, clofilium (15 mg/kg over 30 min) induced TdP in six of eight rabbits. These results suggests that NIP-142 has little effects on ventricular repolarization and not likely to cause proarrhythmia.

In conclusion, NIP-142 preferentially blocks I_{KACh} and has atrial selective ERP prolonging effects and antiarrhythmic effects in some AF models. This compound appeared to be, therefore, a potential therapeutic agent for the treatment and prevention of AF with lower risk of causing ventricular proarrhythmia than conventional drugs. However, NIP-142 at effective dose in AF model significantly decreased blood pressure. Because tertiapin had no significant effects on blood pressure, it was caused by the effects on other target except I_{KACh}. NIP-142 has some blocking effects on I_{CaL} and I_{Na} (Hashimoto et al., 2007), so the effect on blood pressure might be due to the blockade of these channels.

3.3 Pharmacological profile of NIP-151, a novel I_{KACh} channel blocker

We modified the chemical structure of NIP-142 and found a more potent and selective I_{KACh} channel blocker, NIP-151. The compound showed good bioavailability in dogs and rats, almost same as that of NIP-142. The pharmacological profiles of NIP-142 and NIP-151 are shown in Table 4. NIP-151 blocks I_{KACh} 400 times more potently than NIP-142, but the effects on I_{CaL} and I_{Na} were less and about 7 times more potent than those of NIP-142, respectively. As a result, NIP-151 had no significant effects on blood pressure at the dose (0.3 mg/kg) that the compound prolonged atrial ERP by 38 ms under VNS. In contrast, NIP-142 decreased blood pressure by about 40% at the dose (3 mg/kg) that the compound prolonged ERP by 20 ms under VNS.

Compound	Effects on ion channels (IC_{50}; μmo/L)			Effects on anesthetized dogs	
	I_{KACh}	I_{Na}	I_{CaL}	Atrial ERP prolongation	Blood pressure
NIP-142	0.65	45	44	20 ms	-38%
				(3 mg/kg)	
NIP-151	0.0016	6.6	>100	38 ms	-5%
				(0.3 mg/kg)	

Table 4. The pharmacological profile of NIP-142 and NIP-151

3.3.1 Effects of NIP-151 on ion channels

The effects of NIP-151 on I_{KACh} and I_{Kr} were examined using HEK293 cells expressing human GIRK1/GIRK4 channel and hERG channel, respectively by voltage clamp analyses (Hashimoto et al., 2008). NIP-151 at 0.1-100 nmol/L concentration-dependently inhibited the GIRK1/GIRK4 channel current (Fig. 3): NIP-151 at 0.1, 1, 10 and 100 nmol/L inhibited the current at -120 mV by 13.7 ± 24.8%, 42.0 ± 12.2%, 73.1 ± 4.1% and 87.2 ± 1.5%, respectively. The IC_{50} value for the inhibition of GIRK1/GIRK4 channel current was 1.6 nmol/L. NIP-151 at 1, 10 and 100 μmol/L inhibited the tail current of hERG-channel current on repolarization by 15.3 ± 1.5%, 23.9 ± 3.4% and 73.3 ± 2.4%, respectively. The IC_{50} value for the inhibition of hERG channel current was 57.6 μmol/L. In our preliminary experiments, this compound had little effects (less than 50% inhibition at 10 μmol/L) on other components of the delayed rectifier potassium currents, I_{Kur} and I_{Ks}. NIP-151 was extremely selective for GIRK1/GIRK4 channel current over other repolarizing currents.

The mechanism of I_{KACh} blockade by NIP-151 remains unclear. We evaluated the effects of NIP-151 on muscarinic M_2 receptor and adenosine A_1 receptor using radioligands binding assay. NIP-151 had slight inhibitory effects on radio ligand binding to these receptors, but the effect was much weaker than that on I_{KACh}: the IC_{50} on M_2 and A_1 receptors were 57.1 μmol/L and 89.9 μmol/L, respectively. In addition, NIP-151 blocked I_{KACh} in HEK293 cells or xenopus oocyte expressing GIRK1/GIRK4 only (not coexpressing these receptors). These results suggest that NIP-151 directly blocked I_{KACh} channel or inhibited the downstream signaling pathway of these receptors.

We also evaluated the NIP-151 on the various types of GIRK channel subtypes. Cardiac-type and brain-type brain type GIRK channels are composed of GIRK1/GIRK4 and GIRK1/GIRK2 heteromultimeric subunits, respectively. NIP-151 preferentially blocked GIRK1/ GIRK4 channel current over GIRK1/GIRK2 current. In contrast, tertiapin blocked both currents at almost same potency (Matsumoto et al., 2008). The pathophysiological role of GIRK1/GIRK2 channel remains unclear, but seizure activity has been reported in GIRK2 null mice (Siqnorini et al., 1997). Thus, GIRK1/GIRK2 blocker might induce some

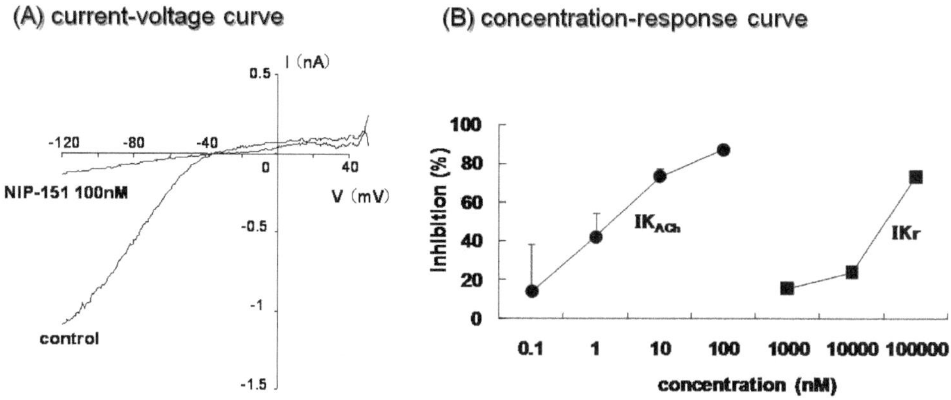

Fig. 3. Effects of NIP-151 on GIRK1/GIRK4 and hERG channel currents. (A) Typical GIRK1/GIRK4-channel current in the absence (control) and presence of NIP-151 at 100 nmol/L. (B) Concentration-response relationship for blockade by NIP-151 of the GIRK1/GIRK1 channel current at 120 mV (solid circle) and the tale current of hERG-channel current (solid square). Data are shown as mean ± SEM from three to five experiments (Hashimoto et al., 2008).

adverse effects on neural activity, such as seizure. Thus, inhibitory effects on GIRK1/GIRK4 channel current over GIRK1/GIRK2 current might be preferable profile for anti AF agents.

3.3.2 Effects of NIP-151 on paroxysmal AF models

We examined the effects of NIP-151 on canine paroxysmal AF models and atrial and ventricular ERP, and compared against those of a standard class III agent dofetilide (Roukoz & Saliba 2007), which is clinically used for the management of AF. NIP-151 (15-30 µg/kg/min) converted AF to sinus rhythm in canine VNS- and aconitine-induced AF models (Table 5, Fig. 4). The compound at the same doses (15-75 µg/kg/min) prolonged atrial ERP significantly, thus the AF termination effects were associated with the atrial ERP prolongation (Hashimoto et al., 2008). In contrast, a selective I_{Kr} blocker dofetilide, which had little effects on GIRK1/GIRK4 channel current, represented significant ERP prolongation both in the atrium and ventricle, but it was not effective in the VNS-induced and aconitine-induced AF models (Table 5).

The reason why dofetilide did not show positive effects on AF models would be mainly due to reverse use dependency. In our preliminary study, dofetilide (0.3 µg/kg) prolonged atrial ERP by 29 ± 7 ms at a basic cycle length of 300 ms, but had slight prolongation (5 ± 5 ms) at a basic cycle length of 200 ms. Nattel et al. (1998) also have shown that dofetilide had limited efficacy in VNS-induced AF model, because of reverse use dependent ERP prolongation, compared with azimilide, which increased atrial ERP in a frequency-independent manner. Alternatively, NIP-151 (0.3 mg/kg) significantly prolonged atrial ERP by 41± 7 ms and 27 ± 5 ms at basic cycle lengths of 300 and 200 ms, respectively. These results suggest that the reverse use dependency of NIP-151 is less significant than that of IKr blockers such as dofetilide and consequently effective under the AF (high frequent) condition.

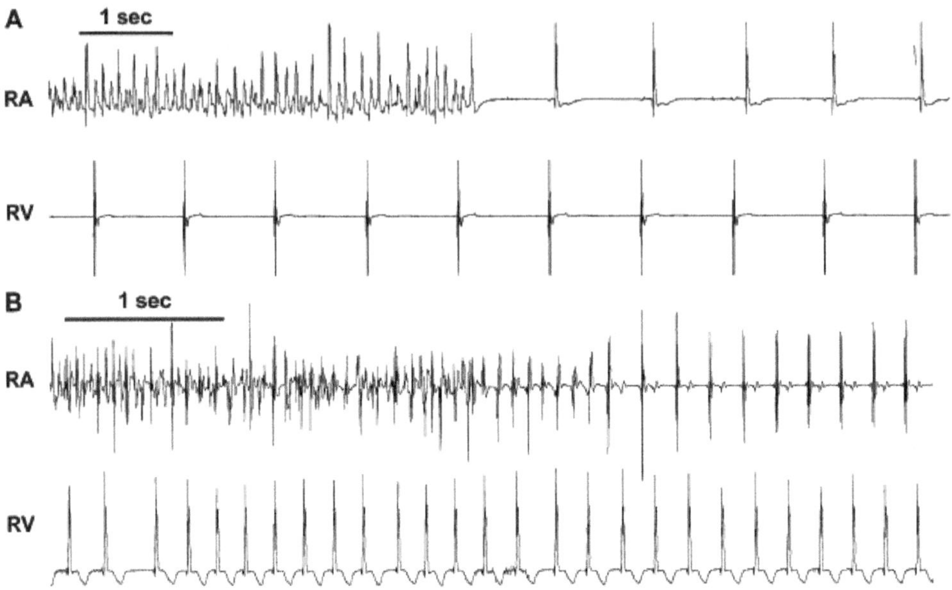

Fig. 4. Representative examples of atrial fibrillation (AF) termination with NIP-151. Electrograms from right atrium (RA) and right ventricular free wall (RV) were recorded. (A) Termination of vagal nerve stimulation-induced AF with NIP-151 at 15 μg/kg/min. (B) Termination of aconitine-induced AF with NIP-151 at 100μg/kg. (Hashimoto et al., 2008)

	VNS-induced AF model				*aconitine-induced AF model*		
	dose (μg/kg/min)	termination of AF	time to AF termination(s)	AF reinduction	dose (μg/kg)	termination of AF	time to AF termination(s)
vehicle	-	1/10	98	1/1	-	0/5	-
NIP-151	5	4/5*	525 ± 25	3/4	10	0/5	-
	15	5/5**	372 ± 38	1/5	30	4/5*	85 ± 23
					100	5/5**	76 ± 15
dofetilide	3	1/4	793	1/1	100	0/4	-
	10	0/4	-	-			

Time to AF termination data were expressed as mean ±SEM
**P<0.01, *P<0.05 vs vehicle-treated group

Table 5. Effects of NIP1-151 and dofetilide in terminating vagal nerve stimulation (VNS)-induced and aconitine-induced atrial fibrillation (AF). (Hashimoto et al., 2008)

We also evaluated the effects of NIP-151 in canine atrial flutter model with Y-shaped right atrial incision. Intravenous infusion of NIP-151 (75 μg/kg/min over 10 min) did not terminated atrial flutter in this model (0 of four dogs), although the compound slightly prolonged atrial flutter cycle length. This result suggests that the I_{KACh} blocker might have weak efficacy on macro-reentry type atrial flutter.

3.3.3 Low proarrhythmic risk with NIP-151

We found that NIP-151 had little effects on hemodynamic (blood pressure, left ventricular systolic pressure and maximum left ventricular developed pressure increased rate) and electrophysiological values (PQ, QRs, QT and corrected QT) in isoflurane-anesthetized dogs, even when the drug was administrated at doses that 20- to 60- fold higher than the effective dose in the VNS-AF model. NIP-151 also represented no changes in action potential parameters (Vmax and APD) in beagle dog ventricular muscle, and no proarrhythmic effects in the methoxamine-sensitized rabbit model (Carlsson model). In contrast, dofetilide prolonged the QTc interval in anesthetized dogs and APD in beagle dog ventricular muscle, and it induced TdP in Carlsson model (Hashimoto et al., 2008). These results suggest that NIP-151 is expected to be devoid of a ventricular proarrhythmic effects rather than a clinically available class III drug.

3.4 The effect of I_{KACh} blockers in remodeled heart

It is clinically observed that the recurrent episode of paroxysmal AF often progresses more persistent forms of AF. Wijffels et al. (1995) reported this phenomenon as "AF begets AF". They found continuous rapid atrial pacing in the goat heart lead to progress shortening of atrial ERP and increased duration of AF once it is induced. This phenomenon was found to be associated with structural and electrical remodeling. Structural remodeling, characterized by fibrosis and hypertrophy, affects excitation pattern of atria and creates a substitute for AF development and maintenance (Ehrlich et al., 2006). Electric remodeling is accompanied by alterations in the expression and/or function of various ion channels in a way that promotes rapid and irregular activation of atria (Wijffels et al., 1995; Nattel et al., 2007). The ion channels affected by electrical remodeling include I_{Na} and I_{Kr}, which are targets of conventional antiarrhthmic agents. The expressions and activities of these channels are significantly decreased after atrial tachypacing, thus the conventional drugs have limited efficacies in the remodeled hearts of persistent AF patients. Thus, the development of a new drug which is effective in persistent AF patients is highly desirable.

We evaluated the I_{KACh} blockers on the canine atrial tachypacing model to predict the efficacy in persistent AF patients. The atrial tachypacing model was established by 7-10 days right atrial pacing at 400 bpm. In this model, the atrial ERP was significantly decreased by about 40 ms at a basic cycle length of 300 ms. Intravenous administration of NIP-151 (0.3 mg/kg) prolonged atrial ERP by 15 ± 2 ms and 44 ± 8 ms at a basic cycle length of 300 ms before and after the atrial tachypacing, respectively. Tertiapin (12 nmol/kg) also prolonged atrial ERP by 7 ± 1 ms and 20 ± 1 ms at a basic cycle length of 300 ms before and after the atrial tachypacing, respectively (Fig. 5). The atrial ERP prolonging effects by these I_{KACh} blockers was significantly potentiated after the atrial tachypacing. Interestingly, the atrial ERP prolongation by these I_{KACh} blockers did not significant show use-dependency. The atrial ERP prolongations by NIP-151 (0.3 mg/kg) after the atrial tachypacing were 40 ± 6 ms, 44 ± 8 ms and 32 ± 5 ms at basic cycle length of 400 ms, 300 ms and 200 ms. A selective I_{Kr} blocker, E-4031 prolonged atrial ERP before and after atrial tachypacing, but the prolonging effect was significantly decreased from 46 ± 7 ms to 25 ± 5 ms after atrial tachypacing (Fig. 5). These results suggest that I_{KACh} blockers might have better efficacy in persistent AF patients than conventional I_{Kr} blockers.

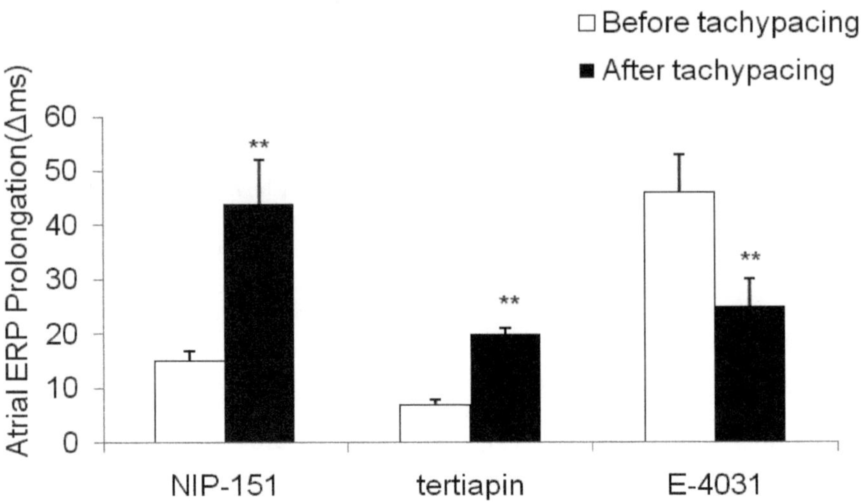

Fig. 5. Effects of NIP-151, tertiapin and E-4031 on atrial effective refractory period (ERP) prolongation in atrial tachypacing model. The ERP was mesuared at the basic sysle length of 300 ms. Data are shown as mean ± s.e.m. (n=4-5). **P<0.01 compared with before tachypacing.

To clarify the activation mechanism of I_{KACh} in this model, we evaluated the effects of a muscarinic M_2 receptor antagonist, AF-DX116 and an adenosine A_1 receptor antagonist, DPCPX. AF-DX 116 (0.3 mg/kg) slightly prolonged atrial ERP (~10 ms) before and after atrial tachypacing, but the prolonging effect was unchanged between before and after the pacing. DPCPX (0.3 mg/kg) had little effects on atrial ERP both before and after the atrial tachypacing. These results suggest the I_{KACh} activation in the model would be associated with non-receptor regulated mechanism. As discussed above, constitutively I_{KACh} is activated in the persistant AF patients and dogs with atrial tachypacing (Dobrev et al., 2005, Ehrlich et al., 2004). The potentiated ERP prolongation by NIP-151 and tertiapin after the atrial tachypacing might be associated with the blockade of constitutively active I_{KACh} channel.

4. Clinical implication

Currently available anti-arrhythmic agents such as sodium channel blockers and potassium channel blockers have not only limited efficacy but also severe side effects such as proarrhythmia and reduced cardiac function (Li et al., 2009). Considerable attention has recently focused on atrial-selective AF drug. I_{KACh} channel has been thought to be a good target for AF treatment, because the channel is important for atrial, but not for ventricular repolarization and AF susceptibility (Nattel & Carlsson, 2006). Paroxysmal AF occurring at night, at rest, and/or consuming meals or alcohol is caused at least partly by the activation of ligand-operated I_{KACh} channel (Coumel, 1999). In addition, our results from atrial tachypacing model suggested that electrical remodeling increased the density of constitutively active I_{KACh} that is activatedd in atrial cells through muscarinic receptor or adenosine receptor-independent mechanism. The constitutively active I_{KACh} channel is observed in cardiomyocytes from patients with persistent AF (Dobrev et al., 2005). These observations suggest that I_{KACh} blockers would be effective not only in paroxysmal AF but also persistent AF treatment.

Agonist-activated inward rectifier potassium current are lager in left than right atria of patients with paroxysmal AF (Voigt et al., 2010). The left-to-right gradient in inward rectifier background current may contribute to the left-to-right atrium dominant frequency gradients in paroxysmal AF patients, accelerating frequency and stability of reentry-promoting rotors. I_{KACh} blockers might modify not only atrial refractoriness but also AF -promoting reentrant sources in the experimental models described.

The contribution of I_{KACh} channel activation to the development and maintenance of AF in patients remains unknown, because a highly selective I_{KACh} blocker has not been clinically available. As with all animal experiments or human tissue studies, it might be difficult to predict whether the efficacy can be directly extrapolated to patients because the AF is complex and has varied manifestations. From this perspective, the clinical assessment to verify the importance of I_{KACh} channel and to ascertain the therapeutic utility of a selective I_{KACh} blocker is required.

We have shown that the highly safe profile of I_{KACh} blocker in cardiovascular systems, but there is little information about the adverse effects of the blockers on extracardiac organs. GIRK1/GIRK4 channel is mainly located in atrium, but other subtypes such as GIRK1/GIRK2, GIRK1/GIRK3, and GIRK2/GIRK3 are located in some types of neurons (Saenz del Burgo et al., 2008). The physiological roles of these subtypes have not been cleared, but seizure activity has been reported in GIRK2 null mice (Siqnorini et al., 1997). Before conducting clinical study, we have to examine fully the extracardiac effects of I_{KACh} blockers.

5. Conclusion

Recent studies clearly showed that I_{KACh} channel has a crucial role in the development and maintenance of AF. This channel would be a novel target for the treatment both in paroxysmal and persistent AF patients. I_{KACh} blockers terminated AF in some canine AF models with atrial-specific ERP prolongation. This profile is thought to be ideal for anti-AF agent, because the blockers have minimum risk of ventricular proarrhthmia such as TdP. Some drug candidates that block I_{KACh} are under clinical or preclinical stages (Machida et al., 2011; Ehrlich & Nattel, 2009; Voigt et al, 2009). The clinical efficiency of the blockers will be clarified in the near future.

6. References

Bosch, R.F., Zeng, X., Grammer, J.B., Popovic, K., Mewis, C., Kühlkamp, V. (1999). Ionic mechanisms of electrical remodeling in human atrial fibrillation. *Cardiovasc. Res.*, 44(1), pp. 121-31. ISSN 0008-6363

Brundel, B.J., Van Gelder, I.C., Henning, R.H., Tieleman, R.G., Tuinenburg, A.E., Wietses, M., Grandjean, J.G., Van Gilst, W.H., Crijns, H.J. (2001a). Ion channel remodeling is related to intraoperative atrial effective refractory periods in patients with paroxysmal and persistent atrial fibrillation. Circulation, 103(5), pp. 684-90. ISSN 0009-7322

Brundel, B.J., Van Gelder, I.C., Henning, R.H., Tuinenburg, A.E., Wietses, M., Grandjean, J.G., Wilde, A.A., Van Gilst, W.H., Crijns, H.J. (2001b). Alterations in potassium channel gene expression in atria of patients with persistent and paroxysmal atrial fibrillation: differential regulation of protein and mRNA levels for K+ channels. *J. Am. Coll. Cardiol.*, 37(3), pp. 926-32. ISSN 0735-1097

Carlsson, L., Almgren, O., Duker, G. (1990). QTU-prolongation and torsades de pointes induced by putative class III antiarrhythmic agents in the rabbit: etiology and interventions. *J. Cardiovasc. Pharmacol.*, 16(2), pp. 276-85. ISSN 0160-2446

Cha, T.J., Ehrlich, J.R., Chartier, D., Qi, X.Y., Xiao, L., Nattel, S. (2006). Kir3-based inward rectifier potassium current: potential role in atrial tachycardia remodeling effects on atrial repolarization and arrhythmias. *Circulation,* 113(14), pp. 1730-7. ISSN 0009-7322

Chen, Y.J., Chen, S.A., Tai, C.T., Wen, Z.C., Feng, A.N., Ding, Y.A., Chang, M.S. (1998). Role of atrial electrophysiology and autonomic nervous system in patients with supraventricular tachycardia and paroxysmal atrial fibrillation. *J. Am. Coll. Cardiol.*, 32(3), pp. 732-8. ISSN 0735-1097

Coumel, P. (1996) Autonomic influences in atrial tachyarrhythmias. *J. Cardiovasc. Electrophysiol.*, 7(10), pp. 999-1007. ISSN 1045-3873

Dobrev, D., Graf, E., Wettwer, E., Himmel, H.M., Hála, O., Doerfel, C., Christ, T., Schüler, S., Ravens, U. (2001). Molecular basis of downregulation of G-protein-coupled inward rectifying K(+) current (I(K,ACh) in chronic human atrial fibrillation: decrease in GIRK4 mRNA correlates with reduced I(K,ACh) and muscarinic receptor-mediated shortening of action potentials. *Circulation*, 104(21), pp. 2551-7. ISSN 0009-7322

Dobrev, D., Wettwer, E., Kortner, A., Knaut, M., Schüler, S., Ravens, U. (2002). Human inward rectifier potassium channels in chronic and postoperative atrial fibrillation. *Cardiovasc. Res.*, 54(2), pp. 397-404. ISSN 0008-6363

Dobrev, D., Friedrich, A., Voigt, N., Jost, N., Wettwer, E., Christ, T., Knaut, M., Ravens, U. (2005). The G protein-gated potassium current I(K,ACh) is constitutively active in patients with chronic atrial fibrillation. *Circulation,* 112(24), pp. 3697-706. ISSN 0009-7322

Drici, M.D., Diochot, S., Terrenoire, C., Romey, G., Lazdunski, M. (2000). The bee venom peptide tertiapin underlines the role of I(KACh) in acetylcholine-induced atrioventricular blocks. *Br. J. Pharmacol.*, 131(3), pp. 569-77. ISSN

Ehrlich, J.R., Cha, T.J., Zhang, L., Chartier, D., Villeneuve, L., Hébert, T.E., Nattel, S. (2004). Characterization of a hyperpolarization-activated time-dependent potassium current in canine cardiomyocytes from pulmonary vein myocardial sleeves and left atrium. *J. Physiol.*, 557(Pt 2), pp. 583-97. ISSN 0022-3751

Ehrlich, J.R., Hohnloser, S.H., Nattel, S. (2005). Role of angiotensin system and effects of its inhibition in atrial fibrillation: clinical and experimental evidence. *Eur. Heart. J.* 27(5), pp. 512-8. ISSN 0195-668X

Ehrlich, J.R. & Nattel, S. (2009). Novel approaches for pharmacological management of atrial fibrillation. *Drugs,* 69(7), pp. 757-74. ISSN 0019-9419

Ellenbogen, K.A., Clemo, H.F., Stambler, B.S., Wood, M.A., VanderLugt, J.T. (1996). Efficacy of ibutilide for termination of atrial fibrillation and flutter. *Am. J. Cardiol.*, 78(8A), pp. 42-5. ISSN 0002-9149

Falk, R.H., Pollak, A., Singh, S.N., Friedrich, T. (1997). Intravenous dofetilide, a class III antiarrhythmic agent, for the termination of sustained atrial fibrillation or flutter. Intravenous Dofetilide Investigators. *J. Am. Coll. Cardiol.*, 29(2), pp. 385-90. ISSN 0735-1097

Furberg, CD., Psaty, BM., Manolio, T.A., Gardin, J.M., Smith, V.E., Rautaharju, P.M. (1994). Prevalence of atrial fibrillation in elderly subjects (the Cardiovascular Health Study). *Am. J. Cardiol.*, 74(3), pp. 236-41, ISSN 0002-9149

Go, A.S., Hylek, E.M., Phillips, K.A., Chang, Y., Henault, L.E., Selby, J.V., Singer, D.E. (2001). Prevalence of diagnosed atrial fibrillation in adults: national implications for rhythm management and stroke prevention: the AnTicoagulation and Risk Factors in Atrial Fibrillation (ATRIA) Study. *J.A.M.A.*, 285(18), pp. 2370-5. ISSN 0098-7484

Goldstein, R.N & Stambler, B.S. (2005). New antiarrhythmic drugs for prevention of atrial fibrillation. *Prog. Cardiovasc. Dis.* 48(3), pp. 193-208. ISSN 0033-0620

Guillemare, E., Marion, A., Nisato, D., Gautier, P. (2000). Inhibitory effects of dronedarone on muscarinic K+ current in guinea pig atrial cells. *J. Cardiovasc. Pharmacol.*, 36(6), pp. 802-5. ISSN 0160-2446

Hashimoto, N., Yamashita, T., Tsuruzoe, N. (2006). Tertiapin, a selective IKACh blocker, terminates atrial fibrillation with selective atrial effective refractory period prolongation. *Pharmacol. Res.* 54(2), pp. 136-41. ISSN 1043-6618

Hashimoto, N., Yamashita, T., Fujikura, N., Tsuruzoe, N. (2007). NIP-141, a multiple ion channel blocker, terminates aconitine-induced atrial fibrillation and prevents the rapid pacing-induced atrial effective refractory period shortening in dogs. *Europace*, 9(4), pp. 246-51. ISSN 1099-5129

Hashimoto, N., Yamashita, T., Tsuruzoe, N. (2008). Characterization of in vivo and in vitroelectrophysiological and antiarrhythmic effects of a novel IKACh blocker, NIP-151: a comparison with an IKr-blocker dofetilide. *J. Cardiovasc. Pharmacol.*, 51(2), pp. 162-9. ISSN 0160-2446

Huang, C.L., Feng, S., Hilgemann, D.W. (1998). Direct activation of inward rectifierpotassium channels by PIP2 and its stabilization by Gbetagamma. *Nature*, 391(6669), pp. 803-6. ISSN 0028-0836

Jin, W. & Lu, Z. (1998). A novel high-affinity inhibitor for inward-rectifier K+ channels. *Biochemistry*, 37(38), pp. 13291-9. ISSN 0006-2960

Kabell, G., Buchanan, L.V., Gibson, J.K., Belardinelli, L. (1994). Effects of adenosine on atrial refractoriness and arrhythmias. *Cardiovasc. Res.*, 28(9), pp. 1385-9. ISSN 0008-6363

Kannel, W.B., Wolf, P.A., Benjamin, E.J., Levy, D. (1998). Prevalence, incidence, prognosis, and predisposing conditions for atrial fibrillation: population-based estimates. *Am. J. Cardiol.* 82(8A), pp. 2N-9N. ISSN 0002-9149

Kim, D., Watson, M., Indyk, V. (1997). ATP-dependent regulation of a G protein-coupled K+ channel (GIRK1/GIRK4) expressed in oocytes. *Am. J. Physiol.*, 272(1 Pt 2), pp. H195-206. ISSN 0002-9513

Kim, D. & Pleumsamran, A. (2000). Cytoplasmic unsaturated free fatty acids inhibit ATP-dependent gating of the G protein-gated K(+) channel. *J Gen Physiol.*, 115(3), pp. 287-304. ISSN 0002-9513

Kitamura, H., Yokoyama, M., Akita, H., Matsushita, K., Kurachi, Y., Yamada, M. (2000). Tertiapin potently and selectively blocks muscarinic K(+) channels in rabbit cardiac myocytes. *J. Pharmacol. Exp. Ther.*, 293(1), pp. 196-205. ISSN 0022-3565

Kovoor, P., Wickman, K., Maguire, C.T., Pu, W., Gehrmann, J., Berul, CI., Clapham, D.E. (2001). Evaluation of the role of I(KACh) in atrial fibrillation using a mouse knockout model. *J. Am. Coll. Cardiol.* 37(8), pp. 2136-43. ISSN 0735-1097

Krapivinsky, G., Krapivinsky, L., Velimirovic, B., Wickman, K., Navarro, B., Clapham, D.E. (1995). The cardiac inward rectifier K+ channel subunit, CIR, does not comprise the ATP-sensitive K+ channel, IKATP. *J. Biol. Chem.*, 270(48), pp. 28777-9. ISSN 0021-9258

Kubo, Y., Reuveny, E., Slesinger, P.A., Jan, Y.N., Jan, L.Y. (1993). Primary structure and functional expression of a rat G-protein-coupled muscarinic potassium channel. *Nature*, 1993 364(6440), pp. 802-6. ISSN 0028-0836

Li, D., Sun, H., Levesque, P. (2009). Antiarrhythmic drug therapy for atrial fibrillation: focus on atrial selectivity and safety. *Cardiovasc. Hematol. Agents. Med. Chem.* 7, pp. 64-75. ISSN 1871-5257

Liu, L. & Nattel, S. (1997). Differing sympathetic and vagal effects on atrialfibrillation in dogs: role of refractoriness heterogeneity. *Am. J. Physiol.*, 273(2 Pt 2), pp. H805-16. ISSN 0002-9513

Machida, T., Hashimoto, N., Kuwahara, I., Ogino, Y., Matsuura, J., Yamamoto, W., Itano, Y., Zamma, A., Matsumoto, R., Kamon, J., Kobayashi, T., Ishiwata, N., Yamashita, T., Ogura, T., Nakaya, H. (2011). Effects of a highly selective acetylcholine-activated K+ channel blocker on experimental atrial fibrillation. *Circ. Arrhythm. Electrophysiol.*, 4(1), pp. 94-102. ISSN 0009-7322

Matsuda, T., Masumiya, H., Tanaka, N., Yamashita, T., Tsuruzoe, N., Tanaka, Y., Tanaka, H., Shigenoba, K. (2001). Inhibition by a novel anti-arrhythmic agent, NIP-142, of cloned human cardiac K+ channel Kv1.5 current. *Life Sci.*, 68(17), pp. 2017-24. ISSN 0024-3205

Matsuda, T., Takeda, K., Ito, M., Yamagishi, R., Tamura, M., Nakamura, H., Tsuruoka, N., Saito, T., Masumiya, H., Suzuki, T., Iida-Tanaka, N., Itokawa-Matsuda, M., Yamashita, T., Tsuruzoe, N., Tanaka, H., Shigenobu, K. (2005) Atria selective prolongation by NIP-142, anantiarrhythmic agent, of refractory period and action potential duration inguinea pig myocardium. *J Pharmacol Sci.* 98(1), pp. 33-40. ISSN 0021-5198

Matsuda, T., Ito, M., Ishimaru, S., Tsuruoka, N., Saito, T., Iida-Tanaka, N., Hashimoto, N., Yamashita, T., Tsuruzoe, N., Tanaka, H., Shigenobu, K. (2006). Blockade by NIP-142, an antiarrhythmic agent, of carbachol-induced atrial action potential shortening and GIRK1/4 channel. *J. Pharmacol. Sci.*, 101(4), pp. 303-10. ISSN 0021-5198

Matsumoto, R., Hashimoto, N., Ishiwata, N., Yamashita, T., Tsuruzoe, N. and Nakaya, H. (2008). Comparison of GIRK channel blocking effects of NIP-151 and Tertiapin. *J Pharmacol Sci.*, 106(suppl 1), pp. 265. ISSN 0021-5198

Mori, K., Hara, Y., Saito, T., Masuda, Y., Nakaya, H. (1995). Anticholinergic effects of class III antiarrhythmic drugs in guinea pig atrial cells. Different molecular mechanisms. *Circulation*, 91(11), pp. 2834-43. ISSN 0008-6363

Nagasawa, H., Fujiki, A., Fujikura, N., Matsuda, T., Yamashita, T., Inoue, H. (1999). Effects of a novel class III antiarrhythmic agent, NIP-142, on canine atrial fibrillation and flutter. *Circ. J.*, 66(2), pp. 185-91. ISSN 1346-9843

Nattel, S, Liu, L, St-Georges, D. (1998). Effects of the novel antiarrhythmic agent azimilide on experimental atrial fibrillation and atrial electrophysiologic properties. *Cardiovasc Res.*, 37(3), pp. 627-35. ISSN 0008-6363

Nattel, S. (1999). The molecular and ionic specificity of antiarrhythmic drug actions. *J Cardiovasc. Electrophysiol.* 10(2), pp. 272-82. ISSN 1045-3873

Nattel, S. & Carlsson, L. (2006). Innovative approaches to anti-arrhythmic drug therapy. *Nat. Rev. Drug. Discov.* 5(12), pp. 1034-1049. ISSN 1474-1776

Nattel, S., Maguy, A., Le Bouter, S., Yeh, Y.H. (2007). Arrhythmogenic ion-channel remodeling in the heart: heart failure, myocardial infarction, and atrial fibrillation. *Physiol. Rev.*, 87(2), pp. 425-56. ISSN 0031-9333

Okishige, K., Fukunami, M., Kumagai, K., Atarashi, H., Inoue, H. (2006). Pilsicainide Suppression Trial for Persistent Atrial Fibrillation II Investigators. Pharmacological conversion of persistent atrial fibrillation into sinus rhythm with oral pilsicainide: pilsicainide suppression trial for persistent atrial fibrillation II. *Circ.* J., 70, pp. 657-61. ISSN 0363-6135

Roukoz, H & Saliba W. (2007). Dofetilide: a new class III antiarrhythmic agent. *Expert Rev. Cardiovasc. Ther.* 5(1), pp. 9-19. ISSN

Saenz del Burgo, L., Cortes, R., Mengod, G., Zarate, J., Echevarria, E., Salles, J. (2008). Distribution and neurochemical characterization of neurons expressing GIRK channels in the rat brain. *J. Comp. Neurol.*, 510(6), pp. 581-606. ISSN 1096-9861

Signorini, S., Liao, Y.J., Duncan, S.A., Jan, L.Y., Stoffel, M. (1997). Normal cerebellar development but susceptibility to seizures in mice lacking G protein-coupled, inwardly rectifying K+ channel GIRK2. *Proc. Natl. Acad. Sci. U. S. A.* 94(3), pp. 923-7. ISSN 0027-8424

Stewart, S., Hart, C.L, Hole, D.J. & McMurray, J.J. (2002). A population-based study of the long-term risks associated with atrial fibrillation: 20-year follow-up of the Renfrew-Paisley study. Am. J. Med., 113, pp. 359–354, ISSN 0002-9343

Sui, J.L., Chan, K.W., Logothetis, D.E. (1996). Na+ activation of the muscarinic K+ channel by a G-protein-independent mechanism. *J Gen Physiol.*, 108(5), pp. 381-91. ISSN 0022-1295

Tanaka, H. & Hashimoto, N. (2007). A multiple ion channel blocker, NIP-142, for the treatment of atrial fibrillation. Cardiovasc. Drug Reviews, 25(4), pp. 342-356. ISSN 0897-5957

Thomsen, M.B., Volders, P.G., Stengl, M., Spätjens, R.L., Beekman, J.D., Bischoff, U., Kall, M.A., Frederiksen, K., Matz, J., Vos, M.A. (2003). Electrophysiological safety of sertindole in dogs with normal and remodeled hearts. *J. Pharmacol. Exp. Ther.* 307(2), pp. 776-84. ISSN 0022-3565

Thomsen, M.B., Verduyn, S.C., Stengl, M., Beekman, J.D., de Pater, G., van Opstal, J., Volders, P.G., Vos, M.A. (2004). Increased short-term variability of repolarization predicts d-sotalol-induced torsades de pointes in dogs. *Circulation*, 110(16), pp. 2453-9. ISSN 0009-7322

Torp-Pedersen, C., Møller, M., Bloch-Thomsen, P.E., Køber, L., Sandøe, E., Egstrup, K., Agner, E., Carlsen, J., Videbaek, J., Marchant, B., Camm, A.J. (1999). Dofetilide in patients with congestive heart failure and left ventricular dysfunction. Danish Investigations of Arrhythmia and Mortality on Dofetilide Study Group. *N. Engl. J. Med.*, 341(12), pp. 857-65. ISSN 0028-4793

Voigt, N., Maguy, A., Yeh, Y.H., Qi, X., Ravens, U., Dobrev, D., Nattel, S. (2007). Changes in I K, ACh single-channel activity with atrial tachycardia remodelling in canine atrial cardiomyocytes. *Cardiovasc Res.*, 77(1), pp. 35-43. ISSN 0008-6363

Voigt, N., Rozmaritsa, N., Trausch, A., Zimniak, T., Christ, T., Wettwer, E., Matschke, K., Dobrev, D., Ravens, U. (2009). Inhibition of IK,ACh current may contribute to clinical efficacy of class I and class III antiarrhythmic drugs in patients with atrial fibrillation. *Naunyn. Schmiedebergs. Arch. Pharmacol.*, 381(3), pp. 251-9. ISSN 0028-1298

Voigt, N., Trausch, A., Knaut, M., Matschke, K., Varró, A., Van Wagoner, D.R., Nattel, S., Ravens, U., Dobrev, D. (2010). Left-to-Right Atrial Inward-Rectifier Potassium Current Gradients in Patients with Paroxysmal Versus Chronic Atrial Fibrillation. *Circ. Arrhythm. Electrophysiol.* 3(5), pp. 472-80. ISSN 0009-7322

Vos M.A. (2004). Atrial-specific drugs: the way to treat atrial fibrillation? *J. Cardiovasc. Electrophysiol.*. 15(12), pp. 1451-2. ISSN 1045-3873

Waldo, A.L., Camm, A.J., deRuyter, H., Friedman, P.L., MacNeil, D.J., Pauls, J.F., Pitt, B., Pratt, C.M., Schwartz, P.J., Veltri E.P.(1996). Effect of d-sotalol on mortality in patients with left ventricular dysfunction after recent and remote myocardial infarction. The SWORD Investigators. Survival With Oral d-Sotalol. *Lancet*, 348(9019), pp. 7-12. ISSN 0140-6736

Wijffels, M.C., Kirchhof, C.J., Dorland, R., Allessie, M.A. (1995). Atrial fibrillation begets atrial fibrillation. A study in awake chronically instrumented goats. *Circulation*, 92(7), pp. 1954-68. ISSN 0009-7322

Wirth, K.J., Paehler, T., Rosenstein, B., Knobloch, K., Maier, T., Frenzel, J., Brendel, J., Busch, A.E., Bleich, M. (2003). Atrial effects of the novel K(+)-channel-blocker AVE0118 in anesthetized pigs. *Cardiovasc Res.*, 60(2), pp. 298-306. ISSN 0008-6363

Part 5

Specific Populations and Complications

19

Atrial Fibrillation in Children

Thomas C. Martin and Sean C. Hagenbuch
University of Vermont College of Medicine, Burlington, Vermont,
Division of Pediatric Cardiology, Department of Pediatrics,
Eastern Maine Medical Center, Bangor, Maine
USA

1. Introduction

Atrial fibrillation is a relatively uncommon arrhythmia in childhood which is seen in a variety of pediatric clinical settings and continues to challenge health care providers.Atrial fibrillation may be seen at any age during childhood. Recent advances have allowed for prenatal diagnosis and treatment. Perinatal atrial fibrillation has been described, often in the absence of obvious structural or electrophysiological cardiac abnormality. In childhood, atrial fibrillation may be seen occasionally in association with cardiac tumors, myocarditis or cardiomyopathy. Certain medications and drug exposures may precipitate atrial fibrillation in children. Several congenital defects may be associated with atrial fibrillation in early adulthood, if left unrepaired or repaired or palliated with surgical or catheter intervention. The clinical significance of atrial fibrillation may range from trivial to life threatening, depending on the clinical setting and underlying electrophysiological or structural substrate. Recent research into the origins of atrial fibrillation, new drug therapy, interventional catheter and surgical procedures offer new treatment options for children or young adults at risk. This chapter reviews the recent advances in genetic, structural, electrophysiological, pharmacological, medical and surgical observations and the impact on understanding and management of this arrhythmia in children.

2. Atrial embryology

Atrial fibrillation is a relatively rare arrhythmia in the pediatric age group. But the antecedents for atrial fibrillation in adulthood are often the consequence of alterations in the developmental genetics, anatomy, function and electrical properties of the developing heart. Most of the information regarding the developing atrial conduction system comes from animal studies (Gourdie et al., 2003; Ho & Anderson, 1990; Jongbloed et al., 2004). The most useful model for the developing human cardiac conduction system concerns the rings of specialized tissue separating the five components of the primitive heart tube (at the juncture of the venous sinus, primitive atrium, inlet and outlet portions of the ventricular segment and the arterial segment). These rings form the primordial conduction system, a concept that can be extended to account for the ectopic distribution in malformed hearts (Gourdie et al., 2003; Ho & Anderson, 1990; Jongbloed et al., 2004). Among the atrial structures of the conduction system, the sinoatrial node is recognizable as early as the first stage of cardiac looping, at the juncture of the superior caval vein and the right atrium (Boyett, 2009;

Gourdie et al., 2003; Ho & Anderson, 1990; Jongbloed et al., 2004). The histologically discrete nodal cells are set in a connective tissue matrix, which increases in size toward birth. The remainder of the sinoatrial junction is infolded to form the valves of the venous sinus (Boyett, 2009; Gourdie et al., 2003; Ho & Anderson, 1990; Jongbloed et al., 2004). The sinus node was first identified by Sir Arthur Keith (suspected perpetrator of the Piltdown fraud) in 1907 (Boyett, 2009). Although textbooks show the sinoatrial node as a discrete nodule, electrophysiologic data and newer anatomic techniques suggest a more variable and extensive structure extending from the superior vena cava toward the inferior vena cava (Boyett, 2009; Dobrzynski et al., 2005; Scheussler et al., 1996).

There is debate about whether significant connections exist between the sinoatrial nodal tissues and the atrioventricular node (Mommersteeg et al., 2009; Platanov, 2007; Sherf & James, 1979). Although illustrated in prior works, the circumferential muscle bundle located at the anterior wall of the left atrium connecting the right and left atrial appendages was named after George Bachmann, who described its participation in the interatrial propagation of electrical impulses in 1916 (Sherf & James, 1979). Recent embryologic studies in mice suggest that arrhythmogenic areas such as Bachmann's bundle, the pulmonary veins and sinus venosus are intranodal structures which demonstrate lacZ gene expression, a characteristic of specialized conduction tissue (Boyett, 2009; Jongbloed et al., 2004; Mommersteeg, 2009; Platanov 2007).

The atrioventricular node development is quite complex (Boyett, 2009; Gourdie et al., 2003; Ho & Anderson, 1990; Jongbloed et al., 2004). The ring of specialized tissue at the atrioventricular junction forms the primordium of the atrioventricular node. It is initially sandwiched between the atrioventricular sulcus and the endocardial cushion tissue (Boyett, 2009; Gourdie et al., 2003; Ho & Anderson, 1990; Jongbloed et al., 2004). The conduction tissue on the inlet and apical trabecular components of the ventricular septum are brought together to form a continuous ventricular conduction axis. The endocardial cushions gradually regress, bringing the conduction bundle into direct contact with the inferior rim of the atrial septum (Boyett, 2009; Gourdie et al., 2003; Ho & Anderson, 1990; Jongbloed et al., 2004). The atrial tissues immediately around the contact region become the transitional cell zone, while the end of the bundle becomes the compact atrioventricular node (Boyett, 2009; Gourdie et al., 2003; Ho & Anderson, 1990; Jongbloed et al., 2004). The atrioventricular node was first described in 1906 by Sunao Tawara working in Ludwig Aschoff's laboratory in Germany (Boyett, 2009). Recent genetic work in animals and human beings suggest that mutations in the transcription factor Nkx2.5 may be associated with conduction system developmental abnormalities (Gittenberger-De Groot et al., 2007; Jay et al., 2004).

The atrial and ventricular working myocardial cells are similar in characteristics but different in anatomic arrangement (Boyett, 2009; Gourdie et al., 2003;Ho & Anderson, 1990). These cells are characterized by a greater degree of depolarization at rest, no spontaneous pacemaker activity and rapid impulse conduction (Boyett, 2009; Gourdie et al., 2003;Ho & Anderson, 1990). Differentiation of conduction system elements from working atrial myocardial cells involves switching on and off controlling genes (Boyett, 2009). The transcription factor Tbx3 is expressed in the developing conduction system tissues and is usually turned off in working atrial myocytes (Boyett, 2009; Hoogaars et al., 2007). Working atrial myocardial cells have more efficient electrical coupling due to expression of genes controlling the connexion Cx43 in creating more and larger gap junctions (Boyett, 2009, Chandler et al., 2009). Cardiac conduction system cells have fewer and smaller gap junctions and express the connexion Cx45 instead (Boyett, 2009, Chandler et al., 2009). An examination of messenger ribonucleic acid (mRNA) from human hearts show that sinoatrial and atrioventricular nodal cells have increased expression of hyperpolarization-activated cyclic nucleotide-gated channels, HCN4, (controlling I_f current) and decreased expression of K_{ir} channel genes, especially $K_{ir}2.1$ (controlling $I_{K,1}$ current) resulting in decreased resting potential, slower conduction and spontaneous depolarization through other ion channels (Boyett, 2009; Chandler et al., 2009; Hoogaars et al., 2007). The cardiac sodium channel, $Na_v1.5$, (controlling I_{Na} current) is abundantly expressed in working myocardial cells but not in nodal tissue (Boyett, 2009). Genetic issues, such as persistence of Tbx3 activity or acquired genetic alterations in ion channel function, may underlie the propensity to develop atrial fibrillation later in life (Hoogaars et al., 2007; Roberts & Gollob, 2010).

3. Atrial genetics

Recent reports suggest that channelopathies play a part to play in the development of atrial fibrillation (Darbar et al., 2008; Johnson et al., 2008; Kaufman, 2009; Patel & Pavri, 2009; Thejus & Francis, 2009). Atrial fibrillation may be associated with genes resulting in either ion channel gain-of-function or loss-of-function (Darbar et al., 2008; Johnson et al., 2008; Kaufman, 2009;Patel & Pavri, 2009;Thejus & Francis, 2009) and may be seen in 2% of patients with long QT syndrome, 10% of patients with Brugada syndrome and 30% of patients with short QT syndrome (Johnson et al., 2008; Patel & Pavri, 2009; Roberts & Gollob, 2010, Thejus & Francis, 2009). Familial atrial fibrillation has also been associated with identified channelopathies (Benito et al., 2008; Darbar et al., 2008; Johnson et al., 2008; Kaufman 2009;Patel & Pavri, 2009;Roberts & Gollub, 2010; Thejus & Francis, 2009). Mutations involving ion transport associated with atrial fibrillation include SCN5A, KCNH2, KCNQ1, KCNJ2, KCNE2, KCNA5, HERG + MiRP1, KCNE1 and probably others (Benito et al., 2008; Darbar et al., 2008; Johnson et al., 2008; Kaufman 2009;Patel & Pavri, 2009;Thejus & Francis, 2009). Although these mutations affect cardiac myocyte action potential height and duration, cellular repolarization duration and cardiac impulse conduction speed, the exact relation of ion channel abnormalities to atrial fibrillation development is unknown. The fact these genetic variants have been identified in families of patients with atrial fibrillation may facilitate new approaches to the diagnosis, prevention and treatment (Otway et al., 2007).
Mechanisms other than enhanced atrial action potential repolarization (from gain-of-function mutations) and delayed atrial action potential repolarization (from loss-of-function mutations) may be inherited. There has been a recent focus on hormonal control of atrial electrophysiology, including genes controlling atrial natriuretic peptide levels and mineralocorticoid receptor expression, in patients with atrial fibrillation (Hodgson-Zingman et al., 2008; Roberts & Gollob, 2010; Tsai et al., 2010). Re-expression of dormant fetal genes may be one mechanism associated with the development of atrial fibrillation in adults, as was demonstrated by the appearance of the fetal ssTnI isoform of troponin in patients with atrial fibrillation (Thijssen et al., 2004). These changes could be primary causes of atrial fibrillation or may represent secondary changes related to other changes in myocardial metabolism, function or distension.

4. Atrial fibrillation in the fetus

Atrial fibrillation in the fetus is rare, but not unheard of. Depending on the report, fetal atrial flutter or fibrillation accounts for somewhere between 20-33% of all fetal tachyarrythmias

(Azancot-Benistry et al., 1992; Belhassen et al., 1982; Silverman et al., 1985; Simpson et al., 1998)and may be detected on routine obstetrical examination as an irregular or rapid fetal heart rate. In general, any congenital heart disease may predispose to development of atrial fibrillation in this period, but several specific entities are generally considered higher risk. The Wolff-Parkinson-White (WPW) syndrome was first noted to have intrauterine atrial fibrillation and several other observations have come as fetal echocardiography has developed into a fully accepted clinical technique. Atrial septal defects, ventricular septal defects, atrioventricular canal, Ebstein anomaly, cor triatriatum and any single ventricular anatomy (most prominently hypoplastic left heart) are all felt to be higher than average risk for fetal atrial tachyarrythmia. The most common arrythmia defined in several series is premature atrial contractions, which is most often benign, but has the potential to convert to an atrial tachyarrythmia (Belhassen et al., 1982; Silverman et al., 1985). Detection of fetal arrhythmia is primarily done clinically using ultrasound in most settings, and is well validated in multiple reports. Physiologic correlations have been demonstrated, the most severe of which is hydrops fetalis (Azancot-Benistry et al., 1992; Frohn-Mulder et al., 1995; Hajdu et al., 1997; Hansmann et al., 1991; Jaeggiet al., 1998; Kleinman et al., 1999; Matta et al., 2010; Naumburg et al., 1997; Reed et al., 1987; Soyeur D, 1996; Szabo et al., 1997; van Engelen et al., 1994; Zielinskyet al., 1998). As discussed above, familial atrial fibrillation has been noted to occur prenatally in the absence of hereditary structural heart disease, and may be indication for referral for high risk obstetrical screening (Aburawi et al., 2006; Bertram et al., 1996; Soyeur, 1996; Tikanoja et al., 1998).

As the common pathway of hydrops fetalis is a devastating and often fatal diagnosis, early detection of fetal atrial flutter and other fetal supraventricular tachyarrhythmias is essential to prevention. The published mortality that has generally been attributed to fetal atrial flutter is in the 8-10% range, and while some have theorized that it is both harder to control and more likely to lead to fetal demise secondary to this phenomenon, a recent meta-analysis of published data has shown that the overall risk of atrial flutter is similar to all other types of atrial tachyarrhythmia when taken together (Krapp et al., 2003).

As fetal ultrasonography is essentially a mechanical observation of a presumed electrical phenomenon based upon our knowledge of extrauterine life, much research has been ongoing to refine techniques that will allow us to noninvasively monitor a fetus with suspected arrhythmia. One of the more exciting advances has been fetal magnetocardiography. As magnetic resonance imaging (MRI) technology has advanced, cardiac MRI has become a viable field for extrauterine evaluation of the heart. To date, the motion artifacts associated with fetal movement have conspired to render fine detailed anatomic evaluation of the fetal cardiac structures as just a goal, but the physics of detecting the magnetic signature of the fetal electrical impulses have proven to be very promising, if somewhat cumbersome (Kahler et al., 2001; Wakai et al., 2003). Fetal magnetocardiography (fMCG) has advanced by leaps and bounds in recent years, and can be reliably performed beginning at 20 weeks gestation in the correct setting. The technique essentially takes advantage of the physical fact that electrical movement generates a magnetic field, and that when this magnetic field is affected by a second, focused and known magnetic field like an MRI scanner, the final vectors can be transformed to give an approximation similar to a surface ECG, which can then be interpreted similarly. This is a simplification of complex concepts and may give the impression that this technique should be readily and widely available. However, this technique, while promising, is currently only investigatory. It is,

however, one of the few areas under investigation that would give us a potential leap forward in both detecting and understanding fetal arrhythmias.
Many different treatments have been attempted and recommended for fetal atrial flutter and fibrillation, and this condition may be the most accurate representation of the medical truism that the greater the number of potential treatments, the less likely any one is to be successful. The paradigm that is currently held is that any fetal tachycardia that is intermittent, present less than roughly half the time, and without obvious impact to the fetus, is followed closely but otherwise left untreated. (Cuneo & Strasburger, 2000).If treatment is indicated due to cardiac or valve dysfunction potentially leading to hydrops, the current mainstay of therapy at this time in the United States is digoxin. It has excellent ability to cross the placenta and has generally demonstrated good efficacy. For the same indications in Europe, the intervention of choice has become flecainide (Strasburger & Wakai, 2010). For atrial flutter or fibrillation resistant to digoxin or flecainide in the absence of ventricular dysfunction, the current recommendation is to attempt to control the arrhythmia with sotalol and amiodarone (Cuneo & Strasburger, 2000;Srinivasan &Strasburger, 2008; Strasburger et al., 2004; Strasburger&Wakai, 2010).
There have been several reports of alternative methods to maternal oral administration with varying degrees of success (Hallak et al., 1991; Parilla et al., 1996; Weiner et al, 1988), but most of these have been met without much general enthusiasm for the increased risk when the success rate of traditional therapy is in excess of 90% (Cuneo & Strasburger, 2000; Kleinman & Nehgme, 2004; Maeno et al., 2009; Srinivasan & Strasburger, 2008; Strasburger et al., 2004; Strasburger & Wakai, 2010). A recent report suggests that neurodevelopmental outcome for babies who experience fetal arrhythmias is very good (Lopriore et al., 2009).

5. Atrial fibrillation in neonates

The diagnosis of atrial fibrillation in the neonate is simpler than in the fetus due to the convenience of direct access to the patient. A 12-lead electrocardiogram can obtained and diagnostic accuracy greatly increased. Rarely is a neonatal invasive electrophysiological study indicated, but esophageal monitoring and pacing may be performed relatively easily. Additionally, the transition from the fetal circulation to the neonatal circulation puts added stretch and stress on the left atrium (and the pulmonary veins) due to lower pulmonary resistance and increased pulmonary blood flow. (Estlin et al., 1998; Larmay & Strasberger, 2004). Two iatrogenic causes of atrial fibrillation or flutter may be seen in newborn infants. The most common of these is due to introduction of an umbilical venous catheter (UVC) into the right atrium. It is not uncommon to find that even a carefully measured UVC line will end up in the right atrium and cause premature atrial contractions, atrial flutter or atrial fibrillation that will be intermittent and spontaneously resolve when the catheter is repositioned to outside of the atrium (da Silva & Waisberg, 2010; Sinha et al., 2005). A second major cause is exposure to the stress of surgical interventions in the neonatal period. If the neonate has structural heart disease, the incidence of atrial flutter or fibrillation is significantly higher, but less intuitive is the structurally normal heart of the infant that must undergo anesthesia and surgical correction of other conditions. Several case reports emphasize the variability with regard to underlying anatomic and electrophysiologic substrate and response to intervention (Bronzetti et al., 2009; Larmay & Strasburger, 2004; Mainzer et al., 2008). The sudden shifts in volume and potential cardiac effects of both inhaled and parenteral anesthetics associated with surgical intervention can easily overtax even the normal neonatal heart and lead to arrhythmias, including atrial flutter and fibrillation. Intrathoracic procedures may add to this risk, with incidental mechanical contact with the neonatal atria triggering an arrhythmia.(Estlin et al., 1998; Gilbert-Barness & Barness 2006;Texter et al., 2006).

The increased risk with neonates is not just limited to their small size and relative fragility, however. It is felt that the immature myocardium, and specifically the atrioventricular node, is also more suited to conduct rapidly, and therefore set the neonate at particularly high risk for rapid ventricular response of any atrial tachyarrythmia, which in turn puts the infant at high risk for a sudden and precipitous drop in cardiac output. If the resultant cardiac output is insufficient for tissue oxygen delivery, the affected infant will then be at significant risk for both developing an irrecoverable rhythm and having end organ damage if the rhythm is not converted in a timely fashion.The largest study of neonates to date identified 50 children over a 25 year period that entered into atrial flutter (seen more often than atrial fibrillation in neonates) with no prior cardiac surgery and only an atrial septal defect found as an associated congenital defect (Texter et al., 2006). There were excellent results with electrical cardioversion (20 of 23, 87%), moderate success with transesophageal pacing (7of 22, 32%), and only 7 of 50 (14%) who required chronic antiarrhythmic therapy. Of those experiencing recurrence of atrial flutter (6 of 50, 12%), all developed an additional supraventricular arrhythmia. Most of the initial atrial flutter (36 of 50, 72%) presented within the first 48 hours of life, and the vast majority (5 of 6, 83%) of recurrent atrial flutter occurred within 24 hours of initial cardioversion. There were an additional five infants who did not experience recurrent atrial flutter (10%) who developed a second supraventricular rhythm (Texter et al., 2006).

Drugs which do not cross the placenta easily are now available for use in newborns if primary electrical cardioversion fails or the infant is in stable arrhythmia and the clinical decision to attempt chemical cardioversion as first line therapy is made. Adenosine may be useful in slowing the ventricular response (which may help identify the underlying arrhythmia) but may not be useful in terminating an atrial tachyarrhythmia. Ventricular rate may be slowed with beta blockade but hypotension and hypoglycemia are even more prevalent in the neonate than in older patients, and should be monitored closely when initiating therapy. Regardless of initial therapy choice, atrialtachyarrhythmias may be difficult to control, and often may require trial and error prior to arriving at either the correct therapeutic drug or drug combination. Once arrhythmia control is established, these patients may be allowed to "outgrow" their medication regimens after careful weight adjustment and monitoring as an outpatient for several months. As they mature, and the atrial conduction system matures, a large number of them have no reported recurrence.

6. Atrial fibrillation in children with myocarditis, cardiomyopathy and cardiac tumors

Infants and children make up a small percentage of patients presenting with atrial fibrillation (Martin, 2001). The seminal report of Radford and Izukawa on atrial fibrillation in children examined the spectrum of conditions associated with this arrhythmia (Radford & Izukawa, 1977). In the 35 cases of atrial fibrillation in children reported, associated conditions included rheumatic heart disease, cardiomyopathy, atrial tumors, infective endocarditis, Marfan syndrome, endocardial fibroelastosis and structural congenital heart disease (Radford & Izukawa, 1977). Cardiomyopathy (six patients), cardiac tumors (three patients), myocarditis and endocarditis (four patients) accounted for 37% of their reported series. One specific type of myocarditis, acute rheumatic fever and subsequent rheumatic heart disease, has decreased to very low levels in developed countries, and will not be discussed in this review.

Myocarditis, cardiomyopathy and cardiac tumors all can present with atrial fibrillation. Myocarditis is often the most difficult of these to diagnose and often requires a high level of clinical suspicion. Fulminant myocarditis can progress to a potentially fatal cardiac failure, often heralded by difficult to control arrhythmias, including atrial fibrillation (Ichikawa et al., 2011). The acute onset and probable viral etiology are keys in the history, but often myocarditis may present with only sudden onset atrial tachyarrhythmia. Resolution is often just as sudden if inflammation recedes and no myocardial scarring occurs. This is particularly the case if the inflamed myocardium is limited to the posterior left atrium. These children would have no findings other than the atrial fibrillation or flutter, possibly with clinical or laboratory evidence of a viral syndrome. Even myocardial biopsies may be negative as they are rarely if ever taken from the atria due the extreme risk of this maneuver. Myocarditis may be suggested on pathological specimens (Chimenti et al., 2010; Frustaci et al., 1997). It is possible that cardiac MRI may be prove useful in the noninvasive diagnosis of myocarditis. There has been some controversy recently surrounding the generally held precept that atrial fibrillation in the setting of myocarditis is caused by the inflammation that is the hallmark of the disease. The potential exists that the arrhythmias are not caused by the active inflammation, but by the remodeling and healing process that comes after the inflammation recedes (Boos et al., 2006; Boos & Lip, 2008; McCabe et al., 2008; Hoyano et al., 2010; Yap, 2009). The progressive nature of atrial structural remodeling appears to underlie the progression of atrial fibrillation in other settings (de Vos et al, 2010; Wolf et al., 2009).

Myocarditis in the setting of other structural or electrophysiologic abnormalities may present special issues. It has been postulated that atrial myocarditis and atrial tachyarrhythmias in the setting of ventricular pre-excitation may cause of sudden death in susceptible children and young adults (Basso et al., 2001). Myocarditis carries a higher risk for some children with congenital heart disease. Children with single ventricular physiology tend to be more reliant on atrial contraction to maintain cardiac output, and may have experienced extensive cardiac surgery. Atrial scarring also characterizes those having undergone atrial switch procedures. Extensive suture lines, atrial scarring, chronic stretch would increase the risk of inflammation and remodeling associated with myocarditis. Treating the underlying myocarditis may be needed to control persistent arrhythmia (Korantzopoulos et al., 2005).

Myocarditis and cardiomyopathy may be linked with acute inflammation leading to chronic myocardial dysfunction. There are many cases of cardiomyopathy that do not follow myocarditis, however. Uncontrolled atrial tachyarrhythmias, particularly with rapid ventricular responses, can cause tachycardia-mediated cardiomyopathy. The genetics of cardiomyopathy and the genetics of atrial fibrillation are intertwined in complicated ways that are being identified. Some recent studies have shown links between cardiomyopathy and arrhythmia (Banwell et al., 1999; Karst et al., 2008; McNair et al., 2011). All types of cardiomyopathy have the potential for arrhythmia. Similar to children with single ventricle physiology, those with cardiomyopathy are dependent on upon atrial contraction for cardiac output. As atrial pressure, stretch, and remodeling occur with deterioration in ventricular function, the frequency of atrial fibrillation increases. The stress on the atrial chamber increases the potential for atrial inflammation and progression to a noninfectious atrial myocarditis (Hsu, 2010). Atrial fibrillation has been shown to be a major clinical risk factor for morbidity in hypertrophic cardiomyopathy (Kubo et al., 2009).

Cardiac tumors are both easier to understand and diagnose. The infamous "tumor plop" may be present on physical exam. They may obstruct flow into the ventricular cavity, or become caught in the atrioventricular valve causing significant regurgitation. Tumors are easily recognizable using echocardiography by their distinct appearance. Depending on the type and location of the tumor, symptoms will vary. Intracardiac tumors which are myxomatous may be pedunculated and mobile, and may swing wildly around the affected atria, potentially bouncing off the interior walls and inciting atrial fibrillation by this contact (Vermeulen et al., 2009; Yu et al., 2006). The treatment for these tumors is predominantly surgical, and reasonable success has been obtained in this manner (Chuaratanaphong et al., 1995; Ipek et al., 2005).Cardiac rhabdomyomas are a hallmark of tuberous sclerosis, and their natural history is that they recede from the time of birth onward. They rarely require intervention unless they are so large that they obstruct the flow of blood, typically by encompassing so much of the myocardium that they impede filling of the ventricles. These can easily be detected prenatally if they are of sufficient size. Atrial tachyarrhythmias may occur when the tumors involve the atrial walls. They may interfere with atrial depolarization or conduction leading to atrial flutter or fibrillation (Yamashita et al., 1987).

Tumors involving the heart, but not originating there, may be associated with atrial fibrillation. Cardiac effects may be due the high output states, inflammatory or chemotherapeutic processes, or direct tumor infiltration of cardiac chambers of the myocardium. Hypercoagulability may be associated with neoplasia, and combined with atrial fibrillation may predisposes to embolic phenomenon from potential mural wall thrombus formation or murantic endocarditis. Benign tumors that arise in the pericardium may also cause mechanical pressure on the atria due to the limited space available to them to grow. All of these may lead to atrial fibrillation, and the resulting clinical impact (Chen et al., 1992; Cooper et al., 1994; Radford & Izukawa, 1977).

7. Atrial fibrillation in children without structural heart disease

Radford and Izukawa noted that atrial fibrillation in childhood may occur at any age, with nearly 50% of those reported by presenting after age 10 years (Radford & Izukawa, 1977). In describing the children with this arrhythmia, they described four cases of atrial fibrillation associated with supraventricular tachycardia (without structural heart disease) and one case of "lone" atrial fibrillation (Radford & Izukawa, 1977). Atrial fibrillation in the absence of structural heart disease, or "lone" atrial fibrillation, accounted for 6% of the older children in this series. Recent reports in adolescents and young adults suggests that "lone" atrial fibrillation may be associated with an abnormal atrial electrophysiologic substrate, and may not be as "lone" as previously suspected (Holmqvist et al., 2011; Korantzopoulos et al., 2009; Stiles et al., 2009). One case of lone atrial fibrillation with complete heart block in a ten year old boy has been reported, suggesting the possibility of more generalized conduction system dysfunction (Krishna Kumar et al., 1991). In a report of nine adolescents with "lone" atrial fibrillation, irregular rapid atrial tachycardias in the region of the pulmonary veins, left atrium and crista terminalis were noted (Nanthakumar et al., 2004), suggesting the possibility of congenital abnormalities in impulse initiation or conduction in these areas. Recently, a single nucleotide polymorphism has been identified that is associated with prolonged atrial conduction and lone atrial fibrillation in young adults (Goodloe et al., 2011)

Atrial fibrillation has also been reported in adolescents without known cardiac disease experiencing the "holiday heart" phenomenon (Koul et al., 2005; Thorton, 1984). The holiday heart consists of atrial fibrillation occurring after binge alcohol consumption in young people without underlying disease or cardiac abnormalities (Koul et al., 2005; Thorton, 1984). Chronic alcohol consumption is also associated with an increased risk of atrial fibrillation and has been reported in some adolescents (Kodama et al., 2011). The use of alcohol with other illicit drugs has also been linked with atrial fibrillation in young adults (Krisnamoorthy et al., 2009). The use of highly caffeinated beverages by adolescents, a popular new phenomenon, is another reported association (Di Rocco et al., 2011). Obesity appears to be a risk factor for atrial fibrillation in younger adults, and the epidemic of obesity in children may represent an increasing risk factor (Guglin, et al., 2011; Niemann, et al. 2011). Additional types of mayhem have been linked to atrial fibrillation in adolescents. There was one report of atrial fibrillation after Taser exposure in an adolescent who tested positive for marijuana (Multerer et al., 2009). Scorpion bite has been linked to cardiac disorders including atrial fibrillation (Alan et al., 2004).

Prescribed medication use may be associated with atrial fibrillation in children without structural heart disease. The use of corticosteroids, taken orally and inhaled, has been linked to atrial fibrillation in children (Huerta et al., 2005; Oteri et al., 2010; Ueda et al., 1988; Yamamura et al., 2011). There is one report of a child with hyperthyroidism presenting with atrial fibrillation (Perry & Hung, 1971). The low frequency of these reported associations would suggest that a genetic propensity toward atrial fibrillation may have been present in the affected individuals.

Atrial fibrillation associated with the WPW syndrome may be life threatening (Paul et al., 1990; Piertersen et al., 1992). Conduction from the fibrillating atria via an accessory atrioventricular connection with a short refractory period may lead to ventricular fibrillation (Brembilla-Perrot et al., 2010; Paul et al., 1990; Piertersen et al., 1992; Sarubbi, 2006). One of the difficulties is determining which of the children with pre-excitation on their electrocardiograms are at risk. In one reported series, spontaneous atrial fibrillation was seen in 4% of children with WPW syndrome, with 22% of children demonstrating atrial fibrillation during electrophysiologic study (Lee et al., 2004). Degeneration of supraventricular tachycardia into atrial fibrillation was seen in 51% of 53 young patients with WPW syndrome, with 34% having a rapid ventricular response rate (Harahsheh et al., 2008). In another study of 62 asymptomatic children with pre-excitation on their electrocardiogram, supraventricular tachycardia was initiated in 58% and atrial fibrillation was observed in 13% (Sarubbi et al., 2005). In a prospective study of asymptomatic children with WPW syndrome, arrhythmias were seen in 51 of 184 patients, 19 of which were life-threatening including three patients with syncope and three with cardiac arrest (Santinelli et al., 2009). Risk factors for life-threatening arrhythmias included a short antegrade effective refractory period for the accessory atrioventricular connection ($\leq$ 240 msec) and multiple accessory atrioventricular connections (Santinelli et al., 2009). Most pediatric electrophysiologists recommend invasive electrophysiologic testing to stratify risk and assess the need for radiofrequency or cryotherapy catheter ablation of the accessory atrioventricular connection in asymptomatic children with manifest pre-excitation (Campbell et al., 2003, Lee et al., 2006; Santinelli et al., 2006). Some children presenting with recurrent atrial fibrillation have supraventricular tachycardia unrelated to pre-excitation or the WPW syndrome as a triggering event and they may be successfully treated by catheter ablation of their supraventricular tachycardia substrate (Streiper et al., 2010).

8. Atrial fibrillation in children with structural heart disease

Nearly half of the cases of atrial fibrillation in children and young adults are associated with congenital heart disease (Radford & Izukawa, 1977). Congenital heart defects may be associated with atrial arrhythmias either before or after surgical correction (Attenhofer Jost et al., 2005; Berger et al., 2005; Bouchardy et al., 2009; Chatzis et al., 2008; Chauvaud et al 2001; Collins, 2009; Hallioglu et al., 2004; Hayashi et al, 2006; Kammeraad et al., 2004; Kaseno et al., 2008; Khairy et al., 2010;Khositeth et al., 2004; Luciani et al., 2008; Marelli et al;, 2010; Massin et al., 2010; Porter & Garson, 1993; Radford & Izukawa, 1977; Saul, 2008; Spies et al., 2008; Sugimoto et al., 2001, Trojnarska et al., 2009). Those congenital heart defects occurring in conjunction with atrial fibrillation include those associated with abnormalities in the development of the cardiac conduction system, abnormalities in the development of atrial structure, abnormalities in flow resulting in atrial enlargement, abnormalities in impulse initiation or conduction from surgical atrial scarring. The risk factors for developing atrial fibrillation originate in early in life but not become manifest until adulthood.

Congenital heart defects that are most often associated with atrial fibrillation include atrial septal defect, Ebstein anomaly, anomalies in pulmonary venous drainage, transposition of the great arteries, single ventricle, tetralogy of Fallot and Marfan syndrome (Attenhofer Jost et al., 2005; Berger et al., 2005; Bouchardy et al., 2009; Chatzis et al., 2008; Chauvaud et al 2001; Collins, 2009; Hallioglu et al., 2004; Hayashi et al, 2006; Kammeraad et al., 2004; Kaseno et al., 2008; Khairy et al., 2010; Khositeth et al., 2004; Luciani et al., 2008; Marelli et al;, 2010; Martin et. al., 1983; Massin et al., 2010; Porter & Garson, 1993;Radford & Izukawa, 1977; Saul, 2008;Spies et al., 2008; Sugimoto et al., 2001; Trojnarska et al., 2009). Atrial fibrillation has also been seen following heart transplantation in pediatric patients (Collins et al., 2003). Risk factors for atrial fibrillation in congenital heart disease include age at operation, atrial dilatation from intra-cardiac shunting, atrial dilatation from valve insufficiency, extensive atrial suture lines and ventricular myocardial dysfunction. Recent advances in pediatric heart disease management include repair of congenital defects at younger ages, percutaneous catheter and device intervention to avoid complications of cardiac bypass, modifications of surgery to avoid atrial scarring and more aggressive management of residual regurgitant valve lesions. The hope is that these changes will decrease the burden of atrial fibrillation associated with congenital heart disease.

9. Management of atrial fibrillation in children

The diagnosis of atrial fibrillation in childhood is not difficult in most instances. Intravenous adenosine and transesophageal electrode recording can be used to assist in the diagnosis (Fazio et al., 2008; Gewitz & Woolf, 2006; Kaltman & Shah, 2004). Guidelines are available for treatment of atrial fibrillation in adults, and with modifications, provide a framework for treating children with the arrhythmia (American College of Cardiology/American Heart Association/European Society of Cardiology, 2006; American College of Cardiology Foundation/American Heart Association/Heart Rhythm Society (ACCF/AHA/HRS), 2011). Emergency management of children with significant hemodynamic compromise would include electrical cardioversion (Gewitz & Woolf, 2006; Kaltman & Shah, 2004). In more stable children, the use of intravenous beta-adrenergic blocker (eg, esmolol, propranolol) or calcium channel blocker (eg. verapamil, diltiazem) could be used to slow the ventricular response rate (Fazio et al, 2008; Gewitz & Woolf, 2006; Kaltman & Shah, 2004). See table for a listing of useful drugs in the management of atrial fibrillation in children. Intravenous digoxin or amiodarone could be used emergently and continued on a chronic

Drug	Dose	Effect	Indication
Adenosine	Child: 0.1-0.2 mg/kg IV Adolescent (> 50 kg): 6mg IV	Slow AV conduction	Rapid ventricular response Diagnosis Afib
Amiodarone	Child: 5 mg/kg IV 5-15 mg/kg po qd Adolescent: 600 mg/1.73 m² IV 200-1600 mg po qd	Slow AV conduction Prevent AFib recurrence Slow WPW conduction	Rapid ventricular response Persistent or recurrent AFib
Atenolol	Child: 0.5-1 mg/kg po qd Adolescent: 25-100 mg po qd	Slow AV conduction	Rapid ventricular response
Digoxin	Infant: 15-30 mcg/kg IV qd: load 20-35 mcg/kg po qd: load 4-8 mcg/kg IV qd: maintenance 5-10 mcg/kg po qd: maintenance Child: 20-40 mcg/kg IV qd: load 30-50 mcg/kg po qd: load 6-9 mcg/kg IV qd: maintenance 8-12 mcg/kg po qd: maintenance Adolescent (> 10 y, < 100 kg): 8-12 mcg/kg IV qd: load 10-15 mcg/kg po qd: load 2-3 mcg/kg IV qd: maintenance 2.5-5 mcg/kg po qd: maintenance	Slow AV conduction Improve contractility	Rapid ventricular response Avoid in WPW
Diltiazem	Child: 1.5-2 mg/kg po tid or qid Adolescent: 30-120 mg/kg po tid or qid 120-300 mg/kg po qd or bid (SR)	Slow AV conduction	Rapid ventricular response Avoid in WPW
Dofetilide	Adolescent (≥ 18 y): 125-500 mcg/kg po bid	Prevent Afib recurrence	Persistent or recurrent Afib
Esmolol	Child & Adolescent: 100-500 mcg/kg IV: load 25-100 mcg/kg/min IV: infusion Titrate: 50-1000 mcg/kg/min	Slow AV conduction	Rapid ventricular response
Flecainide	Child: 1-2 mg/kgpo bid Adolescent: 25-150 mg po bid	Prevent Afib recurrence Slow WPW conduction	Persistent or recurrent Afib Rapid ventricular response
Heparin	Child: 75 U/kg IV: load 18-28 U/kg/h IV: infusion 75-100 U/kg q 4 h IV: intermittent Adolescent: 50-100 U/kg IV: load 15-25 U/kg/h IV: infusion 75- 125 U/kg q 4 h IV: intermittent	Anticoagulation	Persistent or recurrent Afib Prior to cardioversion
Ibutilide	Adolescent (≥ 18 y) < 60 kg: 0.01 mg/kg IV ≥60 kg: 1 mg IV	Prevent Afib recurrence Slow WPW conduction	Persistent or recurrent Afib Rapid ventricular response
Procainamide	Child: 2-15 mg/kg IV: load 20-80 mcg/kg/min IV: infusion 15-50 mg/kg/24 h q 3-6 h po Adolescent: 50-100 mg IV: load Titrate to 1-6 mg/min IV 250-500 mg po q 3-6 h 500-1000 mg q 6 h (SR)	Prevent Afib recurrence Slow WPW conduction	Persistent or recurrent Afib Rapid ventricular response
Propafenone	Adolescent (≥ 18 y): 150-300 mg po tid	Prevent Afib recurrence Slow WPW conduction	Persistent or recurrent Afib Rapid ventricular response
Propranolol	Child: 0.01-0.1 mg/kg IV Max: 1 mg infants; 3 mg child 0.5-1 mg/kg/24 h po q 6-8 h Adolescent: 1 mg/kg IV; max 5 mg 10-20 mg po tid or qid	Slow AV conduction	Rapid ventricular response
Verapamil	Child: 0.1-0.3 mg/kg IV Max: 5-10 mg 4-8 mg/kg/24 h tid or qid Adolescent: 5-10 mg IV 240-480 mg po tid or qid 240-480 mg/kg bid or qd (SR)	Slow AV conduction	Rapid ventricular response Avoid in WPW
Warfarin	Child: 0.2 mg/kg po qd Max: 5 mg po qd Titrate to INR 2-3 Adolescent: 5-10 mg po qd	Anticoagulant	Persistent or recurrent A fib

Afib = atrial fibrillation; AV = atrioventricular; bid = 2 times per day; h = hours; IV = intravenously; kg = kilogram mcg = micrograms; mg = milligrams; min = minutes; po = by mouth; qid = 4 times per day; qd = daily; tid = 3 times per day; WPW = Wolff Parkinson White syndrome.
Drug recommendations and dosages are subject to change, check prior to administration.
Table adapted from Taketomo, et al., 2010; Lee, et al., 2009 & Manzi, 2006.

Table 1. Useful drugs in the management of atrial fibrillation in infants and children.

basis if needed (Fazio et al, 2008; Gewitz & Woolf, 2006; Kaltman & Shah, 2004). Other drugs available for the management of acute and chronic atrial fibrillation in children include sotalol, propafenone, procaineamide, flecainide, ibutilide, and dofetilide (Gewitz & Woolf, 2006; Kaltman & Shah, 2004; Fazio et al, 2008). In patients with WPW syndrome, digoxin and verapamil should not be used due to tendency to increase antegrade conduction via the accessory atrioventricular connection (Byrum et al, 1982; Fazio et al, 2008; Gewitz & Woolf, 2006; Kaltman & Shah, 2004; Rowland, 1983). If elective cardioversion is needed, transeosophageal or transthoracic echocardiography will be needed to assess the need for anticoagulation prior to the procedure (ACC/AHA/ESC, 2006; Fazio et al, 2008; Gewitz & Woolf, 2006; Horenstein et al, 2004; Kaltman & Shah, 2004). Long term oral anticoagulation with coumadin may be need in high risk pediatric patients with chronic or recurrent atrial fibrillation.

The demonstrated success of the Maze procedure for the surgical treatment of atrial fibrillation (Cox et al., 1991; Cox, 2010) and the development of subsequent percutaneous catheter ablation techniques (Haissaguerre et al., 1998; Weerasooriya et al., 2011) have led to new options in the management of atrial fibrillation. Arrhythmia surgery has been successful in children with and without congenital heart disease (Deal et al, 2003). Congenital heart defects associated with arrhythmias have been successfully treated with combined surgical and ablative procedures (Deal et al., 2003; Fujita et al., 2009; Greason et al., 2003; Mavroudis et al., 2008; Stulak et al., 2006; Therrien et al., 2001). These new techniques allow for an individual approach tailored to the needs of specific patients (Brenyo & Aktas, 2011). Recurrence of atrial fibrillation following surgical or catheter ablation remains a risk and the need for oral anticoagulation is being debated (Themistoclakis et al, 2010). Newer drugs (eg, dabigatran) for long-term anticoagulation may be useful in some childhood cases of atrial fibrillation (Dahl & Huisman, 2010).

10. Prognosis

No prospective long-term follow-up is reported in children with atrial fibrillation. Children in the newborn period with no underlying disease have an excellent prognosis, as do those older patients with a triggering event or disease which is reversible. Lone atrial fibrillation in older children and young adults has a good outcome. Patients with atrial fibrillation associated with abnormal cardiac structural, functional or electrophysiologic substrate have a variable outcome. Newer drugs offer clinical improvement on a short term basis but long-term outcomes, especially for children, are not available. Surgical and catheter management techniques continue to offer a new alternative, but no long-term follow-up in young patients is available.

11. Conclusions

Atrial fibrillation is a relatively uncommon arrhythmia in childhood. It may be associated with genetic, electrophysiologic and structural variables that are present from the prenatal period. It may become manifest early in life under conditions of infection, neoplasia, structural, functional or electrical cardiac disease. It may be seen in the absence of cardiac disease in metabolic, infectious or systemic disease. Drug or alcohol exposure, electric shock or scorpion envenomation may precipitate an attack. Diagnosis and treatment will vary with age, electrophysiologic and anatomic substrate and clinical status. Newer diagnostic tools, pharmacologic therapies, surgical and catheter procedures allow for individualized approach in this interesting group of patients.

12. Acknowledgements

This work is dedicated to Angela C. Gilladoga, MD, FACC, pediatric cardiologist at Eastern Maine Medical Center. Her dedication to the care of pediatric cardiology patients in eastern and northern Maine for the past 30 years is recognized and appreciated.

13. References

Aburawi, E.; Thomson, J. &Blackburn, M. (2006)Familial idiopathic atrial fibrillation with fetal bradycardia.*ActaPaediatr*;Vol.95, pp. 1700-1702.

Akinci, E.; Alp, M. & Yakut C. (2005)Surgical management of cardiac myxoma. *J Card Surg*, May-Jun, Vol. 20, No. 3, pp. 300-304.

Alan, S.; Ulgen, M.S.; Soker, M.; Geyik, F.; Karabulut, A. & Toprak. N. (2004) Electrocardiologic and echocardiographic features of patients exposed to scorpion bite. *Angiology*, Vol.55, No.1, pp. 79-84.

American College of Cardiology/American Heart Association /European Society of Cardiology 2006 Guidelines for the management of patients with atrial fibrillation: a report of the American College of Cardiology/American Heart Association Task Force on Practice Guidelines and the EuropeanSociety of Cardiology Committee for Practice Guidelines (Writing Committee to Revise the 2001Guidelines for Management of Patients With atrial Fibrillation).(2006)*Circulation*, Vol.114:pp. e257-354.2011

American College of Cardiology Foundation/American Heart Association/Heart Rhythm Society focused update on the management of patients with atrial fibrillation (updating the 2006 guideline):a report of the American College of Cardiology Foundation/ American Heart Association Task Force on Practice Guidelines.(2011)*J Am Coll Cardiol*, Vol.57, No.2, pp. 223-242.

Attenhofer Jost, C. H.; Connolly, H. M.; Danielson, G. K.; Bailey, K. R.; Schoff, H. V.; Shen, W. K.; Warnes, C. A.; Seward, J. B.; Puga, F. J. & Talik, A. J. (2005) Sinus venosus atrial septal defect: long-term postoperative outcome for 115 patients. *Circulation*, Vol.11, No.13, pp. 1953-1958.

Azancot-Benistry, A; Jacqz-Aigrain, E.; Guirgis, N. M.; Decrepy, A.; Oury, J. F. & Blot, P. (1992) Clinical and pharmacologic study of fetal supraventricular tachyarrhythmias. *J Pediatr*, Vol.121, pp. 608–613.

Banwell, B.L.; Becker, L. E.; Jay, V.; Taylor, G. P. & Vajsar, J. (1999)Cardiac manifestations of congenital fiber-type disproportion myopathy. *J Child Neurol*, Vol.14, No.2, pp. 83-87.

Basso, C.; Corrado, D.; Rossi, L. & Thiene, G. (2001) Ventricular preexcitation in children and young adults: atrial myocarditis as a possible trigger of sudden death. *Circulation*, Vol.103,pp. 269–275.

Belhassen, B.; Pauzner, D.; Bleiden, L.; Sherez, J.; Zinger, A.; David, M.; Muhlbauer, B. & Laniado, S. (1982) Intrauterine and postnatal atrial fibrillation in the Wolff-Parkinson-White syndrome.*Circulation*, Vol.66, pp. 1124-1128

Benito, B.; Brugada, R.; Perich, R.M.; Lizotte, E.; Cinca, J.; Mont, L.; Berruezo, A.; Tolosana, J. M.; Freixa, X.; Brugada, P. & Brugada, J. (2008) A mutation in the sodium channel is responsible for the association of long QT syndrome and familial atrial fibrillation. *Heart Rhythm*,Vol.5, No.10, pp. 1434-1440.

Berger, F.; Vogel, M.; Kretschmar, O.; Dave, H.; Pretre, R. & Dodge-Khatami A.(2005) Arrhythmias in patients with surgically treated atrial septal defects. *Swiss Med Wkly* Vol.135. No.11-12, pp. 175-178.

Bertram, H.; Paul, T.; Beyer, F. & Kallfelz, H. C. (1996) Familial idiopathic atrial fibrillation with bradyarrhythmia. *Eur J Pediatr*, Vol.155. No.1, pp. 7-10.

Boos, C. J.; Anderson, R. A. & Lip, G. Y. (2006)Is atrial fibrillation an inflammatory disorder? *Eur Heart J*, Jan, Vol.27, No.2, pp. 136-149.

Boos, C. J. & Lip, G.Y. (2008) Inflammation and atrial fibrillation: cause or effect? *Heart*, Vol.94, No.2, pp. 133-134.

Bouchardy, J.; Therrien, J.; Pilote, L.; Ionescu-Ittu, R.; Martucci, G.; Bottega, N. & Marelli, A. J. (2009) Atrial arrhythmias in adults with congenital heart disease. *Circulation*, Vol.120, pp. 1679-1686.

Boyett, M. R. (2009;) 'And the beat goes on' The cardiac conduction system: the wiring system of the heart. *Exp Physiol,*, Vol94, No.10, pp. 1035-1049.

Brembilla-Perrot, B.; Tater, C. & Suty-Selton, C. (2010) Risk factors of adverse presentation as the first arrhythmia in Wolff-Parkinson-White syndrome. *Pacing Clin Electrophysiol*, Vol.33, No.9, pp. 1074-1081.

Brenyo, A. J. & Aktas, M. K. (2011).Non-pharmacologic management of atrial fibrillation.*Am J Cardiol*, Vol.108, pp. 317-325.

Bronzetti, G.; D'Angelo, C.; Angelini, A.; Picchio, F. M. & Boriani, G. (2009) Resolution of atrial thrombosis with heparin in a newborn with atrial flutter. *Acta Paediatr,* Vol.8, pp. 1211-1214.

Byrum, C. J.; Wahl, R. A.; Behrendt, D.M. & Dick, M. (1982) Ventricular fibrillation associated with the use of digitalis in a newborn infant with Wolff-Parkinson-White syndrome. *J Pediatr*, Vol.101, pp. 400-403.

Campbell, R. M.; Strieper, M. J.; Frias, P.A.; Collins, K. K.; Van Hare, G. F. & Dubin, A. M. (2003) Survey of current practice of pediatric electrophysiologists for asymptomatic Wolff-Parkinson-White syndrome. *Pediatrics*, Vol.111, No.3, e245-e247.

Chandler, N. J.; Greener, I.D.; Tellez, J. O.; Inada, S.; Musa, H.; Molenaar, P.; DiFrancesco, D.; Baruscotti, M.; Longhi, R.; Anderson, R. H.; Billeter, R.; Sharma, V.; Sigg, D.C.; Boyett, M.R. & Dobrzynski, H. (2009) Molecular architecture of the human sinus node – insights into the function of the cardiac pacemaker. *Circulation*;119:1562-1575.

Chatzis, A. C.; Giannopoulos, N. M.; Milonakis, M.; Contrafouris, C.A.; Tsoutsinos, A.; Kolettis, T.; Panagiotou, C.; Zavaropoulos, P.; Maraki, P.; Koussi, T.; Sofianidou, J.; Kirvassilis, G.V. & Sarris, G. E. (2008) Mid-term results following surgical treatment of congenital cardiac malformations in adults. *Cardiol Young*, Vol.18, No.5, pp. 461-466.

Chauvaud, S. M.; BranCaccio, G. & Carpentier, A. F. (2001) Cardiac arrhythmias in patients undergoing surgical repair of Ebstein's anomaly. *Ann Thorac Surg*, Vol.71, No.5, pp. 1547-1552.

Chen, H. Z.; Jiang, L.; Rong, W.H.; Wang, J. S.; Shen, C.; Shi, Y. F. & Pu, S. Y. (1992) Tumors of the heart. An analysis of 79 cases. Chin Med J (Engl). Feb, Vol.105, No.2, pp. 153-158.

Chimenti, C.; Russo, M. A.; Carpi, A. & Frustaci, A. (2010) Histological substrate of human atrial fibrillation. *Biomed Pharmacother*, Mar, Vol.64, No.3, pp. 177-83.

Collins, K. K. (2009)The spectrum of long-term electrophysiologic abnormalities in patients with univentricular hearts. *Congenit Heart Dis*, Vol.4, No.5, pp. 310-317.

Collins, K. K.; Thiagarajan, R. R.; Chin, C.; Dubin, A. M.; Van Hare, G. F.; Robbins, R. C.; Mayer, J. E.; Bernstein, D.: Berul, C. I. &Blume, E. D. (2003;)Atrial tachyarrhythmias and permanent pacing after pediatric heart transplantation. *J Heart Lung Transplant*, Vol.22, No.10, pp. 1126-1133.

Cooper, M. J.; deLorimier, A. A.; Higgins, C. B.; Van Hare, G. F. &, Enderlein, M. A. (1994) Atrial flutter-fibrillation resulting from left atrial compression by an intrapericardial lipoma. *Am Heart J*. Apr Vol.127, No.4 Pt 1, pp 950-951.

Cox, J. L. (2010) The longstanding, persistent confusion surrounding surgery for atrial fibrillation. *J Thorac Cardiovasc Surg*, Vol.139, pp. 1374-1386.

Cox, J. L.; Scheussler, J. B.; D'Agostino, H. J. Jr.; Stone, C. M.; Chang, B.C.; Cain, M. E.; Corr, P. B. & Boineau, J. P. (1991) The surgical treatment of atrial fibrillation III: development of a definitive surgical procedure. *J Thorac Cadiovasc Surg*, Vol101, No.4, pp. 569-583.

Cuneo, B. F. & Strasburger, J. F. (2000) Management strategy for fetal tachycardia. *Obstet Gynecol.*, Vol.96, pp. 575–581.

Dahl, O. E. & Huisman, M. V. (2010) Dabigatran etexilate: advances in anticoagulation therapy. *Expert Rev Cardiovasc Ther*, Vol.8, No.6, pp. 771-774.

Darbar, D.: Kannankeril, P. J.; Donahue, B. S.; Kucera, G.; Stubblefield, T.; Haines, J. L.; George, A.L.; Roden DM. (2008) Cardiac sodium channel (*SCN5A*) variants associated with atrial fibrillation. *Circulation*, Vol.117, pp. 1927-1935.

da Silva, P. S. & Waisberg, J. (2010) Induction of life-threatening supraventricular tachycardia during central venous catheter placement: an unusual complication. *J Pediatr Surg*, Aug, Vol.45, No.8, pp. E13-E16

Deal, B. J.; Mavroudis, C. &Backer C. L. (2003) Beyond Fontan conversion: surgical therapy of arrhythmias including patients with associated complex congenital heart disease. *Ann Thorac Surg*, Vol.76, No.2, pp. 542-553.

de Vos, C. B.; Pisters, R.; Nieuwlaat, R.; Prins, M. H.; Tieleman, R.G.; Coelen, R.-J. S., van den Heijkant, A. C.; Alessie, M. A. & Crijns, H. J. G. M. (2010) Progressionfrom paroxysmal to persistent atrial fibrillation. *J Am Coll Cardiol*, Vol.55, pp. 725-731.

Di Rocco, J. R.; During, A.; Morelli, P. J.; Heyden, M. & Biancaniello, T. A. (2011) Atrial fibrillation in healthy adolescents after highly caffeinated beverage consumption: two case reports. *J Med Case Reports*, Vol.5, No.1, p.18.

Dobrzynski, H.; Li, J.; Tellez, J.; Greener, I. D.: Nikolski, V. P.; Wright, S. E.; Parson, S. H.; Jones, S. A.; Lancaster, M. K.; Yamamoto, M.; Honjo, H.; Takagishi, Y.; Kodama, I.; Efimov, I.R: Billeter, R. & Boyett, MR. (2005) Computer three-dimensional reconstruction of the sinoatrial node.*Circulation*, Vol.111, 846-854.

Estlin, E. J.; Bennett, M. K.; Skinner, J. R.; Milligan, D. W. & Wren, C. (1998) Atrial fibrillation with neonatal pulmonary lymphangiectasia. *Acta Paediatr*, Dec, Vol.87, No.12, pp. 1304-1306.

Fazio, G.; Visconti, C.: D'Angelo, L.; Novo, G.; Barbaro, G. & Novo, S. (2008) Pharmacological therapy in children with atrial fibrillation and atrial flutter. *Curr Pharm Des*, Vol.14, No.8, pp. 770-775.

Frohn-Mulder, I.M.: Stewart, P. A.; Witsenburg, M.; Den Hollander, N. S.; Wladimiroff, J. W. & Hess, S. (1995)The efficacy of flecainide versus digoxin inthe management of fetal supraventricular tachycardia. *Prenat Diagn*, Vol.15, pp. 1297–1302.

Frustaci, A.: Chimenti, C.; Bellocc,i F.; Morgante, E.; Russo, M. A. & Maseri, A. (1997) Histological substrate of atrial biopsies in patients with lone atrial fibrillation. *Circulation*, Vol.96, pp. 1180–1184.

Fujita, S.; Takahashi, K.; Takeuchi, D.; Manaka, T.; Shoda, M.; Hagiwara, N.; Kurosawa, H& Nakanisha, T. (2009) Management of late atrial tachyarrhythmias long after Fontan operation. *J Cardiol*, Vol. 53 No.3, 410-416.

Gewitz, M. H. & Woolf, P.K. (2006)Cardiac emergencies. In: *Textbook of Pediatric Emergency Medicine*, 5th ed., Fleister, G. R.: Ludwig, S.; Henretig, F.M., eds., Lippincott Willliams & Wilkins, Philadelphia PA, pp. 717-758.

Gilbert-Barness, E. &Barness, L. A. (2006)Pathogenesis of cardiac conduction disorders in children genetic and histopathologic aspects. *Am J Med Genet A*.Oct 1, Vol.140, No.19, pp. 1993-2006.

Gittenberger-De Groot, A. C.; Mahtab, E. A. F.; Hahurij, N. D.; Wisse, L. J.; DeRuiter, M. C.; Wijffels, M.C. E. F. & Poelman, R. E. (2007) Nkx2.5-negative myocardium of the posterior heart field and its correlation with podoplanin expression in cells from the developing cardiac pacemaking and conduction system. *Anat Rec*, Vol.290, pp 115-122.

Goodloe, A, H.; Herron, K. J. & Olson, T. M. (2011) Uncovering an intermediate phenotype associated with rs2200733 at 4q25 in lone atrial fibrillation. *Am J Cardiol*, Vol.107, pp. 1802-1805.

Gourdie, R. G.; Harris, B. S.; Bond, J.; Justus, C.; Hewett, K. W.; O'Brien, T. X.; Thompson, R. P. & Sedmera, D. (2003) Development of the cardiac pacemaking and conduction system.*Birth Defects Research (Part C)*, Vol.69, pp. 46-57.

Greason, K.L.; Dearan,i J. A.; Theodoro, D. A.; Porter, C. B.; Warnes, C. A. & Danielson, G. K. (2003) Surgical management of atrial tachyarrhythmias associated with congenital cardiac anomalies: Mayo Clinic experience. *Semin Thorac Cardiovasc Surg Pediatr Card Surg Annu*, Vol.6, pp. 59-71.

Guglin, M.; Maradia, K.; Chen, R. & Curtis, A. B. (2011) Relation of obesity to recurrence rate and burden of atrial fibrillation. *Am J Cardiol*, Vol.107, pp. 579-582.

Haissaguerre, M.: Jais, P.; Shah, D. C.; Takahashi, A.; Hosini, M.; Quinou, G.; Garrique, S.; Le Mouroux, A.; Le Metayer, D. &Clementy, J. (1998) Spontaneous initiation of atrial fibrillation by ectopic beats originating in the pulmonary veins. *N Engl J Med*, Vol.339, No.10, pp. 659-666.

Hajdu, J.; Szabo, I.; Papp, C.; Gorbe, E.; Cesko, I. & Papp, Z.(1997) [Treatment of haemodynamically significant fetal arrhythmias].*Orv Hetil*, Vol.138,pp. 2335–2338.

Hallak, M.; Neerhof, M.G.; Perry, R.; Nazir, M. & Huhta, J. C. (1991) Fetal supraventricular tachycardia and hydrops fetalis: combined intensive, direct, and transplacental therapy. *Obstet Gynecol*, Vol.78 (Pt 2) pp. 523–525.

Hallioglu, O.; Aytemir, K. & Celiker, A. (2004) The significance of P wave duration and P wave dispersion for risk assessment of atrial tachyarrhythmias in patients with corrected tetralogy of Fallot. *Ann Noninvasive Electrocardiol* ,Vol.9,No.4, pp. 339-344.

Hansmann, M .; Gembruch, U.; Bald, R.;Manz, M. & Redel, D. A.(1991) Fetal tachyarrhythmias: transplacental and directtreatment of the fetus - a report of 60 cases. *Ultrasound Obstet Gynecol*, Vol.1, pp. 162–70.

Harahsheh, A.: Du, W.; Singh, H. & Karpawich, P. P. (2008) Risk factors for atrioventricular tachycardia degenerating into atrial flutter or fibrillation in the young with Wolff-Parkinson-White. *Pacing Clin Electrophysiol*, Vol.31, No.10, pp 1307-1312.

Hayashi, G.; Kurosaki, K.; Echigo, S.; Kado, H.; Fukushima, N.; Yokota, M.; Niwa, K.; Shinohara, T. & Nakazawa M. (2006) Prevalence of arrhythmias and their risk factors mid- and long-term after the arterial switch operation. *Pediatr Cardiol*, Vol.27, No.6, pp. 689-694.

Ho, S.Y. & Anderson, R. H. (1990) Embryology and anatomy of the normal and abnormal conduction system. In: *Pediatric Arrhythmias: Electrophysiology and Pacing*. Gillette, P. C. & Garson, A. Jr., eds. W. B. Saunders Company, Philadelphia PA, pp. 2-27.

Hodgson-Zingman, D. M.; Karst, M. L.; Zingman, L. V.; Heublein, D. M.; Darbar, D,: Herron, K. J.; Ballew J. D.; de Andrade, M.; Burnett, J.C. Jr. & Olson, T. M. (2008) Atrial natriuretic peptide frameshift Mutation in familial atrial fibrillation.*N Engl J Med*, Vol.359, pp. 158-165.

Holmqvist. F.; Olesen, M. S.; Tveit, A.; Enger, S.; Topanainen, J.; Jurkko, R.; Havmoller, R.; Haimso, S.; Carlson, J.; Svendsen, J.H. & Platanov, P. G. (2011) Abnormal atrial activation in young patients with loneatrial fibrillation. *Europace*, Vol.13, pp. 188-192.

Hoogaars, W. M. H.; Engel, A.; Brons, J. F.; Verkerk, A. O.; de Lange, F. J.; Wong, L. Y. E.; Bakker, M. L.; Clout, D. E.; Wakker, V.; Barnett, P.; Ravesloot, J. H.; Moorman, A. F. M; Verheijck, E. E. & Christoffels, V. M. (2007). Tbx3 controls the sinoatrial gene program and imposes pacemaker function on the atria. *Genes Dev*, Vol.21, pp. 1098-1112.

Horenstein, M. S.; Karpawich, P. P.; Epstein, M. L. & Singh, T. P. (2004) Transthoracic echocardiography for precardioversion screening during atrial flutter/fibrillation in young patients. *Clin Cardiol*, Vol.27, No.7, pp. 413-416.

Hoyano, M.; Ito, M.; Kimura, S.; Tanaka, K.; Okamura, K.; Komura, S.; Mitsuma, W.; Hirono, S.; Chinushi, M.; Kodama; M. & Aizawa, Y. (2010) Inducibility of atrial fibrillation depends not on inflammation but on atrial structural remodeling in rat experimental autoimmune myocarditis. *Cardiovasc Pathol*, Sep-Oct, Vol.19, No.5, pp. e149-e157.

Hsu, D. T. (2010) Cardiac manifestations of neuromuscular disorders in children.*Paediatr Respir Rev*, Mar, Vol.11, No.1, pp. 35-38.

Huerta, C.; Lanes, S. F. & Garcia Rodriguez, L. A. (2005) Respiratory medications and risk of cardiac arrhythmia. *Epidemiology*, Vol.16, No.3, pp. 360-366.

Ichikawa, R.; Sumitomo, N.; Komori, A.; Abe, Y.; Nakamura, T.; Fukuhara, J.; Matsumura, M.; Miyashita, M; Kanamaru, H.; Ayusawa, M. & Mugishima, H. (2011) The follow-up evaluation of electrocardiogram and arrhythmias in children with fulminant myocarditis. *Circ J*, Apr, Vol.75, No.4, pp. 932-938.

Ipek, G.; Erentug, V.; Bozbuga, N.; Polat, A.; Guler, M.; Kirali, K.; Peker, O.; Balkanay, M.;Chuaratanaphong, S.; Songthanasak, T.; Nawarawong, W. & Asavapiyanond, S. (1995) The surgical treatment of atrial myxomas: clinical experience in 6 patients. *J Med Assoc Thai.*, Aug, Vol. 78, No.8, pp. 415-418.

Jaeggi, E.; Fouron, J. C. & Drblik, S.P. (1998) Fetal atrial flutter: diagnosis, clinical features, treatment, and outcome. *J Pediatr*, Vol.132, pp. 335–339.

Jay, P. Y.; Harris, B. S.; Buerger, A.; Rozhitskaya, O.; Maguire CT, Barbosky, LA.; McCusty, E.; Berul, C. I.; O'Brien, T. X.; Gourdie, R. G. & Izumo, S. (2004) Function follows form: cardiac conduction system defects in Nkx2.5 mutation. *Anat Rec Part A*, Vol.280A, pp. 966-972.

Johnson, J. N.; Tester, D. J.; Perry, J.; Salisbury, B.A,.;Reed, C. R. & Ackerman, M. J. (2008) Prevalence of early-onset atrial fibrillation in congenital long QT syndrome. *Heart Rhythm*, Vol.5, No.5, pp. 704-709.

Jongbloed, M. R. M.; Schalij, M.J.; Poelmann, R. E.; Blom, N. A. Fekkes, M. L.; Wang, Z.; Fishman, G. I. & Gittenberger-DeGroot, A. C. (2004;) Embryonic conduction tissue: a special correlation with adult arrhythmogenic areas. *J Cardiovasc Electrophysiol* Vol.15, No.3, pp. 349-365.

Kahler, C.; Grimm, B.; Schleussner, E.; Schneider, A.; Schneider, U.; Nowak, H.; Vogt, L. & Seewald, H. J. (2001)The application of fetal magnetocardiography (FMCG) to investigate fetal arrhythmias and congenital heart defects (CHD). *Prenat Diagn*, Vol.21, No.3, pp. 176-182.

Kaltman, J. & Shah, M. (2004) Evaluation of the child with an arrhythmia. *Pediatr Clin N Am*, Vol.51, pp. 537-1551.

Kammeraad, J. A.; van Deurzen, C. H.; Sreeram, N.; Bink-Boelkins, M. T.; Ottenkamp,J.; Helbing, W. A.; Lam, J.; Sobotka-Plojhar, M. A.; Daniels, O. & Balaji, S. (2004) Predictors of sudden death after Mustard or Senning repair for transposition of the great arteries. *J Am Coll Cardiol*, Vol.44, No.5, pp. 1095-1102.

Karst, M. L.; Herron, K.J & Olson, T. M. (2008) X-linked nonsyndromic sinus node dysfunction and atrial fibrillation caused by emerin mutation. *J Cardiovasc Electrophysiol*, Vol.19, No.5, pp. 510-515.

Kaseno, K.; Tada, H.; Koyama, K.; Jingu. M.; Hiramatsu, S.; Yokokawa, M.; Goto, K.; Naito, S.; Oshima, S. & Taniguchi, K. (2008;) Prevalence and characterization of pulmonary vein variants in patients with atrial fibrillation determined using 3-dimensional computed tomography. *Am J Cardiol*, Vol.101, No.11, pp. 1638-1642.

Kaufman. E. S. (2009) Mechanisms and clinical management of inherited channelopathies: long QT syndrome, Brugada syndrome, catecholaminergic polymorphic ventricular tachycardia, and short QT syndrome.*Heart Rhythm;*, Vol.6, No.8 Suppl, pp. S51-S55.

Khairy, P.; Aboulhosn, J.; Gurvitz, M.Z.; Opotowsky, A. R.; Mongeon, F. P.; Kay, J.; Valente, A. M.; Earing,M. G.; Lui, G.; Gersony, D. R.; Cook, S.; Ting, J. G.; Nickolaus, M. J.; Webb, G.; Landzberg, M. J. & Broberg CS. (2010) Alliance for Adult Research in Congenital Cardiology. Arrhythmia burden in Adultswith surgically repaired tetralogy of Fallot: a multi-institutional study. *Circulation*, Vol.122, No.9. pp. 868-875.

Khositeth, A.; Danielson, G.K.; Dearani, J. A.; Munger, T. M. & Porter, C. J. (2004) Supraventricular tachyarrhythmias in Ebstein's anomaly: management and outcome. *J Thorac Cardiovasc Surg*, Vol.128, No.6, pp. 826-833.

Klein, G. J.; Bashore, I. M.; Sellers, T. D.; Prichett, E. L.; Smith, W. M. & Gallagher, J. J. (1979) Ventricular fibrillation in the Wolff-Parkinson-White syndrome. *N Engl J Med*, Vol.301, pp. 1080-1085.

Kleinman, C. S. & Nehgeme, R. A. (2004) Cardiac arrhythmias in the human fetus.*Pediatr Cardiol*, Vol.25, No.3, pp. 234-251.

Kleinman, C. S.; Nehgeme, R. & Copel, JA.(1999) Fetal cardiac arrhythmias: diagnosis and therapy. In: Creasy, R. K. & Resnik, R., eds.,*Maternal-Fetal Medicine,* 4th ed. Philadelphia: PA, WB Saunder Co, pp. 301–318.

Kodama, S.; Saito, K.; Tanaka, S.; Horikawa, C.; Saito, A.; Heianza, Y.; Anasako, Y.; Nishigaki, Y.; Yachi, Y.; Iida, K. T.; Ohashi, Y. & Yamada, N. (2011) Alcohol consumption and risk of atrial fibrillation.*J AmColl Cardiol* Vol.57, pp. 427-436.

Korantzopoulos, P.; Kolettis, T. M. & Kountouris, E. (2005) Inflammation and anti-inflammatory interventions in atrial fibrillation. *Int J Cardiol,* Oct, Vol.10, No.104(3), pp. 361-362.

Korantzopoulos, P.; Liu, T.; Milionis, H. J.; Li, G. & Goudevenos JA.(2009) 'Lone' atrial fibrillation: hunting for the underlying causes and links. *Int J Cardiol,* Vol.131, No.2, pp. 180-185.

Koul, P. B.; Sussmane, J.B.; Cunil-De Sauta, B. & Minarek, M. (2005) Atrial fibrillation associated with alcohol ingestion in adolescence: holiday heart in pediatrics. *Pediatr Emerg Care,* Vol.21, No.1, pp. 38-39.

Krapp, M.; Kohl, T.,; Simpson,J. M. ; Sharland, G. K;Katalinic, A. & Gembruch, U. (2003) Review of diagnosis,treatment, and outcome of fetal atrial flutter compared with supraventricular tachycardia. *Heart,* Vol.89, pp. 913–917.

Krishna Kumar, R.; Saxena, A. & Talwar, K. K. (1991) Lone atrial fibrillation with complete heart block in a child. *Int J Cardiol,* Vol.30, No.3, pp. 349-351.

Krishnamoorthy, S.; Lip, G. Y. & Lane, D. A. (2009) Alcohol and illicit drug use as precipitants of atrial fibrillation in young adults: a case series and literature review. *Am J Med,* Vol.122, No.9, pp. 851-856.e3.

Kubo, T.; Kitaoka, H.; Okawa, M.; Hirota. T.; Hayato, K.; Yamasaki, N.; Matsumura, Y.; Yabe, T.; Takata, J. & Doi, Y. L. (2009) Clinical impact of atrial fibrillation in patients with hypertrophic cardiomyopathy.Results from Kochi RYOMA Study. *Circ J,*Sep,Vol.73, No.9, pp. 1599-1605.

Larmay, H. J. & Strasburger, J. F. (2004) Differential diagnosis and management of the fetus and newborn with an irregular or abnormal heart rate. *Pediatr Clin North Am,* Vol.51, No.4, pp. 1033-1050.

Lee, C.; Custer, J. W. & Rau, R. E. (2009).Drug doses. In: *The Harriet Lane Handbook: A Manual for Pediatric House Officers.*18th ed.,Custer, J. W. & Rau, R. E., eds., Elsevier Mosby, Philadelphia PA, pp. 717-1029.

Lee, P. C.; Hwang, B.; Chen, Y. J.; Tai, C. T.; Chen, S.A. & Chiang, C.E. (2006) Electrophysiologic characteristics and radiofrequency catheter ablation in children with Wolff-Parkinson-White syndrome. *Pacing Clin Electrophysiol, Vol.*29, No.5, pp. 490-495.

Lee, P. C.; Hwang, B.; Tai, C. T.; Chiang, C.E.; Yu, W. C. & Chen, S. A.(2004) The different electrophysiologic characteristics in children with Wolff-Parkinson-White syndrome between those with and without atrial fibrillation. *Pacing Clin Electrophysiol,* Vol.27, No.2, pp. 235-239.

Lopriore, E.; Aziz, M. I.; Nagel, H. T.; Blom, N. A.; Rozendaal, L.; Kanhai, H. H. H. &Vandenbussche, F. P. H. A. (2009) Long-term neurodevelopmental outcome after fetal arrhythmia.*Am J Obstet Gynecol,* Vol. 4, pp. e1-e5.).

Luciani, G. B.; Viscardi, F.; Pilati, M.; Crepaz, R.; Faggian, G. &Mazzucco, A. (2008) Age at repair affects the very long-term outcome of sinus venosus defect. *Ann Thorac Surg, Vol.*86, No.1, pp. 153-159.

Maeno, Y.; Hirose, A.; Kanbe, T. & Hori, D. (2009) Fetal arrhythmia: prenatal diagnosis and perinatal management. *J Obstet Gynaecol Res*, Vol.35, No.4, pp. 623-629.

Mainzer, G.; Khoury, A.; Gelernter-Yaniv, L. & Lorber, A. (2008) Neonatal atrial fibrillation after surgical repair of tracheoesophageal fistula with esophageal atresia. *Pediatr Cardiol*, Vol.29, No.1, pp. 150-152.

Manzi, S. F. (2006) Appendix B: Emergency Drug Compendium. In: *Textbook of Pediatric Emergency Medicine* 5th ed., Flaisher, G. R.; Ludwig, S. & Henretz F. M., eds. Lippincott Williams & Wilkins, Philadelphia PA, pp. 1963-1993.

Marelli, B.M.; Marelli, A.J.; Pilote, L.; Bouchardy, J.; Bottega, N.; Martucci, G. & Therrien, J. (2010) Atrial arrhythmias in adult patients with right- versus left-sided congenital heart disease anomalies. *Am J Cardiol*, Vol.106, No.4, pp. 547-551.

Martin, T.C.; Smith, L.; Hernandez, A. & Weldon, C. (1983) Dysrhythmias following the Senning operation for d-transposition of the great arteries. *J Thorac Cardiovasc Surg*, Vol.85, pp. 928-933

Martin, T.C. (2001) Echocardiographic findings in a contemporary Afro-Caribbean population referred for evaluation of atrial fibrillation or flutter. *West Ind Med J*,Vol.50, pp. 294-298.

Matta, M.J & Cuneo, B. F. (2010) Doppler echocardiography for managing fetal cardiac arrhythmia. *Clin Obstet Gynecol*, Vol.53, No.4, pp. 899-914.

Massin, M. M.; Dessy, H.; Malekzadeh-Milani, S. G.; Van Aerschot, I. & Verbeet, T. (2010) Prevalence of preoperative arrhythmias in children with delayed treatment of severe congenital heart disease. *Acta Cardiol*, Vol.65, No.1, pp. 37-42.

Mavroudis, C.; Deal, B. J.; Backe,r C. L. & Tsao, S. (2008) Arrhythmia surgery in patients with and without congenital heart disease. *Ann Thorac Surg*, Vol.86, No.3, pp. 857-868.

McCabe, J. M.; Smith, L. M.; Tseng, Z. H.; Badhwar, N.; Lee, B. K.; Lee, R. J.; Scheinman, M. M.; Olgin, J. E. & Marcus, G. M. (2008) Protracted CRP elevation after atrial fibrillation ablation.*Pacing Clin Electrophysiol*, Sep, Vol.31, No.9, pp. 1146-1151.

McNair, W. P.; Sinagra, G.; Taylor, M. R. G.; Di Lenarda, A.; Ferguson, D.A.; Salcedo, E. E.; Slavov, D.; Zhu, X.; Caldwell, J. H. & Mestroni, L. and the Familial Cardiomyopathy Registry Research Group. (2011) *SCN5A* mutations associate with arrhythmic dilated cardiomyopathy and commonly localize to the voltage-sensing mechanism. *J Am Coll Cardiol*, Vol.57, pp. 2160-2168.

Mommersteeg, M. T.: Christoffels, V. M.; Anderson, R. H. & Moorman, A. F. (2009) Atrial fibrillation: a developmental point of view. *Heart Rhythm,*Vol.6, No.12, pp. 1818-1824.

Multerer, S.; Berkenbosch, J. W.; Das, B. & Johnsrude, C. (2009)Atrial fibrillation after Taser exposure in a previously healthy adolescent. *Pediatr Emerg Care* Vol.25, No.12, pp. 851-853.

Nanthakumar, K.; Lau, Y. R.; Plumb, V. J.; Epstein, A. E. & Kay, G. N. (2004) Electrophysiological findings in adolescents with atrial fibrillation who have structurally normal hearts. *Circulation*, Vol.110, pp. 117-123.

Naumburg, E.; Riesenfeld, T. & Axelsson, O. (1997) Fetal tachycardia: intrauterine and postnatal course. *Fetal Diagn Ther*, Vol.12, pp. 205–209.

Niemann, B.; Chen, Y.; Teschner, M.; Li, L.; Silber, R.-E.& Rohrbach, S. (2011) Obesity induces signs of premature aging in younger patients. The role of mitochondria.*J Am Coll Cardiol*, Vol.57, 577-585.

Oteri, A.: Bussolini, A.; Sacchi, M.; Clementi, E.; Zuccotti, G.V. & Radice, S. (2010) A case of atrial fibrillation induced by inhaled fluticasone propionate. *Pediatrics*, Vol.126, pp. e1237-e1241.

Otwa,y R.; Vandenberg, J. I. & Fatkin, D. (2007) Atrial fibrillation - a new cardiac channelopathy. *Heart Lung Circ*,Vol.16, No.5, pp. 356-360.

Parilla, B.V.; Strasburger, J. F. & Socol, M. L. (1996) Fetal supraventricular tachycardia complicated by hydrops fetalis: a role for direct fetal intramuscular therapy. *Am J Perinatol*, Vol.13, pp. 483-486.

Patel, U. & Pavri, B. B. (2009) Short QT syndrome: a review. *Cardiol Rev*, Vol.17, No.6, pp. 300-303.

Paul, T.; Guccione, P. & Garson, A. Jr. (1990) Relation of syncope in young patients with Wolff-Parkinson-White syndrome to rapid ventricular response during atrial fibrillation.*Am J Cardiol*, Vol.65, No.5, pp. 318-321.

Perry, L. W. & Hung, W. (1971) Atrial fibrillation and hyperthyroidism in a 14-year-old boy. *J Pediatr*, Vol.79, No.4, pp. 668-671.

Piertersen, A. H.; Andersen, E. D. & Sandoe, E. (1992) Atrial fibrillation in the Wolff-Parkinson-White syndrome. *Am J Cardiol*, Vol.70, No.5, pp. 38A-43A.

Platanov, P. G. (2007) Interatrial conduction in the mechanisms of atrial fibrillation: from anatomy to cardiac signals and new treatment modalities. *Europace* Vol.9, pp. vi10 vi16.

Porter, C. J & Garson, A. Jr. (1993) Incidence and management of dysrhythmias after Fontan procedure. *Herz*, Vol.18, No.5, pp. 318-327.

Radford, D. J. & Izukawa, T. (1977)Atrial fibrillation in children. *Pediatrics*, Vol.59, pp. 250-256.

Reed, K. L.; Sahn, D. J.; Marx, G. R.; Anderson, C. F. & Shenker, L. (1987)Cardiac Doppler flows during fetal arrhythmias: physiologic consequences. *Obstet Gynecol*, Vol.70, No.1, pp.1-6.

Roberts, J. D. & Gollob, M. H. (2010) Impact of genetic discoveries on the classification of lone atrial fibrillation. *J Am Coll Cardiol*, Vol.55, pp. 705-712.

Rowland, T. W. (1983) Augmented ventricular rate following verapamil treatment for atrial fibrillation with Wolff-Parkinson-White syndrome.*Pediatrics*, Vol.72, pp. 245-246.

Sarubbi, B. (2006) The Wolff-Parkinson-White electrocardiogram pattern in athletes: how to evaluate the risk for dangerous arrhythmias. The opinion of a paediatric cardiologist.*J Cardiovasc Med (Hagerstown)*, Vol.7, No.4, pp. 271-278.

Sarubbi, B.; D'Alto, M.; Vergara, P.; Calvanese, R.; Mercurio, B.; Russo, M. G. & Calabro, R. (2005) Electrophysiologic evaluation of asymptomatic ventricular pre-excitation in children and adolescents. *Int J Cardiol*, Vol.98, No.2, pp. 207-214.

Saul, J. P. (2008) Mechanism and treatment of the single ventricle patient: focus on intraatrial reentry. *Heart Rhythm*, Vol.5, No.11, pp. 1615-1618.

Scheussler, R.B.; Boineau, J. P. & Bromberg, B. I. (1996) Origin of the sinus impulse.*J Cardiovasc Electrophysiol*, Vol.7, pp. 263-274.

Sherf, L. & James, T. N. (1979) Fine structure of cells and their histologic organization within intranodal pathways of the heart: clinical and electrocardiographic implications. *Am J Cardiol,*Vol.44, No.2, pp. 345-369.

Silverman, N. H.; Enderlein, M.A.; Stanger, P.; Teitel, D. F.; Heymann, M.A. & Golbus, M. S. (1985) Recognition of fetal arrhythmias by echocardiography.*J Clin Ultrasound,* Vol.13, No.4, pp. 255-263.

Simpson, J. M. & Sharland, G. K. (1998) Fetal tachycardias: management and outcome of 127 consecutive cases. *Heart,* Vol.79, pp. 576–581.

Sinha, A.; Fernandes, C. J.; Kim, J. J.; Fenrich, A. L. Jr.,& Enciso, J. (2005) Atrial flutter following placement of an umbilical venous catheter. *Am J Perinatol,* Jul, Vol.22, No.5, pp. 275-277.

Soyeur, D. (1996) Atrial flutter in the human fetus: diagnosis, hemodynamic consequences, and therapy. *J Cardiovasc Electrophysiol,* Vol.7, pp. 989–999.

Spies, C.; Khandelwal, A.; Timmermanns, I. & Schrader, R. (2008) Incidence of atrial fibrillation following transcatheter closure of atrial septal defects in adults. *Am J Cardiol,* Vol.102, pp. 902-906.

Srinivasan, S. & Strasburger, J. (2008) Overview of fetal arrhythmias.*Curr Opin Pediatr,* Vol.20, No.5, pp.522-531.

Stiles, M.K.; John, B.; Wong, C. X.; Kuklik, P.; Brooks, A. G.; Lau, D. H.; Dimitri, H.; Roberts-Thomson, K. C.; Wilson, L.; De Sciscio, P.; Young, G. D. &Sanders, P. (2009) Paroxysmal lone atrial fibrillation is associated with an abnormal atrial substrate: characterizing the "second factor". *J Am Coll Cardiol* Vol.53. No.14, pp. 1182-1191.

Strasburger, J. F.: Cuneo, B. F.; Michon, M. M.; Gotteiner, N. L.; Deal, B. J.; McGregor, S. N.; Oudijk, M. A.; Meijboom, E. J.; Feinkind, L.; Hussey, M. & Parilla, B. V. (2004) Amiodarone therapy for drug-refractory fetal tachycardia. *Circulation,* Jan 27 Vol.109, No.3, pp. 375-379.

Strasburger, J. F & Wakai, R. T. (2010) Fetal cardiac arrhythmia detection and in utero therapy. *Nat Rev Cardiol,* Vol.7, No.5, pp. 277-290.

Strieper, M. J.; Frias, P.; Fischbach, P.; Costello, L. & Campbell, R. M. (2010) Catheter ablation of primary supraventricular tachycardia substrate presenting as atrial fibrillation in adolescents. *Congenit Heart Dis,* Vol.5, No.5, pp. 65-69.

Stulak, J. M.; Dearani, J. A.; Puga, F. J.; Zehr, K. J.; Schaff, H. V. & Danielson, G. K. (2006) Right-sided Maze procedure for atrial tachyarrhythmias in congenital heart disease. *Ann Thorac Surg,* Vol.81, No.5, pp.1780-1784.

Sugimoto, S.; Takagi, N.; Hachiro, Y. & Abe, T. (2001) High frequency of arrhythmias after Fontan operation indicates earlier anticoagulant therapy. *Int J Cardiol,* Vol.78, No.1, pp. 33-39.

Taketomo, C. K.; Hurlburt Hodding, J. & Kraus, D. M. (2010) *Pediatric Dosage Handbook,* 17th ed., American Pharmacists Association, Lexi-Comp, Inc. Hudson, OH.

Texter, K. M.; Kertesz, N.J.; Friedman, R. A. & Fenrich, A.L.Jr. (2006) Atrial flutter in infants. *J Am Coll Cardiol,* Sep 5, Vol.48, No.5, pp.1040-1046.

Thejus, J. & Francis, J. (2009) Atrial fibrillation in cardiac channelopathies. *Indian Pacing Electrophysiol J* Vol.9, No.6, pp. 342-350.

Therrien, J.; Siu, S. C.; Harris, L.; Dore, A.; Niwa, K.; Janousek, J.; Williams, W. G.; Webb, G & Gatzoulis, M. A. (2001) Impact of pulmonary valve replacement on arrhythmia propensity late after repair of tetralogy of Fallot. *Circulation,* Vol.103, No.20, pp. 2489-2494.

Themistoclakis, S.; Corrado, A.; Marchlinski, F. E.; Jais, P.; Zado, E.; Rossillo, A.; Di Biase, L.; Schweikert, R. A.; Saliba, W. I.; Horton, R.; Mohanty, P.; Patel, D.; Burkhardt, D. J.; Wazni, O.M.; Bonso, A.; Callans, D. J.; Haissaguerre, M.; Raviele, A. & Natale, A. (2010) The risk of thromboembolism and need for oral anticoagulation after successful atrial fibrillation ablation. *J Am Coll Cardiol,* Vol.55, pp. 735-743.

Thijssen, V. L. J. L.; Ausma, J.; Gorza, L.; van der Velden, H. M. W.; Allessie, M. A.; Van Gelder, I. C.; Borgers, M. & van Eys, G. J. J. M. (2004) Troponin I isoform expression in human and experimental atrial fibrillation. *Circulation*;110:770-775.

Thorton, J. R. (1984) Atrial fibrillation in healthy non-alcoholic people after an alcohol binge. *Lancet,* Vol.2(8410), pp. 1013-1015.

Tikanoja, T.; Kirkinen, P.; Nikolajev, K.; Eresmaa, L. & Haring, P. (1998) Familial atrial fibrillation with fetal onset. *Heart,* Vol.79, No.2, pp. 195-197.

Trojnarska, O.; Grajek, S.; Kramer, L. & Gwizdala, A. (2009) Risk factors of supraventricular arrhythmia in adults with congenital heart disease. *Cardiol J*Vol.16, No.3, pp. 218-226.

Tsai, C.-T.; Chiang. F.-T.; Tseng, C.-D.; Hwang, J.-J.; Kuo, K.-T.; Wu, C.-K.; Yu, C.-C.; Wang, Y.-C.; Lai, L.-P. & Lin J-L.(2010) Increased expression of mineralocorticoid receptor in human atrial fibrillation and a cellular model of atrial fibrillation. *J Am Coll Cardiol,* Vol.55, pp. 758-770.

Ueda, N.; Yoshikawa, T.; Chihara, M.; Kawaguchi, S.; Niinomi, Y. & Yasaka, T. (1988) Atrial fibrillation following methylprednisolone pulse therapy. *Pediatr Nephrol,* Vol.2, No.1, pp. 29-31.

van Engelen, A.D.; Weijtens, O.; Brenner, J. I.;Kleinman, C. S.; Copel, C.A.; Stoutenbeek, P, & Meijboom, E. J.(1994) Management, outcome and follow-up of fetal tachyarrhythmia.*J Am Coll Cardiol* Vol.24, pp. 1371–1375.

Vermeulen, T.; Conraads, V. M.; Vrints, C. & Rodrigus, IE.(. 2009) Recurrent left ventricular myxoma presenting as cerebrovascular accidents in a teenage girl. *Acta Cardiol* Dec,Vol.64, No.6, pp. 811-814.

Wakai, R. T.; Strasburger, J. F.; Li, Z.; Deal, B. J. & Gotteiner, N. L. (2003) Magnetocardiographic rhythm patterns at initiation and termination of fetal supraventricular tachycardia. *Circulation,* Vol.107, No.2, pp. 307-312.

Weerasooriya, R.; Khairy, P.; Litalien, J.; Macle, L.; Hocini, M.; Sacher, F.; Lellouche, N.; Knecht, S.; Wright, M.; Nault, I.; Miyazaki, S.; Scavee, C.; Clemency, J.; Haissaguerre, M. & Jais, P. (2011) Catheter ablation foratrial fibrillation: are results maintained at 5 years of follow-up? *J Am Coll Cardiol,* Vol.57, pp.160-166.

Weiner, C. P. & Thompson, M. I. (1988) Direct treatment of fetal supraventricular tachycardia after failed transplacental therapy. *Am J Obstet Gynecol,* Vol.158 (Pt 1), pp. 570–573.

Wolf, C. M.; Seslar, S. P.; den Boer, K.; Juraszek, A. L.; McGowan, F. X.; Cowan, D. B.; Del Nido, P.; Triedman, J. K.; Berul C. I. & Walsh, E. P. (2009) Atrial remodeling after the Fontan operation.*Am J Cardiol*Vol.104, pp. 1737-1742.

Yamamura, K.; Ohga, S.; Nishiyama, K.; Doi, T.; Tsutsumi, Y.; Ikeda, K.; Fujishima, A.; Takada, H. & Hara, T. (2011) Recurrent atrial fibrillation after high-dose methylprednisolone therapy in a girl with lupus-associated hemophagocytic syndrome. *Lupus*, Mar 17 [Epub ahead of print].

Yamashita, H.; Nagaoka, H.; Matsushima, R.; Nakayama, I.; Goto, K.; Ogawa, T. & Fujii, H. (1987) Cardiac rhabdomyoma associated with tuberous sclerosis. An autopsy case of newborn infant died of cardiac failure. *Acta Pathol Jpn.* Apr, Vol.37, No.4, pp. 645-653.

Yap, Y. G. (2009) Inflammation and atrial fibrillation: cause or para-phenomenon? *Europace*Aug, Vol.11, No.8, pp. 980-981.

Yu, S. H.; Lim, S.H.; Hong, Y. S.; Yoo, K.J.; Chang, B. C. & Kang, M. S. (2006) Clinical experiences of cardiac myxoma. *Yonsei Med J*, Jun 30, Vol.47, No., pp. 367-371.

Zielinsky, P.; Dillenburg, R. F.: de Lima, G. G. & Zimmer, L. P. (1998) [Fetal supraventricular tachyarrhythmias. Experience of a fetal cardiology reference center]. *Arq Bras Cardiol*, Vol.70, pp. 337–340.

20

Mitral Regurgitation and Atrial Fibrillation: The Contribution of Impaired Left Atrial Appendage Function to Atrial Thrombogenesis

Burak Pamukcu[1] and Atilla Bitigen[2]
[1]*Bayrampasa Medical Centre, Istanbul,*
[2]*Medical Park Hospital, Fatih, Istanbul,*
Turkey

1. Introduction

1.1 Epidemiology of atrial fibrillation

Atrial fibrillation (AF) is the commonest sustained cardiac arrhythmia which affects 1 to 2 % of the entire adult population [1]. Current studies indicate that the prevalence of AF will be doubled in a few decades [2]. As a major source of public health problem, atrial fibrillation increases the risk of stroke (up to 18 fold especially in patients with valvular AF), long term disability, hospitalizations, cardiovascular mortality and healthcare costs [3-4]. The prevalence of atrial fibrillation and its complications are more common among patients with rheumatic heart disease especially in patients with mitral stenosis and regurgitation. Stroke is one of the most common and disabling complication of atrial fibrillation. Recent studies indicated that age, presence of hypertension, diabetes, heart failure and/or previous stroke or transient ischemic attack (TIA) as pivotal contributor risk factors to generation of stroke in AF patients [5-8]. Although the presence of these factors increases the risk of stroke in non-valvular AF patients, the absolute risk of stroke is much higher in patients with valvular AF [9].

2. Mitral valve disease and atrial fibrillation

In patients with rheumatic mitral regurgitation (MR) major anatomic changes comprise annular dilatation and prolapse of the anterior mitral valve leaflet due to elongation of chordae tendinea [10]. However, retractile fibrosis of leaflets and chordae tendinea that leads loss of coaptation is the main pathologic finding in patients with chronic rheumatic MR [11]. In the early phases of rheumatic disease the most frequent echocardiographic finding is the enlargement of left atrium in patients on sinus rhythm. However, paroxysmal or permanent atrial fibrillation ultimately affects 50% of patients within 10 years of diagnosis in sinus rhythm [12]. Left atrial enlargement causes impaired mitral apparatus function and loss of coaptation causes mitral regurgitation. On the other hand, left atrial enlargement contributes to the generation of atrial re-entry and atrial fibrillation. Progressive left atrial enlargement increases the risk of AF development. New onset AF occurs in 10 to 20% of patients with myocardial infarction due to ischemia of atria or sinus node [13]. Atrial fibrillation is more common among older and hypertensive patients with mitral regurgitation and enlarged left atria [13].

3. Left atrial appendage as a source of thrombi and stroke

The left atrial appendage (LAA), a blind-ended complex structure that is embryologically distinct from the body of the left atrium, is been identified as the major source of cardiac systemic embolic events in patients with AF [14]. The atrium and the LAA compensate for the age-induced changes in LV diastolic properties by increasing active atrial contraction (a-wave) [15]. An experimental study and a clinical study showed the presence of an inverse relationship between LA filling pressure and LAA emptying function (inverse correlation between capillary wedge pressure and LAA active emptying a-wave) [16, 17]. Due to its compliance, the LAA is acting as a modulator of LA pressure.

It has been demonstrated that more than 15% of strokes originate from the heart, and especially from the LAA [18]. A recent study showed the presence of thrombi in the left atrial cavity in 1.9% of the AF patients. In the same study, the incidence of LAA thrombi was reported 6.6-fold that of left atrial cavity thrombi. Of note, AF was also determined in most of the patients with LAA thrombi [19].

4. Left atrial appendage function in atrial fibrillation

LAA has hemodynamic roles and contributes to atrial function. Impaired LAA function is been shown to lead increased thrombosis in left atrium [19].

Another previous study evaluated LAA function in 60 patients with severe rheumatic MR on both sinus rhythm and atrial fibrillation. Impaired LAA functions were determined in patients with severe mitral regurgitation having AF, whereas LAA was preserved in patients with normal sinus rhythm compared to controls [20]. Another study which aimed to compare LAA functions before and after percutaneous balloon mitral valvuloplasty (PBMV) by tissue wave Doppler imaging enrolled 20 patients with symptomatic rheumatic mitral stenosis [21]. LAA functions were evaluated by the measurement of; LAA late filling (LAALF) velocity, LAA late emptying (LAALE) velocity, and percent area change of the LAA [21]. No significant difference was reported in LAALF velocity and area percent change of the LAA after PBMV [21] while LAALE velocity was found increased after PBMV compared to baseline values ($p=0.005$). In the same study increased late emptying, systolic, and diastolic wave values were determined by tissue Doppler imaging after PBMV when compared to basal measurements ($p=0.023$, $p=0.002$, and $p=0.002$, respectively). Of note, significant improvement was determined in left atrial spontaneous echo-contrast after PBMV and LAA functions [21].

The functions of LAA have been evaluated in patients with severe rheumatic mitral regurgitation both in AF or sinus rhythm [22]. Impairment of LAA functions is been shown to contribute to thrombogenic processes and it is been often determined among AF patients when compared to those in sinus rhythm. Recent studies indicated that the LAA flows were strongly affected by the type of atrial arrhythmia. For example, the average emptying flow velocity was found weaker in AF than in sinus rhythm, and it was found greater in atrial flutter than in AF [23].

5. Markers of left atrial appendage function

The role of different markers that can be associated with LAA function has been evaluated in recent studies. One of these studies investigated the expression of proteins associated with the cytoskeleton, energetic metabolism, and cardiac cytoprotection between left atrial appendages (LAA) and right atrial appendages (RAA) obtained from patients with mitral valve disease both in sinus rhythm and in permanent atrial fibrillation. Similar levels of protein expression is been reported both in RAA and LAA samples. However, expression of cardiac alpha-actin isotypes 1 and 2, tropomyosin alpha and beta-chains, and myosin light chain embryonic muscle/atrial isoform in LAA from AF patients was found increased when compared to those from SR patients [24]. Another potential contributor to atrial remodelling, cardiac endothelin-1 (ET-1), is expressed as a response to wall stress and can promote myocyte hypertrophy and interstitial fibrosis [25]. Elevated atrial ET-1 level is been found associated with increased LA size, AF prevalence, hypertension, and heart failure [25]. An association between ET-1 and atrial dilatation, fibrosis, and hypertrophy is been reported. Endothelin-1 is suggested as a contributing factor to AF persistence [25].
Although both mitral stenosis and MR are strongly associated with AF, the prevalence of AF in mitral stenosis patients is much higher than MR patients. Approximately 29% of the patients with isolated mitral stenosis develop AF while only 16% of the patents with isolated MR [26, 27].

6. Atrial remodelling in atrial fibrillation

A recent study aimed to assess the relationship between atrial structural remodelling in AF patients with different types of mitral valve diseases [28]. The study recruited 24 patients undergoing mitral valve surgery with different diagnoses. Left atrial appendage tissue samples were obtained from patients with mitral valve disease either in sinus rhythm or AF. Masson's trichrome staining and immunohistochemical staining were performed to assess the extent of the fibrosis. The authors reported significantly increased fibrosis in patients with AF when compared to patients in sinus rhythm ($p=0.023$) [28]. The collagen volume fraction of fibrosis was also significantly increased in patients with mitral stenosis and atrial fibrillation when compared to patients with mitral regurgitation and atrial fibrillation ($p=0.043$) [28]. Collagen Type I levels were also significantly increased in AF patients with mitral stenosis when compared to patients with mitral regurgitation and AF ($p=0.043$). Of note, different collagen volume fraction of Matrix MetalloProteinases-2 (MMP2) was determined between the patients with mitral stenosis and sinus rhythm and patients with mitral stenosis and AF ($p=0.001$). The authors concluded that heart rhythm status and type of underlying mitral valve disease influence

atrial structural remodelling and different atrial structural remodelling may contribute to the development of AF [28].
The remodelling processes involving atrial fibrosis and atrial dilatation in AF patients also recruit angiotensin II mediated pathways and MMPs. There are evidences showing that patients with mitral stenosis and AF have significantly larger atria than patients with mitral stenosis but sinus rhythm [29]. Fibrosis was found increased in mitral stenosis patients in AF and SR in the left atria, but only in mitral stenosis patients with AF in the right atria. Furthermore, MMP-1 was reported to be down-regulated in left atria of mitral stenosis patients ($p=0.02$) both in sinus rhythm or AF [29]. Although there is no evidence showing that AF contributes to altered fibrosis or MMP-expression in the left atria, atrial remodelling appears to recruit changes in MMP-expression in patients with mitral valve disease either in sinus rhythm or AF [29].
Interestingly, mitral regurgitation can provide protective effects against left atrial blood stasis. The relationship between the severity of MR and thromboembolic risk has been clarified in patients with AF. A recent study indicated a protective effect of MR against thromboembolic risk over reducing LA blood stasis but only limited to patients with severe MR [30].

7. Mitral valve disease, atrial fibrillation and thrombosis

The association between mitral valve disease and atrial fibrillation appears to constitute a vicious cycle. Different dynamics including changes in LAA functions affect the generation and persistence of atrial fibrillation. The severity of mitral valve regurgitation has pivotal influence on left atrial flow dynamics and LAA stasis which appears to be the major determinant of thrombus generation [31].
The mechanisms of thrombogenesis in patients with MR or aortic stenosis (AS) have been investigated in patients both in sinus rhythm and AF. Patients with MR or AS have been shown to have higher plasma fibrinogen levels when compared to healthy people and also lower plasma fibrin D-dimer levels suggesting decreased intravascular clotting has been reported [32]. Furthermore, the presence of immunoreactive von Willebrand factor (vWF) in the endocardial endothelium and its relationship to thrombogenesis in the human atrial appendage has been investigated [33]. Immunoreactive vWF in the endocardial endothelium was found increased in overloaded human atrial appendage, which was supposed to be a local predisposing factor for intraatrial thrombogenesis [33].
Another study investigated the contribution of plasma D-dimer levels to thrombogenesis in 89 patients with mitral valve disease and 21 subjects with AF but normal valves, and 15 healthy controls. Plasma D-dimer levels correlated with the embolic risk in mitral valve disease and non-valvular AF. The highest levels were found in patients with MS and AF and non-valvular AF. Severe MR decreased the D-dimer levels in MS and/or AF to control levels [34].
Transmitral pressure gradient is supposed to be another parameter that may influence the development of AF and thrombogenesis in patients with rheumatic heart disease [26]. However, patients' age and left atrial diameter has been shown to be the major parameters that predict the occurrence of AF in patients with rheumatic heart disease [26].

8. Conclusions

Atrial fibrillation is the most common sustained cardiac arrhythmia and a severe public health problem. The prevalence of AF increases while the population is ageing. Mitral valve diseases, including mitral stenosis and mitral regurgitation increase AF prevalence. There are strong associations between severe mitral valve disease and the development of atrial fibrillation. Once atrial fibrillation starts it causes impaired LAA function and leads to increased intraatrial thrombogenesis. Left atrial thrombi and especially LAA thrombi are shown to be the commonest causes of embolic stroke. Management of this complex situation should comprise several steps including restoration of impaired LAA function, prevention of thrombogenesis and maintenance of sinus rhythm whenever it is feasible.

9. References

[1] Stewart S, Hart CL, Hole DJ, McMurray JJ. Population prevalence, incidence, and predictors of atrial fibrillation in the Renfrew/Paisley study. Heart 2001; 86: 516-21.

[2] Go AS, Hylek EM, Phillips KA, Chang Y, Henault LE, Selby JV, Singer DE. Prevalence of diagnosed atrial fibrillation in adults: national implications for rhythm management and stroke prevention: the AnTicoagulation and Risk Factors in Atrial Fibrillation (ATRIA) Study. JAMA 2001; 285: 2370-5.

[3] Kirchhof P, Auricchio A, Bax J, Crijns H, Camm J, Diener HC, Goette A, Hindricks G, Hohnloser S, Kappenberger L, Kuck KH, Lip GY, Olsson B, Meinertz T, Priori S, Ravens U, Steinbeck G, Svernhage E, Tijssen J, Vincent A, Breithardt G. Outcome parameters for trials in atrial fibrillation: executive summary. Recommendations from a consensus conference organized by the German Atrial Fibrillation Competence NETwork (AFNET) and the European Heart Rhythm Association (EHRA). Eur Heart J 2007; 28: 2803-17.

[4] Thrall G, Lane D, Carroll D, Lip GY. Quality of life in patients with atrial fibrillation: a systematic review. Am J Med 2006; 119: 448 e1–e19.

[5] Benjamin EJ, Levy D, Vaziri SM, D'Agostino RB, Belanger AJ, Wolf PA. Independent risk factors for atrial fibrillation in a population-based cohort. The Framingham Heart Study. JAMA 1994; 271: 840-4.

[6] Stroke Risk in Atrial Fibrillation Working Group. Comparison of 12 risk stratification schemes to predict stroke in patients with non-valvular atrial fibrillation. Stroke 2008; 39: 1901–10.

[7] Lip GYH, Nieuwlaat R, Pisters R, Lane DA, Crijns HJGM. Refining clinical risk stratification for predicting stroke and thromboembolism in atrial fibrillation using a novel risk factor-based approach: The Euro Heart Survey on Atrial Fibrillation. Chest 2010; 137: 263–72.

[8] Kannel WB, Wolf PA, Benjamin EJ, Levy D. Prevalence, incidence, prognosis, and predisposing conditions for atrial fibrillation: population-based estimates. Am J Cardiol 1998; 82(8A): 2N-9N.

[9] Fuster V, Rydén LE, Cannom DS, et al. American College of Cardiology/American Heart Association Task Force on Practice Guidelines; European Society of Cardiology

Committee for Practice Guidelines; European Heart Rhythm Association; Heart Rhythm Society. ACC/AHA/ESC 2006 Guidelines for the Management of Patients with Atrial Fibrillation: a report of the American College of Cardiology/American Heart Association Task Force on Practice Guidelines and the European Society of Cardiology Committee for Practice Guidelines (Writing Committee to Revise the 2001 Guidelines for the Management of Patients With Atrial Fibrillation): developed in collaboration with the European Heart Rhythm Association and the Heart Rhythm Society. Circulation 2006; 114:e257-354. Erratum in: Circulation 2007; 116: e138.

[10] Marcus RH, Sareli P, Pocock WA, Barlow JB. The spectrum of severe rheumatic mitral valve disease in a developing country. Correlations among clinical presentation, surgical pathologic findings, and hemodynamic sequelae. Ann Intern Med 1994;120:177–83.

[11] Acar C, de Ibarra JS, Lansac E. Anterior leaflet augmentation with autologous pericardium for mitral repair in rheumatic valve insufficiency. J Heart Valve Dis 2004;13:741–6.

[12] Enriquez-Sarano M, Tajik AJ, Schaff HV, et al. Echocardiographic prediction of left ventricular function after correction of mitral regurgitation: results and clinical implications. J Am Coll Cardiol 1994; 24: 1536-43.

[13] Krahn AD, Manfreda J, Tate RB, Mathewson FAL, Cuddy TE. The natural history of atrial fibrillation: Incidence, risk factors, and prognosis in the Manitoba follow-up study. Am J Med 1995; 98: 476-84.

[14] Goldman ME, Pearce LA, Hart RG, et al. Pathophysiologic correlates of thromboembolism in nonvalvular atrial fibrillation: Reduced flow velocity in the left atrial appendage (the Stroke Prevention in Atrial Fibrillation [SPAF-III] study). J Am Soc Echocardiogr 1999; 12:1080-7.

[15] Thomas L, Boyd A, Thomas SP, et al. Atrial structural remodelling and restoration of atrial contraction after linear ablation for atrial fibrillation. Eur Heart J 2003; 24:1942-51.

[16] Hondo T, Okamoto M, Yamane T, et al. The role of the left atrial appendage: a volume loading study in open-chest dogs. Jpn Heart J 1995; 36: 225-34.

[17] Tabata T, Oki T, Fukuda N, et al. Influence of left atrial pressure on left atrial appendage flow velocity patterns in patients in sinus rhythm. J Am Soc Echocardiogr 1996; 9: 857-64.

[18] Kaneko K, Hirono O, Fatema K, et al. Direct evidence that sustained dysfunction of left atrial appendage contributes to the occurrence of cardiogenic brain embolism in patients with paroxysmal atrial fibrillation. Intern Med 2003; 42:1077-83.

[19] Jaber, WA, Prior, DL, Thamilarasan, M, et al Efficacy of anticoagulation in resolving left atrial and left atrial appendage thrombi: a transesophageal echocardiography study. Am Heart J 2000; 140: 150-6.

[20] Bitigen A, Bulut M, Tanalp AC, Kirma C, Barutçu I, Pala S, Erkol A, Boztosun B. Left atrial appendage functions in patients with severe rheumatic mitral regurgitation. Int J Cardiovasc Imaging 2007; 23: 693-700.

[21] Effect of Percutaneous Mitral Balloon Valvuloplasty on Left Atrial Appendage Function: A Doppler Tissue Study. Karakaya O, Turkmen M, Bitigen A, Sağlam M, Barutcu I, Esen AM, Bulut M, Turkyilmaz E, Kirma C. Journal of the American Society of Echocardiography 2006; 19: 434-7.

[22] Donal E, Yamada H, Leclercq C, Herpin D. The left atrial appendage, a small, blind-ended structure: a review of its echocardiographic evaluation and its clinical role. Chest 2005; 128: 1853-62.

[23] Santiago D, Warhofsky M, Mandri GL, et al. Left atrial appendage function and thrombus formation in atrial fibrillation-flutter: a transesophageal echocardiographic study. J Am Coll Cardiol 1994; 24:159-64.

[24] Modrego J, Maroto L, Tamargo J, Azcona L, Mateos-Cáceres P, Segura A, Moreno-Herrero R, Pérez-Castellanos N, Delpón E, Pérez-Villacastín J, Rodríguez E, Macaya C, López-Farré AJ. Comparative expression of proteins in left and right atrial appendages from patients with mitral valve disease at sinus rhythm and atrial fibrillation. J Cardiovasc Electrophysiol 2010; 21: 859-68.

[25] Mayyas F, Niebauer M, Zurick A, Barnard J, Gillinov AM, Chung MK, Van Wagoner DR.Association of left atrial endothelin-1 with atrial rhythm, size, and fibrosis in patients with structural heart disease. Circ Arrhythm Electrophysiol 2010; 3: 369-79.

[26] Diker E, Aydogdu S, Ozdemir M, Kural T, Polat K, Cehreli S, Erdogan A, Göksel S. Prevalence and predictors of atrial fibrillation in rheumatic valvular heart disease. Am J Cardiol 1996; 77: 96-8.

[27] Schwartz R, Myerson RM, Lawrence T, Nichols HT. Mitral stenosis, massive pulmonary hemorrhage, and emergency valve replacement. N Eng J Med 1966; 275: 755-88.

[28] Qian Y, Meng J, Tang H, Yang G, Deng Y, Wei D, Xiang B, Xiao X. Different structural remodelling in atrial fibrillation with different types of mitral valvular diseases. Europace 2010; 12: 371-7.

[29] Anné W, Willems R, Roskams T, Sergeant P, Herijgers P, Holemans P, Ector H, Heidbüchel H. Matrix metalloproteinases and atrial remodeling in patients with mitral valve disease and atrial fibrillation. Cardiovasc Res 2005; 67: 655-66.

[30] Kranidis A, Koulouris S, Filippatos G, Kappos K, Tsilias K, Karvounis H, Exadaktylos N. Mitral regurgitation protects from left atrial thrombogenesis in patients with mitral valve disease and atrial fibrillation. Pacing Clin Electrophysiol 2000; 23: 1863-6.

[31] Fukuda N, Hirai T, Ohara K, Nakagawa K, Nozawa T, Inoue H. Relation of the severity of mitral regurgitation to thromboembolic risk in patients with atrial fibrillation. Int J Cardiol 2011; 146: 197-201.

[32] Lip GY, Rumley A, Dunn FG, Lowe GD. Thrombogenesis in mitral regurgitation and aortic stenosis. Angiology. 1996; 47: 1117-25.

[33] Fukuchi M, Watanabe J, Kumagai K, Katori Y, Baba S, Fukuda K, Yagi T, Iguchi A, Yokoyama H, Miura M, Kagaya Y, Sato S, Tabayashi K, Shirato K. Increased von Willebrand factor in the endocardium as a local predisposing factor for thrombogenesis in overloaded human atrial appendage. J Am Coll Cardiol 2001; 37: 1436-42.

[34] Cevik C, Otahbachi M, Nugent K, Ozkan M. Mitral regurgitation reduces systemic coagulation activity in patients with rheumatic heart disease. J Heart Valve Dis 2009; 18: 278-83.

21

New Onset Atrial Fibrillation in Critically Ill Patients

M. E. Sleeswijk[1], T. van Noord[2] and J. G. Zijlstra[3]
[1]*Flevoziekenhuis, Almere / Department of Critical Care,*
[2]*Scheperziekenhuis, Emmen / Department of Critical Care,*
[3]*University Medical Center Groningen,*
University of Groningen / Department of Critical Care,
The Netherlands

1. Introduction

New onset atrial fibrillation is the most common rhythm disturbance in critically ill patients. Although it is frequently seen in critically ill patients, data regarding the aetiology and treatment are scarce. Extrapolating treatment regimes from non-critically ill patients is not recommended since there is a difference in aetiology of the arrhythmia. In this chapter we will discuss the pathophysiology and treatment strategies of new onset atrial fibrillation in medical- and non-cardiac surgery critically ill patients, based on the latest available evidence.

2. Pathophysiology

In critically ill patients the underlying mechanism for developing atrial fibrillation might differ from the outpatients clinic. Electrolyte disorders, rapid fluid changes like bleeding on one site and fluid overload by rapid filling in case of sepsis on the other site are present in excess and perfect triggers that induce atrial fibrillation. Reduced left ventricular function is also associated with atrial fibrillation. In critically ill patients, especially patients with sepsis, myocardial depression can occur, therefore inducing heart failure and, as a consequence, a higher risk of atrial fibrillation. Also underlying cardiac ischemia, for example the results of tremendous physically exercise which sepsis is, but also as a results of previously known or unknown coronary artery disease, can induce atrial fibrillation.
Recent studies have shown that elevated inflammatory biomarkers are associated with the development of atrial fibrillation. Inflammatory markers like C-reactive protein (CRP), high-sensitivity CRP (hs-CRP) an interleukin-6 are elevated in both patients with paroxysmal as persistent atrial fibrillation (Chung et al 2001 Dernellis et al 2001, Gaudino et al 2003). Atrial fibrillation is also common in septic patients, (Salman et al 2008, Christians et al 2008) the incidence is even higher in patients with septic shock. 46% of patients with septic shock developed new onset atrial fibrillation, often with an increase in C-reactive protein (CRP) levels before the onset of atrial fibrillation. (Meierhenrich et al 2010) As most critically ill patients have elevated inflammatory markers, they, therefore might be at risk for the development of atrial fibrillation (Sequin et al 2006). Furthermore, atrial fibrillation is also associated with local inflammation like pericarditis and myocarditis.

3. Treatment

Evidence for the best treatment strategy in critically ill patients is scarce. There are only 4 randomized controlled trials and furthermore 3 prospective follow-up studies who included mainly non-cardiac surgery and medical critically ill patients (table 1). However, since there is heterogeneity in not only patient selection, but also type of atrial arrhythmia and definition of treatment goals, these trials are not comparable and therefore the best treatment strategy based on these trials cannot be recommended. Even the question whether to treat or not critically ill patients with new onset atrial fibrillation has not been answered yet. Placebo controlled trials are lacking and, furthermore, spontaneous conversion is common in new onset atrial fibrillation, even in the setting of critically ill patients.

RCT trials	**Number of patients**	*Rhythm*	**Intervention**
Chapman 1993	24	AT	Amiodarone vs Procainamide
Barranco 1994	30	SVT	Flecainide vs Verapamil
Moran 1995	42	SVT	Magnesium vs Amiodarone
Balser 1998	64	SVT	Esmolol vs Diltiazem
Prospective			
Holt 1989	10	SVT	Amiodarone
Mayr 2003	37	SVT	Direct current cardioversion
Sleeswijk 2008	29	NAF	Magnesium Amiodarone

AT= atrial tachycardia
SVT= supraventricular tachycardia
PSVT= paroxysmal atrioventricular nodal reentrant tachycardia
NAF= new onset atrial fibrillation
A.fib= atrium fibrillation
A.flut= atrium flutter

Table 1.

Despite the lack of evidence, it is common practice to treat atrial fibrillation in the ICU setting. Many physicians feel the need to restore sinus rhythm in critically ill patients with either electrical cardioversion, chemical conversion or a combination of these treatment strategies. These feelings are predominantly based on their experience in non-critically ill patients. However, critically ill patients differ from the general population, therefore, extrapolating treatment regimes and results are not justified and may even harm. For example, DC electrical cardioversion in patients with new onset atrial fibrillation has a success rate of over 90%, while the only study investigating DC electrical cardioversion in critically ill patients yields an initial success rate of 35 % and only 13,5% after 48 hours, (Mayr et al 2003) which data are comparable to control group e.g. spontaneous conversion. Guidelines recommend immediate cardioversion in hemodynamic unstable patients.

Although critically ill patients are often hemodynamic unstable, this is in most cases not directly the results of atrial fibrillation, but on the contrary, atrial fibrillation is often the result of hemodynamic instability. Therefore an approach with direct DC electrical cardioversion may not be suitable in the ICU setting.

Although data are lacking, as mentioned before, most physicians tend to treat atrial fibrillation with rapid ventricular response in some way, therefore, the three cornerstones of treatment for atrial fibrillation include corrections of the underlying condition, rhythm or rate control and prevention of thrombo-embolic complications

3.1 The underlying condition

Whether treatment of the underlying condition may restore sinus rhythm or prevent recurrent atrial fibrillation, is not exactly known. However, treatment of the underlying disease and correction of precipitating factors such as electrolyte disturbances, volume imbalance or hypoxia are part of the general treatment in the ICU setting and are treated anyway. By "simply" treating sepsis lots of triggers that may induce atrial fibrillation will be eliminated and in most cases the arrhythmia will convert spontaneously to sinus rhythm by correcting electrolyte disorders and major fluid changes. However, in some of these patients, atrial fibrillation direct contribute to further hemodynamic deterioration of the patient and therefore should be treated as soon as possible. Since, as mentioned before, triggers are available in excess and also cannot always be removed, conversion to sinus rhythm might be a rather optimistic treatment goal, which means, conversion might be possible, but subsequently remaining sinus rhythm might be the Achilles' heel of this treatment strategy. Therefore, a goal that might be easier to achieve might be rate control to an acceptable ventricular frequency.

3.2 Rhythm or rate control

Based on the studies performed in the general population, (Van Gelder et al 2002, Wyse et al 2002) and postoperative atrial fibrillation, (Soucier et al 2003) and given the fact that a rhythm strategy with DC electrical cardioversion in critically ill cardiac surgery patients failed to show any benefit (Mayr et al 2003) and furthermore, chemical conversion is often accompanied by severe side effects or is contra-indicated, a rhythm control strategy is not recommend in critically ill patients, with the exception of those patients with life threatening cardiovascular collapse due to atrial fibrillation or in a setting of acute coronary syndrome. In these cases it is recommended to add an anti-arrhythmic drug in order to maintain sinus rhythm.

This might introduce another problem, while most anti-arrhythmic drugs lower pressure or are contra-indicated in ischemic heart failure.

Experience with rather new Vaughan-Williams class III anti arrhythmic drugs like ibutilide or nifekalant for chemical conversion is scarce. Ibitulide has been used in a few studies, (Bernard et al 2003, Hennersdorf et al 2002, Varriale et al 2000) but for the fact of limited safety data, we cannot recommend treatment with ibitulide in the ICU setting.

Few studies in critically ill patients have shown that just lowering ventricular rate by drugs that lower AV conduction and thereby contributing to more hemodyamic stability is effective for conversion to sinus rhythm. Amiodarone intravenously is the most common used anti-arrrhythmic drug in this setting.

Amiodarone, a type III anti-arrhythmic drug with also class II and IV effects , is well tolerated in hemodynamic unstable patients. Even patients with compromised left ventricular function can be safely treated with amiodarone. (Kumar 1996) However, the high rate of serious adverse reactions makes amiodarone very unpopular. These adverse reactions are usually seen in prolonged administration although, amiodarone-induced pulmonary toxicity (Daniels et al 1997, Donaldson et al 1997, Laprinsky et al 1993, Van Mieghem et al 1994) and acute liver failure (Bravo et al 2005) may also present within days or weeks. These short terms adverse reactions of amiodarone are not well studied and may be underdiagnosed in clinical trials, especially in critically ill patients, since these patients often have more than one reason to develop (multi) organ failure.

Beta adrenergic receptor blockers or nondihydropyridine calcium channel blockers like verapamil are also widely used for lowering ventricular rate, however, in ICU setting, these drugs may further compromise hemodynamic state in critically ill patients.

The use of magnesium has shown some promising results both in critically ill patients (Sleeswijk et al 2008, Moran et al 1995) as also in the general population presenting with new onset atrial fibrillation. (Gullenstad et al 1993) However, the anti-arrhythmic effect of magnesium is not completely understood. A normal serum level of magnesium does not rule out an absolute magnesium deficiency since magnesium is mainly located intracellular. So, it is difficult to establish whether the anti-arrhythmic effects of magnesium are mainly due to repletion of intracellular hypomagnesiaor the result of the presumed effect on Na-K-ATP-ase (Dyckner 1980, Ebel 1983) or the effect of blocking of calcium channels. (White et al 1989) However, magnesium seems to be effective in patients with both a low and normal level of serum magnesium. (Eray et al 2000) The optimal dosage of magnesium has not yet been establish. There are different regimens used in clinical trials, which may explain the difference in success of the treatment.

The facts that hypomagnesia is frequently seen in critically ill patients (Ryzen et al 1985) and that hypomagnesia is associated with increased mortality (Chernow et al 1989), in combination with the positive effects of magnesium seen on both ventricular and supraventricular arrhythmia, (Toraman et al 2001, Gullenstad et al 1993, Sleeswijk et al 2008, Moran et al 1995, Chiladakis et al 2001, Hays et al 1994, Jensen et al 1997) in the absence of serious adverse effects, and furthermore combined with the low cost, the prophylactic effect on pro-arrhythmia, (Caron et al 2003), the synergistic effect with anti-arrhythmic drugs (Kalus et al 2003) and the reduction for the need of potential toxic anti-arrhythmic, (Sleeswijk et al 2008) justify its use in all critically ill patients with atrial fibrillation. Of course, serum levels should be monitored, especially in those with renal failure, to prevent toxicity of hypermagnesia. Although there are different regimes used in clinical trials, we suggested a treatment regime with a bolus magnesium of 0.037 gram/kg body weight within 15 minutes followed by a continuous infusion of 0.025 gram/kg body weight / hour. (Sleeswijk et al 2008, Moran et al 1995)

Digoxin is one of the oldest anti-arrhythmic drugs with positive inotropic and negative dromotropic effect. However, its dromotropic effect is very disappointing, especially in the critically ill patients probably because the enhanced adrenergic state which is seen in these patients. (Falk et al 1987, Clemo et al 1998, Goldman et al 1975) Furthermore, digoxin has several serious side effects and the combination of rather ineffectiveness with safety matters makes digoxin not recommended in critically ill patients.

Since inflammation plays an important crucial role in the pathophysiology of new onset atrial fibrillation in critically ill patients, it is tempting to use anti-inflammatory agents for the treatment and prevention of atrial fibrillation. Glucocorticoids, (Whitlock et al 2008) statins, angiotensin converting enzyme inhibitor and 3 fatty acids (Guglin et al 2008) may have shown to be effective in preventing or termination atrial fibrillation by modulating the substrate. Due to the limited evidence and safety concerns these agents cannot yet be recommended for the treatment of new onset atrial fibrillation in critically ill patients.

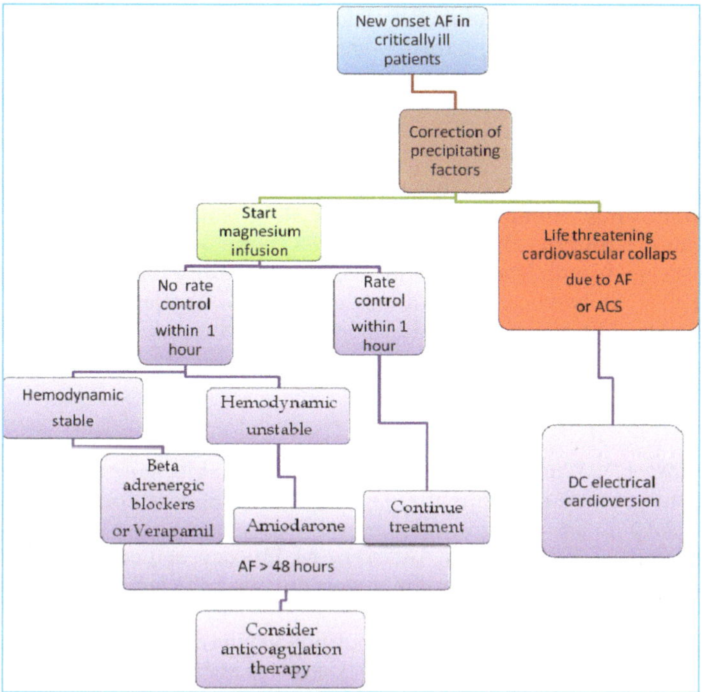

AF= atrial fibrillation
ACS= acute coronary syndrome

Fig. 1. Treatment algorithm for new onset atrial fibrillation in critically ill patients.

In summarize, the treatment of new onset atrial fibrillation in critically ill patients should start with the correction of precipitating factors and is further primarily aimed at a rate control strategy, starting with the infusion of magnesium. If rate control is not achieved we recommend amiodarone for the unstable patients and in hemodynamic stable patients a beta adrenergic receptor blocker of verapamil can be started. With this regime conversion to sinus rhythm will occur within 24 hours in most patients.

4. Prevention of thrombo-embolic complications

The risk for thrombo-embolic complication is increased in patients with atrial fibrillation lasting for more than 48 hours. Critically ill patients are at risk for thrombo-embolic complications due to their underlying disease and immobility. The formation of thrombi in atrial fibrillation is the result of the combination of blood coagulation status, vessel wall related factors and reduced blood flow. All these 3 factors are altered in favor of more easily development of thrombi in critically ill patients. Furthermore, inflammation, usually present in critically ill patients, might enhance development of thrombosis. However, critically ill patients also have a high risk of bleeding complications due to coagulation disorders (Levi et al 2006) or the need for invasive procedures during their stay in the ICU.

In each patient the benefit of stroke prevention must be weighed against the risk of bleeding. Although data are lacking, we tend to mention that the CHADS2 risk calculator for thrombo-embolic complication in atrial fibrillation cannot be applied in the critically ill.

In case of persistent atrial fibrillation for at least 48 hours, one should consider starting anticoagulant therapy in critically patients. Due to the high bleeding risk we recommend treatment with unfractionated heparin or short acting low molecular weight heparin.

5. Prognosis

Treatment with magnesium and or drugs that lower AV node conduction is in most case effective to restore sinus rhythm within 24 hours. Recurrence rate and long term outcome has not been studied in critically ill patients. New onset atrial fibrillation in critically ill patients is associated with increased mortality, morbidity and prolonged ICU stay. (Sleeswijk et al 2007) However, a causal link between atrial fibrillation and mortality has not yet been found. Atrial fibrillation may simply be a marker of severity of illness rather than an independent contributor of mortality.

6. References

Balser JR, Martinez EA, Winters BD, et al: Beta-adrenergic blockade accelerates conversion of postoperative supraventricular tachyarrhythmias. Anesthesiology 1998; 89: 1052-1059

Barranco F, Sanchez M, Rodriguez J, Guerrero M Efficacy of flecainide in patients with supraventricular arrhythmia and respiratory insufficiency. Intensive Care Med. 1994; 20:42–4

Bernard EO, Schmid ER, Schmidlin D, et al: Ibutilide versus amiodarone in atrial fibrillation: A double-blinded, randomized study. Crit Care Med 2003; 31:1031-1034

Bravo AE, Drewe J, Schlienger RG, Krahenbuhl S, Pargger H, Ummenhofer W. Hepatotoxicity during rapid intravenous loading with amiodarone: Description of three cases and review of the literature. Crit Care Med. 2005 Jan; 33(1):128-134

Caron MF, Kluger J, Tsikouris JP, Ritvo A, Kalus JS, White CM Effects of intravenous magnesium sulfate on the QT interval in patients receiving ibutilide.Pharmacotherapy. 2003 Mar; 23(3):296-300

Chapman MJ, Moran JL, O'Fathartaigh MS, et al: Management of atrial tachyarrhythmias in the critically ill: A comparison of intravenous procainamide and amiodarone. Intensive Care Med 1993; 19:48-52

Chernow B, Bamberger S, Stroiko M, et al: Hypomagnesemia in patients in the postoperative intensive care unit. Chest 95:391-397, 1989

Chiladakis JA, Stathopoulos C, Davlouros P, Manolis AS.Intravenous magnesium sulfate versus diltiazem in paroxysmal atrial fibrillation. Int J Cardiol. 2001 Jul; 79(2-3):287-91

Christian SA, Schorr C, Ferchau L, Jarbrink ME, Parrillo JE, Gerber DR. Clinical characteristics and outcomes of septic patients with new-onset atrial fibrillation. J Crit Care. 2008 Dec; 23(4):532-6.

Chung MK, Martin DO, Sprecher D, et al: C-reactive protein elevation in patients with atrial arrhythmias: Inflammatory mechanisms and persistence of atrial fibrillation. Circulation 2001; 104:2886-2891

Daniels CJ, Schutte DA, Hammond S, Granklin WH (1997) Acute pulmonary toxicity in an infant from intravenous amiodarone. Am J Cardiol 80:1113-1116

Dernellis J, Panaretou M: C-reactive protein and paroxysmal atrial fibrillation: Evidence of the implication of an inflammatory process in paroxysmal atrial fibrillation. Acta Cardiol 2001; 56:375-380

Donaldson L, Grant IS, Naysmith MR, Thomas JS (1997) Amiodarone should be used with caution in patients in intensive care (letter). BMJ 314:1832

Dyckner T: Serum magnesium in acute myocardial infarction -Relation to arrhythmias. Acta Med Scand 1980; 207: 59-66

Ebel H: Role of magnesium in cardiac disease. J Clin Chem Clin Biochem 1983; 21: 249-265

Eray O, Akca S, Pekdemir M, Eray E, Cete Y, Oktay C. Magnesium efficacy in magnesium deficient and non deficient patients with rapid ventricular response atrial fibrillation. Eur J Emerg Med. 2000 Dec; 7(4):287-90

Falk RH, Knowlton AA et al. Digoxin for converting recent-onset atrial fibrillation to sinus rhythm: a randomised double-blind trial. Ann Intern Med 1987; 106:503-506

Gaudino M, Andreotti F, Zamparelli R, et al: The -174G/C interleukin-6 polymorphism influences postoperative interleukin-6 levelsand postoperative atrial fibrillation: Is atrial fibrillation an inflammatory complication? Circulation 2003; 108 (Suppl 1):II195-II19

Clemo HF, Wood MA, Gilligan DM, et al: Intravenous amiodarone for acute heart rate control in the critically ill patient with atrial tachyarrhythmias. Am J Cardiol 1998; 81:594-598

Goldman S, Probst P, et al. Inefficacy of therapeutic serum levels of digoxin in controlling the ventricular rate in atrial fibrillation. Am J Cardiol 1975; 35:651655

Guglin M, Garcia M, Yarnoz MJ and Curtis AB. Non-antiarrhythmic medications for atrial fibrillation: From bench to clinical practice. J Interv Card Electrophysiol (2008) 22:119–128

Gullestad L, Birkeland K, Molstad P, Hoyer MM, Vanberg P, Kjekshus J. The effect of magnesium versus verapamil on supraventricular arrhythmias. Clin Cardiol. 1993 May; 16(5):429-34

Hays JV, Gilman JK, Rubal BJ. Effect of magnesium sulfate on ventricular rate control in atrial fibrillation. Ann Emerg Med. 1994 Jul; 24(1):61-4

Hennersdorf M, Stefan M. Perings, Christian Zühlke, Ulrich E. Heidland, Christian Perings Matthias P. Heintzen, Bodo E. Strauer, Conversion of recent-onset atrial fibrillation or flutter with ibutilide, after amiodarone has failed Intensive Care Med (2002) 28:925-929

Holt AW: Hemodynamic responses to amiodarone in critically ill patients receiving catecholamine infusions. Crit Care Med 1989; 17:1270-1276

Jensen BM, Alstrup P, Klitgard NA. Magnesium substitution and postoperative arrhythmias in patients undergoing coronary artery bypass grafting Scand Cardiovasc J. 1997; 31(5):265-9

Kalus JS, Spencer AP, Tsikouris JP, Chung JO, Kenyon KW, Ziska M, Kluger J, White CM. Impact of prophylactic i.v. magnesium on the efficacy of ibutilide for conversion of atrial fibrillation or flutter.Am J Health Syst Pharm. 2003 Nov 15;60(22):2308-12

Kumar A. Intravenous amiodarone for therapy of atrial fibrillation and flutter in critically ill patients with severely depressed left ventricular function. South Med J. 1996 Aug;89(8):779-85.

Laprinsky SE, Mullen JB, Baller MS (1993) Rapid pulmonary phospholipid accumulation induced by intravenous amiodarone. Can J Cardiol 9:322-324

Levi M and Opal SM. Coagulation abnormalities in critically ill patients. Crit Care 2006; 10(4):222

Mayr A, Ritsch N, Knotzer H, et al: Effectiveness of direct-current cardioversion for treatment of supraventricular tachyarrhythmias, in particular atrial fibrillation, in surgical intensive care patients. Crit Care Med 2003; 31:401-405

Meierhenrich R, Steinhilber E, Eggermann C, Weiss M, Voglic S, Bögelein D, Gauss A, Georgieff M, Stahl W

Incidence and prognostic impact of new-onset atrial fibrillation in patients with septic shock: a prospective observational study. Crit Care. 2010; 14(3):R108. Epub 2010 Jun 10.

Moran JL, Gallagher J, Peake SL, et al: Parenteral magnesium sulfate versus amiodarone in the therapy of atrial tachyarrhythmias:A prospective, randomized study. CritCare Med 1995; 23:1816-1824

Ryzen E, Wagers PW, Singer FR, et al: Magnesium deficiency in a medical ICU population. Crit Care Med 13:19-21, 1985

Salman S, Bajwa A, Gajic O, Afessa B. Paroxysmal atrial fibrillation in critically ill patients with sepsis. J int care med. 2008:23(3):178-183

Seguin P, Laviolle B, Maurice A, Leclercq C, Mallédant Y. Atrial fibrillation in trauma patients requiring intensive care. Intensive Care Med. 2006 Mar; 32(3):398-404. Epub 2006 Jan 27

Sleeswijk ME, Tulleken JE, Noord van T, Meertens JHJM, Ligtenberg JJM and Zijlstra JG. Efficacy of Magnesium-Amiodarone Step-Up Scheme in Critically Ill Patients with new-onset atrial fibrillation: A Prospective Observational Study. J Int Care Med 2008; 23; 61-66

Sleeswijk ME, Noord van T, Tulleken JE, Ligtenberg JJM, Girbes ARJ and Zijlstra JG. Clinical review: Treatment of new-onset atrial fibrillation in medical intensive care patients - a clinical framework. Critical Care 2007, 11:233;

Soucier R, Silverman D, Abordo M, Jaagosild P, Abiose A, Madhusoodanan KP, Therrien M, Lippman N, Dalamagas H, Berns E. Propafenone versus ibutilide for post operative atrial fibrillation following cardiac surgery: neither strategy improves outcomes compared to rate control alone (the PIPAF study). Med Sci Monit. 2003 Mar; 9(3):PI19-23

Toraman F, Karabulut EH, Alhan HC, Dagdelen S, Tarcan S.Magnesium infusion dramatically decreases the incidence of atrial fibrillation after coronary artery bypass grafting. Ann Thorac Surg. 2001 Oct;72(4):1256-61; discussion 1261-2

Van Gelder IC, Hagens VE, Bosker HA, Kingma JH, Kamp O, Kingma T,et al. Rate Control versus Electrical Cardioversion for Persistent Atrial Fibrillation (RACE) Study Group. N Engl J Med 2002; 347:1834-40.

Van Mieghem W, Coolen L, Malysse I, Lacquet LM, Deneffe GJD, Demedts MGP (1994) Amiodarone and the development of ARDS after lung surgery. Chest 105:1642-1645

Varriale P, Sedighi A: Acute management of atrial fibrillation and atrial flutter in the critical care unit: Should it be ibutilide? Clin Cardiol 2000; 23:265-268

White RE, Hartzell HC: Magnesium ions in cardiac function. Regulator of ion channels and second messengers. Biochem Pharmacol 1989; 38: 859-867

Whitlock RP, Chan S, Devereaux PJ, Sun J, Rubens FD, Thorlund K, Teoh KH. Clinical benefit of steroid use in patients undergoing cardiopulmonary bypass: a meta-analysis of randomized trials. Eur Heart J. 2008 Nov; 29(21):2592-600. Epub 2008 Jul 28.

Wyse DG, Waldo AL, DiMarco JP, Domanski MJ, Rosenberg Y, Schron EB, et al. The Atrial Fibrillation Follow-up Investigation of Rhythm Management (AFFIRM) Investigators. A comparison of rate control and rhythm control in patients with atrial fibrillation. N Engl J Med 2002; 347:1825-33.

22

Stroke and Dementia in Atrial Fibrillation

Miljenka-Jelena Jurašić, Sandra Morović,
Sonja Antić, Iris Zavoreo and Vida Demarin
University Department of Neurology, Sestre milosrdnice University Hospital Centre, Croatia

1. Introduction

1.1 Incidence and prevalence

Atrial fibrillation (AF) and its consequences are today's main epidemiologic concerns. Two most important population based studies, the Framingham Study and the Rotterdam Study, report a lifetime risk of developing AF as one in four people after the age of 40 years. This is opposed to breast cancer which affects one in eight women, or heart failure affecting every fifth individual. (Lloyd-Jones et al., 2004, Mattace-Raso et al., 2006) With aging population, both AF prevalence and incidence are also increasing. (Lakatta & Levy, 2003b) AF represents the most common, highly prevalent cardiac arrhythmia which is the strongest risk factor for ischemic stroke, currently affecting 4,5 to 6 million Europeans and 2,3 to 5,1 million Americans. The prevalence of AF ranges from 2,5% in individuals over 40 yrs of age, 6% in those older than 65, to 12-16% in those over 75 yrs. (Lloyd-Jones et al., 2004; Stewart et al., 2002; Wolf et al., 1991; Kannnel et al., 2008; Miyasaka et al., 2006) AF affects more than 1% of the population in total, and 70% of AF patients are aged between 65 and 85 yrs. (Phillips et al., 1990) This number is expected to double in the next 30 years. (Miyasaka et al., 2006; Savelieva & Camm, 2001; Go et al., 2008).

1.2 AF burden

AF also represents a great burden both for the patient and the society. AF symptoms (palpitations, fatigue, chest pain, dizziness, light headedness, syncope and dyspnoea) have a strong negative impact on patients' quality of life, regardless of their frequency or duration. (Fuster et al., 2006; Van den Berg et al., 2005) Studies have shown that 68% of patients find AF symptoms disruptive, and 30% suffer an associated anxiety or depression. (Hamer et al., 1994; Thrall et al., 2007) AF accounts for more hospitalizations than any other arrhythmia. Society wise, AF represents a great public health issue which is expected to increase over the next decades due to aging population and improved cardiac disease management. In 1995, there were more than 1,6 million consultations, and more than 59000 hospitalizations due to AF. (Stewart et al., 2002) In Denmark alone, this number has increased by 60% in the last 20 years. (Friberg et al., 2003).

2. AF – risk for stroke and dementia occurrence

AF is the commonest sustained cardiac rhythm disorder, and is encountered in everyday clinical practice. Irrespective of whether we use a rate-control or rhythm-control strategy, stroke prevention with appropriate thromboprophylaxis still remains central to the management of this common arrhythmia. When strokes occur in AF patients, the risk of mortality and disability, as well as recurrent stroke is substantially much higher. (Lip & Halperin, 2010)

Additionally, AF as the most common arrhythmia in the elderly is becoming more frequently evaluated in various studies. Furthermore, Leibovitch has pointed out, in his review article, that the most important issues to treat in the very elderly are hypertension and AF. (2008)

AF is a potentially dangerous condition for the development of two very serious neurological conditions: stroke and dementia. Those two conditions are the leading causes of mortality and disability in the developed countries and also in the developing world as estimated in 2010 by World Health Organizations. (Shirwany et Zou, 2010)

The risk of stroke is increased five-fold in individuals with AF. (Wolf et al., 1991) However, it often passes on unnoticed until its gloomy consequences are discovered. Appearently, about 20% of ischemic stroke patients have AF, based on their admission electrocardiogram (ECG). (Kimura et al., 2004; Liao et al., 2007) Additionally, AF seems to be even more important than hypertension in stroke aetiology of the very old. (Marengoni et al., 2009; Ratcliffe et Wilcock, 1985) And, silent or asymptomatic AF unfortunately carries the same long-term risk for stroke, just like for symptomatic patients. (Page et al., 2003) Continuous ECG monitoring can register up to 40% of cases, where a pacemaker reading can reveal as much as 88% of cases. Namely, a Scottish population study showed that for both women and men, there was a significant increase in all-cause mortality, cardiovascular events, fatal or nonfatal stroke, and heart failure. (Stewart et al., 2002; Benjamin et al., 1998) Regardless whether it is paroxysmal or persistent AF, risk of stroke is similar (Atrial Fibrillation Investigators, 1994) since there is a high risk of recurrence and conversion of paroxysmal to persistent AF. (Allessie et al., 2001) The increasing risk of fatal AF consequences comes from the fact that AF is asymptomatic in more than one third of the patients. (Israel et al., 2004)

The presence of AF worsens the prognosis in patients with cardiovascular comorbidities, increasing their risk for cardiovascular events, stroke, and hospitalization due to heart failure (RR 1,88-4,96). (Wachtel et al., 2005; Pizzetti et al., 2001; Wang et al., 2003) New onset AF has shown to be an independent predictor of in-hospital mortality, longer intensive care unit stay, and longer overall hospital stay. (Rivero-Ayerza et al., 2008) Additionally, in a hospital setting, AF as a comorbidity indicates worse metabolic status and poor clinical outcome for patients with dementia, stroke or heart failure. (Fumagalli et al., 2010)

The road from AF to cognitive impairment and dementia can be either direct or via stroke as an intermediate. Silent or asymptomatic strokes are valuable predictors for clinical strokes and dementia, as well. The Rotterdam study showed a 3 fold risk increase for stroke, and 2,3 fold risk increase for dementia with a steeper decline in cognitive function. (Vermeer et al, 2003a; Vermeer et al., 2003b) Concerning pre and post stroke dementia burden, it was analyzed recently by Pendlebury and Rothwell in a meta-analysis that there are 10% of demented patients before first stoke, 10% of dementia occurred soon after first stroke and more that 30% after recurrent stroke. (2009)

Lastly, it is thought that other often underdiagnosed vascular conditions like hypertension and ischemic heart disease or depression in the elderly will eventually lead to dementia development, as well. (Collerton et al., 2009).

3. AF and stroke

3.1 AF and increase in stroke risk

Non-valvular atrial fibrillation (NVAF) is associated with a prothrombotic state which carries an increased risk for thromboembolic events. Studies show that levels of coagulation markers are still elevated even during anticoagulation therapy. Patients with chronic AF were found to have a higher prevalence of chronic heart failure and history of stroke, but the prevalence of high D-dimer levels of these patients was comparable to those with paroxysmal AF. (Sadanaga et al., 2010) Recent data also link the hypercoagulability of AF with decreased renal function in NVAF patients. By yet unclear mechanism, the reduction in residual renal function enhances hypercoagulability in NVAF patients. (Tanaka et al., 2009) Predictors for thrombombolic events in NVAF are established, and they include recent heart failure, hypertension, advanced age, diabetes mellitus, previous thromboembolic events, echocardiographic evidence of left ventricular disfunction and left atrial enlargement. (Stroke Prevention in Atrial Fibrillation Investigators, 1992) Increased concentrations of hemostatic markers TAT and D-dimer were found in patients with NVAF, linking hypercoagulability and AF. Both of these markers have high molecular weights, ensuring very limited excretion from the kidneys. Therefore, their concentrations accurately reflect intravascular fibrin formation and lysis, and not accumulation as a result of renal failure. Several recent studies have established a relationship between elevation of these markers and subsequent thromboembolic events in patients with NVAF. (Enata et al., 2004; Nozawa et al., 2006) Therefore, elevation of D-dimer levels despite proper anticoagulant treatment can predict thromboembolic and cardiovascular events in patients with AF. Whether these events can be prevented by increasing anticoagulant intensity still needs to be discovered. (Sadanaga et al., 2010)

The risk for thromboembolic events is present even during the non-paroxysmal period in patients with paroxysmal AF. Plasma markers of thrombin activity (thrombin-antithrombin III complex-TAT), active fibrinolysis (plasmin-alpha 2-plasmin inhibitor complex-PIC), and platelet activity (platelet factor 4-PF4) were evaluated in the left atria (LA) of patients with paroxysmal AF (pAF) during the non-paroxysmal period. The results of this study showed elevated coagulation activity in LA of patients with pAF, even during the non-paroxysmal period. This is the first study to report hypercoagulability in the LA of pAF patients during sinus rhythm. (Motoki et al., 2009) Experiments demonstrated two coagulation mechanisms, one being endothelial dysfunction caused by AF, (Fukuchi et al., 2001) and oxidative stress induced in the LA by AF. (Dudley et al., 2005; Kim et al., 2005) This study also has clinical relevance since it showed increased cogulation activity in LA in pAF patients, but without increased platelet activity, making anticoagulation, rather than antiplatelet, a therapy of choice.

3.2 AF and stroke – the studies and surveys

Stroke is probably the most devastating complication of AF. AF is the cause of 15-20% of all ischemic strokes, (Go, 2005) and it increases the risk for stroke fivefold. (Wolf et al., 2001) Cardioembolic stroke, most of which is due to AF, is the most lethal subtype of ischemic stroke and has a higher risk of disability than other stroke subtypes. (Simpson et al., 2010)

AF is also an independent risk factor for stroke severity and recurrence. (Penado et al., 2003) Not only do AF patients have increased post-stroke mortality and stroke recurrence, but they also suffer more severe strokes than their age-matched counterparts suffering strokes due to other aetiologies. (Marini et al., 2005; Dulli et al., 2003) AF should be considered when assessing cryptogenic strokes, which account for about one third of first ever ischemic strokes. Most likely 25% to 50% of cryptogenic strokes could be attributed to undetected AF, and therefore are of cardioembolic origin. (Petty et al., 1999) Unrecognized AF can also cause cryptogenic transient ischemic attack (TIA). (Malik et al., 2011) Namely, following prolonged monitoring of asymptomatic patients, 85% of AF episodes lasted less than 30 seconds. (Tayal et al., 2008) To support this thesis, a magnetic resonance (MR) study was performed on more than 2000 asymptomatic subjects. In 10,7% of participants at least one silent cerebral infarction could be detected; the risk for silent brain infarct is doubled in subjects with AF in comparison to those without AF. The Framingham Offspring Study of prevalence and correlates of silent cerebral infarcts (SCI) was the first one to demonstrate a significant relationship between AF and SCI, which has been associated with increased risk of incident stroke and cognitive impairment. (Das et al., 2008) As previously mentioned, silent strokes are, also, predictors of less favourable cognitive outcome and dementia occurrence. (Vermeer et al, 2003a; Vermeer et al., 2003b) For all the above mentioned reasons, it seems wise to develop a risk score, such as that derived from the Framingham Heart Study, that could help to identify risk of atrial fibrillation for individuals in the community, assess technologies or markers for improvement of risk prediction, and target high-risk individuals for preventive measures. (Schnabel et al., 2009)

When a stroke occurs in patients with AF, the severity of the stroke is generally much greater, as is mortality and disability compared to those patients in sinus rhythm. Additionally, it seems that arrhythmia progression in isolated AF is a marker of increased risk for adverse cardiovascular events. (Potpara et al., 2011) Unsurprisingly, the biggest challenge facing physicians caring for patients with AF is the prevention of stroke and thromboembolism, whether as primary or secondary prevention.

In the Euro Heart Survey, prescription of antithrombotic therapy was based on the type of AF and availability of warfarin monitoring clinics, rather than the stroke risk profile per se. (Nieuwlaat et al., 2007) However, the type of AF should not be taken into consideration, given that paroxysmal AF has a similar stroke risk to persistent or permanent AF in the presence of risk factors - therefore such patients would derive much benefit from anticoagulation prescription. (Tay et al., 2009)

The National Acute Israeli Stroke Survey (NASIS) examined the potential effect of preadmission anticoagulation on stroke severity and outcome in patients with AF. Data showed that effective anticoagulation therapy is associated with decreased stroke severity, improved functional outcome, and better survival in patients with AF admitted with acute brain ischemia. Another important finding of this study showed that the effective anticoagulation was not associated with an increased risk of symptomatic hemorrhagic transformation during hospitalization. (Schwammenthal et al., 2010) Rietbrock et al. evaluate stroke incidence by examining the United Kingdom General Practice Research Database from 1987 onwards in routine clinical practice among >51,000 chronic AF patients aged 40 years who were taking either aspirin or warfarin. Virtually all the patients had been treated with warfarin or aspirin, and almost 10,000 patients had received both: concomitantly or separately. Compared to no warfarin use, current and past use were both associated with a significant reduction in stroke rate, by 67% (RR 0,33, 95% CI 0,30–0,35) and 44% (RR 0,56, 95% CI 0,50–0,63), respectively. The benefits were more evident amongst the elderly, whereby the risk of stroke was reduced by 45% in elderly warfarin users (aged 75 years or older) and by 14% in younger users. In contrast, there was no difference in the stroke rate between current and past aspirin use (RR 1,04, 95% CI 0,94 - 1,15). Thus, all AF patients with one or more risk factors (that is, the "moderate risk" and "high risk" categories) should all be seriously considered for warfarin, whilst those with no risk factors at all (essentially, the "low risk" category) could be considered for aspirin or no antithrombotic therapy. Another interesting observation from the study is that the stroke-risk reduction was only apparent after 6–12 months of treatment, possibly reflecting poor INR control in the first six months. (2009)

Further important issue concerning AF and acute ischemic stroke is the destiny of patients who are causally treated with rtPA (recombinant tissue plasminogen activator) intravenous thrombolysis within the first 3 hours after the acute stroke onset. Previous results showed poor rate of early recanalization with a low rate of early major neurological improvement after rtPA administration. (Kimura et al., 2008) In contrast, recent encouraging results were reported by the Czeck multidisciplinary medical researchers. It appears that no initial statistical differences existed between the treated versus non-treated groups when 24 hour and 7 day clinical improvement or rate of achieved recanalizations were compared. However, AF patients had significantly poorer 90-day clinical outcome than non-AF patients using modified Rankin scale for comparison (median mRS 2,5 vs. 1,0). It is speculated that this is most likely due to more severe baseline neurological deficits or the greater number of arterial occlusions witnessed by the MRA before the use of intravenous thrombolysis. The other explanation is the physiology of clot dissolution, which depends on size, site of occlusion, clot composition, surface area of the clot exposed to the blood flow, and penetration of rtPA into the clot structure. Fresh and old clots form in the left atrium, but old and large thrombi may be more resistant to thrombolytic therapy than fresh and small ones. Therefore, it appears that AF stroke patients are more likely to have old and large thrombi, which are resistant to thrombolytic therapy. (Sanak et al., 2011)

4. When to treat AF patients in order to prevent future neurological complications?

The size of expected AF affected TIA and stroke patients is 15%. It seems that the most important factors that need to be evaluated in these patients regarding AF screening are age and left atrial diameter. Using this protocol about 47% of TIA and stroke patients can be excluded from further protocol. (Malik et al., 2011)

Judicious use of antithrombotic therapy importantly reduces stroke for most patients who have atrial fibrillation. Absolute increases in major extracranial hemorrhage associated with antithrombotic therapy were less than the absolute reductions in stroke. Adjusted-dose warfarin and antiplatelet agents reduce stroke by approximately 60% and by approximately 20%, respectively, in patients who have atrial fibrillation. Warfarin is substantially more efficacious (by approximately 40%) than antiplatelet therapy. (Hart et al., 2007)

4.1 Patient selection

Over the last 15 years of so, the various published stroke risk schema only have modest predictive value for thromboembolism, with no improvement in predictive ability over the years. (Lip & Halperin, 2010) Many stroke risk assessment schema classify a large proportion of subjects into the 'moderate risk' category where treatment guidelines recommend either warfarin or aspirin, and risk stratification schema that result in classification of a large proportion of AF subjects into the 'moderate risk' category could potentially be less useful in everyday clinical practice, since current treatment guidelines recommend the use of either warfarin or aspirin in such patients, causing confusion over which therapy should really be prescribed. Alternatively, classification as 'moderate risk' is often used as an excuse not to give anticoagulation, since the guidelines 'allow' aspirin.

Given the modest predictive ability for identifying 'high risk' subjects and the availability of new oral anticoagulant drugs that overcome the shortcomings of warfarin, stroke risk

stratification schema perhaps need to focus more on identifying the 'truly low risk' category of patients where no antithrombotic therapy may even be an option, given the increasing debate over the effectiveness of aspirin and potential for harm. (Sato et al., 2006) This concept was first proposed by van Walraven et al. and more recently revisited by Lip and Halperin. (van Walraven et al., 2003; Lip & Halperin, 2010)
In selecting the appropriate strategy to prevent stroke in an individual patient with AF, clinicians must consider the patients' risk of stroke, their risk of bleeding, concomitant indications for either anti-platelet medications or oral anticoagulants (OAC), anticipated challenges with INR control and patient preference. One of the most frequently used assessment tools by American Cardiologists is the $CHADS_2$ score grouping the patients into low- (score 0 to 1), intermediate- (score 2 to 3), or high- (score 4 to 6) risk category. However, European Society of Cardiology prefers the use of CHA_2DS_2-VASc score. Its components are as follows: C - congestive heart failure/LV dysfunction, H - hypertension, A - age ≥ 75 years, D - diabetes mellitus, S - stroke (TIA/ thromboembolism - TE), V - vascular disease, A - age 65-74 years and S - sex (female); and lower case numbers representing items with greater weight. The second score is more sensitive to a greater number of vascular risk factors and lowers the cut off value for treatment initiation making it therefore a future strategy for more refined stroke risk lowering schema: those at truly low risk (CHA_2DS_2-VASc = 0) who need not be prescribed any antithrombotic therapy, while all others (CHA_2DS_2-VASc score ≥1) can be considered for anticoagulation.(Table 1.)

$CHADS_2$	*Score*	*CHA_2DS_2-VASc*	*Score*
Congestive heart failure	1	Congestive heart failure/LV dysfunction	1
Hypertension	1	Hypertension	1
Aged ≥75 years	1	Aged ≥75 years	2
Diabetes mellitus	1	Diabetes mellitus	1
Stroke/TIA/TE	2	Stroke/TIA/TE	2
Maximum score	6	Vascular disease (prior MI, PAD, or aortic plaque)	1
		Aged 65-74 years	1
		Sex category (i.e. female gender)	1
		Maximum score	10

Table 1. The $CHADS_2$ and CHA_2DS_2-VASc score table

Not less important, is the need to select those patients who are truly at low bleeding risk, and therefore a HAS-BLED (Hypertension, Abnormal renal/liver function, Stroke, Bleeding history or predisposition, Labile International Normalized Ration, Elderly, Drugs/alcohol concomitantly) simple risk assessment score was proposed where score over 3 points indicates „high risk" requiring regular and more frequent check-ups. (Lip, 2011)

4.2 Oral anticoagulation therapy

Weighing all of these, anti-platelet therapy is the most appropriate strategy for many patients. Using either of the two aforementioned scales, OAC are advised if the score is ≥ 2. Furthermore, recent study reported that significantly elevated plasma C-reactive protein levels were noted in the high-risk group compared to those in the intermediate- and low-risk groups; and the use of transoesophageal echocardiography, the incidence of left atrial spontaneous echo contrast and left atrial thrombus increased with an increasing $CHADS_2$ score. (Maehama et al., 2010)

As for AF treatment and stroke, strokes due to AF are largely preventable with warfarin therapy, and that results in a 64% relative risk reduction. (Hart et al., 2007) Furthermore, recent observational study found out that it is even more beneficial if the INR was maintained at 1,8 (range 1,5-2,0) than at the standard target of 2,5. (Pengo et al., 2010) In addition to its established benefit for stroke prevention, effective anticoagulation therapy is associated with decreased stroke severity and better functional outcome and survival in patients with AF presenting with acute brain ischemia. (Schwammenthal et al., 2010) Sadly, many times anticoagulation for stroke prevention was found underused in general for patients with AF, and even in such high-risk groups as patients with stroke. However, participation in special quality improvement programs, like Get-With-The-Guidelines-Stroke (GWTG-S) was associated with improved adherence for patients with ECG-documented AF; still patients with a history of AF alone were largely untreated. (Lewis et al., 2009)

Additional oral treatment choices may soon be available for patients with AF, which would be particularly useful for patients in whom OAC is not used because of poor INR control, inability to comply with INR monitoring or drug-interactions. Both oral direct thrombin inhibitors and factor Xa inhibitors, like endoxaban, overcome these limitations of warfarin and may find a role in stroke prevention among these groups of patients, who are typically treated with anti-platelet agents. (Healy, 2009) The advent of novel oral direct-thrombin inhibitors and Factor Xa inhibitors with their more stable pharmacokinetic profiles, removal of the need for INR monitoring, and fewer patient-related barriers (diet, alcohol and drug interactions, INR control, etc.) that currently limit prescription of anticoagulation, may increase the unmet need of anticoagulation and make anticoagulation available and safe to those patients who may stand to derive benefit from it, including those with a $CHADS_2$ score of 1. (Lane & Lip, 2010)

4.3 Antiplatelet therapy

For the 22% of AF patients with a $CHADS_2$ score of 0, the low observed risk of stroke makes aspirin the preferred treatment option. (Lee et al., 2010) Given the slightly higher stroke risk among the 32% of AF patients with a $CHADS_2$ score of 1, aspirin, the combination of aspirin plus clopidogrel and OAC are all appropriate options, with the ultimate choice between therapies hinging on patient preference, bleeding risk and concomitant indications for one of these therapies. For patients who are at higher risk of stroke, but who cannot or will not take OAC; the combination of aspirin plus clopidogrel has now been shown to provide greater protection against stroke than aspirin alone. Finally, for OAC-treated patients who cannot achieve good INR control, combination anti-platelet therapy may be a safer and equally effective alternative to OAC. (Lee et al., 2010)

4.4 Mechanical devices

Recently, Ohara et al. have shown that the severity of blood stasis in the left atrium was greater in chronic AF patients than in paroxysmal AF patients at the comparable risk level and that severity of blood stasis in the LA and aortic atherosclerosis correlates with an accumulation of clinical risk factors for thromboembolism in non-valvular AF patients.

(2010) Furthermore, enhanced coagulation activation appears to be related to a reduction in residual renal function in patients with non-valvular AF patients which suggests that decreased renal function might be a candidate predictor of thromboembolic events in those patients. (Tanaka et al, 2009)
However, since more than 90% of atrial thrombi originate from the left atrial appendage (LAA), the devices that can isolate this structure from the systemic circulation perhaps may obviate the need for long-term anticoagulation therapy. Namely, the PLAATO device (Percutaneous Left Atrial Appendage Transcatheter Occlusion; Appriva Medical, CA, USA), later withdrawn by the manufacturer in 2006 or the WATCHMAN system (Aritech Inc, MN,USA), which is a self-expanding nitinol frame structure. Newer oral anticoagulants (eg, the oral direct thrombin inhibitors) or even the isolated use of antiplatelet therapy is necessary after device implantation, in addition to refinements in stroke and bleeding risk stratification. Still, not all thrombi originate from the LAA, with up to a quarter of strokes in patients with atrial fibrillation caused by cerebrovascular disease and complex atheromatous plaques involving the aorta and carotid arteries, or other cardiac sites. (Wrigley & Lip, 2009) Another important concern is the development of cardioembolic stroke, a serious periprocedural complication of radiofrequency catheter ablation and it may cause long-term neurocognitive and functional impairment resulting in significant disability or mortality on its own. Most periprocedural clinical events occur during or within 48 hours of the procedure with the incidence of 1–6% for focal ablations and up to 7% for linear AF ablations depending on the implemented anticoagulation strategy and the method of assessment. However, once successfully implemented, at 1 year follow-up interval, complete functional and neurocognitive recovery is expected. (Patel et al., 2010)

4.5 Hypertension treatment

Blockade of the renin–angiotensin system is an important approach in managing high blood pressure, and has increasingly been shown to affect cardiovascular disease processes mediated by angiotensin II throughout the cardiovascular and renal continua. It seems that new-onset AF and associated stroke were significantly reduced by losartan- compared to atenolol-based antihypertensive treatment with similar blood pressure reduction in the LIFE study. (Wachtel et al., 2005) Additionally, clinical evidence was found in favor of telmisartan and reduction of left ventricular hypertrophy, arterial stiffness and the recurrence of atrial fibrillation, as well as renoprotection. (Galzerano et al., 2010)

4.6 Inflammation

In recent years data to support the notion that inflammation plays a role in the pathogenesis of AF are increasing. Many ongoing studies are attempting to attenuate these inflammatory processes in patients with AF by novel therapeutic strategies, such as the use of glucocorticoids. However, systemic glucocorticoid use itself has been linked to increased risk of AF. Therefore, more research is necessary to determine whether these drugs are a potential treatment or risk factor for AF. (Rienstra & Van Gelder, 2010)

4.7 Quality of life surveys

Lastly, but not least important is, side to side with therapeutic effects, the health-related quality of life considered by the patient (HRQoL) at baseline and after potential therapeutic intervention. Most often this is achieved with the use of Short-Form health survey-36 items that does not seem to be proficient enough and formation of standardized AF-specific questionnaires is warranted. So far, two main therapeutic options follow either rate-control or rhythm-control and neither has been proven significantly better than the other, yet both improve HRQoL, so the choice of which pharmacologic agent to prefer could be personally tailored to each patient by such questionnaire. (Fuster & Mearns, 2010)

5. AF and dementia

Dementia prevalence increases with age, from 5-8% over 65 years of age to 25-50% over the age of 85 years. (Collerton et al., 2009; Luchsinger, 2010) The Rotterdam Study showed that dementia occurred twice as common in subjects with AF (more so if subject age was less than 75 years of age and if they were women), and a significant positive association between cognitive impairment and AF was confirmed (no age association was discovered). And, even though AF proved to be commonly discovered in AD and VAD patients, it is more strongly associated with AD incidence. (Ettore et al., 2009) The greatest reason for missing AF diagnosis is that a single ECG is usually ordered for acute stroke patients, thereby causing those with paroxysmal AF to elude from screening and diagnosis. (Kamel et al., 2009). There is no evidence of putative mechanisms of direct relation between dementia and AF, because AF is found in all types of dementia-vascular, Alzheimer and mixed types of dementia which are results of different pathomorphological and pathophysiological mechanisms.

The onset of dementia goes unnoticed in the early stages, sometimes symptoms such as cognitive and intellectual impairment as well as carrying out everyday activities may became apparent only in the mid-to-late stages. Symptoms of dementia include: memory loss, confusion, forgetfulness, poor concentration, inability to cope with everyday activities, language impairment, slurred speech, inability to follow simple instructions, inappropriate laughing and crying, behavioral changes, impaired social skills, eating problems, a shuffling or jerky gait, incontinence and/or lack of bowel control. Lateralizing signs such as hemiparesis, bradykinesia, hyperreflexia, ataxia, pseudobulbar palsy, and gait and swallowing difficulties may also be observed. (Vermeer et al., 2003; Velandai et al., 2006)

Several specific diagnostic criteria can be used to diagnose vascular dementia: Diagnostic and Statistical Manual of Mental Disorders, Fourth Edition (DSM-IV) criteria, International Classification of Diseases, Tenth Edition criteria, National Institute of Neurological Disorders and Stroke- Association International pour la Recherché & L'Enseignement en Neurosciences (NINDS-AIREN) criteria, The Alzheimer's Disease Diagnostic and Treatment Center criteria, The Hachinski ischemic score. In evaluation of dementia patients neuroimaging methods should, also, be included as well as evaluation of specific serum and cerebrospinal fluid markers for AD. A number of neuroimaging candidate markers are promising, such as hippocampal and enthorinal cortex volumetry, basal forebrain nuclei assessment, cortical thickness, deformation based and voxel based morphometry, diffusion tensor imaging tractography and functional magnetic resonance imaging. For example, combined measurements of the cerebrospinal fluid (CSF) t-tau, Aβ42 and p-tau profile and regional flow or mediotemporal lobe atrophy demonstrate higher predictive power than either diagnostic approach alone in cognitive impairment evaluation. Differential diagnosis between AD and vascular dementia seems promising by using the ratio of Aβ42 and p-tau, between AD and Lewy bodies dementia by using the ratio of Aβ peptides of varying lengths (Aβ42/ Aβ38 and Aβ42/ Aβ37) and tau protein. Other interesting novel biomarker candidates derived from blood and CSF are being currently proposed (phase I or II of multicenter studies).

Magnetic resonance imaging (MRI) can provide a detailed image of the brain and cerebrovascular system. However, the structural changes detected with MRI as well as the biomarkes do not accurately predict the clinical manifestation of cognitive impairment so cognitive testing is imperative. (Rockwood et al., 2009)

5.1 Dementia syndromes

Progression of Alzheimer dementia (AD) is highly variable. Most estimates derive from convenience samples from dementia clinics or research centers where there is substantial potential for survival bias and other distortions. Nowadays, there is a growing rise in public health concern due to lack of effective curative treatment and raising prevalence with variable survival rate of the two most frequent dementia syndromes (gloomy results report survival rate for men with AD 4,1 years and for women 4,6 years; while five year survival rate for VAD is 39%). (Tschantz et al., 2011)

AF in connection with dementia is usually analyzed through most common types of dementia: Alzheimer's disease (AD), vascular dementia (VAD) and mixed dementia (MD). When AF is regarded in the pathophysiology of stroke or dementia, it must be said that AF can result in either cardiac thromboembolism or reduced cardiac output and cerebral hypoperfusion with main neuroradiological manifestation such as white matter lesions (WML). WML are a frequent finding in patients with vascular cognitive impairment, AD and VAD. WML are reported to be up to three-fold more prevalent in patients with AD. (Vermeer et al., 2003a) Furthermore, lacunar state, in which numerous lacunae indicate the presence of severe widespread small vessel disease, is another observed manifestation in AF patients. (Vermeer et al., 2003b)

By far, the most common type of dementia is AD accounting for 60-80% of all dementia patients, and having the greatest prevalence among all neurological diseases. AD is defined by the World Health Organization (WHO) as a degenerative brain syndrome characterized by progressive decline in memory, thinking, comprehension, calculation, language, learning capacity and judgment sufficient to impair personal activities of daily living. Today, it is believed to be associated with excessive extracellular beta-amyloid and intracellular hyperphosphorylated tau protein accumulation eventually leading to the loss of cholinergic neurons and relative glutamate excess. (Rocchi et al., 2009)

VAD, accounting for 10-20% of all dementia patients, is characterized by a stepwise deteriorating course and a patchy distribution of neurologic deficits (affecting some functions and not others) caused by cerebrovascular disease. It is not a single disease, but rather a group of syndromes relating to different vascular mechanisms. Common risk factors for VAD are the ones already recognized for cerebrovascular disease – non-modifiable risk factors such as age, gender, race/ethnicity, genotype, previous myocardial infarction, and TIA or stroke; and modifiable risk factors like diabetes, hyperlipidemia, arterial hypertension, atrial fibrillation, coronary and or peripheral artery disease, obesity, physical inactivity, stress, alcohol consumption, and smoking. (Luchsinger, 2010; Llewellyn et al., 2008)

Subtypes of vascular dementia include: mild cognitive impairment, multi-infarct dementia (MID), strategic infarct dementia, subcortical ischemic dementia, ischemic-hypoxic dementia, and haemorrhagic dementia. (Grand et al., 2011)

The term mild cognitive imparement (MCI) refers to a transitional stage between cognitive changes of normal aging and vascular dementia. At this stage, cognitive decline is not severe enough to constitute dementia, but also it is beyond the cognitive functioning deficit which is expected in normal aging. Patinets with MCI have subjective memory complains which are relative to age and education norms, but essentially normal general function as well as activities of daily living. Patients with MCI progress to dementia at a rate of 10-15% per year, far higher than the baseline rate of 1-2% per year in normal elderly. In cases of MCI an elderly patient will come in complaining of memory lapses, and will want to know if they have "normal" age related memory loss or something more serious. In everyday evaluation of cognitive changes most neurologists and psychiatrists rely on the Folstein Mini Mental State Exam (MMSE). But the MMSE has some serious limitations- it is quite sensitive at picking up moderate to severe dementia, it is very poor at screening for patients with MCI. Both, normal and MCI patients will typically score 26 or above, the usual cut-off point for cognitive impairment. The Montreal Cognitive Assessment (MoCA) appears to work much better in such cases. The test was developed specifically to better diagnose MCI, it is a more challenging version of the MMSE. It is quick to administer (about 10 minutes) and has a maximum of 30 points. In a study comparing the MMSE with the MoCA, the MMSE had a sensitivity of only 18% to detect MCI (meaning it missed 82%, while the MoCA detected 90% of MCI subjects). As always, though, high sensitivity comes at the price of somewhat lower specificity- the specificity for MCI was 87%, meaning that 13% of actually normal people will be falsely labeled as impaired -- still quite accurate. (Nasreddine ZS, 2005: Dong Y et al., 2010)

MD is dementia consisting of features proving the coexistence of AD and VAD either clinically or based on neuroimaging evidence of cerebral ischemic lesions. It is thought that vascular processes in both disorders mutually induce each other. To support such thesis, the following shared risk factors are secluded: hypertension, adult onset diabetes mellitus, atherosclerosis, AF and smoking. Lastly, MD is more common among the old elderly (85+), and can be definitely proven solely on autopsy. (Ferriet al., 2005; Collerton et al., 2009)

5.2 Vascular cognitive impairment

Apart from the three previously mentioned dementia syndromes, newly arising topic concerning dementia is vascular cognitive impairment (VCI) that inclines toward substituting "Alzhemerized" dementia concept in the setting of cerebrovascular disease with a spectrum of cognitive deficits that are all of vascular origin. The pyramid of cognitive decline in this setting initiates with condition known as the "brain at risk", perisymptomatic changes, VCI, white matter lesions (WML) and lacunae, and, lastly, VAD. It is important to acknowledge that vascular diseases can cause focal (usually due to thrombosis or embolism) or diffuse (usually due to hypertension) effects on the brain that may eventually lead to cognitive decline. However, both mechanisms are frequently present in the same patient.

Unfortunately, up to date there are no resolute clinical criteria for VCI, still the common clinical finding is progressive gait alteration and incontinence. (Battistin & Cagnin, 2010) And recently, there is a growing interest in the clinical and scientific area involving the elderly community in investigation of elderly fallers. Interestingly, recurrent fallers had lower MMSE scores than single fallers or non-fallers. (Vassalo et al., 2002) Areas of higher cortical function that showed the most deterioration were: attention and calculation, registration (short term memory), recall and praxis (visuospatial perception). (Chen et al., 2010) Chen et al. have isolated independent factors to be history of dementia, stroke or AF or prolonged hospital stay (> 5 weeks). (2010)

5.3 AF, stroke and dementia

Reported estimates of the prevalence of dementia are consistent: 10% of patients had dementia before first stroke, 10% developed new dementia soon after first stroke, and more than a third had dementia after recurrent stroke. The strong association of post-stroke dementia with multiple strokes and the prognostic value of other stroke characteristics highlight the central causal role of stroke itself as opposed to the underlying vascular risk factors and, thus, the likely effect of optimum acute stroke care and secondary prevention in reducing the burden of dementia. (Pendlebury & Rothwel, 2009)

Pendlebury and Rothwel, stated that stroke characteristics determined patient's predisposition towards dementia rather than the underlying vascular risk factors. Namely, most important risk factors in prestroke dementia were medial temporal lobe atrophy, female sex and family history of dementia; while in poststroke dementia the most important was the presence of multiple cerebral lesions in time and place. (2009) Vascular risk factors for AD include stroke, hypertension, diabetes, homocysteine, smoking, hypercholesterolemia, heart failure and AF; it is possible that these can trigger cerebrovascular dysfunction and AD pathology. Explanations for these associations include the coincidence of common disorders in the elderly where vascular and cerebrovascular disease can precipitate AD, implying that the onset of dementia disease is determined by a synergistic combination of risk factors. (de Toledo Ferraz Alves et al., 2010) Additionally, many vascular risk factors for AD, such as atherosclerosis, stroke and cardiac disease in the aging individual, could result in cerebrovascular dysfunction and trigger AD pathology. A major vascular susceptibility factor gene is the apolipoprotein E gene, found to be associated with sporadic late-onset AD cases. Another interesting vascular susceptibility gene is angiotensin converting enzyme (ACE). Other possible genes include VLDL-R, LRP, NOS3, CST3, OLR1, MTHFR, PON1 and VEGF, but many of the related studies have shown conflicting results. (Rocchi et al., 2009)

Some strokes are clinically detected, while others go undetected. Silent strokes are, also, associated with higher age, elevated blood pressure and AF. (Vermeer et al., 2003a) It is important to stress that apart from silent strokes, AF itself can, also, occur silently thus posing great threat to our aging society. (Aliot, 2009) The presence of AF increases the risk for stroke, about 20% of all embolic strokes are associated with it. (Ratcliffe & Wilcock, 1985) There is increasing evidence that AF is associated with an increased risk of asymptomatic or silent cerebral infarction and as a result may confer an increased risk of progressive cognitive impairment. Most cases of AF are now of non-rheumatic or non-valvular (NVAF) aetiology. NVAF confers a fivefold increased risk of clinically apparent stroke compared to those patients, still in sinus rhythm. Silent cerebral infarctions are not associated with the nature (chronic/paroxysmal) or duration of atrial fibrillation. This may be so due to the fact that the risk of stroke for people with silent brain infarcts is comparable with the risk of TIA patients, of whom approximately 20% develop stroke within 4 years. (Vemeer et al., 2003)

Recently, AF was associated with the hazard ratio of 1.8 (95%CI, 1,0-3,4) for first-ever stroke, but not significantly associated with dementia or AD. (Marengoni et al., 2009) However, brain reserve appears to be protective in case of stroke with favourable outcome measures such as younger age, higher premorbid IQ, no AF, no dementia, less apathy and fewer intercurrent cerebrovascular events. (Withall et al., 2009)

5.4 Dementia treatment

Treatment of dementia rests on a two-pronged approach: modification of the underlying disease (risk factors) and prevention and treatment of dementia symptoms. Goals of pharmacotherapy should be: primary and secondary prevention of cognitive changes in AF patients, reduction of present cognitive changes with acceptable side effects of pharmacotherapy, and restoration/improvement in functional measures and quality of life.

Various potential risk or preventive factors for vascular dementia have been suggested by epidemiologic research: lifestyle changes, including diet, physical activity and stress reduction as well as pharmacological strategies such as antihypertensive drugs, statins, antiplatelet, anticoagulant therapy, antidiabetic drugs, insulin, hormone replacement therapy, NSAID (nonsteroidal drugs), Ginko biloba, ENADPH, donepezil, galantamine, memantine, rivastigmine, cyclandelate, hyderginepentoxifylline, CDP choline. Meta analyses have shown that long-term use of NSAID reduces risk of dementia, and the type of NSAID is important - the best drugs contain acetylsalicylic acid in low concentrations (75-100 mg). Ginko Biloba was proven to be useful in secondary prevention of cognitive decline. Anticoagulant therapy is recommended in patients with atrial fibrillation.

WARIS II (Warfarin-aspirin reinfarction study) has shown that aspirin is better than warfarin in stroke risk reduction in diabetic patients with recurrent strokes. WASPO (Warfarin versus aspirin for stroke prevention in octogenarians with atrial fibrillation), BAFTA (Birmingham Atrial Fibrillation Treatment of the Aged Study), ACTIVE W (Atrial fibrillation Clopidogrel Trial with Irbesartan for prevention of Vascular events-W) have shown that warfarin is still the best in prevention of vascular events in patients with atrial fibrillation (even in age more 75). RE-LY (Randomized Evaluation of Long Term Anticoagulant Therapy) study has shown that new drug Dabigatran (DTIs) is superior to warfarin with lower number of complication in prevention of CVD. ROCKET AF (Rivaroxaban Once daily oral direct Factor Xa inhibition Compared with vitamin K antagonism for prevention of stroke and Embolism Trial in Atrial Fibrillation) study has shown similar results. (Bowler JB, 2007; Rockwood et al., 2009) Nonaticoagulant strategies to prevent CVD in AF patients should include: left atrial appendage surgical excision, left atrial appendage percutaneous occlusion, catheter ablation or treatment with dronedarone (amiodarone). (Patel D et al., 2010)

5.5 Use of anticoagulants among the demented

Anticoagulation for stroke prevention seems to be underused in elderly patients with nonvalvular AF and those with falls and/or early dementia are thought to be at a particular risk for stroke and hemorrhage. Jacobs et al. have performed a retrospective observational study using $CHADS_2$ score and outcome events at 12 months concluding that geriatric population with chronic AF, including patients with falls and/or dementia, who were prescribed warfarin (85%) and consequently had low rates of stroke, hemorrhage, and death at 12 months despite a low time-in-therapeutic range. However, patients with falls and/or dementia had had a high mortality rate (~45%). (2009)

Additionally, it needs to be said that despite growing evidence linking cognitive impairment to vascular risk factors, only a minority of clinical practice therapeutic guidelines consider cognition as either an adverse outcome or a factor to be considered in their treatment. (Rockwood et al., 2009) Regarding AF treatment, Flaker et al. have recently shown that less effective anticoagulation indicates more vascular events and greater cognitive dysfunction, and that low MMSE scores select those patients that have to apply strict therapeutic regime to improve their outcome. (2010) A study by Ali et al. proved that less than 50% of AD patients taking oral anticoagulation were within therapeutic targets. Furthermore, the presence of AF is associated with poor performance on neuropsychological testing, regardless of the actual duration of AF in a particular patient. Subcutaneus heparin in patients with AF is superior because of its bioavailability, but its mode of administration and long-term risks makes its use non-feasible. Antithrombotic agents such as aspirin or clopidogrel are not widely used, despite proven clopidogrel's greater efficacy, while the two combined in the ACTIVE study caused its premature cessation due to increased number of vascular events incidence.(Ali et al., 2006) Most promising therapeutic agents today seem to be direct thrombin inhibitors (ximelagatran, argatroban and dabigatran) that appear to be at least as effective as warfarine, but require no monitoring while having great bioavailability. (Spinler, 2010)

6. AF and arterial stiffness

Stiffening in the large central arterial system, such as the aortic tree, significantly contributes to cardiovascular diseases in elderly and is positively associated with systolic hypertension, coronary artery disease, stroke, heart failure and AF. (Shirwany & Zou, 2010) Namely, Mitchell et al. have published that increased pulse pressure (reflection of aortic stiffness) increases cardiac pressure load and thus may lead to an increase new-onset AF risk. (2007) It is becoming clear that we need to address the problem of AF detection among patients with transient ischemic attack (TIA) or stroke in order to prevent further clinical events from occurring. The expected size of affected population is about 15% according to Malik et al. (2011) The most important factors that need to be evaluated are: left atrial diameter, age and diagnosis of stroke, while history of smoking seems to be inversely related. Sensitivity of testing was high (85,5%) and specificity rather low (53,1%), but still about 47% of TIA and stroke can be excluded from further AF screening examination using this protocol. (Malik et al., 2011)

Arterial stiffness (AS) as a measurement of altered vascular mechanics is considered to play a key role in the pathophysiology of the cardiovascular system. Clinical conditions mostly predisposing to AS increase are hypertension, dyslipidemia and diabetes with metabolic syndrome that engulfs all of the three mentioned conditions. (Lakatta & Levy, 2003a) There is, also, evidence that elevated homocysteine in hypertensive individuals or those with isolated office hypertension plays an important role; and that aortic stiffness is associated with estrogen receptors alpha (ESR1) and beta (ESR 2), and not with estrogen aromatase (CYP19A1). (Vyssoulis et al., 2010; Peter et al., 2009) Finally, a study by Midei and Matthews discovered that adolescents with higher attachment anxiety and total hostility have greater pulse wave velocity, which is even more apparent among black individuals. (2009)

Important information can be gained through brain CT imaging in which the presence of cortical infarction suggests the presence of severe ipsilateral carotid stenosis or atrial fibrillation thereby modifying clinical classification, patient investigation and prognosis. (Mead et al., 1999) It seems that small striatal infarct and the presence of high levels of brain amyloid will point to those most prone for the development of cognitive impairment and AD dementia development compared to individuals with just one or the other. This increased risk is supported clinically by adult onset of diabetes mellitus, hypertension, atherosclerosis and atrial fibrillation. (Cechetto et al., 2008) Still, severe age related changes in white matter independently and strongly predict rapid global functional decline. (Inzitari et al., 2009)

6.1 Arterial stiffness (AS) indexes

Most repeatedly mentioned indexes of arterial stiffness in the literature are: beta stiffness index, pulse wave velocity, augmentation index and analysis of characteristics of central blood pressure waveform. And, it seems that two most important factors affecting arterial stiffness increase, such as increasing age and blood pressure, affect the fibrotic components of the extracellular matrix, such as elastin, collagen and fibronectin. (Lakatta & Levy, 2003a) Lately, even tissue Doppler measuring left ventricular systolic dysfunction is used to indicate increased arterial wave reflection. (Russo et al., 2011)

Carotid artery stiffness was found not to be an independent risk factor or predictor of vascular events in patients with manifest arterial disease, but it may prove useful for selection of those patients with lesser risk when evaluated together with low systolic blood pressure. (Dijk et al., 2005) A recent study indicated that central arterial stiffness, usually represented by descendent thoracic aorta stiffness and atheroma presence as expressed by beta stiffness index, can be correlated to and represented by radial augmentation index. (Sako et al, 2009) Lastly, vascular stiffness was found to be inversely related to cognitive function, and greater in VaD compared with AD. Using pulse wave velocity may be useful in identifying VaD. (Rabkin & Jarvie, 2011)

Mitchell et al. have recently published that increased pulse pressure (reflection of aortic stiffness) increases cardiac pressure load and may increase AF risk. The association between pulse pressure and AF persisted in models that adjusted for baseline left atrial dimension, left ventricular mass, and left ventricular fractional shortening. Interestingly, in models adjusted for age, sex, and clinical risk factors for AF (elevated body mass index, history of smoking, valvular disease, diabetes mellitus, left ventricular hypertrophy, hypertension treatment, and myocardial infarction or heart failure), mean arterial pressure was unrelated to incident AF.

It seems that ultrasonographic measurement of AS can be chosen as sensitive for detection of vascular damage prior to IMT (intima-media thickness) increase at all ages. (Nunez et al., 2010) Additionally, glycemic status appears to be independently associated with impaired endothelial function and increased arterial stiffness using multivariate analysis, among sensitive population leading to abnormal vessel wall characteristics and more small vessel disease-related cerebrovascular events in stroke survivors. (Gunarathne et al., 2009)

AS indexes may be regarded as quick, undemanding, and bed-side premorbid diagnostic tools, used as markers or predictors, for the assessment of life and disability threatening neurological conditions such as stroke or dementia in the setting of altered vascular mechanics and AF. Furthermore, perfusion enhancement, monitored by AS parameters, seems to produce a favourable and consistent response in AD patients, unlike other more often used dementia therapeutic regimes, offering a new and powerful window for AD treatment. (London et al., 2004; Hirata et al., 2005; Williams et al., 2006)

6.2 Is there treatment for altered arterial stiffness?

Recently, in order to influence cerebral perfusion and consequently arterial stiffness, the most favourable treatments were mentioned: calcium channel blockers, diuretics and ACE inhibitors. (London et al., 2004; Hirata et al., 2005; Williams et al., 2006) Additionally, newer beta blockers, with supplementary vasodilating properties, showing favourable effects on carbohydrate and lipid metabolism, endothelial function and on oxidative stress, also, indicated substantial positive therapeutic effect. (Agabiti-Rosei et al., 2009)

It is important to acknowledge that beta-blockers and diuretics act mostly on macro-vasculature, while ACE inhibitors and calcium entry blockers show microvascular favourable actions along with improvement of large artery mechanics and reduction of central wave reflections. (Rizzoni et al., 2009)

Opposed to this, statins were not proven to have any beneficial effects outside the treatment of hyperlipidemia and atherosclerosis. Sex difference of AD incidences between men and women may be attributed to better pharmacological treatment of men versus women. (Beri et al., 2009)

7. Conclusion

Since vascular disorders are regarded as being preventable, early detection and accurate diagnosis of such conditions are very important clinical issues. AF plays in important role in future stroke risk and dementia risk. Namely, consistent evidence supports an association between AF and increased incidence of dementia in patients with stroke. Still, potential association between AF and incident dementia in mild cognitive impairment requires further investigation. AS provides a tool for vascular mechanics assessment and thus offers a window of opportunity for early treatment and diversion of overt clinical vascular events.

8. References

Agabiti-Rosei, E.; Porteri, E. & Rizzoni, D. (2009) Arterial stiffness, hypertension, and rational use of nebivolol. *Vasc Health Risk Manag*. Vol. 5, No. 1, pp. 353-360, ISSN 1178-2048

Ali, S.; Hong, M.; Antezano, E.S. & Mangat, I. (2006)Evaluation and management of atrial fibrillation. *Cardiovasc Hematol Disord Drug Targets*. Vol. 6, No.4, pp.233-244, ISSN 1871-529X

Aliot, E. (2009) Silent atrial fibrillation. Ann Cardiol Angeiol (Paris). Vol. 58, Suppl 1, pp.S22-24, ISSN 0003-3928

Allessie, M.A; Boyden, P.A.; Camm, A.J. & al. (2001) Pathophysiology and prevention of atrial fibrillation. *Circulation*. Vol. 103, No. 5, pp. 769–777, ISSN 0009-7322

Atrial Fibrillation Investigators. (1994) Risk factors for stroke and efficacy of antithrombotic therapy in atrial fibrillation: analysis of pooled data from five randomized controlled trials. *Arch Intern Med*. Vol. 154, No. 13, pp.1449–1457, ISSN 0003-9926

Battistin, L. & Cagnin, A. (2010)Vascular cognitive disorder. A biological and clinical overview. Neurochem Res. Vol. 35, No. 12, pp.1933-1938, ISSN 0364-3190

Benjamin, E.J.; Wolf, P.A.; D'Agostino, R.B. & al. (1998) Impact of atrial fibrillation on the risk of death: the Framingham Heart Study. Circulation. Vol. 98, No. 10, pp.946-952, ISSN 0009-7322

Beri, A.; Sural, N. & Mahajan, S.B. (2009) Non-atheroprotective effects of statins: a systematic review. *Am J Cardiovasc Drugs*. Vol. 9, No. 6, pp. 361-370, ISSN 1175-3277

Bowler, J.B. & Gorelic, P.B. (2007) Advances in vascular impairement 2006. *Stroke*. Vol. 38, No. 4, pp.241-244, ISSN 0039-2499

Cechetto, D.F.; Hachinski, V. & Whitehead, S.N. (2008) Vascular risk factors and Alzheimer's disease. *Expert Rev Neurother*. Vol. 8, No.5, pp. 743-750, ISSN 1473-7175

Chen, X.; Van Nguyen, H.; Shen, Q. & Chan, D.K. (2010) Characteristics associated with recurrent falls among the elderly within aged-care wards in a tertiary hospital: The effect of cognitive impairment. *Arch Gerontol Geriatr*. September 26. [Epub ahead of print], ISSN 1872-6976

Collerton, J.; Davies, K.; Jagger, C. & al. (2009) Health and disease in 85 year olds: baseline findings from the Newcastle 85+ cohort study. *BMJ*. Vol. 339, pp. b4904, ISSN 0007-1447

Das, R.R.; Seshadri, S.; Beiser, A.S. & al. (2008) Prevalence and Correlates of Silent Cerebral Infarcts in the Framingham Offspring Study. Stroke. Vol. 39, No. 11,pp. 2929-2935, ISSN 0039-2499

de Toledo Ferraz Alves, T.C.; Ferreira, L.K.; Wajngarten, M. & Busatto, G.F. (2010) Cardiac disorders as risk factors for Alzheimer's disease. *J Alzheimers Dis*. Vol. 20, No. 3, pp.749-763, ISSN 1387-2877

Dijk, J.M.; Algra, A.; van der Graaf, Y. & al.; SMART study group. (2005) Carotid stiffness and the risk of new vascular events in patients with manifest cardiovascular disease. The SMART study. *Eur Heart J*. Vol. 26, No.12, pp. 1213-1220, ISSN 0195-668X

Dong, Y.; Sharma, V.K.; Chan, B.P. & al. (2010) The Montreal Cognitive Assessment (MoCA) is superior to the Mini-Mental State Examination (MMSE) for the detection of vascular cognitive impairment after acute stroke. *J Neurol Sci*. Vol. 299, No. 1-2, pp. 15–18, ISSN 0022-510X

Dudley, S.C. Jr.; Hoch, N.E.; McCann, L.A. & al. (2005) Atrial fibrillation increases production of superoxide by the left atrium and left atrial appendage. Role of NADPH and xanthine oxidases. *Circulation*. Vol. 11, No. 9, pp. 1266-1273, ISSN 0009-7322

Dulli, D.A.; Stanko, H. & Levine, R.L. (2003) Atrial Fibrillation Is Associated with Severe Acute Ischemic Stroke. *Neuroepidemiology*. Vol. 22, No. 2, pp. 118-123, ISSN 0251-5350

Enta, K.; Iwade, K.; Aosaki, M. & al. (2004) Predictive value of coagulative molecular markers for thromboembolism in patients with nonvalvular atrila fibrillation: Prospective five year follow-up study. *J Cardiol*. Vol. 44, No. 6, pp. 223-232, ISSN 0914-5087

Ettorre, E.; Cicerchia, M.; De Benedetto, G. & al. (2009) A possible role of atrial fibrillation as a risk factor for dementia. *Arch Gerontol Geriatr*. Vol. 49, Suppl 1, pp. 71-76, ISSN 0167-4943

Ferri, C.P.; Prince, M.; Brayne, C. & al. (2005) Global prevalence of dementia: a Delphi consensus study. *Lancet*. Vol. 366, No. 9503, pp. 2112-2117, ISSN 0099-5355

Flaker, G.C.; Pogue, J.; Yusuf, S. & al.; Atrial Fibrillation Clopidogrel Trial With Irbesartan for Prevention of Vascular Events (ACTIVE) Investigators. (2010) Cognitive function and anticoagulation control in patients with atrial fibrillation. *Circ Cardiovasc Qual Outcomes*. Vol. 3, No. 3, pp. 277-283, ISSN 1941-7713

Friberg, J.; Buch, P.; Scharling, H. & al.(2003) Rising rates of hospital admissions for atrial fibrillation. Epidemiology. Vol. 14, No. 6, pp.666-672, ISSN 1044-3983

Fukuchi, M.; Watanabe, J.; Kumagi, K. & al. (2001) Increased von Willebrand factor in the endocardium as a local predisposing factor for thrombogenesis in overloaded human atrial appendage. *J Am Coll Cardiol*. Vol. 37, No. 5, pp. 1436-1442, ISSN 0735-1097

Fumagalli, S.; Tarantini, F.; Guarducci, L. & al.; GIFA Study Research Group. (2010) Atrial fibrillation is a possible marker of frailty in hospitalized patients: results of the GIFA Study. *Aging Clin Exp Res*. Vol. 22, No. 2, pp. 129-133, ISSN 1594-0667

Fuster, V. & Mearns, B.M. (2010) Global collaboration needed for AF. *Nat Rev Cardiol*. Vol. 7, No. 3, pp. 115-116, ISSN 1759-5002

Fuster, V.; Rydén, L.E.; Cannom, D.S. & al.; Task Force on Practice Guidelines, American College of Cardiology/American Heart Association; Committee for Practice

Guidelines, European Society of Cardiology; European Heart Rhythm Association; Heart Rhythm Society. (2006) ACC/AHA/ESC 2006 guidelines for the management of patients with atrial fibrillation-executive summary: a report of the American College of Cardiology/American Heart Association Task Force on Practice Guidelines and the European Society of Cardiology Committee for Practice Guidelines (Writing Committee to Revise the 2001 Guidelines for the Management of Patients with Atrial Fibrillation). Eur Heart J. Vol. 27, No. 16, pp. 1979-2030, ISSN 0195-668X

Galzerano, D.; Capogrosso, C.; Di Michele, S. & al. (2010) New standards in hypertension and cardiovascular risk management: focus on telmisartan. *Vasc Health Risk Manag*. Vol. 6, pp. 113-133, ISSN 1176-6344

Go, A.S. (2005) The epidemiology of atrial fibrillation in elderly persons: the tip of the iceberg. Am J Geriatr Cardiol. Vol. 14, No. 2, pp. 56-61, ISSN 1076-7460

Go, A.S.; Hylek, E.M.; Phillips, K.A. & al. (2001) Prevalence of diagnosed atrial fibrillation in adults: national implications for rhythm management and stroke prevention: the Anticoagulation and Risk Factors in Atrial Fibrillation (ATRIA) Study. JAMA. Vol. 285, No. 18, pp. 2370-2375, ISSN 0098-7484

Grand, J.H.; Caspar, S. & Macdonald, S.W. (2011) Clinical features and multidisciplinary approaches to dementia care. J Multidiscip Healthc. Vol. 4, pp. 125-1247, ISSN 1178-2390

Gunarathne, A.; Patel, J.V.; Kausar, S. & al. (2009) Glycemic status underlies increased arterial stiffness and impaired endothelial function in migrant South Asian stroke survivors compared to European Caucasians: pathophysiological insights from the West Birmingham Stroke Project. *Stroke*. Vol. 40, No. 7, pp. 2298-2306, ISSN 0039-2499

Hamer, M.E.; Blumenthal, J.A.; McCarthy, E.A. & al. (1994) Quality-of-life assessment in patients with paroxysmal atrial fibrillation or paroxysmal supraventricular tachycardia. Am J Cardiol. Vol. 74, No. 8, pp. 826-829, ISSN 0002-9149

Hart, R.G.; Pearce, L.A. & Aguilar, M.I. (2007) Meta-analysis: antithrombotic therapy to prevent stroke in patients who have nonvalvular atrial fibrillation. *Ann Intern Med*. Vol. 146, No.12, pp. 857– 867, ISSN 0003-4819

Healy, J.S. (2009) Pro:"Anti-platelet therapy is an alternative to oral anticoagulation for atrial fibrillation". *Thromb Haemost* . Vol. 102, No. 5 , pp. 912–913, ISSN 0340-6245

Hirata, K.; Vlachopoulos, C.; Adji, A. & O'Rourke, M.F. (2005) Benefits from angiotensin-converting enzyme inhibitor 'beyond blood pressure lowering': beyond blood pressure or beyond the brachial artery? *J Hypertens*. Vol. 23, No. 3, pp.551–556, ISSN 0263-6352

Inzitari D.; Pracucci, G.; Poggesi, A. & al.; LADIS Study Group. (2009) Changes in white matter as determinant of global functional decline in older independent outpatients: three year follow-up of LADIS (leukoaraiosis and disability) study cohort. *BMJ*. Vol. 339, No. b2477, ISSN 0007-1447

Israel, C.W.; Grönefeld, G.; Ehrlich, J.R. & al. (2004) Long-term risk of recurrent atrial fibrillation as documented by an implantable monitoring device: implications for optimal patient care. J Am Coll Cardiol. Vol. 43, No. 1, pp. 47-52, ISSN 0735-1097

Jacobs, L.G.; Billett, H.H.; Freeman, K.al. (2009) Anticoagulation for stroke prevention in elderly patients with atrial fibrillation, including those with falls and/or early-stage dementia: a single-center, retrospective, observational study. Am J Geriatr Pharmacother. Vol. 7, No. 3, pp. 159-166, ISSN 1543-5946

Kamel, H.; Lees, K.R.; Lyden, P.D. & al.; Virtual International Stroke Trials Archive Investigators. (2009) Delayed detection of atrial fibrillation after ischemic stroke. *J Stroke Cerebrovasc Dis*. Vol. 18, No. 6, pp. 453-457, ISSN 1052-3057

Kannel, W.B. & Benjamin, E.J. (2008) Status of the epidemiology of atrial fibrillation. Med Clin North Am. Vol. 92, No. 1, pp. 17-40, ix, ISSN 0025-7125

Kim, Y.M.; Guzik, T.J.; Zhang, Y.H. & al. (2005) A myocardial Nox2 containing NAD(PH) oxidase contributes to oxidative stress in human atrial fibrillation. *Circ Res*. Vol. 97, No. 7, pp. 629-636, ISSN 0009-7330

Kimura, K.; Iguchi, Y.; Yamashita, S. & al. (2008) Atrial fibrillation as an independent predictor for no early recanalization after IV-t-PA in acute ischemic stroke. J Neurol Sci. Vol. 267, No. 1-2, pp.57-61, ISSN 0022-510X

Kimura, K.; Kazui, S.; Minematsu, K. & Yamaguchi, T. (2004) Analysis of 16,922 patients with acute ischemic stroke and transient ischemic attack in Japan: a hospital-based prospective registration study. *Cerebrovasc Dis*. Vol. 18, No. 1, pp. 47–56, ISSN 1015-9770

Lakatta, E.G. & Levy, D. (2003a) Arterial and cardiac aging: major shareholders in cardiovascular disease enterprises: Part I: aging arteries: a "set up" for vascular disease. *Circulation*. Vol. 107, No. 1, pp. 139-146, ISSN 0009-7322

Lakatta, E.G. & Levy, D. (2003b) Arterial and cardiac aging: major shareholders in cardiovascular disease enterprises: Part II: the aging heart in health: links to heart disease. *Circulation*. Vol. 107, No. 2, pp.346-354, ISSN 0009-7322

Lane, D.A. & Lip, G.Y.H. (2010) Anticoagulation for Atrial Fibrillation Patients with CHADS2 Score of 1. *J Cardiovasc Electrophysiol*. Vol. 21, No. 5 , pp. 508-510, ISSN 1045-3873

Lee, B.H.; Park, J.S.; Park, J.H. & al. (2010) The effect and safety of the antithrombotic therapies in patients with atrial fibrillation and CHADS score 1. J Cardiovasc Electrophysiol. Vol. 21, No. 5, pp. 501-507, ISSN 1045-3873

Leibovitch, E.R. (2008) Hypertension 2008, refining our treatment. *Geriatrics*. Vol. 63, No. 10, pp. 14-15, 17-20, ISSN 0016-867X

Lewis, W.R.; Fonarow, G.C.; LaBresh, K.A. & al. (2009) Differential use of warfarin for secondary stroke prevention in patients with various types of atrial fibrillation. *Am J Cardiol*. Vol. 103, No. 2, pp. 227-231, ISSN 0002-9149

Liao, J.; Zahira, K.; Scallan, C. & al. (2007) Noninvasive cardiac monitoring for detecting paroxysmal atrial fibrillation or flutter after acute ischemic stroke: a systematic review. *Stroke*. Vol. 38, No.11 , pp. 2935–2940, ISSN 0039-2499

Lip, G.Y.H. & Halperin J.L. (2010) Improving stroke risk stratification in atrial fibrillation. *Am J Med*. Vol. 123, No.6 , pp. 483-488, ISSN 0002-9343

Lip, G.Y.H. (2011) Implications of the CHA2DS2-VASc and HAS-BLED scores for thromboprophylaxis in atrial fibrillation. *Am J Med*. Vol. 124, No. 2, pp. 111-114, ISSN 0002-9343

Llewellyn, D.J.; Lang, I.A.; Xie, J. & al. (2008) Framingham Stroke Risk Profile and poor cognitive function: a population-based study. *BMC Neurol*. Vol. 8, p. 12, ISSN 1471-2377

Lloyd-Jones, D.M.; Wang, T.J.; Lelp, E.P. & al. (2004) Lifetime Risk for Development of Atrial Fibrillation-The Framingham Heart Study. *Circulation*. Vol. 110, No. 9, pp. 1042-1046, ISSN 0009-7322

London, G.M., Asmar, R.G., O'Rourke, M.F. & Safar, M.E.; Reason Project Investigators. (2004) Mechanism(s) of selective systolic blood pressure reduction after a low-dose combination of perindopril/indapamide in hypertensive subjects: comparison with atenolol. *J Am Coll Cardiol*. Vol. 43, No.1 , pp. 92–99, ISSN 0735-1097

Luchsinger, J.A. (2010) Diabetes, related conditions, and dementia. *J Neurol Sci*. Vol. 299, No. 1-2, pp. 35–38, ISSN 0022-510X

Maehama, T.; Okura, H.; Imai, K. & al. (2010) Usefulness of CHADS2 score to predict C-reactive protein, left atrial blood stasis, and prognosis in patients with nonrheumatic atrial fibrillation. *Am J Cardiol*. Vol. 106, No. 4, pp. 535-538, ISSN 0002-9149

Marengoni, A.; Qiu, C.; Winblad, B. & Fratiglioni, L. (2011) Atrial fibrillation, stroke and dementia in the very old: A population-based study. *Neurobiol Aging*. Vol. 32, No. 7, pp. 1336-1337, ISSN 0197-4580

Marini, C.; De Santis, F.; Sacco, S. & al. (2005) Contribution of Atrial Fibrillation to Incidence and Outcome of Ischemic Stroke. Results From a Population-Based Study. *Stroke*. Vol. 36, No. , pp. 1115-1119, ISSN 0039-2499

Mattace-Raso, F.U.; van der Cammen, T.J.; Hofman, A. & al. (2006) Arterial stiffness and risk of coronary heart disease and stroke: the Rotterdam Study. *Circulation*. Vol. 113, No. 5, pp. 657-663, ISSN 0009-7322

Mead, G.E.; Lewis, S.C.; Wardlaw, J.M. & al. (1999) Should computed tomography appearance of lacunar stroke influence patient management? *J Neurol Neurosurg Psychiatry*. Vol. 67, No. 5, pp. 682-684, ISSN 0022-3050

Midei, A.J. & Matthews, K.A. (2009) Social relationships and negative emotional traits are associated with central adiposity and arterial stiffness in healthy adolescents. *Health Psychol*. Vol. 28, No. 3, pp. 347-353, ISSN 0278-6133

Mitchell, G.F.; Vasan, R.S.; Keyes, M.J. & al. (2007) Pulse pressure and risk of new-onset atrial fibrillation. *JAMA*. Vol. 297, No. 7, pp. 709-715, ISSN 0098-7484

Mitsias, P. & Silver, B. (2011) Development of a scoring system for atrial fibrillation in acute stroke and transient ischemic attack patients: the LADS scoring system. *J Neurol Sci*. Vol. 301, No. 1-2, pp. 27-30, ISSN 0022-510X

Miyasaka, Y.; Barnes, M.E.; Gersh, B.J. & al. (2006) Secular Trends in Incidence of Atrial Fibrillation in Olmsted County, Minnesota, 1980 to 2000, and Implications on the Projections for Future Prevalence. *Circulation*. Vol. 114, No. 2, pp. 119-125, ISSN 0009-7322

Motoki, H.; Tomita, T.; Aizawa, K. & al. (2009) Coagulation activity is increased in the left atria of patients with paroxysmal atrial fibrillation during the non-paroxysmal period. Comparison with chronic atrial fibrillation. *Circ J*. Vol. 73, No. 8, pp. 1403-1407, ISSN 1346-9843

Nasreddine, Z.S. (2005) The Montreal Cognitive Assessment, MoCA: a brief screening tool for mild cognitive impairment. J Am Geriatr Soc. Vol. 53, No. 4, pp. 695-699, ISSN 0002-8614

Nieuwlaat, R.; Olsson, S.B.; Lip, G.Y., & al; Euro Heart Survey Investigators; The Euro Heart Survey on Atrial Fibrillation. (2007) Guideline-adherent antithrombotic treatment is associated with improved outcomes compared with undertreatment in high-risk patients with atrial fibrillation. *Am Heart J*. Vol. 153, No. 6, pp. 1006–1012, ISSN 0002-8703

Nozawa, T.; Inoue, H.; Hirai, T. & al. (2006) D-dimer level influences thromboembolic events in patients with atrial fibrillation. *Int J Cardiol*. Vol. 109, No. 1, pp. 59-65, ISSN 0167-5273

Núñez, F.; Martínez-Costa, C.; Sánchez-Zahonero, J. & al. (2010) Carotid artery stiffness as an early marker of vascular lesions in children and adolescents with cardiovascular risk factors. *Rev Esp Cardiol*. Vol. 63, No. 11, pp. 1253-1260, ISSN 0300-8932

O'Connell, J.E.; Gray, C.S.; French, J.M. & Robertson, I.H. (1998) Atrial fibrillation and cognitive function: case-control study. *Neurosurg Psychiatry*. Vol. 65, No. 3, pp. 386–389, ISSN 0022-3050

Ohara, K.; Hirai, T.; Fukuda, N. & al. (2009) Relation of left atrial blood statis to clinical risk factors in atrial fibrillation. *Int J Cardiol*. Vol. 132, No. 2, pp. 210-215, ISSN 0167-5273

Page, R.L.; Tilsch, T.W.; Connolly, S.J. & al; Azimilide Supraventricular Arrhythmia Program (ASAP) Investigators. (2003) Asymptomatic or "silent" atrial fibrillation: frequency in untreated patients and patients receiving azimilide. *Circulation*. Vol. 107, No. 8, pp. 1141-1145, ISSN 0009-7322

Patel, D.; Bailey, S.M.; Furlan, A.J. & al. (2010) Long-term functional and neurocognitive recovery in patients who had an acute cerebrovascular event secondary to catheter ablation for atrial fibrillation. *J Cardiovasc Electrophysiol*. Vol. 21, No. 4, pp. 412-417, ISSN 1045-3873

Penado, S.; Cano, M.; Acha, O. & al. (2003) Atrial fibrillation as a risk factor for stroke recurrence. Am J Med. *Vol.* 114, No. 3, pp. 206-210, ISSN 0002-9343

Pendlebury, S.T. & Rothwell, P.M. (2009) Prevalence, incidence, and factors associated with pre-stroke and post-stroke dementia: a systematic review and meta-analysis. *Lancet Neurol*. Vol. 8, No. 11, pp. 1006-1018, ISSN 1474-4422

Pengo, V.; Cucchini, U.; Denas, G. & al. (2010) Lower versus standard intensity oral anticoagulant therapy (OAT) in elderly warfarin-experienced patients with non-valvular atrial fibrillation. *Thromb Haemost*. Vol. 103, No. 2, pp. 442-449, ISSN 1474-4422

Peter, I. Kelley-Hedgepeth, A.; Huggins, G.S. & al. (2009) Association between arterial stiffness and variations in oestrogen-related genes. *J Hum Hypertens*. Vol. 23, No. 10, pp. 636-644, ISSN 0950-9240

Petty, G.W.; Brown, R.D.; Whisnantet, J.P., & al. (1999) Ischemic Stroke Subtypes. A Population-Based Study of Incidence and Risk Factors. *Stroke*. Vol. 30, No. 12, pp. 2513-2516, ISSN 0039-2499

Phillips, S.J.; Whisnant, J.P.; O'Fallon, W.M. & Frye, R.L. (1990) Prevalence of cardiovascular disease and diabetes mellitus in residents of Rochester, Minnesota. Mayo Clin Proc. Vol. 65, No. 3, pp. 344-359, ISSN 0025-6196

Pizzetti, F.; Turazza, F.M.; Franzosi, M.G. & al; GISSI-3 Investigators. (2001) Incidence and prognostic significance of atrial fibrillation in acute myocardial infarction: the GISSI-3 data. *Heart*. Vol. 86, No. 5, pp. 527-532, ISSN 1355-6037

Potpara, T.S.; Stankovic, G.R.; Beleslin, B.D. & al. (2011) A 12-year follow-up study of patients with newly-diagnosed lone atrial fibrillation: Implications of arrhythmia progression on prognosis: The Belgrade Atrial Fibrillation Study. Chest. May 26. [Epub ahead of print], ISSN 0012-3692

Rabkin, S.W. & Jarvie, G. (2011) Comparison of vascular stiffness in vascular dementia, Alzheimer dementia and cognitive impairment. Blood Press. May 31. [Epub ahead of print], ISSN 0803-7051

Ratcliffe, P.J. & Wilcock, G.K. (1985) Cerebrovascular disease in dementia: the importance of atrial fibrillation. *Postgrad Med J*. Vol. 61, No. 713, pp. 201-204, ISSN 0032-5473

Rienstra, M. & Van Gelder, I.C. (2010) Are glucocorticoids a treatment or a risk factor? *Nat Rev Cardiol*. Vol. 7, No. 3, pp. 122-123, ISSN 1759-5002

Rietbrock, S.; Plumb, J. & van Staa, T-P. (2009) How effective are dose-adjusted warfarin and aspirin for the prevention of stroke in patients with chronic atrial? An analysis of the UK General Practice Research Database. *Thromb Haemost*. Vol. 101, No. 3, pp. 527-534, ISSN 0340-6245

Rivero-Ayerza, M.; Scholte Op Reimer, W.; Lenzen, M. & al. (2008) New-onset atrial fibrillation is an independent predictor of in-hospital mortality in hospitalized heart failure patients: results of the EuroHeart Failure Survey. *Eur Heart J*. Vol. 29, No. 13, pp. 1618-1624, ISSN 0195-668X

Rizzoni, D.; Muiesan, M.L.; Porteri, E. & al. (2009) Vascular remodeling, macro- and microvessels: therapeutic implications. *Blood Press*. Vol. 18, No. 5, pp. 242-246, ISSN 0803-7051

Rocchi, A.; Orsucci, D.; Tognoni, G. & al. (2009) The role of vascular factors in late-onset sporadic Alzheimer's disease. Genetic and molecular aspects. *Curr Alzheimer Res*. Vol. 6, No. 3, pp. 224-237, ISSN 1567-2050

Rockwood, K.; Middleton, L.E.; Moorhouse, P.K. & al. (2009) The inclusion of cognition in vascular risk factor clinical practice guidelines. Clin Interv Aging.Vol. 4, pp. 425–433, ISSN 1176-9092

Russo, C.; Jin, Z.; Takei, Y. & al. (2011) Arterial wave reflection and subclinical left ventricular systolic dysfunction. *J Hypertens*. Vol. 29, No. 3, pp. 574-582, ISSN 0895-7061

Sadanaga, T.; Sadanaga, M. & Ogawa, S. (2010) Evidence that D-dimer levels predict subsequent thromboembolic and cardiovascular events in patients with atrial fibrillation during oral anticoagulant therapy. J Am Coll Cardiol. Vol. 55, No. 20, pp. 2225-2231, ISSN 0735-1097

Sako, H.; Miura, S.I.; Kumagai, K. & Saku K. (2009) Associations between augmentation index and severity of atheroma or aortic stiffness of the descending thoracic aorta by transesophageal echocardiography. *Circ J*. Vol. 73, No. 6, pp. 1151 - 1156, ISSN 1346-9843

Sanák, D.; Herzig, R.; Král, M. & al. (2010) Is atrial fibrillation associated with poor outcome after thrombolysis? *J Neurol*. Vol. 257, No. 6, pp.999-1003, ISSN 0340-5354

Sanák, D.; Herzig, R.; Zapletalová, J. & al. (2011) Predictors of good clinical outcome in acute stroke patients treated with intravenous thrombolysis. Acta Neurol Scand. Vol. 123, No. 5, pp. 339-344, ISSN 0001-6314

Sato, H.; Ishikawa, K.; Kitabatake, A. & al; Japan Atrial Fibrillation Stroke Trial Group. (2006) Low-dose aspirin for prevention of stroke in low-risk patients with atrial fibrillation: Japan Atrial Fibrillation Stroke Trial. *Stroke*. Vol. 37, No. 2, pp. 447-451, ISSN 0039-2499

Savelieva, I. & Camm, J. (2008) Update on atrial fibrillation: part I. *Clin Cardiol*. Vol. 31, No. 2, pp. 55-62, ISSN 0160-9289

Savelieva, I. & Camm, J. (2008) Update on atrial fibrillation: part II. *Clin Cardiol*. Vol. 31, No. 2, pp. 102-108, ISSN 0160-9289

Schnabel, R.B.; Sullivan, L.M.; Levy, D. & al. (2009) Development of a risk score for atrial fibrillation (Framingham Heart Study): a community-based cohort. *Lancet*. Vol. 373, No. 9665, pp. 739-745, ISSN 0099-5355

Schwammenthal, Y.; Bornstein, N.; Schwammenthal, E. & al. (2010) Relation of effective anticoagulation in patients with atrial fibrillation to stroke severity and survival (from the National Acute Stroke Israeli Survey [NASIS]). *Am J Cardiol*. Vol. 105, No. 3, pp. 411-416, ISSN 0002-9149

Shirwany, N.A. & Zou, M.H. (2010) Arterial stiffness: a brief review. *Acta Pharmacol Sin*. Vol. 30, No. 10, pp. 1267-1276, ISSN 1671-4083

Simpson, J.R.; Zahuranec, D.B.; Lisabeth, L.D. & al. (2010) Mexican Americans with atrial fibrillation have more recurrent strokes than do non-Hispanic whites. Stroke. Vol. 41, No. 10, pp. 2132-2136, ISSN 0039-2499

Spinler, S.A. (2010) A promising new anticogulant for stroke prevention. *Nat Rev Cardiol*. Vol. 7, No. 1, pp. 10–11, ISSN 1759-5002

Srikanth, V.K.; Quinn, S.J.; Donnan, G.A. & al. (2006) Long-Term Cognitive Transitions, Rates of Cognitive Change, and Predictors of Incident Dementia in a Population-Based First-Ever Stroke Cohort. *Stroke*. Vol. 37, No. 10, pp. 2479-2483, ISSN 0039-2499

Stewart, S.; Hart, C.L.; Hole, D.J. & McMurray, J.J. (2002) A population-based study of the long-term risks associated with atrial fibrillation: 20-year follow-up of the Renfrew/Paisley study. *Am J Med*. Vol. 113, No. 5; pp. 359–364, ISSN 0002-9343

Stewart, S.; Murphy, N.F.; Walker, A. & al. (2004) Cost of an emerging epidemic: an economic analysis of atrial fibrillation in the UK. Heart. Vol. 90, No. 3, pp. 286-292, ISSN 1355-6037

Stroke Prevention in Atrial Fibrillation Investigators.(1992) Predictors of thromboembolism in atrial fibrillation II: Echocrdiographic features of patients at risk. Am Intern Med. Vol. 116, No. 1, pp. 6-12, ISSN 0003-4819

Tanaka, H.; Sonoda, M.; Kashima, K. & al. (2009) Impact of decreased renal function on coagulation and fibrinolysis in patients with non-valvular atrial fibrillation. *Circ J*. Vol. 73, No. 5, pp. 846-850, ISSN 1346-9843

Tanaka, H.; Sonoda, M;, Kashima, K. & al. (2009) Impact of Decreased Renal Function on Coagulation and Fibrinolysis in Patients With Non-Valvular Atrial Fibrillation. *Circ J*. Vol. 73, No. 5 pp. 846-850, ISSN 1346-9843

Tay, K.H.; Lip, G.Y.H. & Lane, D.A. (2009) Atrial fibrillation and stroke risk prevention in real-life clinical practice. *Thromb Haemost*. Vol. 101, No. 3, pp. 415-416, ISSN 0340-6245

Tayal, A.H.; Tian, M.; Kelly, T.M. & al. (2008) Atrial fibrillation detected by mobile cardiac outpatient telemetry in cryptogenic TIA or stroke. *Neurology*. Vol. 71, No. , pp. 1696-1701, ISSN 1080-2371

Thrall, G.; Lip, G.Y.; Carroll, D. & Lane, D. (2007) Depression, anxiety, and quality of life in patients with atrial fibrillation. Chest. Vol. 132, No. 4, pp. 1259-1264, ISSN 0012-3692

Tschanz, J.T.; Corcoran, C.D.; Schwartz, S. & al. (2011) Progression of Cognitive, Functional, and Neuropsychiatric Symptom Domains in a Population Cohort With Alzheimer

Dementia: The Cache County Dementia Progression Study. Am J Geriatr Psychiatry. Vol. 19, No. 6, pp. 532-542, ISSN 1064-7481

van den Berg, M.P.; Ranchor, A.V.; van Sonderen, F.L. & al. (2005) Paroxysmal atrial fibrillation, quality of life and neuroticism. Neth J Med. Vol. 63, No. 5, pp. 170-174, ISSN 0300-2977

van Walraven, C.; Hart, R.G.; Wells, G.A. & al. (2003) A clinical prediction rule to identify patients with atrial fibrillation and a low risk for stroke while taking aspirin. *Arch Intern Med.* Vol. 163, No. 8, pp. 936-943, ISSN 0003-9926

Vassallo, M.; Sharma, J.C. & allen, S.C. (2002) Characteristics of single fallers and recurrent fallers among hospital in-patients. *Gerontology.* Vol. 48, No. 3, pp. 147-150, ISSN ISSN 0304-324X

Vermeer, S.E.; Hollander, M.; van Dijk, E.J. & al. (2003a) Silent Brain Infarcts and White Matter Lesions Increase Stroke Risk in the General Population. The Rotterdam Scan Study. *Stroke.* 34:1126-1129., ISSN 0039-2499

Vermeer, S.E.; Prins, N.D.; den Heijer, T. & al. (2003b) Silent Brain Infarcts and the Risk of Dementia and Cognitive Decline. *N Engl J Med.* Vol. 348, No.13, pp. 1215-1222, ISSN 0028-4793

Vyssoulis, G.; Karpanou, E.; Kyvelou, S.M. & al. (2010) Associations between plasma homocysteine levels, aortic stiffness and wave reflection in patients with arterial hypertension, isolated office hypertension and normotensive controls. *J Hum Hypertens.* Vol. 24, No. 3, pp. 183-139, ISSN 0950-9240

Wachtell, K.; Lehto, M.; Gerdts, E. & al. (2005) New-Onset Atrial Fibrillation and Subsequent Stroke Compared to Atenolol. The Losartan Intervention for End Point Reduction in Hypertension (LIFE) Study. *J Am Coll Cardiol.* Vol. 45, No.5 , pp. 712-719, ISSN 0735-1097

Wang, T.J.; Larson, M.G.; Levy, D. & al. (2003) Temporal Relations of Atrial Fibrillation and Congestive Heart Failure and Their Joint Influence on Mortality. The Framingham Heart Study. *Circulation.* Vol. 107, No. 23, pp. 2920-2925, ISSN 0009-7322

Williams, B.; Lacy, P.S.; Thom, S.M. & al.; CAFE Investigators; Anglo-Scandinavian Cardiac Outcomes Trial Investigators; CAFE Steering Committee and Writing Committee. (2006) Differential impact of blood pressure-lowering drugs on central aortic pressure and clinical outcomes: principal results of the Conduit Artery Function Evaluation (CAFÉ) study. Circulation. Vol. 113, No. 9 pp. 1213–1225, ISSN 0009-7322

Withall, A.; Brodaty, H.; Altendorf, A. & Sachdev, P.S. (2009) Who does well after a stroke? The Sydney stroke study. *Aging Ment Health.* Vol. 13, No. 5, pp. 693-698, ISSN 1360-7863

Wolf, P.A.; Abbott, R.D. & Kannel, W.B. (1991) Atrial fibrillation as an independent risk factor for stroke: the Framingham Study. *Stroke.* Vol. 22, No.8 , pp. 983–988, ISSN 0039-2499

Wrigley, B.J. & Lip, G.Y. (2009) Can the WATCHMAN device truly PROTECT from stroke in atrial fibrillation? *Lancet Neurol.* Vol. 8, No. 10, pp. 877-878, ISSN 1474-4422

Permissions

The contributors of this book come from diverse backgrounds, making this book a truly international effort. This book will bring forth new frontiers with its revolutionizing research information and detailed analysis of the nascent developments around the world.

We would like to thank Jong-Il Choi, MD, PhD, for lending his expertise to make the book truly unique. He has played a crucial role in the development of this book. Without his invaluable contribution this book wouldn't have been possible. He has made vital efforts to compile up to date information on the varied aspects of this subject to make this book a valuable addition to the collection of many professionals and students.

This book was conceptualized with the vision of imparting up-to-date information and advanced data in this field. To ensure the same, a matchless editorial board was set up. Every individual on the board went through rigorous rounds of assessment to prove their worth. After which they invested a large part of their time researching and compiling the most relevant data for our readers. Conferences and sessions were held from time to time between the editorial board and the contributing authors to present the data in the most comprehensible form. The editorial team has worked tirelessly to provide valuable and valid information to help people across the globe.

Every chapter published in this book has been scrutinized by our experts. Their significance has been extensively debated. The topics covered herein carry significant findings which will fuel the growth of the discipline. They may even be implemented as practical applications or may be referred to as a beginning point for another development.

The editorial board has been involved in producing this book since its inception. They have spent rigorous hours researching and exploring the diverse topics which have resulted in the successful publishing of this book. They have passed on their knowledge of decades through this book. To expedite this challenging task, the publisher supported the team at every step. A small team of assistant editors was also appointed to further simplify the editing procedure and attain best results for the readers.

Our editorial team has been hand-picked from every corner of the world. Their multi-ethnicity adds dynamic inputs to the discussions which result in innovative outcomes. These outcomes are then further discussed with the researchers and contributors who give their valuable feedback and opinion regarding the same. The feedback is then collaborated with the researches and they are edited in a comprehensive manner to aid the understanding of the subject.

Apart from the editorial board, the designing team has also invested a significant amount of their time in understanding the subject and creating the most relevant covers. They scrutinized every image to scout for the most suitable representation of the subject and create an appropriate cover for the book.

The publishing team has been involved in this book since its early stages. They were actively engaged in every process, be it collecting the data, connecting with the contributors or procuring relevant information. The team has been an ardent support to the editorial, designing and production team. Their endless efforts to recruit the best for this project, has resulted in the accomplishment of this book. They are a veteran in the field of academics and their pool of knowledge is as vast as their experience in printing. Their expertise and guidance has proved useful at every step. Their uncompromising quality standards have made this book an exceptional effort. Their encouragement from time to time has been an inspiration for everyone.

The publisher and the editorial board hope that this book will prove to be a valuable piece of knowledge for researchers, students, practitioners and scholars across the globe.

List of Contributors

Attila Roka
Hospital of St. Raphael, USA

Thomas H. Everett
Division of Cardiology, Department of Medicine, University of California San Francisco, San Francisco, California, USA

Gerald Fischer and Leonhard Wieser
Institute of Electrical, Electronic and Bioengineering, University for Health Sciences, Medical Informatics and Technology (UMIT), Hall i.T., Austria

Florian Hintringer
Department for Cardiology, Medical University Innsbruck, Austria

Hanan Ahmed Galal Azzam
Mansoura University, Faculty of Medicine, Egypt

Svetlana Nicoulina, Anna Chernova, Vladimir Shulman and Pavel Shesternya
Krasnoyarsk State Medical University, Russia

Doosang Kim
Seoul Veterans Hospital, Korea

Hyuk Ahn
Seoul National University, Korea

Vaclav Kremen and Lenka Lhotska
Department of Cybernetics, Faculty of Electrical Engineering, Czech Technical University in Prague, Czech Republic

Redmond B. Shouldice, Conor Heneghan and Philip de Chazal
BiancaMed, NovaUCD, Belfield Innovation Park, Ireland

Toshiya Kurotobi
Division of Cardiac Rhythm Management, Shiroyama Hospital, Department of Advanced Cardiovascular Therapeutics, Osaka University Graduate School of Medicine, Japan

Keizo Tsuchida
Tsuchida Clinic of Internal Medicine and Cardiology, Japan

Kazuhiko Tanabe
Tanabe Clinic, Japan

Hideki Hayashi and Minoru Horie
Department of Cardiovascular and Respiratory Medicine, Shiga University of Medical Science, Otsu, Shiga, Japan

Michala Pedersen, Daniel Scherr and Mélèze Hocini
Hôpital Cardiologique du Haut-Lévêque & University Bordeaux 2 Victor Segalen, France

Bobby Yanagawa, Khaled D. Algarni and Gideon Cohen
Division of Cardiac and Vascular Surgery, Schulich Heart Centre, Sunnybrook Health Sciences Centre, University of Toronto, Toronto, Ontario, Canada

Yong Zhang, Mei Gao, Jiangrong Wang and Yinglong Hou
Department of Cardiology, Qianfoshan Hospital of Shandong University, Jinan City, China

Hong-Tao Wang, Qiang-Sun Zheng, Xiong-Tao Liu, Jun Li, Fu-Jun Shang, Fei-Fei Su, Bo-yuan Fan and Dong-Bo Ou
Tangdu Hospital, Fourth Military Medical University, Xi' an, China

Hiroshi Kubota, Kenichi Sudo, Hidehito Endo, Hiroshi Tsuchiya and Yusuke Inaba
Dpt of Cardiovascular Surgery, Kyorin University, Tokyo, Japan

Shinichi Takamoto
Mitsui Memorial Hospital, Tokyo, Japan

Akira Furuse
JR Tokyo General Hospital, Tokyo, Japan

Akihiro Yoshimoto and Yu Takahashi

Carlo Rostagno and Maria Brigitte Berioli
Dipartimento Area Critica Università Firenze, Italia

Pier Luigi Stefàno
Cardiochirurgia AOU Careggi Firenze, Italia

Norio Hashimoto
Nissan Chemical America Corporation, USA

Thomas C. Martin and Sean C. Hagenbuch
University of Vermont College of Medicine, Burlington, Vermont, Division of Pediatric Cardiology, Department of Pediatrics, Eastern Maine Medical Center, Bangor, Maine USA

Burak Pamukcu
Bayrampasa Medical Centre, Istanbul, Turkey

Atilla Bitigen
Medical Park Hospital, Fatih, Istanbul, Turkey

M. E. Sleeswijk
Flevoziekenhuis, Almere / Department of Critical Care, The Netherlands

T. van Noord
Scheperziekenhuis, Emmen / Department of Critical Care, The Netherlands

J. G. Zijlstra
3University Medical Center Groningen, University of Groningen / Department of Critical Care, The Netherlands

Miljenka-Jelena Jurašić, Sandra Morović, Sonja Antić, Iris Zavoreo and Vida Demarin
University Department of Neurology, Sestre milosrdnice University Hospital Centre, Croatia